MW01708549

BASIC AND CLINICAL SCIENCE COURSE

Pediatric Ophthalmology and Strabismus

Section 6

2008–2009

(Last major revision 2006–2007)

AMERICAN ACADEMY OF OPHTHALMOLOGY
The Eye M.D. Association

LEO
LIFELONG EDUCATION FOR THE OPHTHALMOLOGIST®

LEO

The Basic and Clinical Science Course is one component of the Lifelong Education for the Ophthalmologist (LEO) framework, which assists members in planning their continuing medical education. LEO includes an array of clinical education products that members may select to form individualized, self-directed learning plans for updating their clinical knowledge. Active members or fellows who use LEO components may accumulate sufficient CME credits to earn the LEO Award. Contact the Academy's Clinical Education Division for further information on LEO.

The American Academy of Ophthalmology is accredited by the Accreditation Council for Continuing Medical Education to provide continuing medical education for physicians.

The American Academy of Ophthalmology designates this educational activity for a maximum of 40 *AMA PRA Category 1 Credits*™. Physicians should only claim credit commensurate with the extent of their participation in the activity.

The Academy provides this material for educational purposes only. It is not intended to represent the only or best method or procedure in every case, nor to replace a physician's own judgment or give specific advice for case management. Including all indications, contraindications, side effects, and alternative agents for each drug or treatment is beyond the scope of this material. All information and recommendations should be verified, prior to use, with current information included in the manufacturers' package inserts or other independent sources, and considered in light of the patient's condition and history. Reference to certain drugs, instruments, and other products in this course is made for illustrative purposes only and is not intended to constitute an endorsement of such. Some material may include information on applications that are not considered community standard, that reflect indications not included in approved FDA labeling, or that are approved for use only in restricted research settings. **The FDA has stated that it is the responsibility of the physician to determine the FDA status of each drug or device he or she wishes to use and to use them with appropriate, informed patient consent in compliance with applicable law.** The Academy specifically disclaims any and all liability for injury or other damages of any kind, from negligence or otherwise, for any and all claims that may arise from the use of any recommendations or other information contained herein.

Printed in Singapore

Basic and Clinical Science Course

Gregory L. Skuta, MD, Oklahoma City, Oklahoma, *Senior Secretary for Clinical Education*
Louis B. Cantor, MD, Indianapolis, Indiana, *Secretary for Ophthalmic Knowledge*
Jayne S. Weiss, MD, Detroit, Michigan, *BCSC Course Chair*

Section 6

Faculty Responsible for This Edition

John W. Simon, MD, *Chair,* Albany, New York
Aazy A. Aaby, MD, Portland, Oregon
Arlene V. Drack, MD, Atlanta, Georgia
Amy K. Hutchinson, MD, Charleston, South Carolina
Scott E. Olitsky, MD, Kansas City, Missouri
David A. Plager, MD, Indianapolis, Indiana
Edward L. Raab, MD, JD, New York, New York
Christie Morse, MD, Concord, New Hampshire
Practicing Ophthalmologists Advisory Committee for Education
Jane Edmond, MD, Consultant, Houston, Texas

Dr. Simon states that he has an affiliation with Alcon and that he receives financial compensation from Diopsys Corporation.

The other authors state that they have no significant financial interest or other relationship with the manufacturer of any commercial product discussed in the chapters that they contributed to this publication or with the manufacturer of any competing commercial product.

Recent Past Faculty

Edward G. Buckley, MD
Mark S. Ruttum, MD
M. Edward Wilson, MD

In addition, the Academy gratefully acknowledges the contributions of numerous past faculty and advisory committee members who have played an important role in the development of previous editions of the Basic and Clinical Science Course.

American Academy of Ophthalmology Staff

Richard A. Zorab, *Vice President, Ophthalmic Knowledge*
Hal Straus, *Director, Publications Department*
Carol L. Dondrea, *Publications Manager*
Christine Arturo, *Acquisitions Manager*
Nicole DuCharme, *Production Manager*
Stephanie Tanaka, *Medical Editor*
Steven Huebner, *Administrative Coordinator*

AMERICAN ACADEMY OF OPHTHALMOLOGY
The Eye M.D. Association

655 Beach Street
Box 7424
San Francisco, CA 94120-7424

Contents

General Introduction

The Basic and Clinical Science Course (BCSC) is designed to meet the needs of residents and practitioners for a comprehensive yet concise curriculum of the field of ophthalmology. The BCSC has developed from its original brief outline format, which relied heavily on outside readings, to a more convenient and educationally useful self-contained text. The Academy updates and revises the course annually, with the goals of integrating the basic science and clinical practice of ophthalmology and of keeping ophthalmologists current with new developments in the various subspecialties.

The BCSC incorporates the effort and expertise of more than 80 ophthalmologists, organized into 13 Section faculties, working with Academy editorial staff. In addition, the course continues to benefit from many lasting contributions made by the faculties of previous editions. Members of the Academy's Practicing Ophthalmologists Advisory Committee for Education serve on each faculty and, as a group, review every volume before and after major revisions.

Organization of the Course

The Basic and Clinical Science Course comprises 13 volumes, incorporating fundamental ophthalmic knowledge, subspecialty areas, and special topics:

1 Update on General Medicine
2 Fundamentals and Principles of Ophthalmology
3 Clinical Optics
4 Ophthalmic Pathology and Intraocular Tumors
5 Neuro-Ophthalmology
6 Pediatric Ophthalmology and Strabismus
7 Orbit, Eyelids, and Lacrimal System
8 External Disease and Cornea
9 Intraocular Inflammation and Uveitis
10 Glaucoma
11 Lens and Cataract
12 Retina and Vitreous
13 Refractive Surgery

In addition, a comprehensive Master Index allows the reader to easily locate subjects throughout the entire series.

References

Readers who wish to explore specific topics in greater detail may consult the references cited within each chapter and listed in the Basic Texts section at the back of the book.

These references are intended to be selective rather than exhaustive, chosen by the BCSC faculty as being important, current, and readily available to residents and practitioners.

Related Academy educational materials are also listed in the appropriate sections. They include books, online and audiovisual materials, self-assessment programs, clinical modules, and interactive programs.

Study Questions and CME Credit

Each volume of the BCSC is designed as an independent study activity for ophthalmology residents and practitioners. The learning objectives for this volume are given on page 1. The text, illustrations, and references provide the information necessary to achieve the objectives; the study questions allow readers to test their understanding of the material and their mastery of the objectives. Physicians who wish to claim CME credit for this educational activity may do so by mail, by fax, or online. The necessary forms and instructions are given at the end of the book.

Conclusion

The Basic and Clinical Science Course has expanded greatly over the years, with the addition of much new text and numerous illustrations. Recent editions have sought to place a greater emphasis on clinical applicability while maintaining a solid foundation in basic science. As with any educational program, it reflects the experience of its authors. As its faculties change and as medicine progresses, new viewpoints are always emerging on controversial subjects and techniques. Not all alternate approaches can be included in this series; as with any educational endeavor, the learner should seek additional sources, including such carefully balanced opinions as the Academy's Preferred Practice Patterns.

The BCSC faculty and staff are continuously striving to improve the educational usefulness of the course; you, the reader, can contribute to this ongoing process. If you have any suggestions or questions about the series, please do not hesitate to contact the faculty or the editors.

The authors, editors, and reviewers hope that your study of the BCSC will be of lasting value and that each section will serve as a practical resource for quality patient care.

Objectives

Upon completion of BCSC Section 6, *Pediatric Ophthalmology and Strabismus*, the reader should be able to

- describe evaluation techniques for young children that provide the maximum gain of information with the least trauma and frustration
- outline the anatomy and physiology of the extraocular muscles and their fascia
- explain the classification, diagnosis, and treatment options for amblyopia
- describe the commonly used diagnostic and measurement tests for strabismus
- classify the various esodeviations and exodeviations, and describe the management of each type
- identify vertical strabismus and special forms of strabismus, and formulate a treatment plan for each type
- list the possible complications of strabismus surgery, and describe guidelines to minimize them
- differentiate among various causes of congenital and acquired ocular infections in children, and formulate a logical plan for the diagnosis and management of each type
- list the most common diseases and malformations of the cornea, lacrimal drainage system, anterior segment, and iris seen in children
- describe the diagnostic findings and treatment options for childhood glaucoma
- identify common types of childhood cataracts and other lens disorders
- outline a diagnostic and management plan for childhood cataracts

- identify appropriate diagnostic tests for pediatric uveitis
- differentiate among various vitreoretinal diseases and disorders found in children
- list the characteristics of ocular tumors and phakomatoses seen in children
- describe the characteristic findings of accidental and nonaccidental childhood trauma

INTRODUCTION

Rapport With Children: Tips for a Productive Examination

Children are not merely small adults. The most common ophthalmologic problems in children are different from the most common problems in adults. The varying developmental levels of children require different approaches to the ophthalmic examination. Proper preparation and attitude can make the ophthalmic examination of pediatric patients both enjoyable and rewarding.

Preparation

If at all possible, have a small room or corner of the waiting area designated for children. Both the parents and adult patients will be relieved by this separation. A small table and chairs, some books, and some toys are sufficient.

A dedicated long pediatric examination lane with different types of distance fixation targets is optimal. Following the *one toy, one look* rule, have several small toys readily available (Fig I-1). Light-colored plastic finger puppets become silent accommodative near targets that can also provide a corneal light reflex if placed over a muscle light or penlight.

Some children fear the white coat. You may choose to enter the room without yours.

The Examination

Examination of the pediatric patient begins with observing children at ease in the play area, as they navigate their way to the lane, and in their parent's arms as you enter the room. This may be the best look you get before children cry and bury their face in the parent's shoulder.

Observe the parents and siblings. Some ophthalmic conditions tend to run in families.

Some children are more comfortable sitting in a parent's lap.

Be relaxed, open, honest, and playfully engaging during the examination. Gaining the child's confidence makes for a faster and better examination, easier follow-up visits, and greater parental support.

Seat yourself at the child's eye level and introduce yourself to the child and the parent.

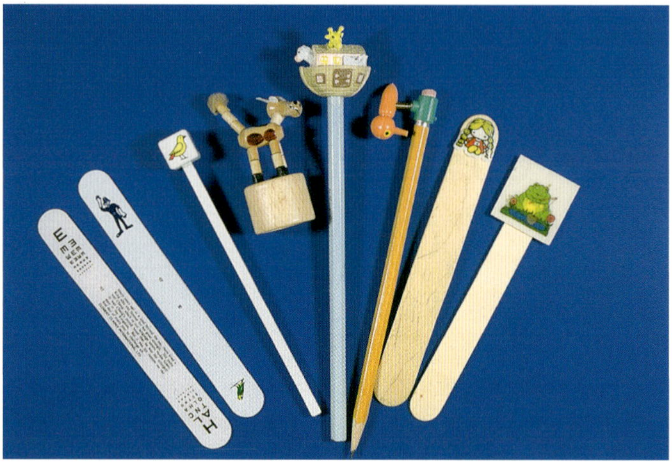

Figure I-1 Small toys, pictures, and reduced letter and E charts are used as near fixation targets. *(Reproduced with permission from Haldi BA, Mets MB. Nonsurgical treatment of strabismus.* Focal Points: Clinical Modules for Ophthalmologists. *San Francisco: American Academy of Ophthalmology; 1997, module 4. Photograph courtesy of Betty Anne Haldi, CO.)*

Establish and maintain eye contact with the child.

Initiate verbal contact by asking children easy questions with simple answers. For example, children enjoy being regarded as "big" and correcting adults when they are wrong. Tell them they look "so grown up"; grossly overestimate their age or grade level and then ask, "Is that right?" A simple joke can relax both child and parent.

To initiate physical contact with children, you can ask them to "give me five" or admire an article of their clothing, such as their shoes. Pushing the "magic button" on the nose of a child as you surreptitiously activate video presentations or mechanical animals with your foot pedal allows you to work close to the child's face while he or she is distracted.

Go where the action is—you may have only a few moments of cooperation, so check what you most need to see at the beginning of the examination.

If fusion is in doubt, check it first before disrupting it with other tests, including those for vision.

While checking vision, make the child feel successful by initially giving him objects he can readily discern; then say, "That's too easy—let's try this one."

Copies of whatever optotypes are appropriate for the child (Allen cards, picture chart, tumbling E) can be given to the parent for at-home rehearsal to help differentiate not seeing the test object from not understanding the test.

Develop a different vocabulary for working with children, such as "I want to show you something special" instead of "I want to examine you." Use "magic sunglasses" for the Polaroid stereo glasses, "special flashlight" for the retinoscope, "funny hat" for the indirect ophthalmoscope, and "magnifying glass" for the indirect lens. Confrontation visual fields can be performed as a counting-fingers game or Simon Says. Talk children into a slit-lamp examination by saying that they can "drive the motorcycle" by having them grab the handles of the slit lamp. Use your imagination to "play" with children as you rapidly proceed with the examination. Children will be more cooperative if you are sharing an experience instead of doing something to them.

Save the most threatening or most unpleasant part of the examination for the end.

The least expensive test you can order is a return office visit. Children who become totally uncooperative can return later to finish the examination.

When dealing with a vision- or life-threatening problem, you must persist with the examination and even use sedation or anesthesia when necessary.

Eyedrops

Almost all children are apprehensive about eyedrops. However, they do not have to *like* the drops; the important thing is to instill them. There are many approaches to giving eyedrops. If possible, someone other than the examining physician should administer the drops. Some practitioners use a cycloplegic spray, some use a topical anesthetic drop first, and some simply use the cycloplegic drop. The drops can be described as being "like a splash of swimming pool water" that will "feel funny for about 30 seconds." Do not give children a long time to think about it. Dark irides are more difficult to dilate. In some cases, the parent can put the cycloplegic drops in at home or an atropine refraction can be performed. (See Table 18-2 in BCSC Section 2, *Fundamentals and Principles of Ophthalmology*, for a complete listing of mydriatics and cycloplegics.)

Use of Anesthesia for Foreign-Body Removal

Procedures that provoke anxiety or are painful are best performed if children know that it is possible to numb the area. For example, the following process to remove foreign bodies can comfort the child:

1. Explain to the child that the eyes can be made numb.
2. Show the child that you have a drop that is cold but that most children say is also comfortable. You can call it a "magic drop." Drop it on the back of the child's hand first, before putting it in the eye. Tell the patient he or she might have felt that first drop but probably won't notice a second drop so much because the eye is already numb.
3. Demonstrate with a second drop that the eye has become numb. Show the child that a soft cotton-tipped applicator with drops on it can touch the eye without hurting or even being felt.
4. Introduce instruments for foreign-body removal in the same way.

Day SH, Sami DA. History, examination, and further investigation. In: Taylor D, Hoyt CS, eds. *Pediatric Ophthalmology and Strabismus.* 3rd ed. Cambridge, MA: Saunders; 2005:66–77.

McKeown CA. The pediatric eye examination. In: Albert DM, Jakobiec FA, eds. *Principles and Practice of Ophthalmology.* 2nd ed. Philadelphia: Saunders; 2000.

Pediatric Ophthalmology Panel. *Pediatric Eye Evaluations.* Preferred Practice Patterns. San Francisco: American Academy of Ophthalmology; 2002.

PART I

Strabismus

CHAPTER 1

Introduction to Strabismus

Terminology

The term *strabismus* is derived from the Greek word *strabismos,* "to squint, to look obliquely or askance." Strabismus means ocular misalignment, whether caused by abnormalities in binocular vision or by anomalies of neuromuscular control of ocular motility. Many terms are employed in discussing strabismus, and unless they are used correctly and uniformly, confusion and misunderstanding can occur.

Orthophoria is the ideal condition of ocular balance. In reality, orthophoria is seldom encountered; a small heterophoria (see below) can be documented in most persons. Some ophthalmologists therefore prefer *orthotropia* to mean correct direction or position of the eyes, even if a small heterophoria is present.

Heterophoria is an ocular deviation kept latent by the fusional mechanism (latent strabismus). *Heterotropia* is a deviation that is manifest and not kept under control by the fusional mechanism *(manifest strabismus).*

A detailed nomenclature has evolved to describe types of ocular deviations. This vocabulary uses many prefixes and suffixes based on the relative positions of the visual axes of both eyes to account for the multiple strabismic patterns encountered.

Prefixes

Eso- The eye is rotated so that the cornea is deviated nasally and the fovea is rotated temporally. Because the visual axes converge, this is also known as *convergent strabismus.*

Exo- The eye is rotated so that the cornea is deviated temporally and the fovea is rotated nasally. Because the visual axes diverge, this is also known as *divergent strabismus.*

Hyper- The eye is rotated so that the cornea is deviated superiorly and the fovea is rotated inferiorly. This is also known as *vertical strabismus.*

Hypo- The eye is rotated so that the cornea is deviated inferiorly and the fovea is rotated superiorly. This is also known as *vertical strabismus.*

Incyclo- The eye is rotated so that the superior pole of the vertical meridian is torted nasally and the inferior pole of the vertical meridian is torted temporally. This is also known as *intorsional strabismus.*

Excyclo- The eye is rotated so that the superior pole of the vertical meridian is torted temporally and the inferior pole of the vertical meridian is torted nasally. This is also known as *extorsional strabismus.*

Suffixes

-phoria A latent deviation (eg, esophoria, exophoria, right hyperphoria) that is controlled by the fusional mechanism so that the eyes remain aligned under normal binocular vision.

-tropia A manifest deviation (eg, esotropia, exotropia, right hypertropia, excyclotropia) that exceeds the control of the fusional mechanism so that the eyes are not aligned.

Usage

It is important to identify the deviating eye, especially when seeking to call attention to the "offending" eye as causing the deviation. This usage is particularly helpful when dealing with vertical deviations, restrictive or paretic strabismus, or amblyopia in a preverbal child.

Classification

No classification is perfect or all-inclusive, and several methods of classifying eye alignment and motility disorders are used.

Fusional Status

Phoria A latent deviation in which fusional control is always present.

Intermittent tropia A deviation in which fusional control is present part of the time.

Tropia A manifest deviation in which fusional control is not present.

Variation of the Deviation With Gaze Position or Fixating Eye

Comitant (concomitant) The deviation does not vary in size more than a few prism diopters with direction of gaze or fixating eye.

Incomitant (noncomitant) The deviation varies in size with direction of gaze or fixating eye. Most incomitant strabismus is paralytic or restrictive. Especially if acquired, incomitant strabismus may indicate neurologic or orbital disease.

Fixation

Alternating Spontaneous alternation of fixation from 1 eye to the other

Monocular Definite preference for fixation with 1 eye

Age of Onset

Congenital A deviation documented prior to 6 months, presumably related to a defect present at birth; the term *infantile* might be more appropriate.

Acquired A deviation with later onset, after a period of apparently normal visual development

Type of Deviation

Horizontal Esodeviation or exodeviation

Vertical Hyperdeviation or hypodeviation

Torsional Incyclodeviation or excyclodeviation

Combined Horizontal, vertical, torsional, or any combination thereof

Abbreviated Designations for Types of Strabismus

E, X, RH, LH Esophoria, exophoria, right hyperphoria, left hyperphoria at distance fixation, respectively. The addition of a prime (′) indicates near fixation (eg, E′, X′, RH′).

ET, XT, RHT, LHT Esotropia, exotropia, right hypertropia, left hypertropia at distance fixation, respectively. The addition of a prime (′) indicates near fixation (eg, ET′, XT′, RHT′).

E(T), X(T), RH(T), LH(T) Intermittent esotropia, intermittent exotropia, intermittent right hypertropia, intermittent left hypertropia at distance fixation, respectively. The addition of a prime (′) indicates near fixation (eg, E(T)′, X(T)′, RH(T)′).

RHoT, LHoT Right hypotropia, left hypotropia at distance fixation, respectively. The addition of a prime (′) indicates near fixation (eg, RHoT′, LHoT′).

O, EX = 0 Orthophoria. The addition of a prime (′) indicates near fixation (eg, O′).

CHAPTER 2

Anatomy of the Extraocular Muscles and Their Fascia

Origin, Course, Insertion, Innervation, and Action of the Extraocular Muscles

There are 7 extraocular muscles: the 4 rectus muscles, the 2 oblique muscles, and the levator palpebrae superioris muscle. Cranial nerve VI (abducens) innervates the lateral rectus muscle; cranial nerve IV (trochlear) innervates the superior oblique muscle; and cranial nerve III (oculomotor) innervates the levator palpebrae, superior rectus, medial rectus, inferior rectus, and inferior oblique muscles. CN III has an upper and a lower division: the upper division supplies the levator palpebrae and superior rectus muscles; the lower division supplies the medial rectus, inferior rectus, and inferior oblique muscles. The parasympathetic innervation of the sphincter pupillae and ciliary muscle travels with the branch of the lower division of cranial nerve III that supplies the inferior oblique muscle. BCSC Section 5, *Neuro-Ophthalmology*, discusses the ocular motor nerves in more detail, and Section 2, *Fundamentals and Principles of Ophthalmology*, extensively illustrates the anatomical structures mentioned in this chapter.

When the eye is directed straight ahead and the head is also straight, the eye is said to be in *primary position*. The *primary action* of a muscle is its major effect on the position of the eye when the muscle contracts while the eye is in primary position. The secondary and tertiary actions of a muscle are the additional effects on the position of the eye in primary position (see also Chapter 3 and Table 3-1). The globe usually can be moved about 50° in each direction from primary position. Under normal viewing circumstances, however, the eyes move only about 15°–20° from primary position before head movement occurs.

Horizontal Rectus Muscles

The horizontal rectus muscles are the medial and lateral rectus muscles. Both arise from the annulus of Zinn. The *medial rectus muscle* courses along the medial orbital wall and inserts 5.5 mm from the limbus. The proximity of the medial rectus muscle to the medial orbital wall means the medial rectus can be injured during ethmoid sinus surgery. The *lateral rectus muscle* inserts 6.9 mm from the limbus after coursing along the lateral orbital wall. In primary position, the medial rectus is an adductor, and the lateral rectus is an abductor. The medial rectus muscle is the only rectus muscle that does not have an oblique muscle running tangential to it. This fact makes surgery on the medial rectus less complicated but also does not offer any landmarks if the surgeon or the muscle is lost during surgery.

Vertical Rectus Muscles

The vertical rectus muscles are the superior and inferior rectus muscles. The *superior rectus muscle* originates from the annulus of Zinn and courses anteriorly, upward over the eyeball, and laterally, forming an angle of 23° with the visual axis of the eye in primary position (Fig 2-1). The superior rectus muscle inserts 7.7 mm from the limbus. In primary position, this muscle's primary action is elevation, secondary action is intorsion (incycloduction), and tertiary action is adduction.

The *inferior rectus muscle* also arises from the annulus of Zinn, and it then courses anteriorly, downward, and laterally along the floor of the orbit, forming an angle of 23° with the visual axis of the eye in primary position. This muscle inserts 6.5 mm from the limbus. In primary position, the inferior rectus muscle's primary action is depression, secondary action is extorsion (excycloduction), and tertiary action is adduction.

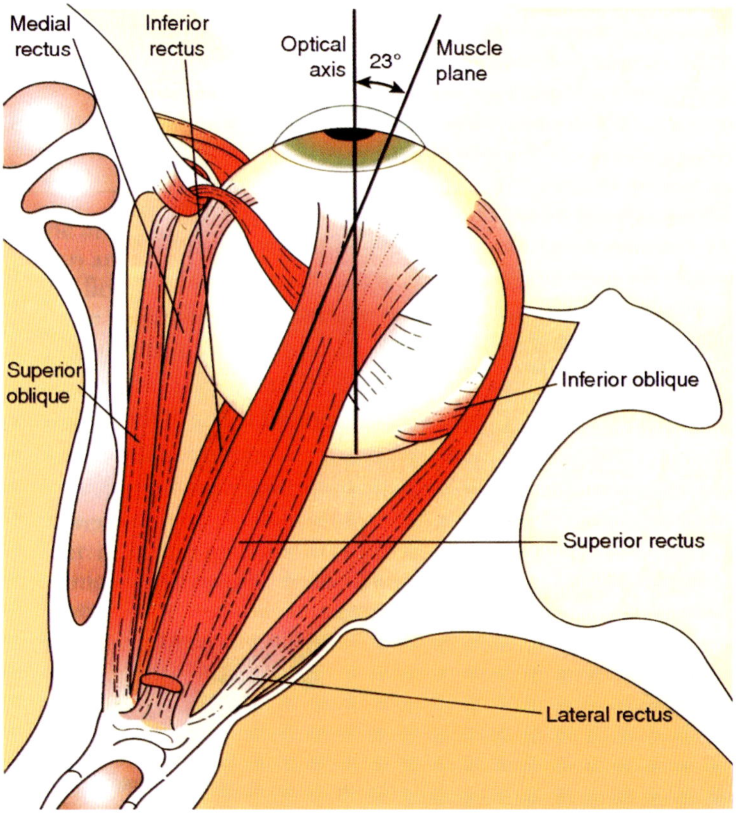

Figure 2-1 The extrinsic muscles of the right eyeball in the primary position, seen from above. The muscles are shown partially transparent. *(Reproduced with permission from Yanoff M, Duker J, eds.* Ophthalmology. *2nd ed. London: Mosby; 2004:549.)*

Oblique Muscles

The *superior oblique muscle* originates from the orbital apex above the annulus of Zinn and passes anteriorly and upward along the superomedial wall of the orbit. The muscle becomes tendinous before passing through the trochlea, a cartilaginous saddle attached to the frontal bone in the superior nasal orbit. A bursa-like cleft separates the trochlea from the loose fibrovascular sheath surrounding the tendon. The discrete fibers of the tendon telescope as they move through the trochlea, the central fibers moving farther than the peripheral ones (Fig 2-2). The function of the trochlea is to redirect the tendon inferiorly, posteriorly, and laterally, forming an angle of 51° with the visual axis of the eye in primary position. The tendon penetrates Tenon's capsule 2 mm nasally and 5 mm posteriorly to the nasal insertion of the superior rectus muscle. Passing under the superior rectus muscle, the tendon inserts in the posterosuperior quadrant of the eyeball, almost or entirely laterally to the midvertical plane or center of rotation. In primary position, the primary action of the superior oblique muscle is intorsion (incycloduction), secondary action is depression, and tertiary action is abduction.

Helveston EM. The influence of superior oblique anatomy on function and treatment. The 1998 Bielschowsky Lecture. *Binocul Vis Strabismus Q.* 1999;14:16–26.

The *inferior oblique muscle* originates from the periosteum of the maxillary bone, just posterior to the orbital rim and lateral to the orifice of the lacrimal fossa. It passes laterally, superiorly, and posteriorly, going inferior to the inferior rectus muscle and inserting under the lateral rectus muscle in the posterolateral portion of the globe, in the

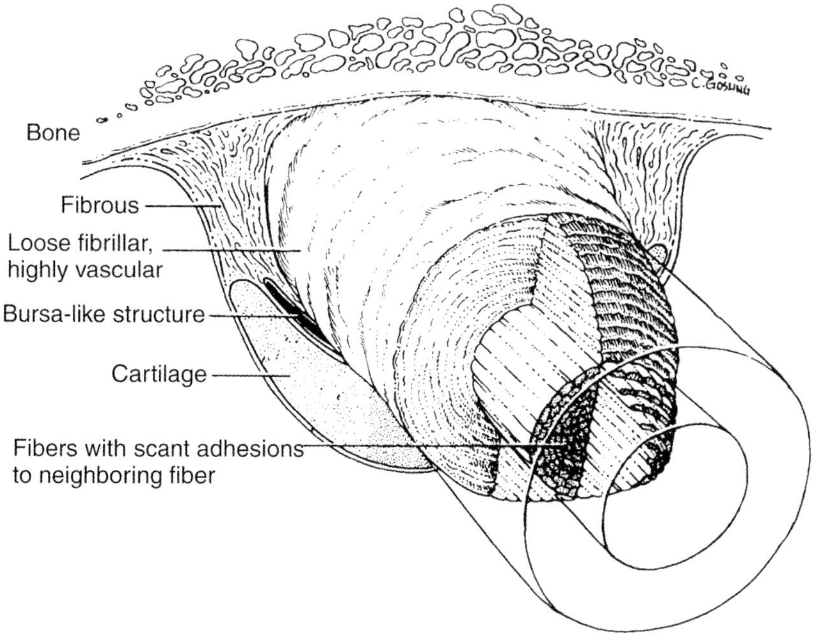

Figure 2-2 Components of the trochlea. *(Reproduced with permission from Helveston EM, Merriam WW, Ellis FD, et al. The trochlea: a study of the anatomy and physiology.* Ophthalmology. *1982;89:124–133.)*

area of the macula. The inferior oblique muscle forms an angle of 51° with the visual axis of the eye in primary position. In primary position, the muscle's primary action is extorsion (excycloduction), secondary action is elevation, and tertiary action is abduction.

Levator Palpebrae Superioris Muscle

The *levator palpebrae superioris muscle* arises at the apex of the orbit from the lesser wing of the sphenoid bone just superior to the annulus of Zinn. The origin of this muscle blends with the superior rectus muscle inferiorly and with the superior oblique muscle medially. The levator palpebrae superioris passes anteriorly, lying just above the superior rectus muscle; the fascial sheaths of these 2 muscles are connected. The levator palpebrae superioris muscle becomes an aponeurosis in the region of the superior fornix. This muscle has both a cutaneous and a tarsal insertion. BCSC Section 7, *Orbit, Eyelids, and Lacrimal System*, discusses this muscle in detail.

Table 2-1 summarizes the characteristics of the extraocular muscles and their relationship to one another (Fig 2-3).

Insertion Relationships of the Rectus Muscles

Starting at the medial rectus and proceeding to inferior rectus, lateral rectus, and superior rectus muscles, the rectus muscle tendons insert progressively farther from the limbus. A continuous curve drawn through these insertions yields a spiral, known as the *spiral of Tillaux* (Fig 2-4). The temporal side of the vertical rectus muscle insertion is farther from the limbus (ie, more posterior) than is the nasal side.

Blood Supply of the Extraocular Muscles

Arterial System

The muscular branches of the ophthalmic artery provide the most important blood supply for the extraocular muscles. The *lateral muscular branch* supplies the lateral rectus, superior rectus, superior oblique, and levator palpebrae superioris muscles; the *medial muscular branch*, the larger of the 2, supplies the inferior rectus, medial rectus, and inferior oblique muscles.

The lateral rectus muscle is partially supplied by the *lacrimal artery;* the *infraorbital artery* partially supplies the inferior oblique and inferior rectus muscles. The muscular branches give rise to the *anterior ciliary arteries* accompanying the rectus muscles; each rectus muscle has 1 to 3 anterior ciliary arteries. These pass to the episclera of the globe and then supply blood to the anterior segment. The superior and inferior rectus muscles carry the bulk of the blood supply.

Venous System

The venous system parallels the arterial system, emptying into the *superior* and *inferior orbital veins.* Generally, 4 *vortex veins* are located posterior to the equator; these are usually found near the nasal and temporal margins of the superior rectus and inferior rectus muscles.

Table 2-1 Extraocular Muscles

Muscle	Approx. Length of Active Muscle (mm)	Origin	Anatomical Insertion	Direction of Pull*	Tendon Length (mm)	Arc of Contact (mm)	Action From Primary Position	Innervation
Medial rectus (MR)	40	Annulus of Zinn	5.5 mm from medial limbus	90°	4.5	7	Adduction	Lower CN III
Lateral rectus (LR)	40	Annulus of Zinn	6.9 mm from lateral limbus	90°	7	12	Abduction	CN VI
Superior rectus (SR)	40	Annulus of Zinn	7.7 mm from superior limbus	23°	6	6.5	Elevation Intorsion Adduction	Upper CN III
Inferior rectus (IR)	40	Annulus of Zinn	6.5 mm from inferior limbus	23°	7	6.5	Depression Extorsion Adduction	Lower CN III
Superior oblique (SO)	32	Orbit apex above annulus of Zinn (functional origin at the trochlea)	Posterior to equator in superotemporal quadrant	51°	26	7–8	Intorsion Depression Abduction	CN IV
Inferior oblique (IO)	37	Behind lacrimal fossa	Macular area	51°	1	15	Extorsion Elevation Abduction	Lower CN III
Levator palpebrae superioris (LPS)	40	Orbit apex above annulus of Zinn	Septa of pretarsal orbicularis and anterior surface of tarsus	—	14–20	—	Eyelid elevation	Upper CN III

* Relative to visual axis in primary position

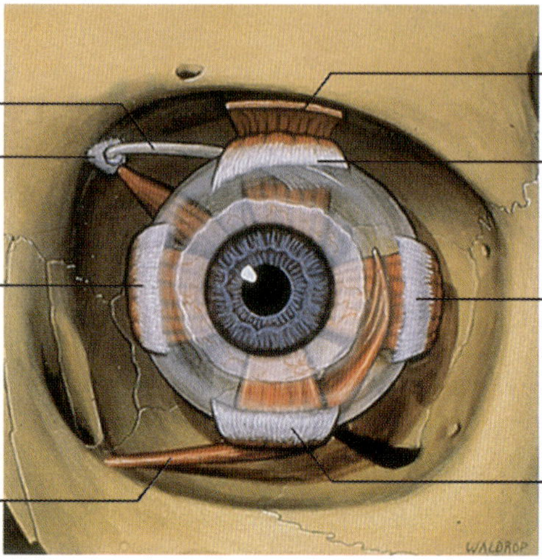

Figure 2-3 Extraocular muscles, frontal composite view, left eye. *(Reproduced with permission from Dutton JJ.* Atlas of Clinical and Surgical Orbital Anatomy. *Philadelphia: Saunders; 1994:23.)*

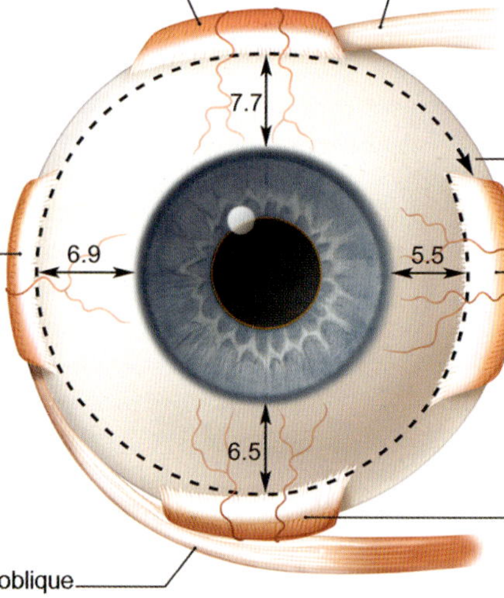

Figure 2-4 Spiral of Tillaux, right eye. *Note:* The distances, given in millimeters, are averages only and may vary greatly in individuals. *(Illustration by Christine Gralapp.)*

Structure of the Extraocular Muscles

Like skeletal muscle, extraocular muscle is voluntary striated muscle. However, developmentally, biochemically, structurally, and functionally, it is different from typical skeletal muscle. The extraocular muscles are richly innervated, with a ratio of nerve fiber to muscle fiber up to 10 times that of skeletal muscle. This difference may allow for more accurate eye movements controlled by an array of systems ranging from the primitive vestibulo-ocular reflex to highly evolved vergence movements.

The extraocular muscles exhibit a distinct 2-layer organization: the outer orbital layer, which acts only on the muscle pulleys, and an inner global layer, which inserts on the sclera to move the globe. The orbital and global muscles can further be divided into groups based on innervation type (single or multiple) and mitochondrial content (red, white, or intermediate). These novel properties of eye muscles lead to differential responses to pharmaceuticals such as botulinum toxin, channel blockers, or local anesthetics, as well as disease processes such as myasthenia gravis and muscular dystrophy.

Orbital and Fascial Relationships

Within the orbit, a complex musculofibroelastic structure suspends the globe, supports the extraocular muscles, and compartmentalizes the fat pads (Fig 2-5). In the past, the

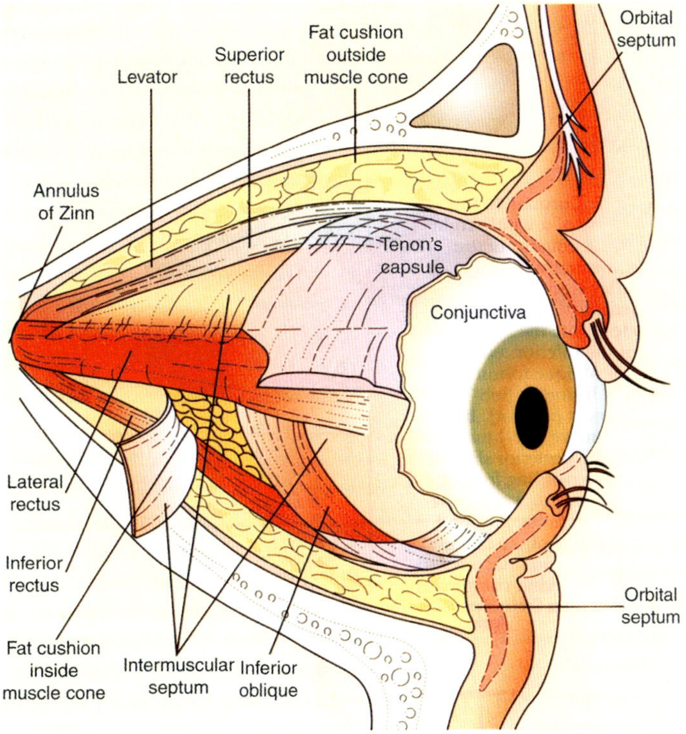

Figure 2-5 The muscle cone contains 1 fat cushion and is surrounded by another, and these 2 fat cushions are separated by the rectus muscles and intermuscular septa. Tenon's capsule anterior to the penetration of the rectus muscles and intermuscular septa is the inner surface of the compartment containing the fat cushion outside the muscle cone. Tenon's capsule posterior to the penetration of the rectus muscles and intermuscular septa is the anterior surface of the compartment containing the fat cushion inside the muscle cone. *(Reproduced with permission from Yanoff M, Duker J, eds.* Ophthalmology. *2nd ed, London: Mosby; 2004:553.)*

distinctness of these layers has been overstated. The extent and complexity of the interconnectedness of the orbital tissues has recently come to light and is still being investigated. Clinically, the consequences of tissue entrapment in blowout fractures and post–retrobulbar hemorrhage fibrosis of delicate fibrous septa illustrate the intense fibrous connections throughout the orbit.

Tenon's Capsule

The bulk of the orbital fascial system is *Tenon's capsule (the fascia bulbi)*, which forms the envelope within which the eyeball moves (Fig 2-6). Tenon's capsule is an envelope of elastic connective tissue that fuses posteriorly with the optic nerve sheath and fuses anteriorly with the intermuscular septum at a position 3 mm from the limbus (Fig 2-7). The posterior portion of Tenon's capsule is thin and flexible, allowing for free movement of the optic nerve, ciliary nerves, and ciliary vessels as the globe rotates, while separating the orbital fat inside the muscle cone from the sclera. At and just posterior to the equator, Tenon's capsule is thick and tough, suspending the globe like a trampoline by means of connections to the periorbital tissues. The extraocular rectus muscles penetrate this thick musculofibroelastic tissue approximately 10 mm posterior to their insertions. This tissue complex forms a sleeve around the penetrating rectus muscles and creates a compliant pulley suspended from the periorbita, which acts as the functional origin of the muscles. The sleeves also extend anteriorly and posteriorly to form slings that stabilize the muscle path, preventing sideslipping or movement perpendicular to the muscle axis (Fig 2-8). Anterior to the equator, the oblique muscles penetrate Tenon's capsule. Tenon's capsule continues forward over all 6 extraocular muscles and separates them from the orbital fat and structures lying outside the muscle cone.

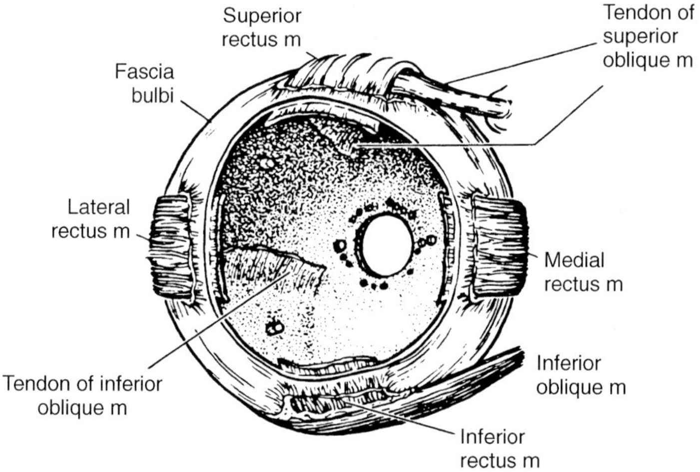

Figure 2-6 Anterior and posterior orifices of Tenon's capsule shown after enucleation of the globe. *(Reproduced with permission from von Noorden GK.* Binocular Vision and Ocular Motility. *6th ed. St. Louis: Mosby; 2002:45.)*

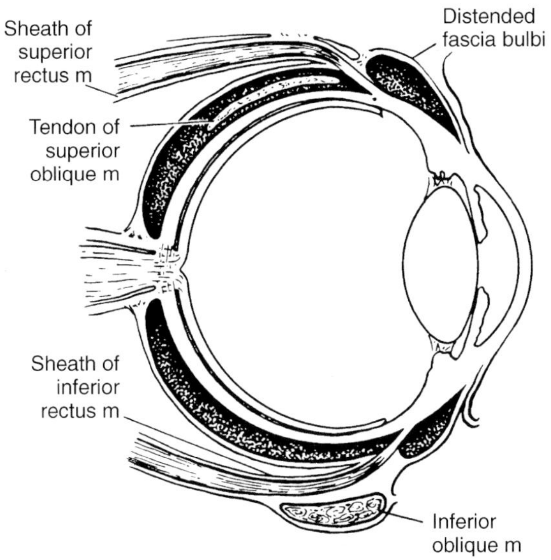

Figure 2-7 Tenon's space shown by injection with India ink. *(Reproduced with permission from von Noorden GK.* Binocular Vision and Ocular Motility. *6th ed. St. Louis: Mosby; 2002:45.)*

Pulley System

Although not as distinct as the trochlea of the superior oblique, there is a pulley system for each of the 4 rectus muscles as well. These pulleys contain smooth muscle, allowing them to contract and relax. The orbital layer of the extraocular muscle inserts on these pulleys, further manipulating their position in the orbit. As the muscle contracts, its pulley must be pulled back so that the distance between the location of the pulley and the insertion of the muscle on the globe is approximately constant.

The adjustability of the pulleys and, therefore, the functional origin of the muscle may play a significant but as yet incompletely defined role in ocular movements. Heterotropia of the pulleys may be responsible for different forms of incomitant strabismus, such as A or V patterns, and may influence the effect of Faden procedures.

Intermuscular Septum

The 4 rectus muscles are connected by a thin layer of tissue that underlies the conjunctiva. This is the *intermuscular septum*, a membrane that spans between rectus muscles and fuses with the conjunctiva 3 mm posterior to the limbus. Posterior to the globe, the intermuscular septum separates the intraconal fat pads from the extraconal fat pads. Numerous extensions from all the extraocular muscle sheaths attach to the orbit and help support the globe.

Lockwood's Ligament

The muscle capsule of the inferior oblique muscle (but not the muscle itself) is bound to the inferior rectus muscle capsule. This fusion is called *Lockwood's ligament*, and it connects to the lower eyelid retractors.

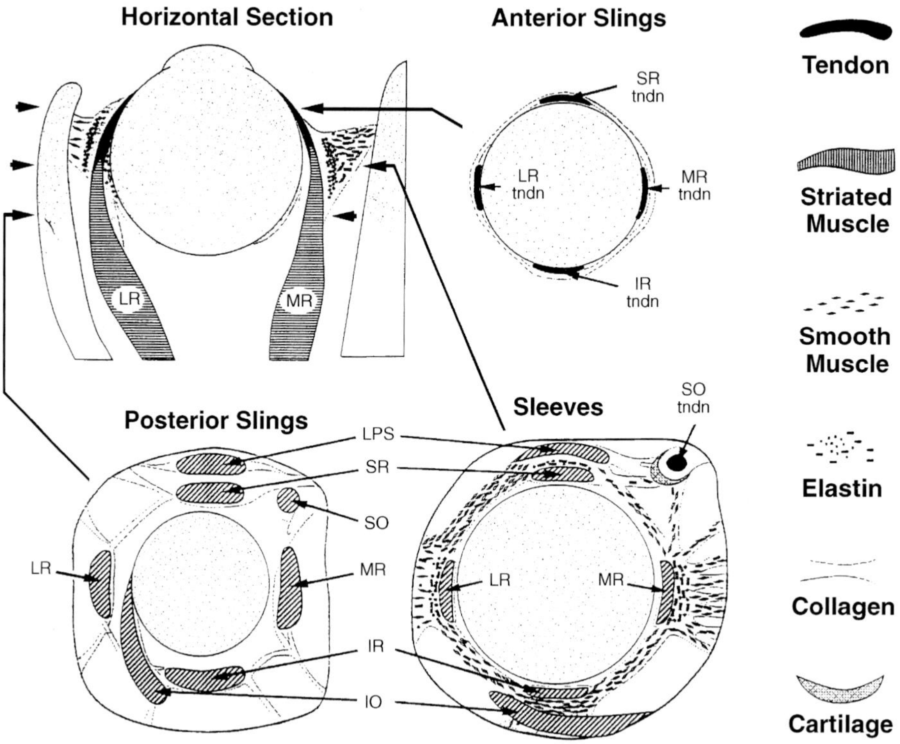

Figure 2-8 Structure of orbital connective tissues. IO, inferior oblique; IR, inferior rectus; LPS, levator palpebrae superioris; LR, lateral rectus; MR, medial rectus; SO, superior oblique; SR, superior rectus. The 3 coronal views are represented at the levels indicated by arrows in horizontal section. *(Reproduced with permission from Demer JL, Miller JM, Poukens V. Surgical implications of the rectus extraocular muscle pulleys.* J Pediatr Ophthalmol Strabismus. *1996;33:208–218.)*

Muscle Capsule

Each rectus muscle has a surrounding fascial capsule that extends with the muscle from its origin to its insertion. These capsules are thin posteriorly, but near the equator they thicken as they pass through the Tenon's capsule sleeve, continuing anteriorly with the muscles to their insertions. Anterior to the equator between the undersurface of the muscle and the sclera there is almost no fascia, only connective tissue footplates that connect the muscle to the globe. The smooth avascular surface of the muscle capsule allows the muscles to slide smoothly over the globe.

Muscle Cone

The muscle cone lies posterior to the equator. It consists of the extraocular muscles, the extraocular muscle sheaths, and the intermuscular membrane. The muscle cone extends posteriorly to the annulus of Zinn at the orbital apex.

Adipose Tissue

The eye is supported and cushioned in the orbit by a large amount of fatty tissue. External to the muscle cone, fatty tissue comes forward with the rectus muscles, stopping about 10 mm from the limbus. Fatty tissue is also present inside the muscle cone, kept away from the sclera by Tenon's capsule (see Fig 2-5).

Anatomical Considerations During Surgery

The nerves to the rectus muscles and the superior oblique muscle enter the muscles about one third of the distance from the origin to the insertion (or trochlea, in the case of the superior oblique muscle) (Fig 2-9). Damaging these nerves during anterior surgery is difficult but not impossible. An instrument thrust more than 26 mm posterior to the rectus muscle's insertion may cause injury to the nerve.

Cranial nerve IV is outside the muscle cone and would not be affected by a retrobulbar block.

The nerve supplying the inferior oblique muscle enters the lateral portion of the muscle, where it crosses the inferior rectus muscle; the nerve can be damaged by surgery in this area. Because the parasympathetic innervation to the sphincter pupillae and ciliary muscle accompanies the nerve to the inferior oblique muscle, surgery in this area may also result in pupillary abnormalities. These nerves and the inferior oblique can be injured by an inferotemporal retrobulbar block.

Maintaining the integrity of the muscle capsules decreases bleeding during surgery and provides a smooth muscle surface with less risk of adhesion formation. If only the muscle capsule is sutured to the globe, the muscle can retract backwards, causing a "slipped muscle."

The intermuscular septum connections, especially between rectus muscles and oblique muscles, can help locate a lost muscle during surgery. Extensive intermuscular septum dissections are not necessary for rectus recession surgery. During resection surgery, the intermuscular septum connections should be severed to prevent, for example, the inferior oblique muscle from being advanced with the lateral rectus muscle.

The inferior rectus muscle is distinctly bound to the lower eyelid by the fascial extension from its sheath. *Recession*, or weakening, of the inferior rectus muscle tends to widen the palpebral fissure with an associated lower lid sag; *resection*, or strengthening, of the inferior rectus muscle tends to narrow the fissure by elevating the lower eyelid. Therefore, any alteration of the inferior rectus muscle may be associated with palpebral fissure change (Fig 2-10).

The superior rectus muscle is loosely bound to the levator palpebrae superioris muscle. The eyelid may be pulled downward following resection of the superior rectus muscle, thus narrowing the palpebral fissure, and pulled upward with a recession, widening the fissure. In hypotropia, a pseudoptosis may be present because the upper eyelid tends to follow the superior rectus (see Fig 2-10).

The blood supply to the extraocular muscles provides almost all of the temporal half of the anterior segment circulation and the majority of the nasal half of the anterior

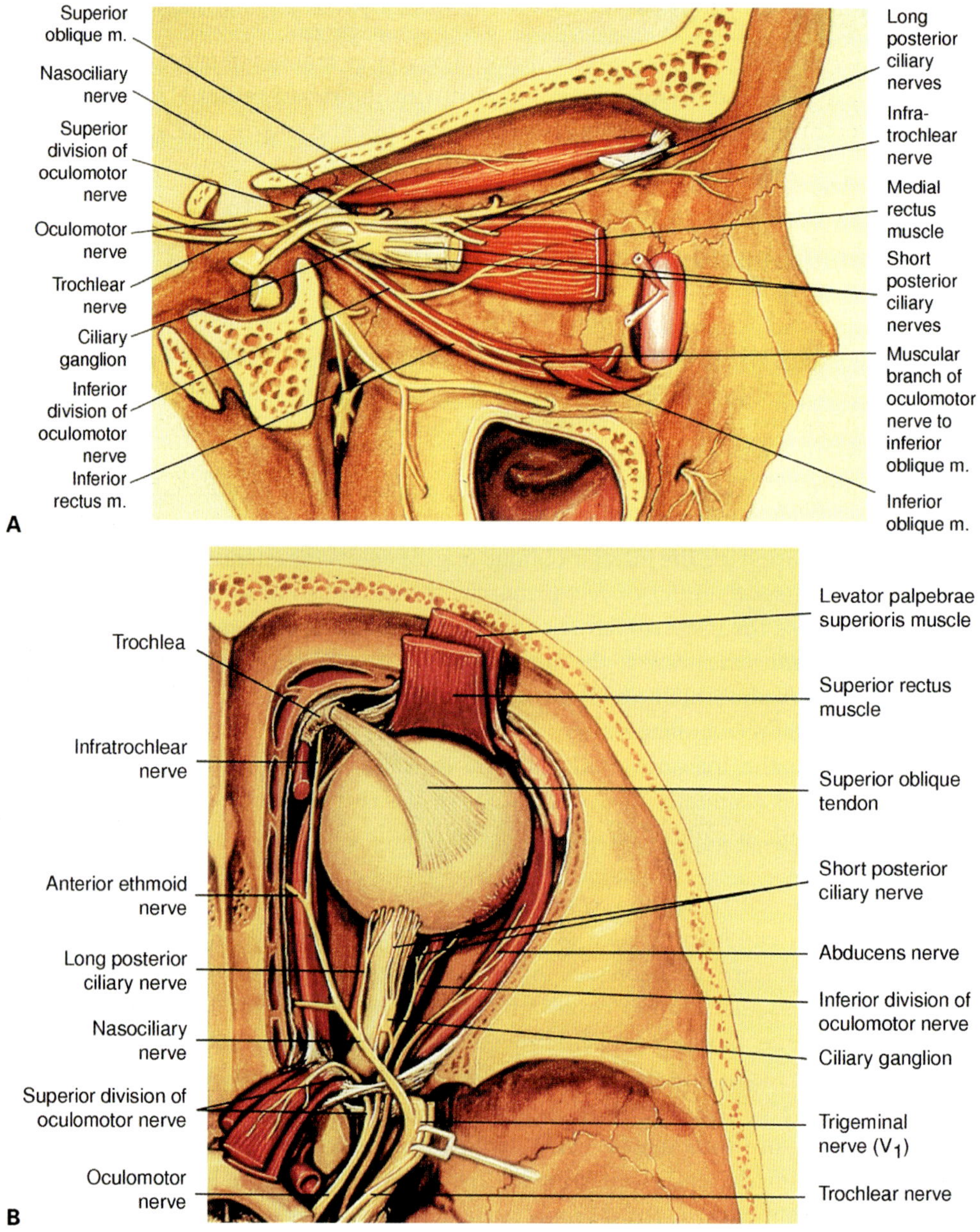

Figure 2-9 The extraocular muscles are innervated by cranial nerves III, IV, and VI. Cutaway views facing nasally **(A)** and down **(B)** show the course of these ocular motor nerves. CN III (oculomotor) branches into a superior and an inferior division in the cavernous sinus or at the superior orbital fissure. The superior division innervates the superior rectus and levator muscles. The inferior division sends branches to the medial rectus, inferior rectus, and inferior oblique muscles, as well as to the ciliary ganglion. CN IV (trochlear) enters the orbit through the superior orbital fissure, crosses over the superior rectus and levator muscle complex, and runs along the external surface of the superior oblique muscle, entering in the posterior third. CN VI (abducens) enters the orbit through the superior orbital fissure and annulus of Zinn to supply the lateral rectus muscle. *(Reproduced with permission from Freedman S, Shields MB, Buckley EG, et al, eds.* Atlas of Ophthalmic Surgery: Strabismus and Glaucoma. *St. Louis: Mosby-Year Book; 1995:11.)*

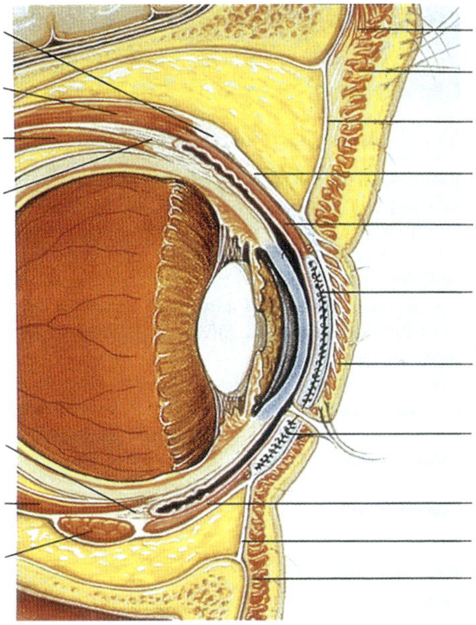

Figure 2-10 Attachments of the upper and lower eyelids to the vertical rectus muscles. Superiorly, the suspensory ligament acts to connect the superior rectus and levator, which facilitates movement of the eyelid on attempted upgaze. Large recessions of the superior rectus muscle can result in upper eyelid retraction, whereas resections can create a ptosis. Surgery on the inferior rectus can also cause changes in position of the lower eyelid because of the presence of Lockwood's ligament. A recession of the inferior rectus muscle can result in lower eyelid retraction, whereas a resection of the inferior rectus muscle can result in advancement of a lower eyelid and a narrowing of the palpebral fissure. *(Reproduced with permission from Freedman S, Shields MB, Buckley EG, et al, eds.* Atlas of Ophthalmic Surgery: Strabismus and Glaucoma. *St Louis: Mosby-Year Book; 1995:15.)*

segment circulation, which also receives some blood from the long posterior ciliary artery. Therefore, simultaneous surgery on 3 rectus muscles may induce anterior segment ischemia, particularly in older patients.

Whenever muscle surgery is performed, special care must be taken to avoid penetration of Tenon's capsule 10 mm or more posterior to the limbus. If the integrity of Tenon's capsule is violated posterior to this point, fatty tissue may prolapse through the capsule and form a restrictive adhesion to sclera, muscle, intermuscular membrane, or conjunctiva, limiting ocular motility.

When surgery is performed near the vortex veins, accidental severing of a vein is possible. The procedures that present the greatest risk for damaging a vortex vein are inferior rectus and superior rectus muscle recession or resection, inferior oblique muscle weakening procedures, and exposure of the superior oblique muscle tendon. Hemostasis can be achieved with cautery or with an absorbable hemostatic sponge.

The sclera is thinnest just posterior to the 4 rectus muscle insertions. This area is the site for most muscle surgery, especially for recession procedures. Therefore, scleral perforation is always a risk during eye muscle surgery. This risk can be minimized by

- using spatulated needles with swedged sutures
- working with a clean, dry, and blood-free surgical field
- using loupe magnification or the operating microscope

Chapter 13 discusses these procedures and complications in greater detail.

Bron AJ, Tripathi RC, Tripathi BJ, eds. *Wolff's Anatomy of the Eye and Orbit.* 8th ed. London: Chapman & Hall; 1997.

Freedman S, Shields MB, Buckley EG, et al, eds. *Atlas of Ophthalmic Surgery: Strabismus and Glaucoma.* St Louis: Mosby-Year Book; 1995.

CHAPTER 3

Motor Physiology

Basic Principles and Terms

Axes of Fick, Center of Rotation, Listing's Plane, and Median Plane

A movement of the eye around a theoretical center of rotation is described with specific terminology. Two helpful concepts are the axes of Fick and Listing's plane (Fig 3-1). The *axes of Fick* are designated as *x, y,* and *z.* The *x-axis* is a transverse axis passing through the center of the eye at the equator; voluntary vertical rotations of the eye occur about this axis. The *y-axis* is a sagittal axis passing through the pupil; involuntary torsional rotations occur about this axis. The *z-axis* is a vertical axis; voluntary horizontal rotations

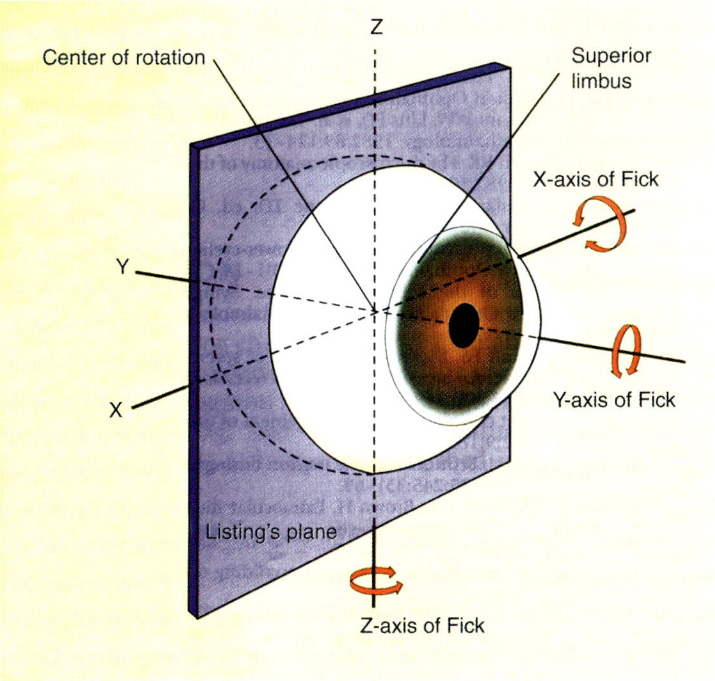

Figure 3-1 Axes of Fick, center of rotation, Listing's plane. *(Reproduced with permission from Yanoff M, Duker J, eds.* Ophthalmology. *2nd ed. London: Mosby; 2004:557.*

occur about this axis. *Listing's equatorial plane* contains the center of rotation and includes the x and z axes. The y-axis is perpendicular to Listing's plane.

Positions of Gaze

Positions of gaze are also discussed in detail in Chapter 6. The following is basic terminology:

- Primary position is straight ahead.
- Secondary positions are straight up, straight down, right gaze, left gaze.
- Tertiary positions are the 4 oblique positions of gaze: up and right, up and left, down and right, down and left.
- Cardinal positions are up and right, up and left, right, left, down and right, down and left (Fig 3-2).

Arc of Contact

The point of effective, or physiologic, insertion is the tangential point where the muscle first contacts the globe. The action of the eye muscle may be considered a vector of force that acts at this tangential point to rotate the eye. The length of muscle actually in contact with the globe constitutes the arc of contact. The traditional concept of arc of contact and muscle plane, based on straight-line 2-dimensional models of orbital anatomy, do not take into account the newly discovered effective muscle pulleys and their effect on linearity of muscle paths. These concepts will need to be modified as the function of the pulleys becomes better known.

Primary, Secondary, and Tertiary Action

With the eye in primary position, the horizontal rectus muscles are purely horizontal movers around the z-axis (the vertical axis), and they have a primary action only. The vertical rectus muscles have a direction of pull that is mostly vertical as their primary action, but the angle of pull from origin to insertion is inclined 23° to the visual axis, giving rise also to torsion, which is defined as any rotation of the vertical corneal meridians. *Intorsion* (also called *incycloduction*) is the secondary action for the superior rectus; *extorsion* (also called *excycloduction*) is the secondary action for the inferior rectus; and *adduction* is the tertiary action for both muscles. Because the oblique muscles are inclined 51° to the visual

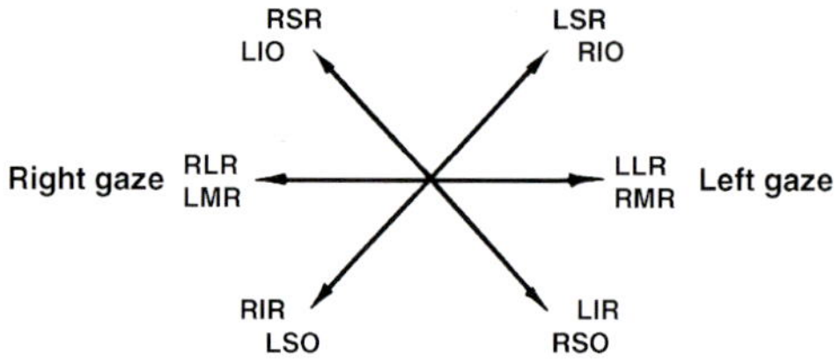

Figure 3-2 Cardinal positions and yoke muscles. RSR, right superior rectus; LIO, left inferior oblique; LSR, left superior rectus; RIO, right inferior oblique; RLR, right lateral rectus; LMR, left medial rectus; LLR, left lateral rectus; RMR, right medial rectus; RIR, right inferior rectus; LSO, left superior oblique; LIR, left inferior rectus; RSO, right superior oblique.

axis, torsion is their primary action. Vertical rotation is their secondary and horizontal rotation their tertiary action (Table 3-1).

Field of Action/Field of Activation

The term *field of action* is used in 2 ways to describe entirely separate and distinct concepts:

1. to indicate the direction of rotation of the eye from primary position if the muscle was the only one to contract
2. to refer to the gaze position in which the effect of the muscle is most readily observed

For the lateral rectus muscle, these 2 movements are both abduction; for the medial rectus, they are both adduction. However, the 2 movements are not the same for all muscles. For example, the inferior oblique muscle, acting alone, is an abductor and elevator, pulling the eye up and out—but its elevation action is best observed in adduction. Similarly, the superior oblique muscle, acting alone, is an abductor and depressor, pulling the eye down and out—but its depression action is best observed in adduction. *Field of activation* may be a better term for defining the muscle's action if it were acting alone.

Thus, evaluation of fields of action must involve 3 separate aspects:

1. plane of the muscle action
2. gaze direction, which increases or decreases the innervation to the muscle
3. vector distribution of the muscle's force (vertical, horizontal, torsional) in various gaze positions

The clinical significance of fields of action is that a deviation (strabismus) that increases with gaze in some directions may result from the weakness of the muscle normally pulling the eye in that direction. For example, an acute left sixth nerve palsy in an adult can be diagnosed by asking the patient with diplopia 3 questions:

1. Is the diplopia horizontal or vertical? *Patient's answer:* Horizontal [eliminating all but the medial and lateral recti].
2. Is the diplopia worse at distance or at near? *Patient's answer:* Distance [implicating the lateral recti, which act more at distance viewing than in convergence].
3. Is the diplopia worse on looking to the left or to the right? *Patient's answer:* Looking to the left [the field of action of the left lateral rectus].

Changing Muscle Action With Different Gaze Positions

The initial gaze position determines the effect of extraocular muscle contractions on the rotation of the eye. The different positions are primary gaze and the 6 cardinal positions (see Fig 3-2). In each of these 6 cardinal positions, each of the 6 extraocular muscles has different effects on the eye rotation based on the relationship between the *visual axis (optical axis, line of sight, y-axis)* of the eye and the orientation of the muscle plane to

Table 3-1 Action of the Extraocular Muscles from Primary Position

Muscle*	Primary	Secondary	Tertiary
Medial rectus	Adduction	—	—
Lateral rectus	Abduction	—	—
Inferior rectus	Depression	Extorsion	Adduction
Superior rectus	Elevation	Intorsion	Adduction
Inferior oblique	Extorsion	Elevation	Abduction
Superior oblique	Intorsion	Depression	Abduction

* The superior muscles are intortors; the inferior muscles are extortors. The vertical rectus muscles are adductors; the oblique muscles are abductors.

the visual axis. Each cardinal position minimizes the angle between the visual axis and the muscle plane of the muscle being tested, thus minimizing the secondary and tertiary actions of the tested muscle. By having the patient move the eyes to the 6 cardinal positions, the clinician can isolate and evaluate the ability of each of the 6 extraocular muscles to move the eye. See also Binocular Eye Movements later in the chapter.

With the eye in primary position, the horizontal rectus muscles share a common horizontal plane that contains the visual axis. Thus, starting from primary position, the horizontal rectus muscles are purely horizontal movers around the z-axis (vertical axis) and have a primary horizontal action only (Fig 3-3). The relative strength of the horizontal rectus muscles can be assessed by observing the horizontal excursion of the eye as it moves medially from primary position to test the medial rectus and laterally to test the lateral rectus.

The muscle actions of the vertical rectus muscles and the oblique muscles are more complex because, in primary position, the muscle axes are not parallel with the visual axis (see Figs 3-4, 3-5, 3-6, 3-7).

In primary position, the superior and inferior rectus muscle planes form an angle of 23° with the visual axis (y-axis) and insert slightly anterior to the z-axis (Figs 3-4, 3-5). Therefore, from primary position, the contraction of the superior rectus has 3 effects: primary elevation around the x-axis, secondary intorsion around the y-axis, and adduction around the z-axis. The relative strength of the superior rectus muscle can be most readily observed by aligning the optical axis parallel to the muscle plane axis—that is, when the eye is rotated 23° in abduction. In this position, the superior rectus becomes a pure elevator and its elevating action is maximal. To minimize the elevation action of the superior rectus, the optical axis should be perpendicular to the muscle axis at a position of 67° of adduction. In this position, the superior rectus would become a pure intorter. Because the globe cannot be adducted this far, there is still a superior rectus elevating action in maximal adduction.

The inferior rectus muscle has analogous action to the superior rectus. Because it is attached to the globe inferiorly, its action from primary position is primarily depression, secondarily extorsion, and tertiarily adduction (see Fig 3-5). Its action as a depressor is maximally demonstrated in 23° of abduction and minimized in adduction.

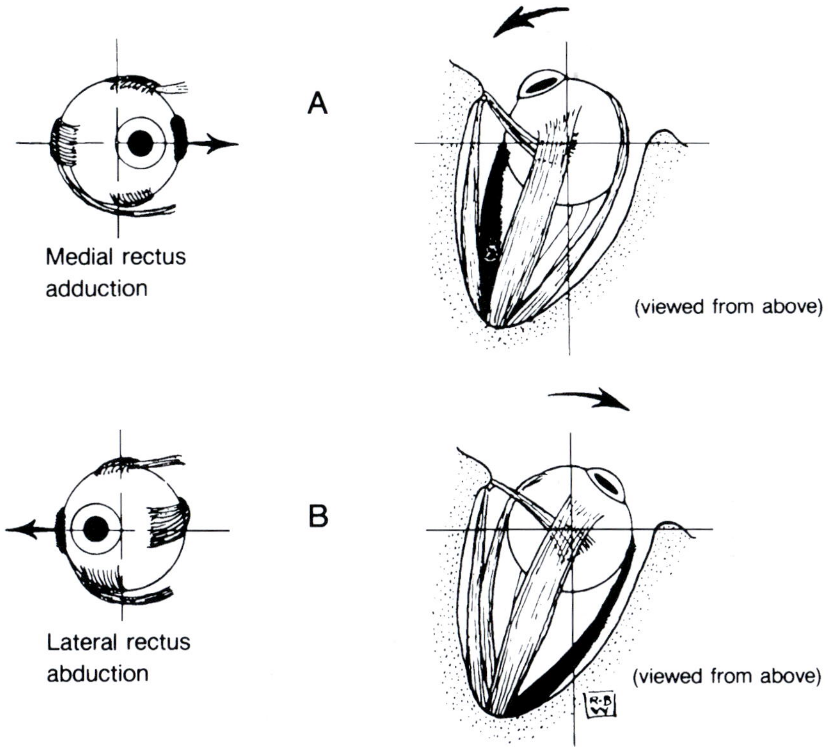

Figure 3-3 The right horizontal rectus muscles. **A,** Right medial rectus muscle. **B,** Right lateral rectus muscle. *(Reproduced with permission from von Noorden GK.* Atlas of Strabismus. *4th ed. St Louis: Mosby; 1983:3.)*

The 2 oblique muscle planes course in a direction from the anteromedial aspect of the globe to the posterolateral, forming an angle of approximately 51° from the visual axis (y-axis) (Figs 3-6, 3-7). Because of the large angle formed in primary position, the primary action of the superior oblique is intorsion, with a secondary depression and tertiary abduction. As the muscle plane is aligned with the visual axis in extreme adduction, the superior oblique muscle action can be seen as a depressor. With abduction of the eye, the visual axis becomes perpendicular to the muscle plane, and the muscle action is one of intorsion.

The action of the inferior oblique is analogous (see Fig 3-7). In primary position, the primary action is extorsion, with secondary elevation and tertiary abduction. Its action as an elevator is best seen in adduction and, as an extorter, in abduction.

Physiology of Muscle

Position of rest

The position of each eye in the orbit without any innervation to the extraocular muscles is described as the position of rest. The position of each eye is slightly divergent in anatomically normal persons.

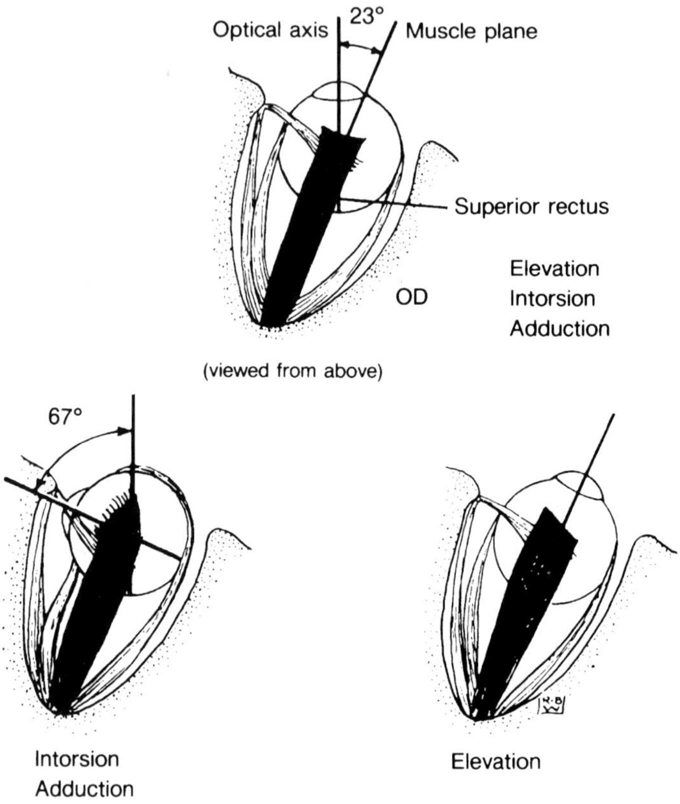

Figure 3-4 The right superior rectus muscle. *(Reproduced with permission from von Noorden GK.* Atlas of Strabismus. *4th ed. St Louis: Mosby; 1983:3.)*

Motor units

An individual motor nerve fiber and its several muscle fibers is a *motor unit. Electromyography* records motor unit electrical activity. An electromyogram is useful in investigating normal and abnormal innervation and can be helpful in documenting paralysis, recovery from paralysis, and abnormalities of innervation in myasthenia gravis and muscle atrophy. However, this test is not helpful in ordinary comitant strabismus.

Recruitment during fixation or following movement

As the eye moves farther into abduction, for example, more and more lateral rectus motor units are activated and brought into play by the brain to help pull the eye. This process is called *recruitment.* In addition, as the eye fixates farther into abduction, the frequency of activity of each motor unit increases until it reaches a peak (for some motor units, several hundred contractions per second).

Saccades

Saccadic movements require a sudden, strong pulse of force from the extraocular muscles in order to move the eye rapidly against the viscosity produced by the fatty tissue and

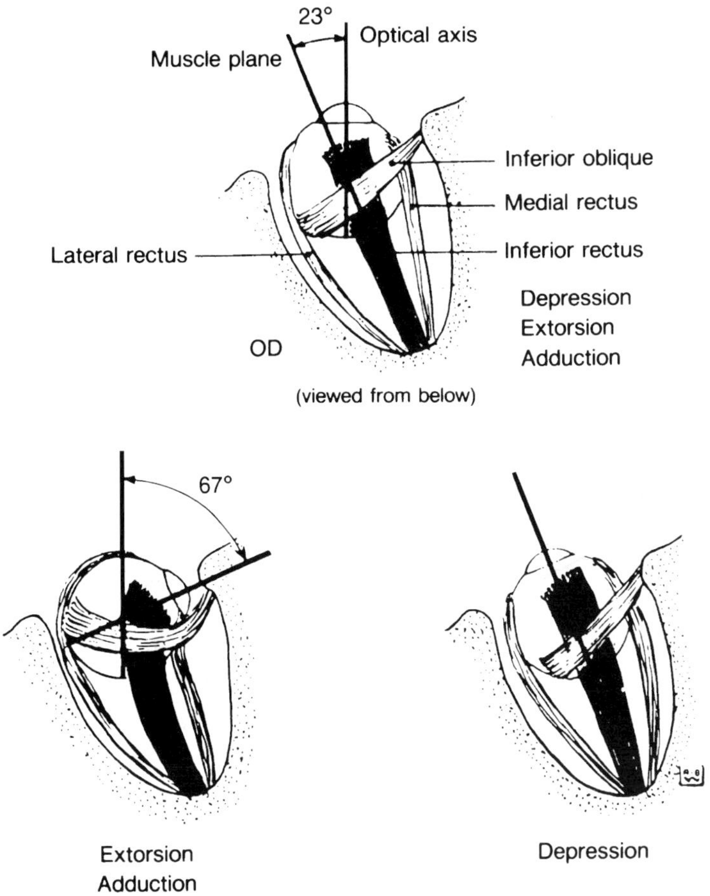

Figure 3-5 The right inferior rectus muscle, viewed from below. *(Reproduced with permission from von Noorden GK.* Atlas of Strabismus. *4th ed. St Louis: Mosby; 1983:5.)*

fascia in which the globe lies. For example, abducting the eye in a saccade requires a sudden great increase in lateral rectus muscle activity to get the eye moving and, at the same time, a total inhibition of the medial rectus muscle until the eye is again stabilized in the new gaze position. Velocity is nearly proportional to the size of the saccade and can be 10°–400°/sec. The velocity of the saccadic movement and the high forces that must be produced are affected by muscle paresis, and study of saccadic velocity is of practical value in determining paresis of muscles and abnormal innervation. BCSC Section 5, *Neuro-Ophthalmology*, discusses saccades in detail.

Goldstein HP, Scott AB. Ocular motility. In: Tasman W, Jaeger EA, eds. *Duane's Foundations of Clinical Ophthalmology.* Vol 2. Philadelphia: Lippincott; 2005:chap 23.

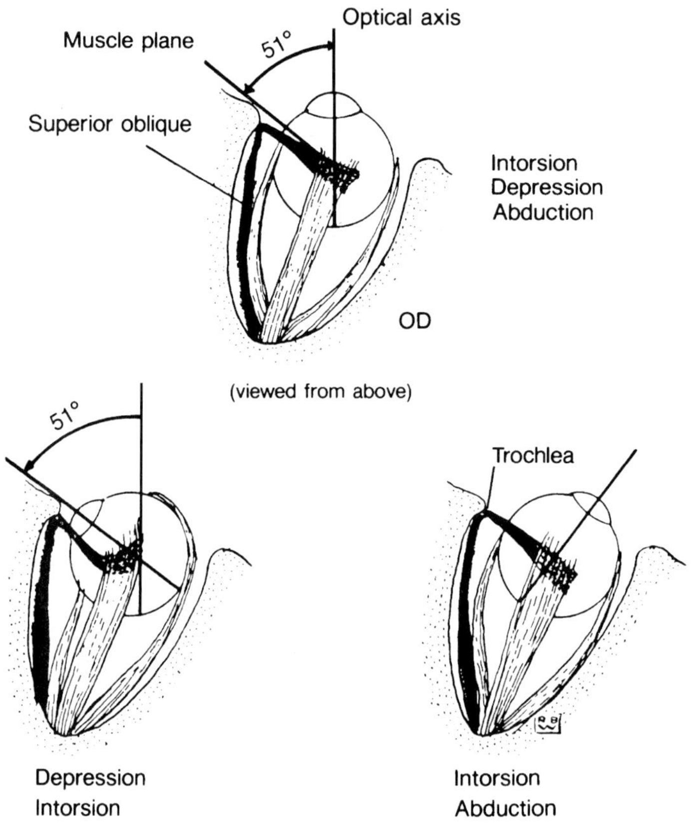

Figure 3-6 The right superior oblique muscle, viewed from above. *(Reproduced with permission from von Noorden GK.* Atlas of Strabismus. *4th ed. St Louis: Mosby; 1983:7.)*

Eye Movements

Monocular Eye Movements

Ductions

Ductions are monocular rotations of the eye. *Adduction* is movement of the eye nasally; abduction is movement of the eye temporally. *Elevation (supraduction or sursumduction)* is an upward rotation of the eye; *depression (infraduction or deorsumduction)* is a downward rotation of the eye. *Intorsion (incycloduction)* is defined as a nasal rotation of the superior portion of the vertical corneal meridian. *Extorsion (excycloduction)* is a temporal rotation of the superior portion of the vertical corneal meridian.

The following terms relating to the muscles used in monocular eye movements are also important:

- *agonist:* the primary muscle moving the eye in a given direction

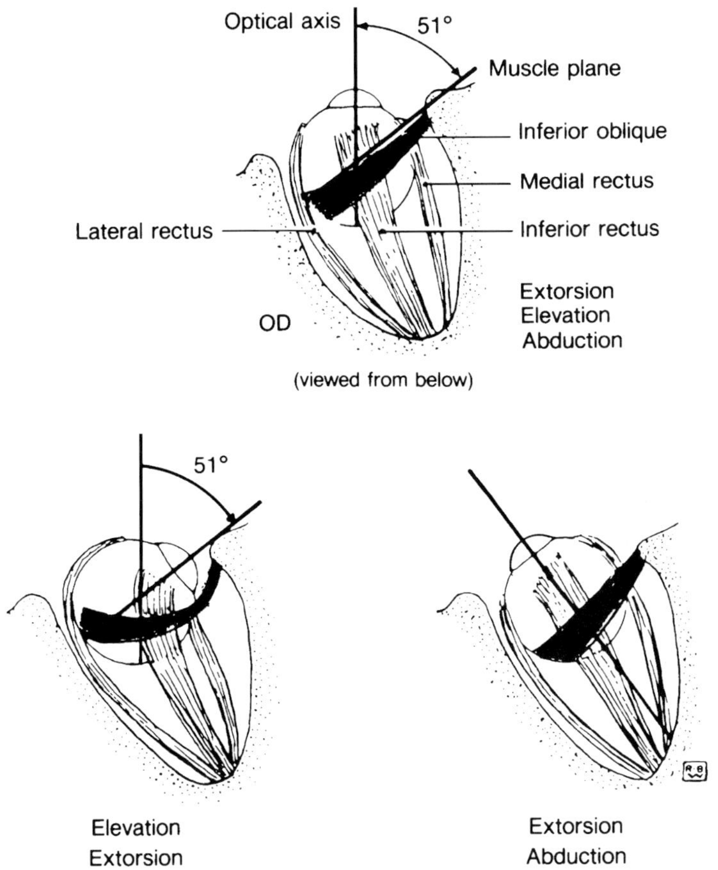

Figure 3-7 The right inferior oblique muscle, viewed from below. *(Reproduced with permission from von Noorden GK.* Atlas of Strabismus. *4th ed. St Louis: Mosby; 1983:9.)*

- *synergist:* the muscle in the same eye as the agonist that acts with the agonist to produce a given movement (eg, the inferior oblique muscle is a synergist with the agonist superior rectus muscle for elevation of the eye)
- *antagonist:* the muscle in the same eye as the agonist that acts in the direction opposite to that of the agonist; the medial rectus and lateral rectus muscles are antagonists

Sherrington's law of reciprocal innervation states that increased innervation and contraction of a given extraocular muscle are accompanied by a reciprocal decrease in innervation and contraction of its antagonist. For example, as the right eye abducts, the right lateral rectus muscle receives increased innervation while the right medial rectus receives decreased innervation.

Binocular Eye Movements

When binocular eye movements are conjugate and the eyes move in the same direction, such movements are called *versions*. When the eye movements are disconjugate and the eyes move in opposite directions, such movements are known as *vergences* (eg, convergence and divergence).

Versions: conjugate binocular eye movements

Right gaze *(dextroversion)* is movement of both eyes to the patient's right. Left gaze *(levoversion)* is movement of both eyes to the patient's left. *Elevation*, or *upgaze (sursumversion)*, is an upward rotation of both eyes; *depression*, or *downgaze (deorsumversion)*, is a downward rotation of both eyes. In *dextrocycloversion*, both eyes rotate so that the superior portion of the vertical corneal meridian moves to the patient's right. Similarly, *levocycloversion* is movement of both eyes so that the superior portion of the vertical corneal meridian rotates to the patient's left.

The term *yoke muscles* is used to describe 2 muscles (1 in each eye) that are the prime movers of their respective eyes in a given position of gaze. For example, when the eyes move or attempt to move into right gaze, the right lateral rectus muscle and the left medial rectus muscle are simultaneously innervated and contracted. These muscles are said to be "yoked" together.

Each extraocular muscle in 1 eye has a yoke muscle in the other eye. Because the effect of a muscle is usually best seen in a given direction of gaze, the concept of yoke muscles is used to evaluate the contribution of each extraocular muscle to eye movement. See Figure 3-2, which shows the 6 cardinal positions of gaze and the yoke muscles whose primary actions are in that field of gaze.

Hering's law of motor correspondence states that equal and simultaneous innervation flows to yoke muscles concerned with the desired direction of gaze. The most useful application of this law is in evaluating binocular eye movements and, in particular, the yoke muscles involved.

Hering's law has important clinical implications, especially when dealing with a paralytic or restrictive strabismus. Because the amount of innervation to both eyes is always determined by the fixating eye, the angle of deviation varies according to which eye is fixating. When the normal eye is fixating, the amount of misalignment is called the *primary deviation.* When the paretic or restrictive eye is fixating, the amount of misalignment is called the *secondary deviation.* The secondary deviation is larger than the primary deviation due to the increased innervation necessary to move the paretic or restrictive eye to the position of fixation.

Hering's law is also necessary to explain the following example. If a patient has a right superior oblique muscle paresis and uses the right eye to fixate an object that is located up and to the patient's left, the innervation of the right inferior oblique muscle required to move the eye into this gaze position is reduced because the right inferior oblique does not have to overcome the normal antagonistic effect of the right superior oblique muscle. Therefore, according to Hering's law, less innervation is also received by the right inferior oblique muscle's yoke muscle, the left superior rectus muscle. This decreased innervation could lead to the incorrect impression that the left superior rectus muscle is paretic (Fig 3-8).

This example is said to involve an inhibitional paresis of the contralateral antagonist when the paretic eye is fixating. However, the term *contralateral antagonist,* when used in conjunction with the concept of inhibitional paresis, is a contradiction. A more accurate description would be an *inhibitional paresis of the antagonist* (left superior rectus

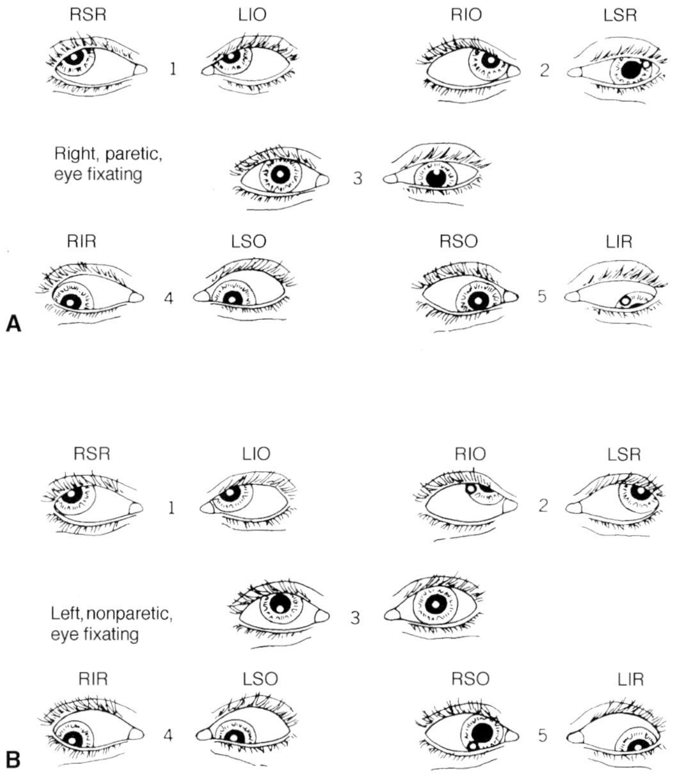

Figure 3-8 Paresis of right superior oblique muscle. **A,** With right paretic eye fixating, little or no vertical difference appears between the 2 eyes in the right (uninvolved) field of gaze (1 and 4). In primary position (3), a left hypotropia may be present because the right elevators require less innervation and thus the left elevators will receive less than normal innervation. When gaze is up and left (2), the RIO needs less than normal innervation to elevate OD because its antagonist, the RSO, is paretic. Consequently, its yoke, the LSR, will be apparently underacting, and pseudoptosis with pseudoparesis of the LSR will be present. When gaze is toward the field of action of the paretic muscle (5), maximal innervation is required to move OD down during adduction, and thus the LIR will be overacting. **B,** With left sound eye fixating, no vertical difference appears in the right field of gaze (1 and 4). In primary position (3), OD is elevated because of unbalanced elevators. When gaze is up and left (2), the RIO shows marked overaction because its antagonist is paretic and there is contracture of the unopposed muscle. The action of the LSR is normal. When gaze is down and left (5), normal innervation required by the fixating normal eye does not suffice to fully move the paretic eye. *(Reproduced with permission from von Noorden GK.* Atlas of Strabismus. *4th ed. St Louis: Mosby; 1983:24–25.)*

muscle) *of the yoke muscle* (left inferior rectus muscle) *of the paretic muscle* (right superior oblique muscle).

Vergences: disconjugate binocular eye movements

Convergence is movement of both eyes nasally relative to a given position; *divergence* is movement of both eyes temporally relative to a given position. *Incyclovergence* is a rotation of both eyes so that the superior portion of each vertical corneal meridian rotates toward the median plane; *excyclovergence* is a rotation of both eyes so that the superior pole of each vertical corneal meridian rotates away from the median plane. *Vertical vergence* movement, although less frequently encountered, can also occur: 1 eye moves upward and the other downward. (See also Chapter 4, Sensory Physiology and Pathology.) Other important terms and concepts related to vergences include the following:

Tonic convergence The constant innervational tone to the extraocular muscles when a person is awake and alert. Because of the anatomical shape of the bony orbits and the position of the rectus muscle origins, the alignment of the eyes under complete muscle paralysis is divergent. Therefore, convergence tone is necessary in the awake state to maintain straight eyes even in the absence of strabismus.

Accommodative convergence of the visual axes Part of the synkinetic near reflex. A fairly consistent increment of accommodative convergence (AC) occurs for each diopter of accommodation (A), giving the *accommodative convergence/accommodation (AC/A) ratio.*

Abnormalities of this ratio are common, and they are an important cause of strabismus. With an abnormally high AC/A ratio, the excess convergence tends to produce esotropia during accommodation on near targets. An abnormally low AC/A ratio tends to make the eyes exotropic when the person looks at near targets. For techniques of measuring this ratio, see the discussion of the AC/A ratio under Convergence in Chapter 6.

Voluntary convergence A conscious application of the near synkinesis.

Proximal (instrument) convergence An induced convergence movement caused by a psychological awareness of near; this movement is particularly apparent when a person looks through an instrument such as a binocular microscope.

Fusional convergence An optomotor reflex to converge and position the eyes so that similar retinal images project on corresponding retinal areas. Fusional convergence is accomplished without changing the refractive state of the eyes and is prompted by bitemporal retinal image disparity.

Fusional divergence The only clinically significant form of divergence. It is an optomotor reflex to diverge and align the eyes so that similar retinal images project on corresponding retinal areas. Fusional divergence is accomplished without changing the refractive state of the eyes and is prompted by binasal retinal image disparity.

Supranuclear Control Systems for Eye Movement

There are 5 supranuclear eye movement systems:

1. The *saccadic system* generates all fast (up to 400°–500°/sec) eye movements, or eye movements of refixation. This system functions to place the image of an object of interest on the fovea or to move the eyes from one object to another. Saccades are initiated by burst cells within the paramedian pontine reticular formation. Activation of burst cells requires suppression of pause cell activity. Pause cells are inhibited by corticobulbar projections from the frontal lobe.
2. The *smooth pursuit system* generates all following, or pursuit, eye movements. Pursuit latency is shorter than for saccades, but the maximum peak velocity of these slow pursuit movements is limited to 30°–60°/sec. The pathway starts with the striate cortex, which receives input from the lateral geniculate bodies. Extrastriate visual areas then receive input and project ipsilaterally to the dorsolateral pontine nuclei. Ultimately, the vestibular nuclei receive the input (probably through the cerebellar flocculus and dorsal vermis) and transmit it to ocular motor nuclei of cranial nerves III, IV, and VI.
3. The *vergence system* controls disconjugate eye movement, as in convergence or divergence. Supranuclear control of vergence eye movements is not yet fully understood.
4. The *position maintenance system* maintains a specific gaze position, allowing an object of interest to remain on the fovea. The site of this system is not known.
5. The *nonoptic reflex systems* integrate eye movements and body movements. The most clinically important system is the *labyrinthine reflex system*, which involves the semicircular canals of the inner ears. Other, less important, systems involve the utricle and saccule of the inner ears. The cervical, or neck, receptors also provide input for this nonoptic reflex control.

These systems are discussed in depth in BCSC Section 5, *Neuro-Ophthalmology.*

von Noorden GK, Campos EC. *Binocular Vision and Ocular Motility: Theory and Management of Strabismus.* 6th ed. St Louis: Mosby; 2002:55.

CHAPTER 4

Sensory Physiology and Pathology

Objective visual space consists of actual visual objects in physical space outside of, and independent of, our visual system. *Subjective visual space* is our conscious awareness of these visual objects and their relationships to us as perceived and interpreted by the brain.

Physiology of Normal Binocular Vision

If an area of the retina is stimulated by any means—externally by light or internally by mechanical pressure or electrical processes—the resulting sensation is always one of light, and the light is subjectively localized as coming from a specific visual direction in space. This directional value of the retinal elements is an intrinsic physiologic property of the retina and the brain. Thus, the stimulation of any retinal area results in a visual sensation from a subjective visual direction relative to the visual direction of the fovea. The visual direction of the fovea is termed the *visual axis*, and normally, with central fixation, it is subjectively localized straight ahead. BCSC Section 12, *Retina and Vitreous*, illustrates and discusses in depth the anatomy and physiology of the retina.

Correspondence

If retinal areas in the 2 eyes share a common subjective visual direction—that is, if their simultaneous stimulation results in the subjective sensation that the stimulating target or targets come from the same direction in space—these retinal areas or points are said to be *corresponding*. If the simultaneous stimulation of retinal areas in the 2 eyes results in the sensation of 2 separate visual directions for a target, or diplopia, these retinal areas or points are said to be *noncorresponding*, or *disparate*. If corresponding retinal areas in the 2 eyes bear identical relationships to the fovea in each eye (eg, both corresponding areas are located equidistantly to the right or left of and above or below the fovea), *normal retinal correspondence (NRC)* exists. Dissimilar relationships between 2 corresponding retinal areas and their respective foveas indicate *anomalous retinal correspondence (ARC)*. (ARC is discussed at length later in the chapter.) Correspondence is necessary for single vision.

If the 2 eyes have NRC and each fovea fixates an identical point, this point is seen singly. Points to both sides of this fixation point likewise fall on corresponding retinal areas and also are seen singly, as long as these points lie on a horizontal construct known as the *Vieth-Müller circle*. This circle passes through the optical centers of each eye and the point of fixation. When attempts are made to duplicate the Vieth-Müller circle experimentally, the locus of all points seen singly falls not on the circle but on a curved surface called the *empirical horopter* (Fig 4-1). The horopter not only exists in 2 dimensions but is actually a 3-dimensional space obtained by rotating the horizontal horopter around an axis connecting the centers of rotation of the 2 eyes. The geometric figure thus formed is a *torus.*

Each fixation point determines a specific horopter. By definition, all points lying on the horopter curve stimulate corresponding retinal elements and thus are seen singly. All points not lying on the horopter fall on disparate retinal elements and would therefore be expected to create double vision. However, double vision does not occur physiologically within a limited area surrounding the horopter curve because the visual system fuses the 2 disparate retinal images, resulting in single binocular vision with stereopsis. The slightly different images caused by the 3-dimensional object stimulate stereoscopic perception.

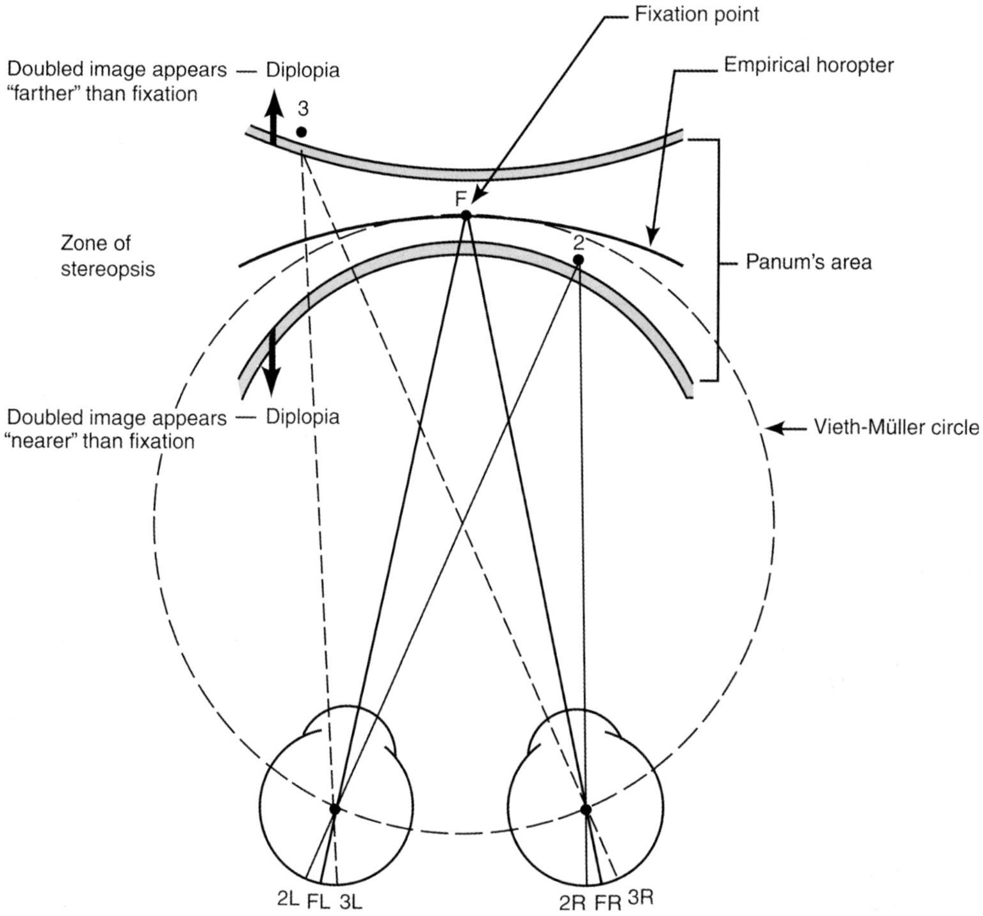

Figure 4-1 Empirical horopter. *F*, Fixation point; *FL* and *FR*, left and right foveas, respectively. Point 2, falling within Panum's area, is seen singly and stereoscopically. Point 3 falls outside of Panum's area and is therefore seen double.

The areas near the fovea allow very little overlap (small receptive fields) before diplopia is elicited, whereas more overlap (larger receptive fields) is tolerated farther toward the periphery of vision. Figure 4-1 shows objects in this space that fall mathematically on disparate retinal areas but are physiologically seen singly. This space is called *Panum's area of single binocular vision.* Objects outside of Panum's area fall on widely disparate retinal areas and are seen as coming from 2 different visual directions, causing physiologic diplopia.

A 3-dimensional object is partly in front of and partly behind the empirical horopter and thus stimulates disparate retinal points and is seen stereoscopically. As long as the 3-dimensional object falls entirely within Panum's area, it is seen singly. Objects that fall outside of Panum's area are seen double because the images are too disparate to be fused cortically into a single image. Stereopsis is a response to horizontally disparate retinal stimulation.

Fusion

Fusion is the cortical unification of visual objects into a single percept that is made possible by the simultaneous stimulation of corresponding retinal areas. For retinal images to be fused, they must be similar in size and shape. Fusion has been artificially divided into sensory fusion, motor fusion, and stereopsis.

Sensory fusion

Sensory fusion is based on the innate orderly topographic relationship between the retinas and the visual cortex, whereby corresponding retinal points project to the same cortical locus, and corresponding adjacent retinal points have adjacent cortical representations.

Motor fusion

Motor fusion is a vergence movement that causes similar retinal images to fall and be maintained on corresponding retinal areas even though natural (eg, phorias) or artificial causes tend to induce disparities. For example, if progressive base-out prism is introduced before both eyes while a target is viewed, the retinal images move temporally over both retinas if the eyes remain in fixed position. However, fusional convergence movements maintain similar retinal images on corresponding retinal areas, and the eyes are observed to converge. This response is called *fusional convergence.* Motor fusion may be thought of as a diplopia avoidance mechanism. Motor fusion is the exclusive function of the extrafoveal retinal periphery. Fusional vergence amplitudes can be measured with rotary prisms, by major haploscopes, and by other devices. Representative normal values are given in Table 4-1. Fusional vergences are also discussed in Chapter 6.

Table 4-1 Average Normal Fusional Amplitudes in Prism Diopters (Δ)

Testing Distance	Convergence Fusional Amplitudes	Divergence Fusional Amplitudes	Vertical Fusional Amplitudes
6 m	14Δ	6Δ	2.5Δ
25 cm	38Δ	16Δ	2.6Δ

Stereopsis

Stereopsis should not be thought of as a form of simple fusion. As discussed, stereopsis occurs when retinal disparity is too great to permit the simple superimposition or fusion of the 2 visual directions but is not great enough to elicit diplopia. Stereopsis, therefore, is a bridge between simple sensory and motor fusion and diplopia. Stereopsis allows a subjective ordering of visual objects in depth, or 3 dimensions. It is the highest form of binocular cooperation, and it adds a new quality to vision.

Stereopsis and depth perception should not be considered synonymous. Monocular clues contribute to depth perception. These monocular clues include object overlap, relative object size, highlights and shadows, motion parallax, and perspective. Stereopsis is a binocular sensation of relative depth caused by horizontal retinal image disparity. Nasal disparity between 2 similar retinal images is interpreted by the brain as farther away from the fixation point, temporal disparity as nearer. At distances farther than 20 feet, we rely almost entirely on monocular clues for depth perception.

Selected Aspects of the Neurophysiology of Vision

The decussation of the optic nerves at the chiasm is essential for the development of binocular vision and stereopsis. With decussation, visual information from corresponding retinal areas from each eye runs via adjacent parallel separate circuits through the lateral geniculate body and optic tracts to the visual cortex, where the information from both eyes is finally commingled and modified by various inputs coming together.

Substantial research has recently focused on the neurophysiology of vision. We will focus on the retinal ganglion cell layer; the *lateral geniculate body (LGB)*, which is classically represented as 6 purely monocular laminae (4 dorsal parvocellular and 2 ventral magnocellular laminae with koniocellular laminae separating them); and the primary visual cortex, also called the *striate cortex, V1*, or *Brodmann area 17*. This retinogeniculocortical pathway provides the neural substrate for visual perception (Fig 4-2).

The LGB is the principal thalamic visual nucleus linking the retina and the striate cortex. Of the approximately 1 million ganglion cells in the retina, approximately 90% of these terminate in the LGB. The LGB contains about 1.8 million neurons, which yields a ratio of ganglion cells to geniculate neurons of approximately 1:2. After a relatively direct transfer through the LGB, the signal activates a unit in the striate cortex containing approximately 1000 processing elements. According to the classic view, the striate cortex performs the basic analysis of geniculate input and then transmits its essence to higher peristriate cortical areas for further interpretation. These areas have been called *Brodmann areas 18* and *19*, or *V2, V3, V3a, V4*, and *V5*.

Retinogeniculocortical Pathway

The *magnocellular (M) system* and the *parvocellular (P) system* are the main neural systems in the retinogeniculocortical pathway. Less is known about the *koniocellular (K) system.* The M system originates with the *parasol retinal ganglion cells.* These cells have large somas with large dendritic fields and large axons; they are rare in the foveal area and increase in number toward the near periphery. They synapse with the magnocellular

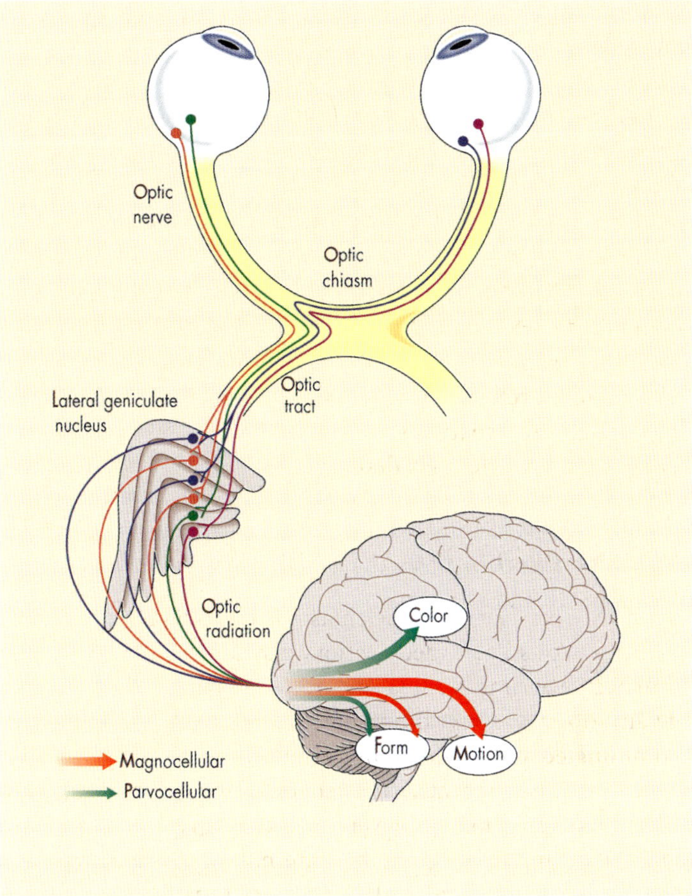

Figure 4-2 Distribution of higher-order visual processing among different cortical areas. The magnocellular system (inferior stream) is concerned generally with the location and motion of objects; the parvocellular system (superior stream) is concerned with the fine resolution (acuity), form, and color of objects. *(Reproduced with permission from Lawton A. The afferent visual system cortical representation of vision. In: Yanoff M, Duker J, eds.* Ophthalmology. *2nd ed. London: Mosby; 2004:1299.)*

neurons in the LGB. The M geniculate axons terminate in the striate cortex (V1) layer 4Cα. The neurons in this system have a fast response time, but these responses decay rapidly when the stimulus is maintained, making the M system especially sensitive to moving stimuli but not to stationary images. The M system is also relatively insensitive to color. In Macaque monkeys and probably also in humans, approximately 10% of the retinal input to the LGB comes from M cells.

The P system originates in the *midget ganglion cells*, which have small somas and small dendritic fields; these cells are of relatively high density in the fovea and decrease in number as retinal eccentricity increases. The P retinal ganglion cells synapse with the parvocellular LGB cells. The P geniculate axons terminate in layer 4Cβ of V1. The P system gives a slow tonic response to visual stimulation, carries high-resolution information about object borders and color contrast, and is important for shape perception and the ability to see standing objects in detail. Approximately 80% of retinal input is from P ganglion cells.

The K system originates in the small, bistratified retinal ganglion cells, which have large dendritic fields. They synapse with the konicellular LGB cells. The geniculate axons terminate in layers 3 and 1 of V1. This system is involved with aspects of color vision, especially blue color.

The fibers of the optic tract terminate in the LGB. Geniculate laminae 1 (parvo), 4 (parvo), and 6 (magno) receive axons from the contralateral nasal retina; laminae 2 (parvo), 3 (parvo), and 5 (magno) receive axons from the ipsilateral temporal retina. This monocular separation of corresponding retinal areas continues through the lateral geniculate laminae into the striate cortex (V1), where the geniculate axon terminals from the right and left eyes are segregated into a system of alternating parallel stripes called *ocular dominance columns* (Fig 4-3). In the P system, these strictly monocular geniculate axons terminate in layer 4Cβ. From there, the paired right and left monocular cells finally converge on the first binocular cells in layers 2 and 3 of V1. In the M system, after the monocular geniculate axons terminate in layer 4Cα, the paired right and left monocular cells converge on the first binocular cells in layer 4B of V1. In the K system, cells send their axons to cortical layers 3B and 1.

Visual Development

In the human retina, most of the ganglion cells are generated between the 8th and 15th weeks of gestation, reaching a plateau of 2.2–2.5 million by week 18. After week 30, the ganglion cell population falls dramatically during a period of rapid cell death that lasts 6–8 weeks. Thereafter, cell death continues at a low rate into the first few postnatal months. The retinal ganglion cell population is reduced to a final count of about 1 to 1.5 million. The loss of about 1 million optic axons may serve to refine the topography and specificity of the retinogeniculate projection by eliminating inappropriate connections.

The neurons of the human LGB are probably formed between the 8th and 11th weeks of gestation. By week 10, the first retinal ganglion cells invade the developing LGB. Segregation of the M, P, and K system retinal ganglion cells occurs on a timetable that parallels the lamination in the LGB. Retinal afferents prune back their axon terminals so that the synaptic connections are preserved only within the appropriate geniculate laminae, which emerge between weeks 22 and 25. It is thought that ganglion cells die if their axons do not successfully synapse with the appropriate targets in the brain. The LGB laminae become so precisely oriented that a properly positioned straight needle passing through all 6 layers would skewer only cells from corresponding retinal areas from each eye.

The cells that will become the striate cortex are probably formed between the 10th and 25th weeks of gestation. Initially, the geniculate afferents representing each eye overlap extensively in layer 4C (Fig 4-4). The maturation of the ocular dominance columns requires thousands of left and right eye geniculate afferents to gradually disentangle their overlapping axon terminals. This segregation transpires during the last few weeks of pregnancy and is almost complete at birth.

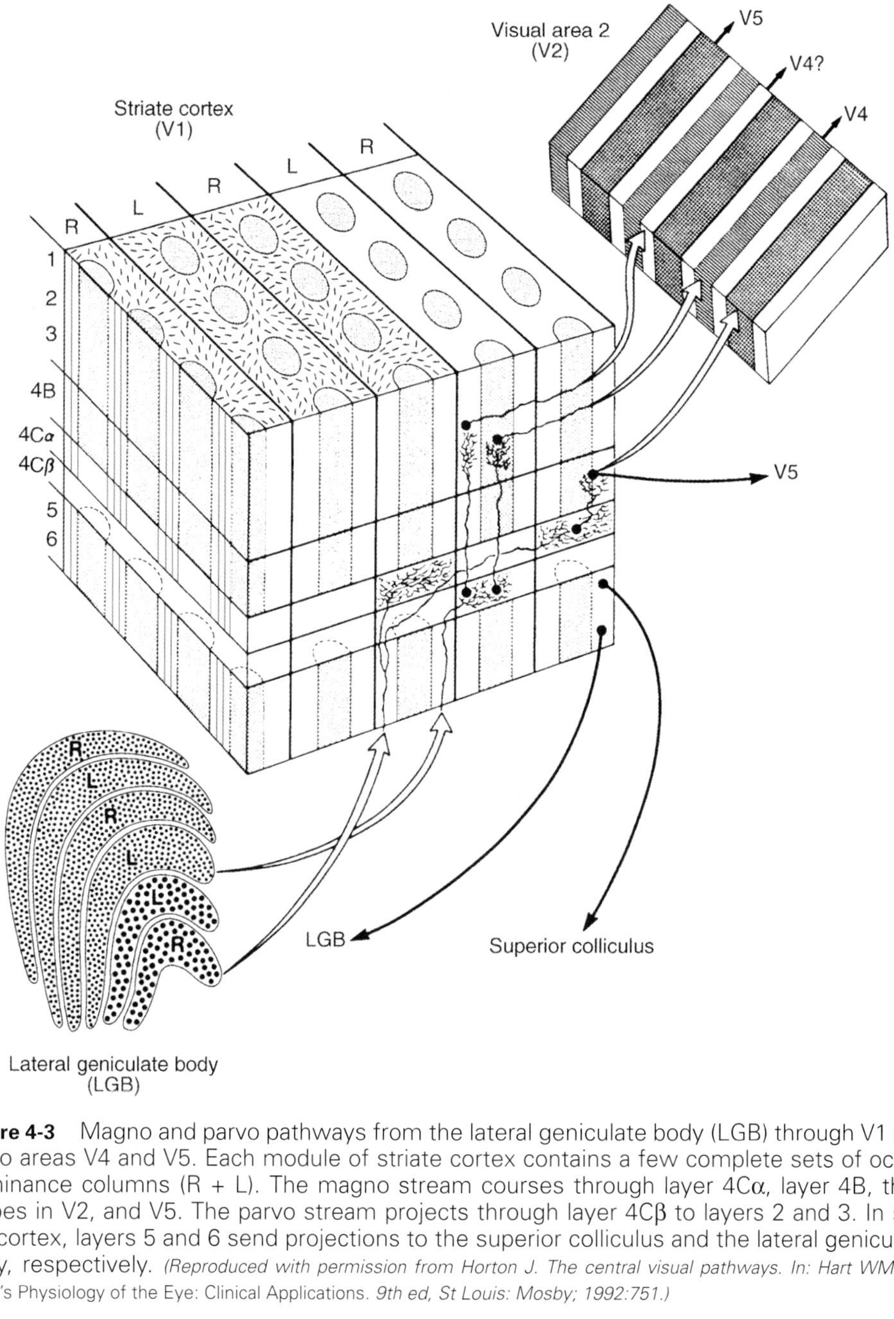

Figure 4-3 Magno and parvo pathways from the lateral geniculate body (LGB) through V1 and V2 to areas V4 and V5. Each module of striate cortex contains a few complete sets of ocular dominance columns (R + L). The magno stream courses through layer 4Cα, layer 4B, thick stripes in V2, and V5. The parvo stream projects through layer 4Cβ to layers 2 and 3. In striate cortex, layers 5 and 6 send projections to the superior colliculus and the lateral geniculate body, respectively. *(Reproduced with permission from Horton J. The central visual pathways. In: Hart WM, ed.* Adler's Physiology of the Eye: Clinical Applications. *9th ed, St Louis: Mosby; 1992:751.)*

The continued development of visual function after birth is accompanied by major anatomical changes occurring simultaneously at all levels of the central visual pathways. The fovea is still covered by multiple cell layers and is sparsely packed with cones, which may account for the estimated visual acuity of 20/400 at birth. During the first years of

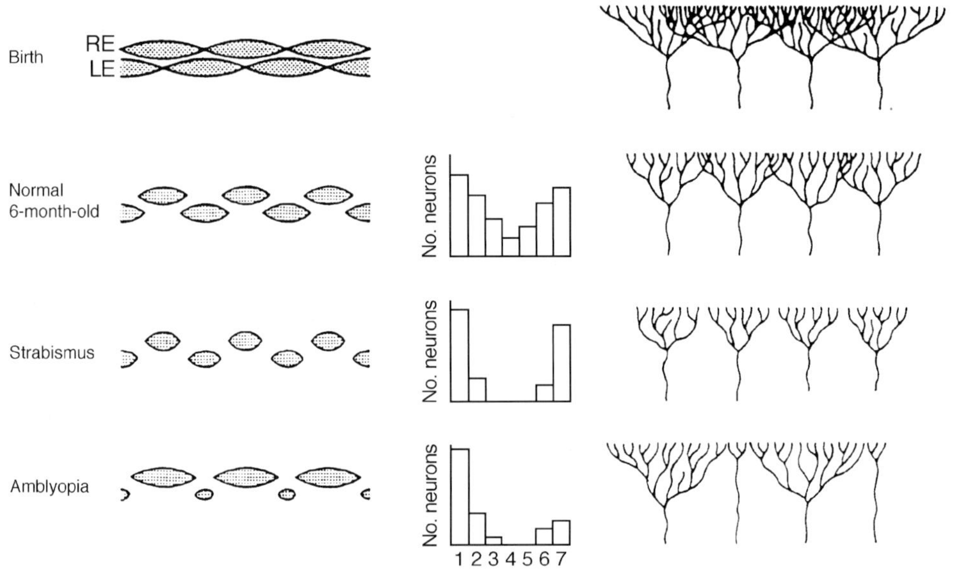

Figure 4-4 Anatomical and physiologic maturation of ocular dominance in lamina 4 of the left primary visual cortex in normal and deprived monkeys. *Birth:* Broad overlap of afferents from the lateral geniculate nucleus to lamina 4, hence little dominance by right *(RE)* vs left *(LE)*. *Normal 6-month-old:* Regression of overlapping afferents from both eyes with distinct areas of monocular dominance. The bar graph shows the classic U-shaped distribution obtained by single-cell recordings from the visual cortex. About half the cells are driven predominantly by the contralateral right eye and the other half by the ipsilateral left eye. A small number are driven equally by the 2 eyes. *1* = driven only by contralateral eye; *7* = driven only by ipsilateral eye; *2–6* = driven binocularly. *Strabismus:* Effect of artificial eye misalignment in the neonatal period on ocular dominance. The monkey alternated fixation (no amblyopia) and lacked fusion. Lack of binocularity is evident as exaggerated segregation into dominance columns. The bar graph shows the results of single-cell recordings obtained from this animal after age 1 year. Almost all neurons are driven exclusively by the right or left eye. *Amblyopia:* Effect of suturing the left eyelid shut shortly after birth. Dominance columns of the normal right eye are much wider than those of the amblyopic left eye. The bar graph shows markedly skewed ocular dominance. *(Reproduced with permission from Tychsen L. Binocular vision. In: Hart WM, ed.* Adler's Physiology of the Eye: Clinical Application. *9th ed. St Louis: Mosby; 1992:810.)*

life, the photoreceptors redistribute within the retina, and peak foveal cone density increases fivefold to achieve the configuration found in the adult retina, with an improvement in visual acuity to the 20/20 level. In newborns, the white matter of the visual pathways is not fully myelinated. For the first 2 years after birth, myelin sheaths enlarge rapidly and then continue at a slower rate through the first decade of life. At birth, the neurons of the LGB are only 60% of their average size. Their volume gradually increases until age 2 years. Striate cortex refinement of synaptic connections continues for many years after birth. The density of synapses declines by 40% over several years to attain final adult levels at about age 10 years.

Physiologic activity in the fetus is vital to the development of normal anatomical connections in the visual system. In utero, mammalian retinal ganglion cells discharge spontaneous action potentials in the absence of any visual stimulation. Abolishing these action potentials with tetrodotoxin prevents the normal prenatal segregation of the retinogeniculate axons into appropriate geniculate laminae and blocks the formation of ocular dominance columns in the striate cortex. Thus, although the functional architecture of the visual system is ordained by genetics, the specificity and refinement are molded by physiologic vision-independent activity occurring in the fetus, as well as by postnatal vision-dependent experience.

Effects of Abnormal Visual Experience on the Retinogeniculocortical Pathway

Abnormal visual experience can powerfully affect retinogeniculocortical development. Abnormal development produced by visual deprivation, anisometropia, or strabismus appears to result in changes in the primary visual cortex, which ceases to be a faithful relay of visual signals. The developing visual system's extreme sensitivity to unequal binocular competition and competitive inhibition is the price to be paid for the mechanisms that use patterns of activity to refine neural connections to a level of high precision.

If a newborn monkey is reared in the dark or with both eyes sutured closed, cells in the striate cortex eventually lose sharp orientation tuning and normal binocular responses. Some of the cells become unresponsive to visual stimulation and activate erratically and spontaneously. The remaining units give sluggish and unpredictable responses, with minimal potential for recovery. Cells in the striate cortex do not recover their normal responses.

Following the postnatal critical period, the visual system becomes impervious to the effects of sensory deprivation. If an adult monkey is visually deprived by the suturing of both eyelids, the cells in the striate cortex remain unaffected.

Single eyelid suturing in baby macaque monkeys usually produces axial myopia but no other significant changes in the eye. There is minor shrinkage of both the M and P cells of the lateral geniculate laminae receiving input from that deprived eye, but these cells respond briskly to visual stimulation, implying that a defect in the LGB is not likely to account for amblyopia. In the striate cortex, monocular visual deprivation causes the ocular dominance columns of the closed eye to appear radically narrowed (see Fig 4-4; Fig 4-5). The explanation is that the 2 eyes compete for synaptic contacts in the cortex. As a result, the deprived eye loses many of the connections already formed at birth with postsynaptic cortical targets. This leads to excessive pruning of the terminal arbors of geniculate cells driven by the deprived eye. In turn, the ocular dominance columns of the deprived eye begin to shrink, which leads to a reduction in the cell size of the LGB cells required to sustain a reduced arbor of axon terminals in layer 4C. The open eye profits by the sprouting of terminal arbors beyond their usual boundaries to occupy territory relinquished by the deprived eye. However, the benefit derived by invading the cortical territory of the deprived eye is unclear because visual acuity does not improve beyond normal. Positron emission testing (PET) has shown a reduction in the cortical blood flow and glucose metabolism during stimulation of the amblyopic eye compared with the normal eye, suggesting the visual cortex as the primary site of amblyopia. This monocular deprivation also devastates binocularity in that few cells can be driven by both eyes.

There is a critical period in which the eye of the macaque monkey is vulnerable to the effects of eyelid suturing. This critical period corresponds to that in which the wiring

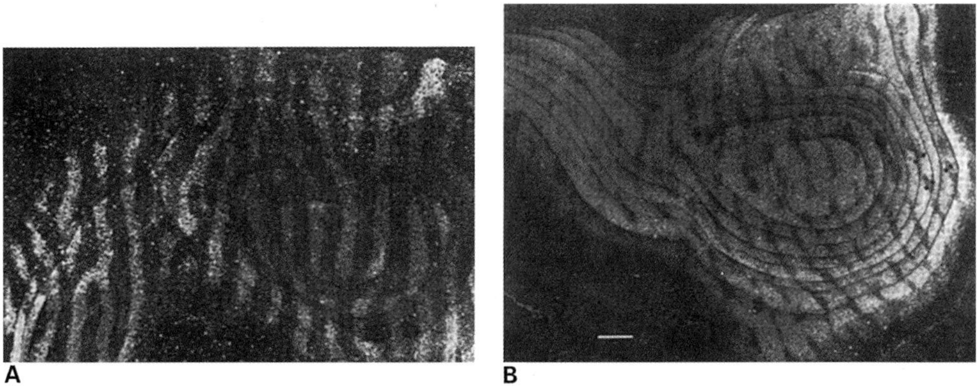

Figure 4-5 Change of ocular dominance columns in macaque monkey visual cortex after monocular deprivation. Radioactive proline was injected into the normal eye and transported to the visual cortex to reveal the projections of that eye. In these sections, cut parallel to the cortical surface, white areas show labeled terminals in layer 4. **A,** Normal monkey. The stripes representing the injected eye (bright) and noninjected eye (dark) have roughly equal spacing. **B,** Monocularly deprived monkey that had 1 eye sutured closed from birth for 18 months. The bright stripes (representing label in layer 4 from the open, injected eye) are widened; the dark ones (closed eye) are greatly narrowed. (Scale bar = 1 mm). *(Reproduced with permission from Kaufman PL, Alm A.* Adler's Physiology of the Eye. *10th ed. St Louis: Mosby; 2003:699. Originally from Hubell DH, Wiesel TN, LeVay S. Plasticity of ocular dominance columns in monkey striate cortex.* Philos Trans R Soc Lond B Biol Sci. *1977;278:377–409.)*

of the striate cortex is still vulnerable to the effects of visual deprivation. During the critical period, the deleterious effects of eyelid closure are correctable by reversal of the eyelid suture—that is, opening the sutured eye and closing the fellow eye. After this reversal, the ocular dominance columns of the initially closed eye appear practically normal, indicating that anatomical recovery of the initially shrunken columns was induced by opening the right eye and penalizing the left eye. However, when the right eye is sewn closed beyond the critical period and then is reopened and the fellow eye closed, the deprived eye columns do not reexpand.

Eyelid suturing in the baby macaque monkey is a good model for visual-deprivation amblyopia. In children, this condition can be caused by any dense opacity of the ocular media or occlusion by the eyelid. Visual deprivation can cause a rapid and profound amblyopia.

Amblyopia in children also has other causes. Optical defocus caused by anisometropia causes the cortical neurons driven by the defocused eye to be less sensitive (particularly to higher spatial frequencies because they are most affected by blur) and to send out a weaker signal. This results in a binocular neural imbalance, resulting in reduced binocular activity, little if any narrowing of the ocular dominance columns, and cell shrinkage in the parvocellular laminae. Only the function of the P system is abnormal in anisometropic amblyopia. Deficits in binocular processing are also more pronounced when tested with stimuli of high spatial frequency.

The critical period for anisometropic amblyopia begins when the unilateral optical blur exceeds the lessening bilateral neural blur, which improves as the visual system develops sensitivity to high spatial frequency. This critical period may have a later onset than strabismic amblyopia and may require a prolonged period of unilateral blur. Meridional (astigmatic) amblyopia does not develop during the first year of life and may not develop until age 3.

Strabismus can be artificially created in monkeys by the sectioning of an extraocular muscle. Some monkeys develop alternating fixation after this procedure; they maintain normal acuity in each eye. Examination of the striate cortex reveals cells with normal receptive fields and an equal number of cells responsive to stimulation of either eye. However, the cortex is bereft of binocular cells (see Fig 4-4; Fig 4-6). After 1 extraocular muscle is cut, some monkeys do not alternately fixate but constantly fixate with the same eye, and the deviating eye develops amblyopia. An important factor in the development of strabismic amblyopia is interocular suppression due to image uncorrelation. Strabismus causes abnormal input to the striate cortex by preventing the synchronous firing provided by simultaneous correlated images from the 2 foveas. Another factor is the optical defocus of the deviated eye. The dominant eye is focused on the object of regard while the deviated eye is pointed in a different direction; for the

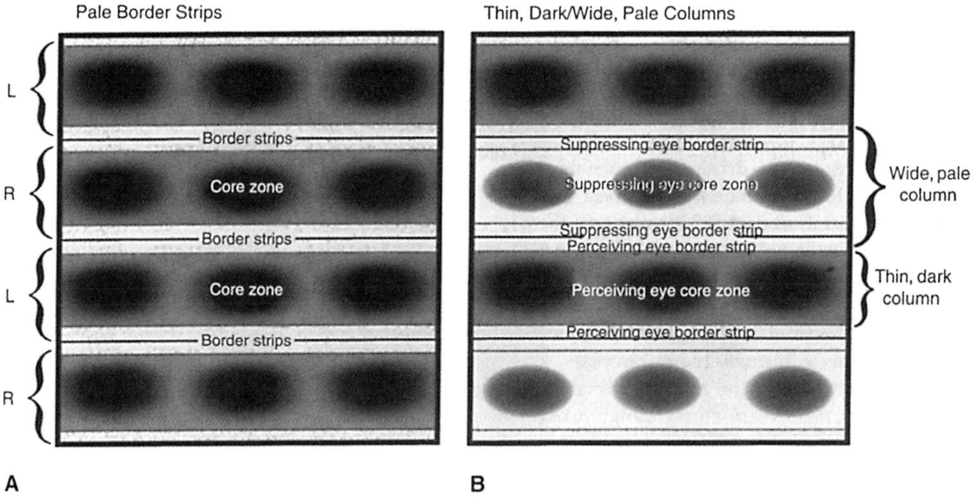

Figure 4-6 Schematic diagrams showing the 2 patterns of cytochrome oxidase (CO) activity induced by experimental strabismus in monkeys. **A,** Pale border strips prevailed in regions of the cortex where CO activity was lost in the binocular border strips from disruption of ocular alignment, but metabolic activity remained strong in the monocular core zones serving each eye. This pattern is seen only in cortex representing the central 15° and in monkeys with a weak fixation preference. **B,** Thin, dark columns alternating with wide, pale columns were seen in cortex where CO activity was reduced in both eyes' binocular border strips and 1 eye's monocular core zones. Presumably, CO was lowered in the suppressed eye's core zones. This pattern was seen throughout the cortex in animals with a strong fixation preference but only in the peripheral cortex of those with a weak fixation preference. *(Reproduced with permission from Kaufman PL, Alm A.* Adler's Physiology of the Eye. *10th ed. St Louis: Mosby; 2003:703. Originally from Horton JC, Hocking DR, Adams DL. Metabolic mapping of suppression scotomas in striate cortex of macaques with experimental strabismus.* J Neurosci. *1999;19:7111–7129.)*

deviated eye, an object may be too near or too far to be in focus. Either mechanism can cause asynchrony or inhibition of 1 set of signals in the striate cortex layer 4C. In strabismic amblyopia, layer 4C, especially the parvocellular recipient layer, appears less active and binocular activity is reduced, but there is little change in the width of the ocular dominance columns.

The critical period for developing strabismic amblyopia appears to begin at approximately 4 months of age, during the time of ocular dominance segregation and sensitivity to binocular correlation.

It is remarkable that abnormal sensory input alone is sufficient to alter the normal anatomy of the visual cortex. Other areas of the cerebral cortex may also depend on sensory stimulation to form the proper anatomical circuits necessary for normal adult visual function. This notion underscores the importance of providing children with an adequate and healthy sensory environment.

Booth R, Fulton A. Amblyopia. In: Albert D, Jakobiec F, eds. *Principles and Practice of Ophthalmology.* 2nd ed. Philadelphia: Saunders; 2000:4340–4354.

Bron A, Tripathi RC, Tripathi BJ, eds. *Wolff's Anatomy of the Eye and Orbit.* 8th ed. London: Chapman & Hall; 1997:551–594.

Matsubara J. Central visual pathways. In: Kaufman P, Alm A, eds. *Adler's Physiology of the Eye: Clinical Application.* 10th ed. St Louis: Mosby; 2003:641–709.

Shan Y, Moster ML, Roemer RA, et al. Abnormal function of the parvocellular visual system in anisometropic amblyopia. *J Pediatr Ophthalmol Strabismus.* 2000;37:73–78.

Abnormalities of Binocular Vision

When a manifest deviation of the eyes occurs, the corresponding retinal elements of the eyes are no longer directed at the same object. This places the patient at risk for 2 different visual phenomena: visual confusion and diplopia.

Confusion

Visual confusion is the simultaneous perception of 2 different objects projected onto corresponding retinal areas. The 2 foveal areas are physiologically incapable of simultaneous perception of dissimilar objects. The closest foveal equivalent is retinal rivalry, wherein the 2 perceived images rapidly alternate (Fig 4-7). Confusion may be a phenomenon of nonfoveal retinal areas only. Clinically significant visual confusion is rare.

Diplopia

Double vision, or *diplopia*, usually results from an acquired misalignment of the visual axes that causes an image to fall simultaneously on the fovea of 1 eye and on a nonfoveal point in the other eye. The object that falls on these noncorresponding points must be outside Panum's area to be seen double. The same object is seen as having 2 different locations in subjective space, and the foveal image is always clearer than the nonfoveal image of the nonfixating eye. The symptoms of diplopia depend on the age at onset, duration, and subjective awareness. The younger the child, the greater the ability to suppress, or inhibit, the nonfoveal image.

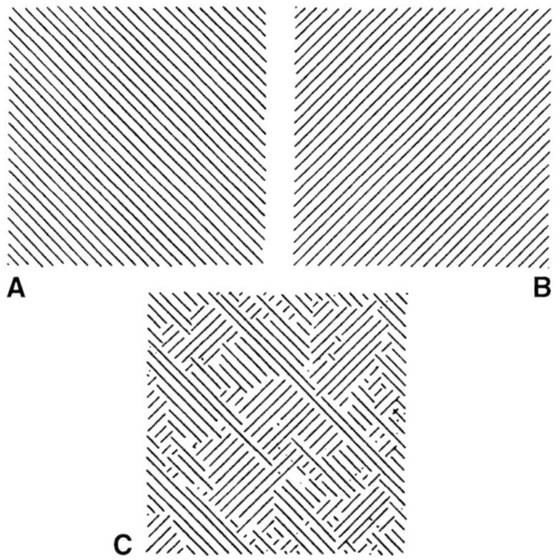

Figure 4-7 Rivalry pattern. **A,** Pattern seen by the left eye. **B,** Pattern seen by the right eye. **C,** Binocular vision. *(Reproduced with permission from von Noorden GK, Campos EC.* Binocular Vision and Ocular Motility: Theory and Management of Strabismus. *6th ed. St Louis: Mosby; 2002:12.)*

Central fusional disruption (horror fusionis) is an intractable diplopia that features the avoidance of bifoveal stimulation, an absence of suppression, and a loss of fusional amplitudes to maintain fusion. The angle of strabismus may be small or may vary. Horror fusionis can occur in a number of clinical settings: after disruption of fusion for a prolonged period; after head trauma; and, rarely, in long-standing strabismus. Management can be challenging.

Lee MC. Acquired central fusional disruption with spontaneous recovery. *Strabismus.* 1998;6:175–179.

Sensory Adaptations in Strabismus

To avoid confusion and diplopia, the visual system can use the mechanisms of suppression and ARC (Fig 4-8). It is important to realize that pathologic suppression and ARC develop only in the immature visual system.

Suppression

Suppression is the alteration of visual sensation that occurs when the images from 1 eye are inhibited or prevented from reaching consciousness. Pathologic suppression results from strabismic misalignment of the visual axes. Such suppression can be seen as an adaptation of a visually immature brain to avoid diplopia. Physiologic suppression is the mechanism that prevents physiologic diplopia (diplopia elicited by objects outside of Panum's area) from reaching consciousness.

The following is a useful classification of suppression for the clinician:

- *Central versus peripheral. Central suppression* is the term used to describe the mechanism that keeps the foveal image of the deviating eye from reaching consciousness,

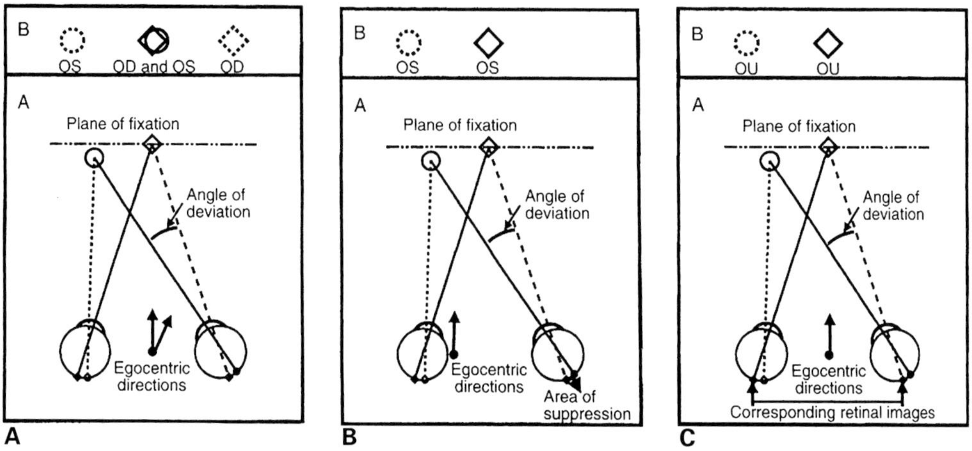

Figure 4-8 Retinal correspondence and suppression in strabismus. **A,** A strabismic patient with normal retinal correspondence (NRC) and without suppression would have diplopia, 2 egocentric directions of single objects (solid and dashed images in **B**) and visual confusion, a common visual direction for 2 separate objects (represented by the superimposition of the images of the fixated diamond and the circle, which is imaged on the fovea of the deviating eye in **B**). **B,** The elimination of diplopia and confusion by suppression of the retinal image of the deviating eye. **C,** The elimination of diplopia and confusion by anomalous retinal correspondence (ARC), an adaptation of visual directions of the deviated eye. *(Reproduced with permission from Kaufman PL, Alm A.* Adler's Physiology of the Eye. *10th ed. St Louis: Mosby; 2003:490.)*

thereby preventing confusion. However, because the 2 foveas cannot simultaneously perceive dissimilar objects, this central scotoma of the nonfixating fovea is considered by many clinicians to be a physiologic form of suppression rather than a pathologic one. In addition, this scotoma of the deviated eye can be documented immediately after the onset of ocular misalignment, even in new-onset strabismus in a visually mature adult. Despite complaints of diplopia, adults with new-onset strabismus fixate with 1 eye at a time and demonstrate a small scotoma of the nonfixating fovea, thus preventing central visual confusion. This response to adult-onset strabismus supports the opinion that central suppression should be classified as physiologic rather than pathologic because pathologic suppression can develop only in an immature visual system. *Peripheral suppression* is the mechanism that eliminates diplopia by preventing awareness of the image that falls on the peripheral retina in the deviating eye, the image that resembles the image falling on the fovea of the fixating eye. This form of suppression is clearly pathologic, developing as a cortical adaptation only within an immature visual system. Adults may be unable to develop peripheral suppression and therefore may be unable to eliminate the peripheral second image of the object viewed by the fixating eye (the object of regard) without closing or occluding the deviating eye.

- *Monocular versus alternating.* If suppression is unidirectional or always causes the image from the dominant eye to predominate over the image from the deviating eye, the suppression is *monocular.* This type of mechanism may lead to the establishment of strabismic amblyopia. If the process is bidirectional or switches over time between the images of the 2 eyes, the suppression is described as *alternating.*

- *Facultative versus obligatory.* Suppression may be considered *facultative* if present only when the eyes are in the deviated state and absent in all other states. Patients with intermittent exotropia, for instance, often experience suppression when the eyes are divergent but may enjoy high-grade stereopsis when the eyes are straight. In contrast, *obligatory* suppression is present at all times, whether the eyes are deviated or aligned. The suppression scotoma in the deviating eye may be either *relative* (in the sense of permitting some visual sensation) or *absolute* (permitting no perception of light).

Tests of suppression

If a patient with strabismus and NRC does not have diplopia, suppression is present provided the sensory pathways are intact. In less clear-cut situations, several simple tests are available for clinical diagnosis of suppression. (See Subjective Testing for Suppression and ARC, later in this chapter.)

Management of suppression

Therapy for suppression often involves the treatment of the strabismus itself:

- proper refractive correction
- occlusion or pharmacologic penalization, to permit equal and alternate use of each eye and to overcome any amblyopia that may be present
- alignment of the visual axes, to permit simultaneous stimulation of corresponding retinal elements by the same object

Orthoptic exercises may be attempted to overcome the tendency of the image from 1 eye to suppress the image from the other eye when both eyes are open. These exercises are designed to make the patient aware of diplopia first, then of simultaneous perception, and then of fusion—both on an instrument and in free space. The role of orthoptics in the therapy of suppression is controversial. In treatment of patients with esotropia, antisuppression therapy can cause intractable diplopia as suppression disappears. Antisuppression therapy is safer in patients with intermittent exotropia, but the results have received mixed reviews. Patients with no fusion potential should never undergo antisuppression therapy.

Anomalous Retinal Correspondence

Anomalous retinal correspondence (ARC) can be described as a condition wherein the fovea of the fixating eye has acquired an anomalous common visual direction with a peripheral retinal element in the deviated eye. The 2 foveas have different visual directions. ARC is an adaptation that restores some sense of binocular cooperation. Anomalous binocular vision is a functional state superior to that prevailing in the presence of total suppression. In the development of ARC, the normal sensory development is replaced only gradually and not always completely. The more long-standing the deviation, the more deeply rooted the ARC may become. The period during which ARC may develop probably extends through the first decade of life.

Paradoxical diplopia can occur when ARC persists after surgery. When esotropic patients whose eyes have been set straight or nearly straight postoperatively report a crossed diplopic localization of foveal or parafoveal stimuli, they are experiencing paradoxical diplopia (Fig 4-9). Clinically, paradoxical diplopia is a fleeting postoperative phenomenon, seldom lasting longer than a few days to weeks. However, in rare cases, this condition has persisted for much longer.

Testing for ARC

Testing in patients with ARC is performed to determine how patients use their eyes in normal life and to seek out any vestiges of normal correspondence. As discussed earlier, ARC is a sensory adaptation to abnormal binocular vision. Because the depth of the sensory rearrangement can vary widely, an individual can test positive for both NRC

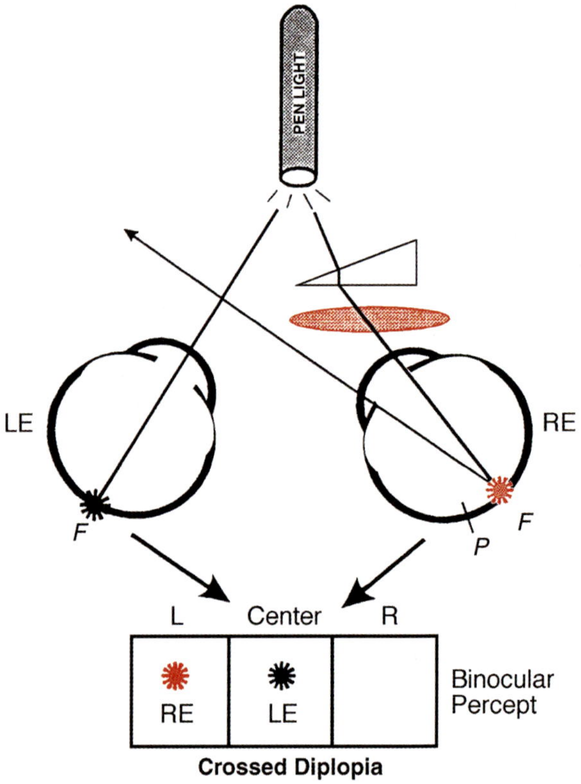

Figure 4-9 Paradoxical diplopia. Diagram of esotropia and ARC, wherein the deviation is being neutralized with a base-out prism. A red glass and base-out prism are placed over the right eye. The prism neutralizes the deviation by moving the retinal image of the penlight temporally, off the pseudofovea *(P)* to the true fovea *(F)*. Because the pseudofovea is the center of orientation, the image is perceived to fall on the temporal retina and is projected to the opposite field, thus resulting in crossed diplopia. *(Reproduced with permission from Wright KW, Spiegel PH.* Pediatric Ophthalmology and Strabismus. *St Louis: Mosby; 1999:219.)*

and ARC. Tests that closely simulate everyday use of the eyes are more likely to give evidence of ARC. The more dissociative the test, the more likely the test will produce an NRC response unless the ARC is deeply rooted. Some of the more common tests, in order of least dissociating to most dissociating, are the Bagolini striated glasses, amblyoscope, red-glass test (dissociation increases with the density of the red filter), Worth 4-dot test, and afterimage test. The farther down this test list the patient gives an anomalous localization response, the greater the depth of ARC. (See Subjective Testing for Suppression and ARC, later in this chapter.)

The tests for ARC can basically be divided into 2 groups: those that stimulate the fovea of 1 eye and an extrafoveal area of the other eye, and those that stimulate the foveal area in each eye. Note that ARC is a binocular phenomenon, tested for and documented in both eyes simultaneously. Eccentric fixation is a monocular phenomenon found on testing 1 eye alone; it is not in any way related to ARC. In eccentric fixation, patients do not fixate with the fovea when the fellow eye is covered. On cover testing, the eye remains more or less deviated, depending on how far the nonfoveolar area of fixation is from the fovea. Because some tests for ARC depend on separate stimulation of each fovea, the presence of eccentric fixation can significantly affect the test results.

Monofixation Syndrome

The term *monofixation syndrome* is used to describe a particular clinical presentation of the 2 preceding sensory adaptations, suppression and ARC. In this syndrome, both a small foveal suppression scotoma and a minute angle of ARC are present. The essential feature of this syndrome is the presence of peripheral fusion without central fusion.

A patient with monofixation syndrome usually has a small-angle esotropia, but there may be exotropia or even no manifest deviation. A small-angle strabismus (usually $<8\Delta$) can often be detected under binocular conditions. These patients are sometimes said to have *microtropias.* A central scotoma and peripheral fusion are present with binocular viewing. Amblyopia is a common finding; usually it is slight, but it may be profound. Fixation can be central or eccentric, stereo acuity is reduced, and horizontal fusional amplitudes are present. ARC is found on some sensory tests.

Patients with monofixation syndrome may have latent phoria in excess of a manifest microtropia. When this occurs, the alternate prism cover test measurement will exceed the simultaneous prism cover test measurement.

Monofixation syndrome may be a primary condition, although it is a favorable consequence of esotropia treatment with glasses, surgery, or both. This syndrome can also result from anisometropia or macular lesions. It can be the cause of unilaterally reduced vision when no obvious strabismus is present. If amblyopia is clinically significant, occlusion therapy is indicated.

Diagnosis

To accurately diagnose monofixation syndrome, the clinician must demonstrate both the absence of central binocular vision *(bifixation)* and the presence of peripheral binocular vision *(peripheral fusion).* Documentation of a macular scotoma in the nonfixating eye during binocular viewing is needed to verify the absence of bifixation. Several binocular perimetric techniques have been described to plot the monofixation scotoma. However, they are rarely used clinically.

Vectographic projections of Snellen letters can be used clinically to document the facultative scotoma of the monofixation syndrome. Snellen letters are viewed through polarized analyzers or goggles equipped with liquid crystal shutters in such a way that some letters are seen with only the right eye, some with only the left eye, and some with both eyes. Patients with monofixation syndrome delete letters that are imaged only in the nonfixating eye.

Testing stereo acuity is an important part of the monofixation syndrome evaluation. Any amount of gross stereopsis confirms the presence of peripheral fusion. Most patients with monofixation syndrome demonstrate 200–3000 sec of arc stereopsis. However, because some patients with monofixation syndrome have no demonstrable stereopsis, other tests for peripheral fusion must be used in conjunction with stereo acuity measurement. Fine stereopsis (better than 67 sec of arc) is present only in patients with bifixation.

Parks MM. The monofixation syndrome. *Trans Am Ophthalmol Soc.* 1969;67:609–657. (This classic thesis outlines early studies of small-angle deviations and central versus peripheral binocular vision. The development of the various terms used to describe these conditions is also covered in detail.)

von Noorden GK, Campos EC. *Binocular Vision and Ocular Motility: Theory and Management of Strabismus.* 6th ed. St Louis: Mosby; 2002:340–345.

Subjective Testing for Suppression and ARC

All tests are tainted by the inability of the testing conditions to reproduce the patient's condition of casual seeing. The more dissociative the test, the less the test simulates everyday use of the eyes. These tests should always be performed in conjunction with a cover test to decide whether a fusion response is due to orthophoria or ARC.

Red-glass test

The *red-glass* (diplopia) *test* involves stimulation of both the fovea of the fixating eye and an extrafoveal area of the other eye. First, the patient's deviation is measured objectively. Then a red glass is placed before the nondeviating eye while the patient fixates on a white light. This test can be performed both at distance and at near. Diplopia is present if the patient notes both a red light (through the glass) and a white light (Fig 4-10A, B). If only 1 light is seen (either red or white), suppression is present (Fig 4-10C). A 5Δ or 10Δ prism base-up in front of the deviated eye can be used to move the image out of the suppression scotoma, causing the patient to experience diplopia. With NRC, the white image will be localized correctly: the white image is seen below and to the right of the left image (Fig 4-10D). With ARC, the white image will be localized incorrectly: it is seen directly below the image (Fig 4-10E).

The following responses are possible with the red-glass test:

- The patient may see a red light and a white light. If the patient has esotropia, the images appear uncrossed (eg, the red light is to the left of the white light with the red glass over the left eye). This response is known as *homonymous*, or *uncrossed, diplopia.* This can easily be remembered because the esotropic patient sees the red

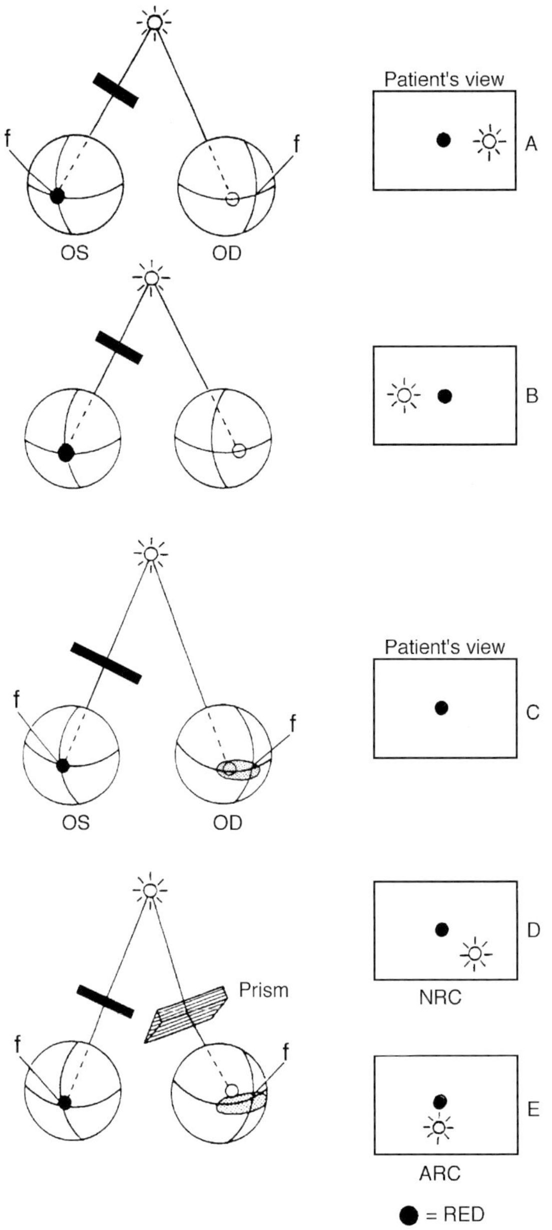

Figure 4-10 Red-glass test for suppression ARC (see text for explanation). *(Reproduced with permission from von Noorden GK, Campos EC.* Binocular Vision and Ocular Motility: Theory and Management of Strabismus. *6th ed. St Louis: Mosby; 2002:223.)*

light on the same side as the red glass (see Fig 4-10A). If the patient has exotropia, the images appear crossed (eg, the red light is to the right of the white light with the red glass over the left eye). This response is known as *heteronymous*, or *crossed, diplopia* (see Fig 4-10B). If the measured separation between the 2 images equals the previously determined deviation, the patient has NRC.

- If the patient sees the 2 lights superimposed so that they appear pinkish despite a measurable esotropia or exotropia, an abnormal localization of retinal points is present. This condition is known as *harmonious anomalous retinal correspondence.*
- If the patient sees 2 lights (with uncrossed diplopia in esotropia and with crossed diplopia in exotropia), but the separation between the 2 images is found to be less than the previously determined deviation, the patient has *unharmonious anomalous retinal correspondence.* Some investigators consider unharmonious ARC to be an artifact of the testing situation.

Worth 4-dot test

In the *Worth 4-dot test*, a red glass is worn in front of 1 eye and a green glass in front of the other (Fig 4-11). The eye behind the red glass can see red light but not green light because the red glass blocks this wavelength. Similarly, the eye behind the green glass can see green light but not red light. If a target consisting of 2 green lights, 1 red light, and 1 white light is viewed, the patient with normal ocular alignment will report a total of 4 lights. The white light is usually reported to undergo color rivalry; however, only 1 light is seen in the position of the white light. If the eye behind the green glass is suppressed, a total of 2 lights is reported. If the eye behind the red glass is suppressed, a total of 3 lights is reported. If the patient reports 5 lights, diplopia is present. A report of more than 5 lights is factitious. A polarized Worth 4-dot test is now available; it is administered and interpreted much like the traditional test except that polarized glasses are worn rather than red and green ones. As with the red-glass test, the Worth 4-dot test can produce a diplopic response in nonsuppression heterotropic NRC and either a diplopic or a fusion response in ARC, depending on the depth of the ARC adaptation. As mentioned earlier, this test must be performed in conjunction with cover testing.

When testing a patient for monofixation syndrome, the Worth 4-dot test can be used to demonstrate both the presence of peripheral fusion and the absence of bifixation. The standard Worth 4-dot flashlight projects onto a central retinal area of 1° or less when viewed at 10 feet, well within the 3°–5° scotoma characteristic of monofixation syndrome. Therefore, patients with monofixation syndrome will report 2 or 3 lights when viewing at 10 feet, depending on their ocular fixation preference. As the Worth 4-dot flashlight is brought closer to the patient, the dots begin to project onto peripheral retina outside the central monofixation scotoma until a fusion response (4 lights) is obtained. This usually occurs between 2 and 3 feet.

Bagolini glasses

Bagolini striated glasses are glasses of no dioptric power that have many narrow striations running parallel in one meridian. These glasses cause the fixation light to appear as an elongated streak, like micro-Maddox cylinders. The lenses are usually placed at 135° in front of the right eye and at 45° in front of the left eye. The advantages of the Bagolini

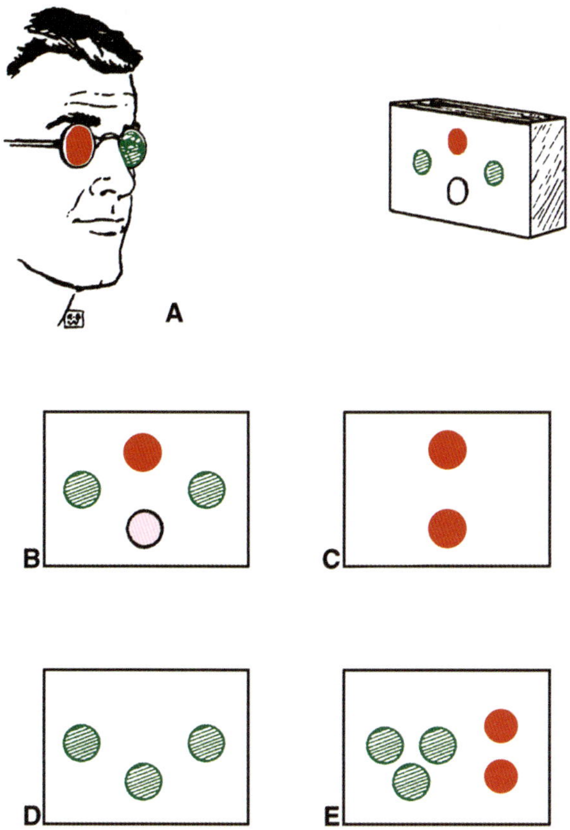

Figure 4-11 The Worth 4-dot test. **A,** Looking through a pair of red and green goggles, the patient views a box with 4 lights (1 red, 2 green, 1 white) at 6 m and at 33 cm (with the 4 lights mounted on a flashlight). The possible responses are given in B to E. **B,** Patient sees all 4 lights: peripheral fusion with orthophoria or strabismus with ARC. Depending on ocular dominance, the light in the 6 o'clock position is seen as white or pink. **C,** Patient sees 2 red lights: suppression in OS. **D,** Patient sees 3 green lights: suppression in OD. **E,** Patient sees 5 lights. The red lights may appear to the right, as in this figure (uncrossed diplopia with esotropia), or to the left of the green lights (crossed diplopia with exotropia). *(Reproduced with permission from von Noorden GK, Campos EC.* Binocular Vision and Ocular Motility: Theory and Management of Strabismus. *6th ed. St Louis: Mosby; 2002:221.)*

glasses are that they afford the most lifelike testing conditions and permit the examiner to perform cover testing during the examination. Figure 4-12 summarizes some of the possible subjective results of this test. Note that in monofixation syndrome, the central scotoma is perceived as a gap in one of the lines surrounding the fixation light.

4Δ base-out prism test

The *4Δ base-out prism test* is a diagnostic maneuver performed primarily to document the presence of a small facultative scotoma in a patient with monofixation syndrome. In this test, a 4Δ base-out prism is quickly placed before 1 eye and then the other during binocular viewing, and motor responses are observed (Fig 4-13). Patients with bifixation

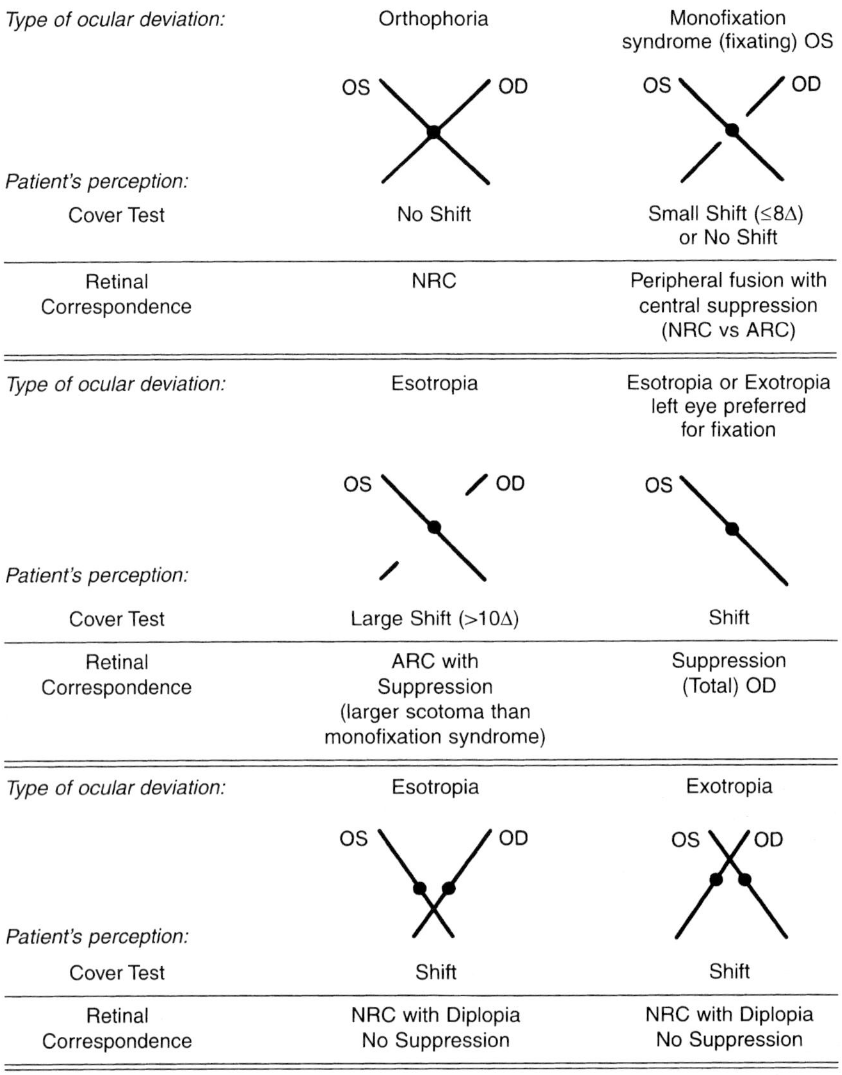

Figure 4-12 Bagolini striated glass test for retinal correspondence and suppression. For these figures, the Bagolini lens is oriented at 135° in front of the right eye and at 45° in front of the left eye. The perception of the oblique lines seen by each eye under binocular conditions is shown. Examples of the types of strabismus in which these responses are commonly found are given.

usually show a version (bilateral) movement away from the eye covered by the prism followed by a unilateral fusional convergence movement of the eye not behind the prism. A similar response occurs regardless of which eye the prism is placed over. Often, no movement is seen in patients with monofixation syndrome when the prism is placed before the nonfixating eye. A refixation version movement is seen when the prism is placed before the fixating eye, but the expected fusional convergence does not occur.

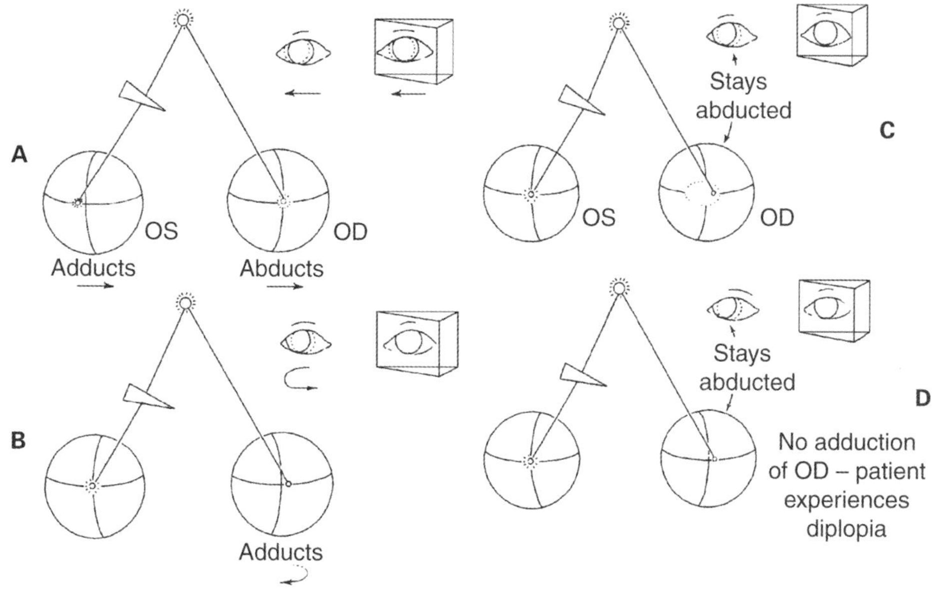

Figure 4-13 The 4Δ base-out prism test. **A,** When a prism is placed over the left eye, dextroversion occurs during refixation of that eye, indicating absence of foveal suppression in the left eye. If a suppression scotoma is present in the left eye, there will be no movement of either eye when placing the prism before the left eye. **B,** A subsequent slow fusional adduction movement of the right eye is observed, indicating absence of foveal suppression in the right eye. **C,** In a second patient, the right eye stays abducted, and the absence of an adduction movement **(B)** indicates foveal suppression in the right eye. **D,** Another cause for absence of the adduction movement is weak fusion, and such patients experience diplopia until refusion occurs spontaneously. *(Reproduced with permission from von Noorden GK, Campos EC.* Binocular Vision and Ocular Motility: Theory and Management of Strabismus. *6th ed. St Louis: Mosby; 2002:220.)*

The 4Δ base-out prism test is the least reliable method used to document the presence of a macular scotoma. An occasional patient with bifixation recognizes diplopia when the prism is placed before an eye but makes no convergence movement to correct for it. Patients with monofixation syndrome may switch fixation each time the prism is inserted and show no movement, regardless of which eye is tested.

Afterimage test

The *afterimage test* is used to determine whether a patient has NRC or ARC. The test can be performed by covering a camera flash with black paper and then exposing only a narrow slit, the center of which is covered with black tape to serve as a fixation point, as well as to protect the fovea from exposure. This test involves stimulation of the macula of each eye. Because the light flash stimulation is done for each eye separately, this test requires good foveal fixation with each eye. The presence of eccentric fixation in 1 eye significantly affects the results. This test involves the stimulation, or labeling, of each eye with a different linear afterimage, 1 horizontal and 1 vertical. Because suppression scotomata extend along the horizontal retinal meridian and may obscure most of a horizontal afterimage, the vertical afterimage is placed on the deviating eye and the horizontal afterimage on the fixating eye simply by having each eye fixate the linear light filament separately.

The central zone of the linear light is occluded to allow the fovea to fixate and remain unlabeled. The patient is then asked to draw the relative positions of the perceived afterimages. Possible perceptions are the following (Fig 4-14):

- If the patient has NRC, the 2 afterimages will be seen as a cross with a single gap (which corresponds to the fovea of each eye) in the center.
- If the patient has an esotropia and ARC, the afterimages from both eyes will be seen as crossed (paradoxical diplopia response).
- If the patient has a left exotropia and ARC, the afterimages from both eyes will be seen as uncrossed (paradoxical diplopia response).

Amblyoscope testing

Amblyoscope testing can also determine whether a patient has NRC or ARC. With the amblyoscope (Fig 4-15A), the examiner determines the objective angle—the angle at which the targets imaged on the 2 foveas produce no movement with alternate target presentation. If the images are seen superimposed, with the angle between the arms of the amblyoscope equal to the objective angle, correspondence is normal—that is, a patient with 20 prism diopters of esotropia will measure 20 prism diopters on the amblyoscope (Fig 4-15A); if not, correspondence is anomalous. The patient is then asked to superimpose the 2 targets. If superimposition occurs with the amblyoscope arms set at zero angle (arms parallel), the patient shows harmonious ARC (Fig 4-15B). If the arms are

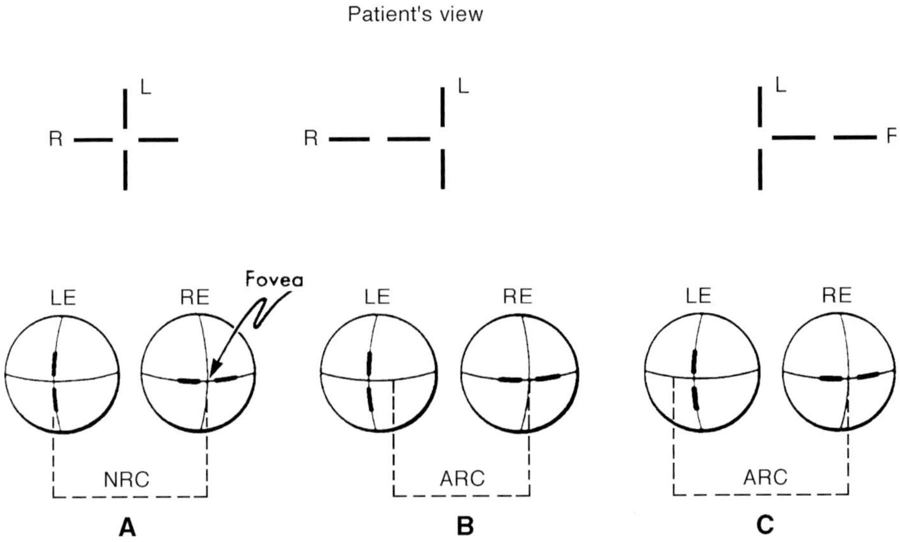

Figure 4-14 Afterimage test. **A,** Normal localization (cross) in normal correspondence (NRC). **B,** Anomalous crossed localization (ARC) in a case of esotropia. **C,** Anomalous uncrossed localization in a case of exotropia. *(Reproduced with permission from von Noorden GK, Campos EC.* Binocular Vision and Ocular Motility: Theory and Management of Strabismus. *6th ed. St Louis: Mosby; 2002:227.)*

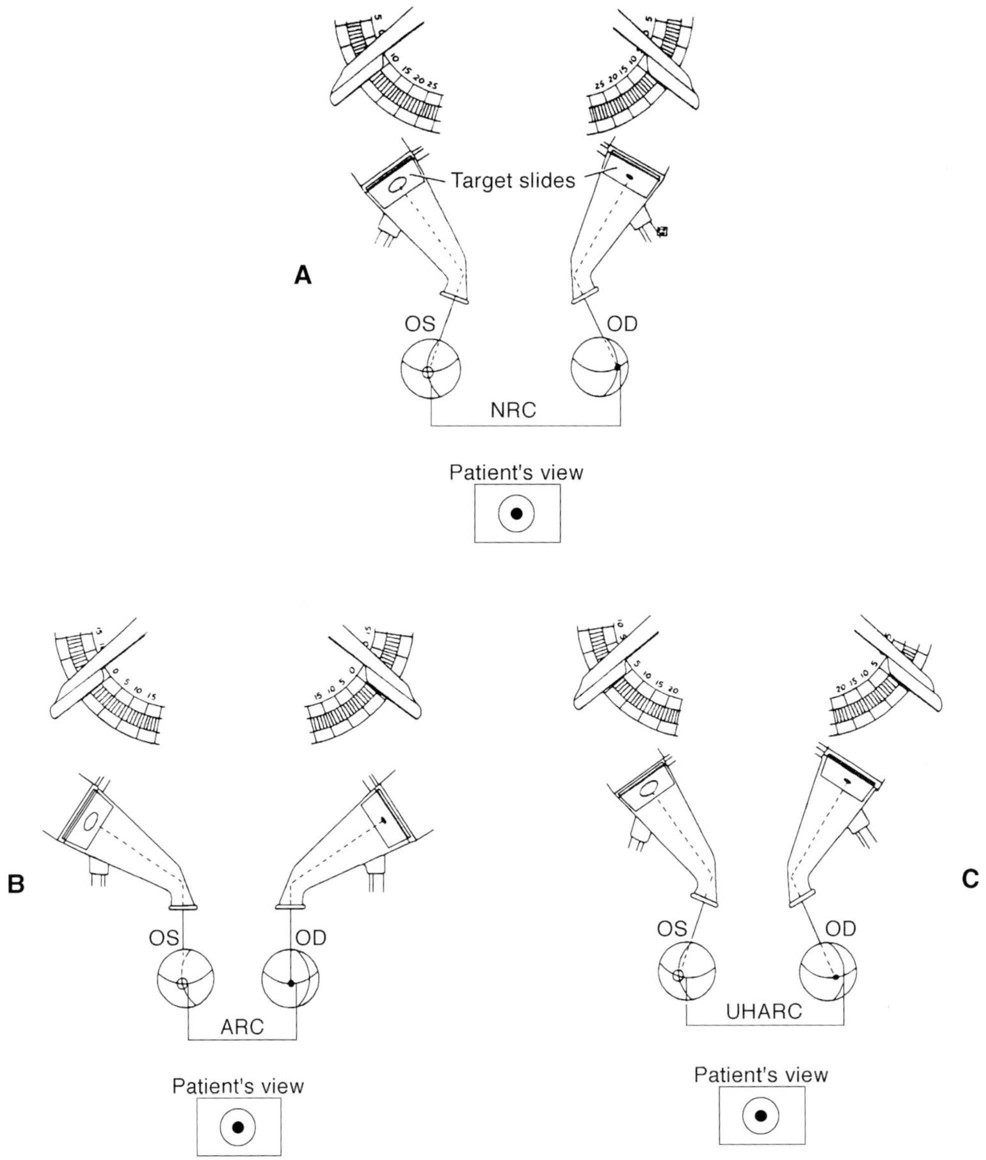

Figure 4-15 Testing with a major amblyoscope for retinal correspondence. (See text for explanation of *A–C*.) NRC, normal retinal correspondence; ARC, anomalous retinal correspondence; UHARC, unharmonious anomalous retinal correspondence. *(Reproduced with permission from von Noorden GK, Campos EC.* Binocular Vision and Ocular Motility: Theory and Management of Strabismus. *6th ed. St Louis: Mosby; 2002:229.)*

set somewhere between zero and the objective angle of squint, unharmonious ARC is theoretically present (Fig 4-15C). The reader is reminded that unharmonious ARC may be an artifact of the testing situation.

CHAPTER 5

Amblyopia

Amblyopia is a unilateral or, less commonly, bilateral reduction of best-corrected visual acuity that cannot be attributed directly to the effect of any structural abnormality of the eye or the posterior visual pathways. Amblyopia is caused by abnormal visual experience early in life resulting from one of the following:

- strabismus
- anisometropia or high bilateral refractive errors (isometropia)
- visual deprivation

Amblyopia is responsible for more unilaterally reduced vision of childhood onset than all other causes combined, with a prevalence of 2%–4% in the North American population. This fact is particularly distressing because, in principle, most amblyopic visual loss is preventable or reversible with timely detection and appropriate intervention. Children with amblyopia or at risk for amblyopia should be identified at a young age, when the prognosis for successful treatment is best. Screening for amblyopia can be performed in the primary care practitioner's office or in community-based vision screening programs. The role of photoscreening to identify amblyogenic risk factors in children who cannot be screened with visual acuity tests is being intensively investigated. A consensus about the best technology and the appropriate age to screen has not yet emerged, however.

Simons K. Photoscreening [editorial]. *Ophthalmology.* 2000;107:1619–1620.

Simons K. Preschool vision screening: rationale, methodology and outcome. *Surv Ophthalmol.* 1996;41:3–30.

Amblyopia is primarily a defect of central vision; the peripheral visual field is usually normal. Experimental studies on animals and clinical studies of infants and young children support the concept of critical periods for sensitivity in developing amblyopia. These critical periods correspond to the period when the child's developing visual system is sensitive to abnormal input caused by stimulus deprivation, strabismus, or significant refractive errors. In general, the critical period for stimulus deprivation amblyopia occurs earlier than that for ocular misalignment or anisometropia. Furthermore, the time necessary for amblyopia to occur during the critical period is shorter for stimulus deprivation than for strabismus or anisometropia.

Although the neurophysiologic mechanisms that underlie amblyopia are far from clear, the study of experimental modification of visual experience in animals and laboratory testing of humans with amblyopia has provided some insights. Animal models have revealed that a variety of profound disturbances of visual system neuron function may result from abnormal early visual experience. Cells of the primary visual cortex can completely lose their innate ability to respond to stimulation of 1 or both eyes, and cells that remain responsive may show significant functional deficiencies. Abnormalities also occur in neurons in the lateral geniculate body. Evidence concerning involvement at the retinal level remains inconclusive; if present, changes in the retina make at most a minor contribution to the overall visual defect.

Several findings from both animals and humans, such as increased spatial summation and lateral inhibition when light detection thresholds are measured using different-sized spots, suggest that the receptive fields of neurons in the amblyopic visual system are abnormally large. This disturbance may account for the *crowding phenomenon* (also known as *contour interaction*), whereby Snellen letters or equivalent symbols of a given size become more difficult to recognize if they are closely surrounded by similar forms, such as a full line or field of letters. The crowding phenomenon sometimes causes the measured "linear" acuity of an amblyopic eye to drop several lines below that measured with isolated letters. For this reason, it is best not to test visual acuity with isolated letters or pictures if possible.

Daw NW. Critical periods and amblyopia. *Arch Ophthalmol.* 1998;116:502–505.

von Noorden GK. Amblyopia: a multidisciplinary approach. Proctor lecture. *Invest Ophthalmol Vis Sci.* 1985;26:1704–1716.

Classification

Amblyopia has traditionally been subdivided in terms of the major disorders that may be responsible for its occurrence.

Strabismic Amblyopia

The most common form of amblyopia develops in the consistently deviating eye of a child with ocular misalignment. Constant, nonalternating tropias (typically esodeviations) are most likely to cause significant amblyopia. *Strabismic amblyopia* is thought to result from competitive or inhibitory interaction between neurons carrying the nonfusible inputs from the 2 eyes, which leads to domination of cortical vision centers by the fixating eye and chronically reduced responsiveness to input by the nonfixating eye. It has been suggested, but not proven, that this same mechanism is responsible for eliminating diplopia in strabismic children through suppression. Amblyopia itself does not as a rule prevent diplopia, however. Older patients with long-standing deviations might develop double vision after strabismus surgery despite the presence of substantially reduced visual acuity from amblyopia.

Several features of typical strabismic amblyopia are uncommon in other forms of amblyopia. In strabismic amblyopia, grating acuity, the ability to detect patterns composed of uniformly spaced stripes, is often reduced considerably less than Snellen acuity. Apparently, the affected eye sees forms in a twisted or distorted manner that interferes more with letter recognition than with the simpler task of determining whether a grating pattern is present. This discrepancy must be considered when the results of tests based on grating detection, such as Teller card preferential looking (a method of estimating acuity in infants and toddlers), are interpreted (Fig 5-1).

When illumination is reduced, the acuity of an eye with strabismic amblyopia tends to decline less sharply than that of an organically diseased eye. This phenomenon is sometimes called the *neutral-density filter effect*, after the device classically used to demonstrate it.

Eccentric fixation refers to the consistent use of a nonfoveal region of the retina for monocular viewing by an amblyopic eye. Minor degrees of eccentric fixation, detectable only with special tests such as visuscopy, are seen in many patients with strabismic amblyopia and relatively mild acuity loss. A visuscope projects a target with an open center surrounded by 2 concentric circles onto the retina, and the patient is asked to fixate on the target. If the target is not directed at the fovea, the degree of eccentric fixation can be measured using the concentric circles as a guide. Many ophthalmoscopes are equipped with a visuscope. Clinically evident eccentric fixation, detectable by observing the noncentral position of the corneal reflection from the amblyopic eye while it fixates a light with the dominant eye covered, generally implies visual acuity of 20/200 or worse. See Chapter 6 for a discussion of clinical testing. Use of the nonfoveal retina for fixation cannot, in general, be regarded as the primary cause of reduced acuity in affected eyes. The mechanism of this interesting phenomenon, long a source of speculation, remains unknown.

Anisometropic Amblyopia

Second in frequency to strabismic amblyopia, *anisometropic amblyopia* develops when unequal refractive error in the 2 eyes causes the image on 1 retina to be chronically defocused. This condition is thought to result partly from the direct effect of image blur on the development of visual acuity in the involved eye and partly from interocular competition or inhibition similar (but not necessarily identical) to that responsible for strabismic amblyopia. Relatively mild degrees of hyperopic or astigmatic anisometropia

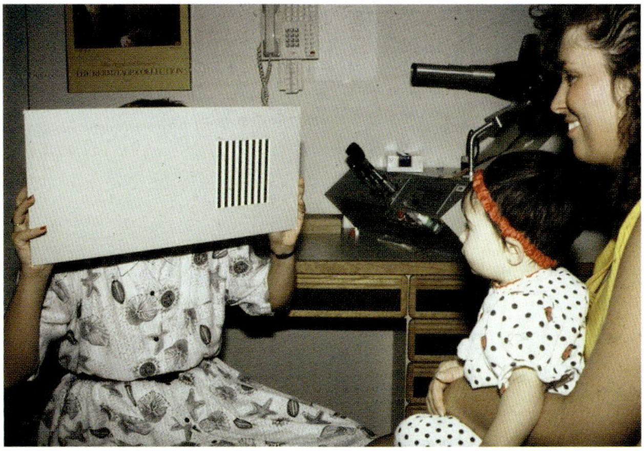

Figure 5-1 Teller acuity card being used to measure the visual acuity in a preverbal child. *(Photograph courtesy of Scott Olitsky, MD.)*

(1–2 D) can induce mild amblyopia. Mild myopic anisometropia (less than –3 D) usually does not cause amblyopia, but unilateral high myopia (–6 D or greater) often results in severe amblyopic visual loss. Unless strabismus is present, the eyes of a child with anisometropic amblyopia look normal to the family and primary care physician, typically causing a delay in detection and treatment.

Ametropic Amblyopia

Ametropic amblyopia, a bilateral reduction in acuity that is usually relatively mild, results from large, approximately equal, uncorrected refractive errors in both eyes of a young child. Its mechanism involves the effect of blurred retinal images alone. Hyperopia exceeding about 5 D and myopia in excess of 10 D carry a risk of inducing bilateral amblyopia. Uncorrected bilateral astigmatism in early childhood may result in loss of resolving ability limited to the chronically blurred meridians *(meridional amblyopia)*. The degree of cylindrical ametropia necessary to produce meridional amblyopia is not known, but most ophthalmologists recommend correction of greater than 2 D of cylinder.

Deprivation Amblyopia

The old terms *amblyopia ex anopsia* and *disuse amblyopia* are sometimes still used for *deprivation amblyopia*, which is caused by obstruction of the visual axis. The most common cause is a congenital or early acquired cataract, but corneal opacities and vitreous hemorrhage may also be implicated. Deprivation amblyopia is the least common but most damaging and difficult to treat. Amblyopic visual loss resulting from a unilateral occlusion of the visual axis tends to be worse than that produced by bilateral deprivation of similar degree because interocular effects add to the direct developmental impact of severe image degradation. Even in bilateral cases, however, acuity can be 20/200 or worse.

In children younger than 6 years, dense congenital cataracts that occupy the central 3 mm or more of the lens must be considered capable of causing severe amblyopia. Similar lens opacities acquired after age 6 years are generally less harmful. Small polar cataracts, around which retinoscopy can be readily performed, and lamellar cataracts, through which a reasonably good view of the fundus can be obtained, may cause mild to moderate amblyopia or may have no effect on visual development. *Occlusion amblyopia* is a form of deprivation amblyopia that may be seen after therapeutic patching.

Diagnosis

Amblyopia is diagnosed when reduced visual acuity cannot be explained entirely on the basis of physical abnormalities and is found in association with a history or finding of a condition known to be capable of causing amblyopia. Characteristics of vision alone cannot be used to reliably differentiate amblyopia from other forms of visual loss. The crowding phenomenon, for example, is typical of amblyopia but is not pathognomonic or uniformly demonstrable. Afferent pupillary defects rarely occur in amblyopia, and then, only in severe cases. Amblyopia sometimes coexists with visual loss directly caused by an uncorrectable structural abnormality of the eye such as optic nerve hypoplasia or coloboma. When such a situation ("organic amblyopia") is encountered in a young child, it is appropriate to undertake a trial of occlusion therapy; improvement in vision confirms that amblyopia was indeed present.

Multiple assessments using a variety of tests or performed on different occasions are sometimes required to make a final judgment concerning the presence and severity of amblyopia. General techniques for visual acuity assessment in children are discussed in Chapter 6, but the clinician trying to determine the degree of amblyopic visual loss in a young patient should keep certain special considerations in mind. The binocular fixation pattern, which indicates strength of preference for 1 eye or the other under binocular viewing conditions, is a test for estimating the relative level of vision in the 2 eyes for preverbal children with strabismus. This test is quite sensitive for detecting amblyopia, but results can be falsely positive, showing a strong preference when vision is equal or nearly equal in the 2 eyes, particularly with small-angle strabismus.

A variety of optotypes can be used to directly measure acuity in children 3–6 years old. Often, however, only isolated letters can be used, which may lead to underestimated amblyopic visual loss. Crowding bars may help alleviate this problem (Fig 5-2). In addition, the young child's brief attention span frequently results in measurements that fall short of the true limits of acuity; these results can mimic bilateral amblyopia or obscure or falsely suggest a significant interocular difference.

Treatment

Treatment of amblyopia involves the following steps:

1. Eliminate (if possible) any obstacle to vision such as a cataract.
2. Correct any significant refractive error.
3. Force use of the poorer eye by limiting use of the better eye.

Cataract Removal

Cataracts capable of producing amblyopia require surgery without unnecessary delay. In young children, amblyopia may develop as quickly as 1 week per age of life. Removal of visually significant congenital lens opacities during the first 2–3 months of life is necessary for optimal recovery of vision. In symmetric bilateral cases, the interval between operations on the first and second eyes should be no more than 1–2 weeks. Acutely developing

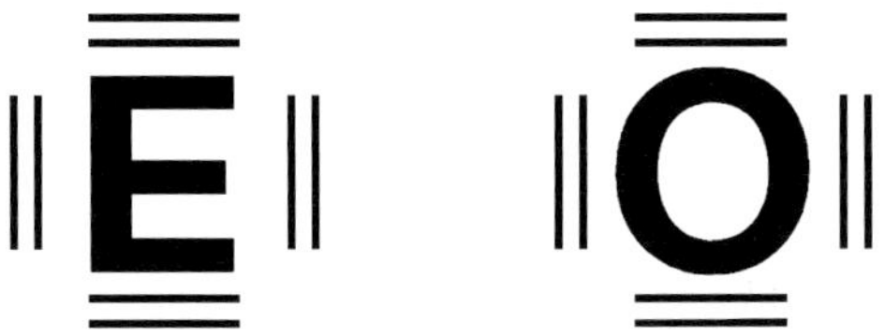

Figure 5-2 Crowding bars, or contour interaction bars, allow the examiner to test crowding phenomenon with isolated optotypes. Bars surrounding the optotype mimic the full row of optotypes to the amblyopic child. *(Reproduced with permission from Coats DK, Jenkins RH. Vision assessment of the pediatric patient.* Refinements. *San Francisco: American Academy of Ophthalmology; 1997,1:1.)*

severe traumatic cataracts in children younger than 6 years should be removed within a few weeks of injury, if possible. Significant cataracts with uncertain time of onset also deserve prompt and aggressive treatment during childhood if recent development is at least a possibility (eg, in the case of an opacity that appears to have originated from a posterior lenticonus deformity). Chapter 22 of this volume and BCSC Section 11, *Lens and Cataract*, discuss the special considerations of cataract surgery in children.

Refractive Correction

In general, optical prescription for amblyopic eyes should be based on the refractive error as determined with cycloplegia. Because an amblyopic eye's ability to control accommodation tends to be impaired, it cannot be relied on to compensate for uncorrected hyperopia as would a normal child's eye. Sometimes, however, symmetric decreases in plus lens power may be required to foster acceptance of spectacle wear by a child. Refractive correction for aphakia following cataract surgery in childhood must be provided promptly to avoid compounding the visual deprivation effect of the lens opacity with that of a severe optical deficit. Both anisometropic and ametropic amblyopia may improve considerably with refractive correction alone over several months.

Occlusion and Optical Degradation

Full-time occlusion of the sound eye, defined as occlusion during all waking hours, thus forcing use of the defective eye, is the most powerful means of treating amblyopia. This treatment is usually performed using commercially available adhesive patches. Spectacle-mounted occluders or special opaque contact lenses can be used as an alternative to full-time patching if skin irritation, inadequate adhesion, or poor compliance proves to be a significant problem, provided that close supervision ensures that the spectacles remain in place consistently. (Most skin-related problems can be eliminated by switching to a different brand of patch or by preparing the skin with tincture of benzoin or ostomy adhesive before application.) Full-time patching should generally be used only when constant strabismus eliminates any possibility of useful binocular vision because full-time patching presents a small risk of perturbing binocularity. Rarely, strabismus may result from full-time patching; it is not known whether strabismus would have occurred with other forms of amblyopia treatment. The child whose eyes are consistently or intermittently straight should be given some opportunity to see binocularly. Modest reductions are employed by many ophthalmologists (removing the patch for an hour or two a day) to reduce the likelihood of occlusion amblyopia or of inducing strabismus.

Part-time occlusion, defined as occlusion for 1–6 hours per day, may achieve the same results as full-time occlusion. The relative duration of patch-on and patch-off intervals should reflect the degree of amblyopia; for moderate to severe deficits, at least 6 hours per day is preferred. The child undergoing part-time occlusion should be kept as visually active as possible when the patch is in place, but no specific visual exercises have been proven to be of particular benefit.

Compliance with occlusion therapy for amblyopia declines with increasing age. The effectiveness of more acceptable part-time patching regimens in older children is being actively investigated. Furthermore, recent studies in older children with amblyopia have shown that treatment can still be beneficial beyond the first decade of life. This is especially true in children who have not previously undergone treatment.

Other methods of amblyopia treatment involve optical degradation of the better eye's image to the point that it becomes inferior to the amblyopic eye's, an approach often called *penalization.* Use of the amblyopic eye is thus promoted within the context of binocular seeing. Recent studies have demonstrated that pharmacologic penalization can be used to successfully treat moderate levels of amblyopia. The improvement in vision has been shown to be similar to that obtained with patching. A cycloplegic agent (usually atropine 1% drops or homatropine 5% drops) is administered daily to the better eye so that it is unable to accommodate. As a result, the better eye experiences blur with near viewing and, if uncorrected hyperopia is present, with distance viewing. This form of treatment has recently been demonstrated to be as effective as patching for mild to moderate amblyopia (visual acuity of 20/100 or better in the amblyopic eye). Depending on the depth of amblyopia and the response to prior treatment, the hyperopic correction of the dominant eye can be reduced to plano to enhance the effect. Regular follow-up of patients whose amblyopia is being treated with cycloplegia is important to avoid reverse amblyopia in the previously preferred eye.

Atropinization offers the particular advantage of being difficult to thwart even if the child objects. Alternative methods of treatment based on the same principle involve prescribing excessive plus-power lenses (fogging) or diffusing filters. These methods avoid potential pharmacologic side effects and may be capable of inducing greater blur. If the child is wearing glasses, application of translucent tape or a Bangerter foil (a neutral-density filter) to the spectacle lens can be tried. Proper utilization (no peeking!) of spectacle-borne devices must be closely monitored.

Another benefit of atropinization and other nonoccluding methods in patients with straight eyes is that the eyes can work together, a great practical advantage in children with latent nystagmus.

The Pediatric Eye Disease Investigator Group. A randomized trial of atropine vs. patching for treatment of moderate amblyopia in children. *Arch Ophthalmol.* 2002;120:268–278.

Complications of Therapy

Any form of amblyopia therapy introduces the possibility of overtreatment leading to amblyopia in the originally better eye. Full-time occlusion carries the greatest risk of this complication and requires close monitoring, especially in the younger child. The first follow-up visit after initiation of treatment should occur within 1 week for an infant and after an interval corresponding to 1 week per year of age for the older child (eg, 4 weeks for a 4-year-old). Subsequent visits can be scheduled at longer intervals based on early response. Part-time occlusion and optical degradation methods allow for less frequent observation, but regular follow-up is still critical. The parents of a strabismic child should be instructed to watch for a switch in fixation preference and to report its occurrence promptly. Iatrogenic amblyopia can usually be treated successfully with judicious patching of the better-seeing eye or by alternating occlusion. Sometimes, simply stopping treatment altogether for a few weeks leads to equalization of vision.

The desired endpoint of therapy for unilateral amblyopia is free alternation of fixation (although 1 eye may still be used somewhat more frequently than the other), linear Snellen acuity that differs by no more than 1 line between the 2 eyes, or both. The time required for completion of treatment depends on the following:

- degree of amblyopia
- choice of therapeutic approach
- compliance with the prescribed regimen
- age of the patient

More severe amblyopia, less complete obstruction of the dominant eye's vision, and older age are all associated with a need for more prolonged treatment. Full-time occlusion during infancy may reverse substantial strabismic amblyopia in 1 week or less. In contrast, an older child who wears a patch only after school and on weekends may require a year or more of treatment to overcome a moderate deficit.

Compliance issues

Lack of compliance with the therapeutic regimen is a common problem that can prolong the period of treatment or lead to outright failure. If difficulties derive from a particular treatment method, a suitable alternative should be sought. Families who appear to lack sufficient motivation should be counseled concerning the importance of the project and the need for firmness in carrying it out. They can be reassured that once an appropriate routine is established and maintained for a short time, the daily effort required is likely to diminish, especially if the amblyopia improves.

The problems associated with an unusually resistant child vary according to age. In infancy, restraining the child through physical methods such as arm splints or mittens or merely making the patch more adhesive with tincture of benzoin may be useful. For children older than 3 years, creating goals and offering rewards tends to work well, as does linking patching to play activities (eg, decorating the patch each day or patching while the child plays a video game). Authoritative words directed specifically toward the child by the doctor may also help. The toddler period (1–3 years) is particularly challenging.

Unresponsiveness

In some cases, even conscientious application of an appropriate therapeutic program fails to improve vision at all or beyond a certain level. Complete or partial unresponsiveness to treatment occasionally affects younger children but most often occurs in patients older than 5 years. Conversely, significant improvement in vision may be achievable with protracted effort even in adolescents. The decision whether to initiate or continue treatment in a prognostically unfavorable situation should consider the wishes of the patient and family. Primary therapy should generally be terminated if there is a lack of demonstrable progress over 3–6 months with good compliance.

Before it is concluded that intractable amblyopia is present, refraction should be rechecked, the pupils carefully reevaluated, and the macula and optic nerve critically inspected for subtle evidence of hypoplasia or other malformation that might have been previously overlooked. Neuroimaging might be considered in cases that inexplicably fail to respond to treatment. Amblyopia associated with unilateral high myopia and extensive myelination of retinal nerve fibers is a specific syndrome in which treatment failure is particularly common.

Recurrence

When amblyopia treatment is discontinued after fully or partially successful completion, approximately 25% of patients show some degree of recurrence, which can usually be reversed with renewed therapeutic effort. Backsliding can be prevented by instituting an acuity maintenance regimen such as patching for 1–3 hours per day, optical penalization with spectacles, or pharmacologic penalization with atropine 1 or 2 days per week. If the need for maintenance treatment is established, it must be continued until stability of visual acuity is demonstrated with no treatment other than regular spectacles. This may require periodic monitoring until age 8–10 years. As long as vision remains stable, intervals of up to 6 months between follow-up visits are acceptable.

Keech RV. Practical management of amblyopia. *Focal Points: Clinical Modules for Ophthalmologists.* San Francisco: American Academy of Ophthalmology; 2000, module 2.

Lambert SR, Boothe RG. Amblyopia: basic and clinical science perspectives. *Focal Points: Clinical Modules for Ophthalmologists.* San Francisco: American Academy of Ophthalmology; 1994, module 8.

Preferred Practice Patterns Committee, Pediatric Ophthalmology Panel. *Amblyopia.* San Francisco: American Academy of Ophthalmology; 2002.

CHAPTER 6

Diagnostic Techniques for Strabismus and Amblyopia

History and Characteristics of the Presenting Complaint

The ophthalmologist should attempt to establish rapport with the patient and, if examining a child, with the parent(s) as well. The motility examination begins with a patient's history. Because children become increasingly impatient during an examination, an experienced ophthalmologist will take advantage of the opportunity to observe the child while taking the history. See Introduction: Rapport With Children: Tips for a Productive Examination at the beginning of this volume for a detailed discussion on examining a child.

When the patient is a child, it is especially important to obtain information regarding the mother's pregnancy, paying close attention to maternal health, gestational age at the time of birth, birth weight, and neonatal history. The physician should also ask about the child's developmental milestones.

It is desirable to document the age of onset of a deviation or symptom. Old photographs are invaluable for this purpose. Baby pictures, grade-school snapshots, graduation photographs, and driver's license pictures can often provide critical information. In addition, the physician should seek to answer the following questions about the deviation or symptom:

- Did its onset coincide with trauma or illness?
- Is the deviation constant or intermittent?
- Is it present for distance, near, or both?
- Is it unilateral or alternating?
- Is it present only when the patient is inattentive or fatigued?
- Does the child close 1 eye?
- Is the deviation associated with double vision?

Earlier treatment should be reviewed, including any previous management such as amblyopia therapy, spectacle correction, use of miotics, orthoptic therapy, or prior eye muscle surgery. While obtaining the history, the physician should observe the patient continually, noting such behaviors as head posturing, head movement, attentiveness, and motor control.

Past and present medications should be recorded, along with drug sensitivities and allergic responses. Any history of thyroid or neurologic problems should be particularly emphasized. It is also important to document previous surgeries, anesthetic methods used and any related problems, and a detailed family history of strabismus or other eye disorders.

Assessment of Visual Acuity

Distance Visual Acuity

Several tests are available for distance visual acuity determination. Snellen letters or numbers, the HOTV test, LEA symbols, the illiterate E test, and Allen pictures are the most commonly used tests for visual acuity. Table 6-1 lists the expected acuity for various tests at different ages.

By convention, visual acuity is determined first for the right eye and then for the left. A patch or occluder is used in front of the left eye as the acuity of the right eye is checked, then vice versa. An adhesive patch is the most effective occluder but the most objectionable from the child's point of view. The line with the smallest figures in which the majority of letters can be read accurately is recorded; if the patient misses a few of the figures on a line, a notation is made. If the patient does not have corrective lenses, a pinhole may be used to estimate the best visual acuity potential. However, the use of pinholes with children is cumbersome and often inconclusive.

Patients with poor vision may need to walk to the chart until they can see the big E or equivalent (20/400 line). In such cases, visual acuity is recorded as the distance in feet (numerator) over the size of the letter (denominator); for example, if the patient is able to read the big E at 5 feet, the acuity would be recorded as 5/400. Because the selection of large figures is limited, it is advisable to confirm measurements slightly closer to the chart using figures that can be changed.

Visual acuity assessment of children is often difficult, and the clinician must resort to various means of evaluation. In preverbal or nonverbal children, acuity can be evaluated by the *CSM method. C* refers to the location of the corneal light reflex as the patient fixates the examiner's light under monocular conditions (opposite eye covered). Normally, the reflected light from the cornea is near the *center* of the cornea, and it should be positioned symmetrically in both eyes. If the fixation target is viewed eccentrically,

Table 6-1 Normal Visual Acuity Using Various Tests in Children

Age (Years)	Vision Test	Normal
0–2	Visual evoked potential (VEP)	20/30 (age 1)
0–2	Preferential looking	20/30 (age 2)
0–2	Fixation behavior	CSM (see text)
2–5	Allen pictures	20/40–20/20
2–5	HOTV	20/40–20/20
2–5	E-game	20/40–20/20
5+	Snellen	20/30–20/20

fixation is termed *uncentral (UC). S* refers to the *steadiness* of fixation on the examiner's light as it is held motionless and as it is slowly moved about. The S evaluation is also done under monocular conditions. *M* refers to the ability of the strabismic patient to *maintain* alignment first with 1 eye, then with the other, as the opposite eye is uncovered. Maintenance of fixation is evaluated under binocular conditions. Inability to maintain fixation with either eye with the opposite eye uncovered is presumptive evidence of a difference in acuity between the 2 eyes. Thus, preverbal or nonverbal patients with strong fixation preference in 1 eye should be suspected of having amblyopia in the other eye. An eye that has eccentric fixation and nystagmoid movements when attempting fixation would have its visual acuity designated *uncentral, unsteady*, and *unmaintained (UC, US, UM).*

In a child with straight eyes, it is impossible to tell if he or she will maintain fixation with either eye unless the *induced tropia test* is used. This test is performed by placing a 10Δ–15Δ base-down prism over 1 eye to induce a vertical deviation. An alternative method includes the use of a prism of greater strength held base-out. The patient is then tested for the ability to maintain fixation with either eye under binocular, albeit dissociated, viewing conditions. It is important to determine whether each eye can maintain fixation through smooth pursuit or a blink; strong fixation preference for 1 eye indicates amblyopia in the nonpreferred eye.

Occasionally, avoidance movements can be demonstrated when the good eye is occluded. The patient may attempt to maneuver around the occluder when the good eye is covered but not when the poorly seeing eye is covered. A child with poor vision in the right eye, for example, might be noted to "fix and follow" (F and F) more poorly using that eye and to object to occlusion of the left eye.

The visual acuity of preschool-age and older children can be tested using the illiterate E test (the *E-game*), letters, numbers, or symbols, all generically referred to as *optotypes.* Children being tested with the E-game are asked to point their hand or fingers in the direction of the E. This test can be difficult to use because of developmental status and confusion of right versus left even among children with good acuity. Visual acuity testing with Snellen letters or numbers requires the child to name each letter or number, whereas visual acuity testing with the HOTV test or with LEA symbols can be done by matching, a cognitively easier task. Whenever possible, a line of optotypes or single optotypes surrounded by *contour interaction bars* ("crowding bars") should be used to prevent the overestimation of visual acuity of an amblyopic eye that often occurs with isolated optotypes (see Chapter 5, Fig 5-2). Allen pictures should be used only if the child cannot be tested with any other class of optotype; Allen pictures do not provide any contour interaction, and their overall size and the width of their underlying components fail to conform to accepted parameters of optotype design.

The type of test used should be identified along with the results to facilitate comparisons with measurements taken at other times. Most pediatric ophthalmologists consider Snellen acuity most reliable, followed by HOTV, LEA symbols, the illiterate E test, Allen pictures, and fixation behavior. The most reliable test that the child can perform should be used. Preferential looking techniques using Teller acuity cards can be a useful adjunctive test for comparing visual acuity between fellow eyes in infants and preverbal children.

Patients with latent nystagmus may show better visual acuity with both eyes together than with 1 eye occluded. To assess distance monocular visual acuity in this situation, it may be helpful to fog the eye not being tested with a lens that is +5 D greater than the refractive error in that eye.

Wright KW, Walonker F, Edelman P. 10-Diopter fixation test for amblyopia. *Arch Ophthalmol.* 1981;99:1242–1246.

Near Visual Acuity

Tests of near visual acuity include reading cards with graduated, small standardized print. With a near card, visual acuity at 14 inches (35 cm) is recorded. Again, both uncorrected and corrected visual acuity are determined. Because of inaccuracy related to viewing distance, near visual acuities should never be compared with distance acuities in children. A measurement of near visual acuity in children with reduced vision is important in helping to determine how they function at school.

Assessment of Eye Movements

Generally, when assessing eye movements, versions are tested first. The examiner should pay particular attention to the movements of both eyes into the 9 diagnostic positions of gaze. Limitations of movement into these positions and asymmetry of excursion of the 2 eyes should be noted. Spinning the child, or provoking the doll's head phenomenon, may be helpful in eliciting the vestibular-stimulated eye movements. If versions are not full, duction movements should be tested for each eye separately. BCSC Section 5, *Neuro-Ophthalmology*, also discusses testing of the ocular motility system.

The examiner must use ingenuity to keep the patient's attention, and such tricks as brightly colored toys, pictures, and storytelling about the objects are essential. A well-prepared examiner always has several toys or pictures at hand (see Introduction: Rapport With Children: Tips for a Productive Examination).

Tests of Ocular Alignment

Ocular alignment tests can be grouped into 4 basic types: cover tests, corneal light reflex tests, dissimilar image tests, and dissimilar target tests.

Cover tests

Eye movement capability, image formation and perception, foveal fixation in each eye, attention, and cooperation are all necessities for cover testing. If a patient is unable to maintain constant fixation on an accommodative target, the results of cover testing may not be valid, and this battery of tests therefore should not be used.

There are 3 types of cover tests: the cover-uncover test, the alternate cover test, and the simultaneous prism and cover test. All can be performed with fixation at distance or near. Some deviations (eg, intermittent exotropia) may be more evident at distance; others (eg, accommodative esotropia) may be more evident at near.

The monocular *cover-uncover test* is the most important test for detecting the presence of manifest strabismus and for differentiating a phoria from a tropia (Fig 6-1). As

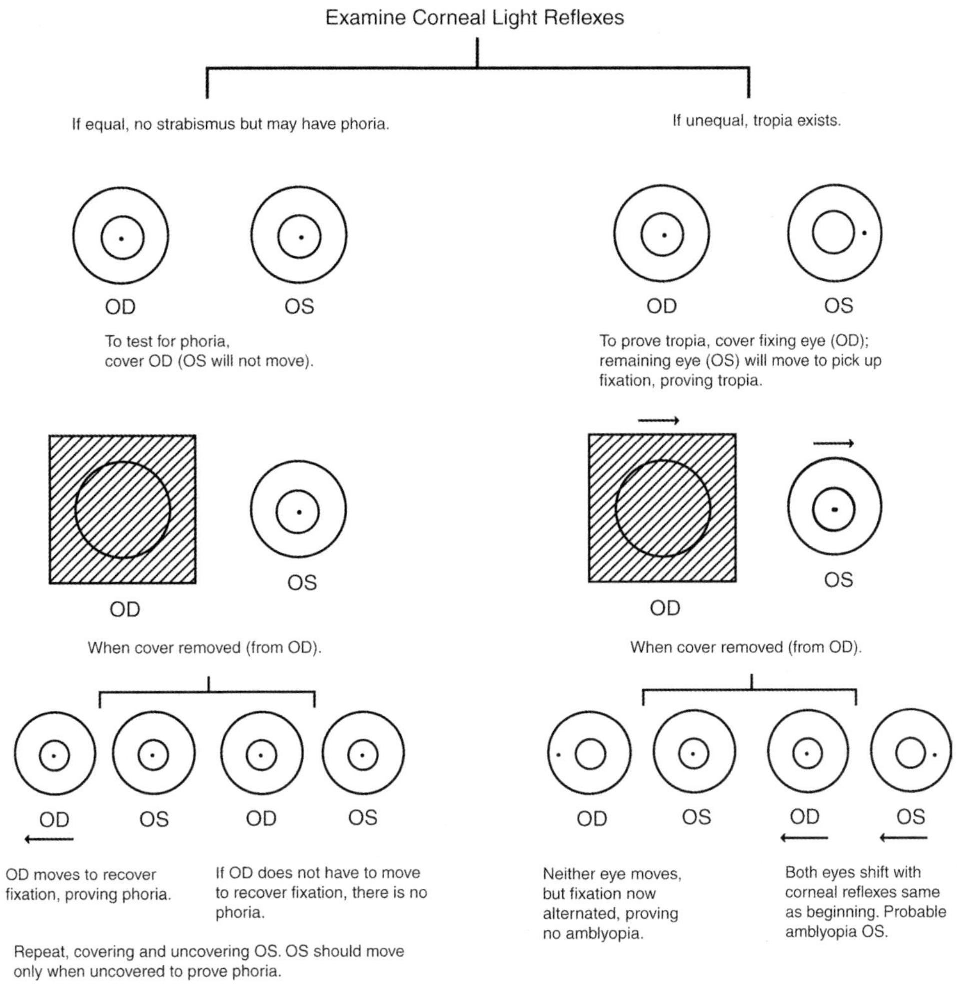

Figure 6-1 The monocular cover-uncover test.

1 eye is covered, the examiner watches carefully for any movement in the opposite, *non-covered* eye; such movement indicates the presence of a tropia. Movement of the *covered* eye in one direction just after the cover is applied and a movement in the opposite direction (a fusional movement) as the cover is removed indicates a phoria that becomes manifest only when binocularity is interrupted. If the patient has a phoria, the eyes will be straight before and after the cover-uncover test; the deviation that appears during the test is a result of interruption of binocular vision and the inability of the fusional mechanism to operate. A patient with a tropia, however, starts out with a deviated eye and ends up (after the test) with either the same or the opposite eye deviated (if the opposite eye is the deviated one, the condition is termed *alternating heterotropia*). Some patients may have straight eyes and start out with a phoria prior to the cover-uncover test; however, after prolonged testing—and therefore prolonged interruption of binocular vision—dissociation into a manifest tropia can occur.

The *alternate cover test (prism and cover test)* measures the total deviation, both latent and manifest (Fig 6-2). This test does not specify how much of each type of deviation is present (ie, it does not separate the phoria from the tropia). The cover is placed alternately in front of each eye several times to dissociate the eyes and maximize the deviation; it is important to quickly transfer the occluder from 1 eye to the other to prevent fusion. This test should be done at both distance and near fixation. Once dissociation is achieved, the amount of deviation is measured using prisms to eliminate the eye movement as the cover is alternately switched from eye to eye. It may be necessary to use both horizontally and vertically placed prisms. The amount of prism power required is the measure of deviation. Two horizontal or 2 vertical prisms should not be stacked on each other because this can induce significant measurement errors. Their values cannot be directly added. A more accurate method for measuring large deviations is to place prisms in front of each eye, although it should be noted that these are not perfectly additive either. However, it is acceptable to stack a horizontal and a vertical prism before the same eye if necessary.

Whereas the alternate cover test measures the total deviation (phoria and tropia), the *simultaneous prism and cover test* is helpful in determining the actual heterotropia when both eyes are uncovered (tropia alone). The test is performed by covering the fixating eye at the same time the prism is placed in front of the deviating eye. The test is repeated using increasing prism powers until the deviated eye no longer shifts. Again, the power of the prism is the measure of the deviation. This test has special application in monofixation syndrome, which may include a small-angle heterotropia. Patients with this condition may reduce the amount of deviation measured in the alternate cover test by exerting at least partial control over a coexisting phoria through peripheral fusion when both eyes are open. In this instance, the simultaneous prism and cover test measures the amount of tropia in a deviation that has a superimposed phoria. This test may be useful in assessing the deviation under real-life conditions with both eyes viewing.

Thompson JT, Guyton DL. Ophthalmic prisms. Measurement errors and how to minimize them. *Ophthalmology*. 1983;90:204–210.

Light reflex tests

Corneal light reflex tests are useful in assessing ocular alignment in patients who cannot cooperate sufficiently to allow cover testing or who have poor fixation. The main tests of this type are the Hirschberg, modified Krimsky, Brückner, and major amblyoscope methods.

The *Hirschberg method* is based on the premise that 1 mm of decentration of the corneal light reflection corresponds to about 7°, or 15Δ, of ocular deviation of the visual axis. Therefore, a light reflex at the pupillary margin is about 2 mm from the pupillary center (with a 4-mm pupil), which corresponds to 15°, or approximately 30Δ, of deviation. A reflex in the mid-iris region is about 4 mm from the pupillary center, which is roughly 30°, or 60Δ, of deviation; similarly, a reflex at the limbus is about 45°, or 90Δ, of deviation (Fig 6-3).

The *Krimsky method* uses reflections produced on both corneas by a penlight. The original method involved placing prisms in front of the deviating eye. More common

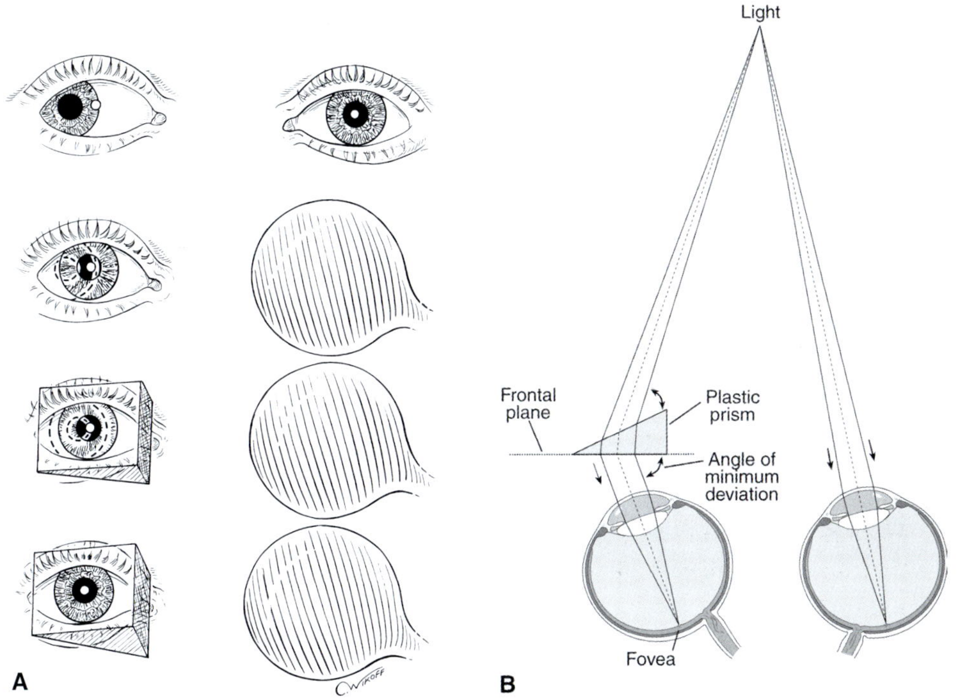

Figure 6-2 **A**, In the top row, the child is seen to have a right exotropia. In the second row, the cover test shows movement of the right eye to fixate when the left eye is covered. In the third row, a small prism introduced before the right eye begins to neutralize the deviation. In the bottom row, the correct prism has been introduced and no more movement is seen when the cover is alternated between eyes. **B**, The diagram shows how the prism eliminates movement on cover testing by aligning rays of light from the fixation target with the fovea in the exotropic right eye. The size of the prism gives a measurement of the exotropia. *(Reproduced with permission from Simon JW, Calhoun JH.* A Child's Eyes: A Guide to Pediatric Primary Care. *Gainesville, FL: Triad Publishing; 1997:72.)*

modifications today involve holding prisms before the fixing eye or split between the 2 eyes. By adjusting the prisms to center the corneal reflection in the deviated eye, it is possible to approximate and quantitate the near deviation (Fig 6-4). The Hirschberg and Krimsky methods can be inaccurate even when used by experienced strabismologists. Therefore, their use is often limited to patients who are uncooperative or have vision that is too poor to allow for a measurement with other techniques.

Choi RY, Kushner BJ. The accuracy of experienced strabismologists using the Hirschberg and Krimsky tests. *Ophthalmology.* 1998;105:1301–1306.

The *Brückner* test is performed by using the direct ophthalmoscope to obtain a red reflex simultaneously in both eyes. If strabismus is present, the deviated eye will have a lighter and brighter reflex than the fixating eye. Note that this test detects, but does not measure, the deviation. This test also identifies opacities in the visual axis and moderate to severe anisometropia. The Brückner test is primarily used by primary care practitioners to screen for strabismus and anisometropia.

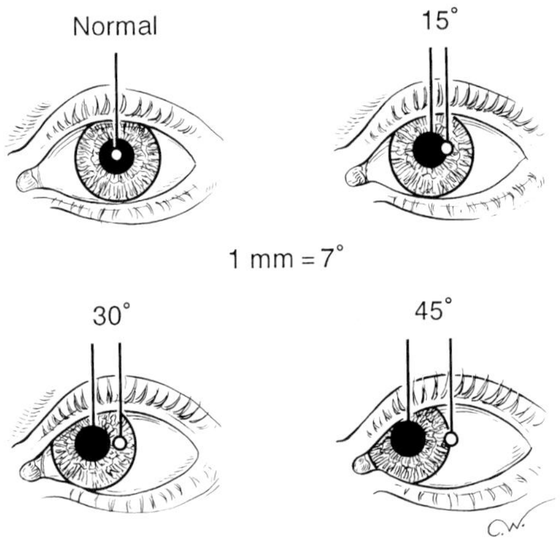

Figure 6-3 Hirschberg test. The extent to which the corneal light reflex is displaced from the center of the pupil provides an approximation of the angular size of the deviation (in this example, a left esotropia). *(Reproduced with permission from Simon JW, Calhoun JH.* A Child's Eyes: A Guide to Pediatric Primary Care. *Gainesville, FL: Triad Publishing; 1997:72.)*

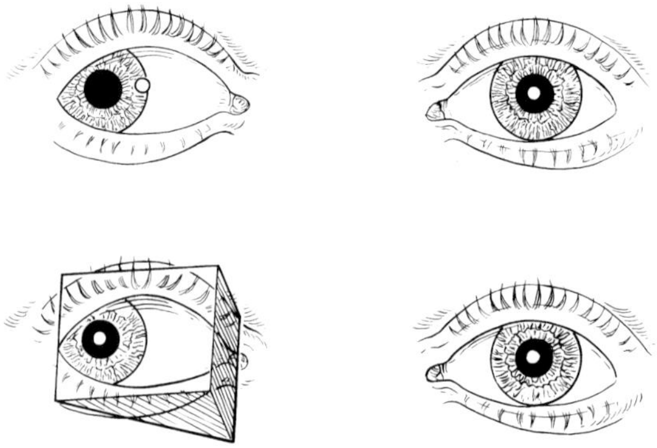

Figure 6-4 Original Krimsky test. The right exotropia is measured by the size of the prism required to center the pupillary reflexes, as shown at bottom. *(Reproduced with permission from Simon JW, Calhoun JH.* A Child's Eyes: A Guide to Pediatric Primary Care. *Gainesville, FL: Triad Publishing; 1997:72.)*

The *major amblyoscope method* uses separate target illumination, which can be moved to center the corneal light reflection. The amount of deviation is then read directly from the scale of the amblyoscope.

Dissimilar image tests

Dissimilar image tests are based on the patient's response to diplopia created by 2 dissimilar images. The 3 major types are the Maddox rod test, the double Maddox rod test, and the red glass test.

The *Maddox rod test* uses a specially constructed device consisting of a series of parallel cylinders that converts a point source of light into a line image. The optical properties of the cylinders cause the streak of light to be situated 90° to the orientation of the parallel cylinders. Because fusion is precluded by the Maddox rod, heterophorias and heterotropias cannot be differentiated. The Maddox rod can be used to test for horizontal and vertical deviations, and, when used in conjunction with another Maddox rod, for cyclodeviations.

To test for horizontal deviations, the Maddox rod is placed in front of the right eye with the cylinders in the horizontal direction. The patient fixates a point source of light and then sees a vertical line with the right eye and a white light with the left eye. If the light superimposes the line, orthophoria is present; if the light is on the left side of the line, an esodeviation is present; and if the light is on the right side of the line, an exodeviation is present. A similar procedure with the cylinders aligned vertically is used to test for vertical deviations. To measure the amount of deviation, the examiner holds prisms of different powers until the line superimposes the point source. The Maddox rod test is not a satisfactory test for horizontal deviations, however, because accommodative convergence cannot be controlled.

The *double Maddox rod test* is used to determine cyclodeviations. A Maddox rod is placed in front of each eye in a trial frame or phoropter with the rods aligned vertically so that the patient sees horizontal line images. The patient or examiner rotates the axes of the rods until the lines are perceived to be parallel. To facilitate the patient's recognition of the 2 lines, it is often helpful to dissociate the lines by placing a small prism base-up or base-down in front of 1 eye. The degrees of deviation and the direction (incyclo or excyclo) can be determined by the angle of rotation that causes the line images to appear horizontal and parallel. Traditionally, a red Maddox rod was placed before the right eye and a white Maddox rod before the left, but recent evidence suggests the different colors can cause fixation artifacts that do not occur if the same color is used bilaterally.

In the *red glass test*, a red glass is placed in front of the right eye. This test is used for the same purpose as the Maddox rod test but is not applicable to cyclodeviations. As in the Maddox rod test, prisms are used to eliminate the horizontal or vertical diplopia, and the amount of deviation is recorded.

Dissimilar target tests

Dissimilar target tests are based on the patient's response to the dissimilar images created by each eye viewing a different target; the deviation is measured first with 1 eye fixating and then with the other. Several tests of this type have been devised, but the 3 most frequently encountered are the Lancaster red-green projection test, the Hess screen test, and the major amblyoscope test.

The *Lancaster red-green test* uses red-green goggles that can be reversed, a red-slit projector, a green-slit projector, and a screen ruled into squares of 7 cm. At a test distance of 2 m, each square subtends 2°. The patient's head is held steady; by convention, the test is begun with the red filter in front of the right eye. The examiner projects a red slit onto the screen, and the patient is asked to place the green slit so that it appears to coincide with the red slit. The relative positions of the 2 streaks are then recorded. The test is repeated for the diagnostic positions of gaze (these positions are discussed later in the chapter), and the goggles are then reversed so that the deviation with the fellow eye fixating can be recorded. The Lancaster red-green test is used primarily for patients with diplopia caused by incomitant strabismus and requires that the patient have normal retinal correspondence.

The *Hess screen test* is also useful in evaluating patients with paretic or paralytic strabismus who have normal retinal correspondence. The test uses red-green goggles, a special screen that has a red dot (or light) in 8 inner positions and 16 outer positions, and a green slit projector. At a test distance of 50 cm, the patient is asked to place the green slit light so that it appears to coincide with the individual red dots (or lights). The relative positions are connected by a straight line; usually, just the 8 inner dots (or lights) and the central point of fixation are plotted. The goggles are then reversed so the deviation with the other eye fixating can be recorded.

The *major amblyoscope test* uses dissimilar targets that the patient is asked to superimpose. If the patient has normal retinal correspondence, the horizontal, vertical, and torsional deviations can be read directly from the calibrated scale of the amblyoscope.

Confounding Factors in Ocular Alignment Assessment

Two potential pitfalls in the evaluation of ocular alignment are the conditions of pseudostrabismus and angle kappa. *Pseudostrabismus* is the appearance of strabismus despite normal alignment. The most common form is pseudoesotropia, which results from coverage of the nasal sclera by the wide, flat nasal bridge and the epicanthal folds so common in infancy. Because no real deviation exists, both light reflex testing and cover testing results are normal. The appearance of crossing should gradually improve during infancy and early childhood. If it does not, repeat examination is warranted.

Angle kappa is the angle between the visual axis and the anatomical pupillary axis of the eye. If the fovea is temporal to the pupillary axis (as is usually the case), the corneal light reflection will be slightly nasal to the center of the cornea. This is termed *positive angle kappa* and simulates exodeviation. If the position of the fovea is nasal to the pupillary axis, the corneal light reflection will be slightly temporal to the center of the cornea. This is termed *negative angle kappa* and simulates esodeviation (Fig 6-5). One cause for a positive angle kappa is retinopathy of prematurity with temporal dragging of the macula. Although affected patients appear to be exotropic, the eye continues to appear abducted even when fixating under monocular conditions.

Positions of Gaze

The *primary position of gaze* is the position of the eyes when fixating straight ahead on an object at infinity. For practical purposes, infinity is considered to be 20 ft (6 m), and for this position the head should be straight. If the patient has vertical strabismus, the definition of primary position is expanded to include the eyes fixating straight ahead on a distant object with the head tilted to the right and to the left (see 3-Step Test, later in the chapter).

Cardinal positions are those 6 positions of gaze in which the prime mover is 1 muscle of each eye, together called *yoke muscles* (see Chapter 3, Fig 3-2). *Midline positions* are straight up and straight down from primary position. These latter 2 gaze positions help determine the elevating and depressing capabilities of the eye, but they do not isolate any 1 muscle because 2 elevator and 2 depressor muscles affect midline gaze positions.

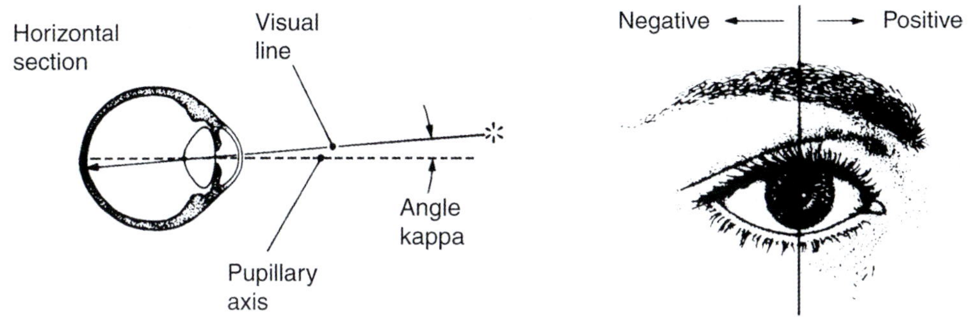

Figure 6-5 Angle kappa. A positive angle kappa simulates exotropia, whereas a negative angle kappa simulates esotropia. *(Reprinted from Parks MM.* Ocular Motility and Strabismus. *Hagerstown, MD: Harper & Row; 1975.)*

The phrase *diagnostic positions of gaze* has been applied to the composite of these 9 gaze positions: the 6 cardinal positions, straight up and down, and primary position. Several schemes have been devised to record the results of ocular alignment and motility in the various diagnostic positions of gaze, as well as those obtained with the head tilted to the right and to the left (Fig 6-6).

A and V patterns should be noted at this point. An *A pattern* refers to an esotropia greatest in upgaze or an exotropia greatest in downgaze; a *V pattern* denotes an esotropia greatest in downgaze or an exotropia greatest in upgaze. The patient should be observed carefully for any chin elevation or depression. See Chapter 9 for a full discussion of A and V patterns.

Convergence

Alignment at near is usually measured at 13 in. (33 cm) directly in front of the patient in the horizontal plane. Comparison of the alignment in the primary position at both distance and near fixation helps assess the accommodative convergence (synkinetic near) reflex. The *near point of convergence* is determined by placing a fixation object at 40 cm in the midsagittal plane of the patient's head. As the subject fixates on the object, it is moved toward the subject until 1 eye loses fixation and turns out. The point at which this action occurs is the near point of convergence. The eye that is able to maintain fixation is considered to be the dominant eye. The normal near point of convergence is 8–10 cm or less.

Accommodative convergence/accommodation ratio

The *accommodative convergence/accommodation (AC/A) ratio* is defined as the amount of convergence measured in prism diopters per unit (diopter) change in accommodation. There are 2 methods of clinical measurement.

1. The *gradient method* arrives at the AC/A ratio by dividing the change in deviation in prism diopters by the change in lens power. An accommodative target must be used, and the working distance (typically at 1/3 m or 6 m) is held constant. Plus or minus lenses (eg, +1, +2, +3, −1, −2, −3) are used to vary the accommodative

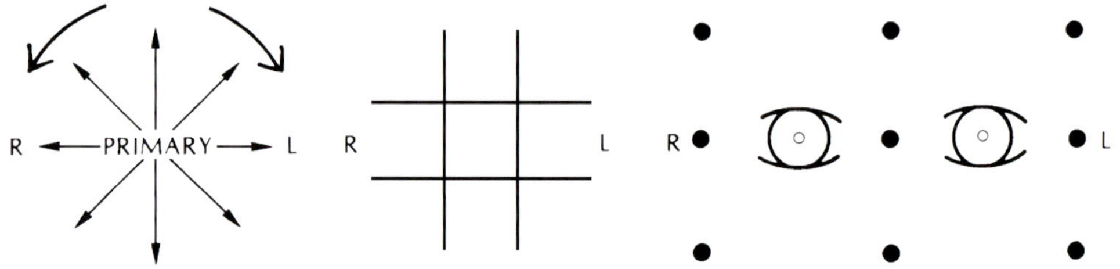

Figure 6-6 Three examples of methods for recording the results of ocular alignment testing.

requirement. This method measures the *stimulus AC/A ratio*, which is not necessarily identical to the *response AC/A ratio*. The latter can be determined only with the use of an optometer that records the change in accommodation actually produced.

2. The *heterophoria method* employs the distance–near relationship, measuring the distance and near deviations. A similar alignment is normally present for distance and near fixation. If the patient is more exotropic or less esotropic at near, too little convergence, or a low AC/A ratio, is present; if the patient is more esotropic or less exotropic at near, a high AC/A ratio is present. In accommodative esotropia, an increase of esotropia of 10Δ or more from distance to near fixation is considered to represent a high AC/A ratio.

An abnormally high AC/A ratio can be managed optically, pharmacologically, or surgically. For example, plus lens spectacles for hyperopia reduce accommodation and therefore reduce accommodative convergence. This principle is the mainstay of the medical management of esotropia. Bifocals reduce or eliminate the need to accommodate for near fixation. This optical management is used for excess convergence at near—that is, an esodeviation greater at near. Underplussed or overminused spectacles create the need for greater-than-normal accommodation. This excess accommodation creates more accommodative convergence and is occasionally used to reduce an exodeviation.

Long-acting cholinesterase inhibitors (eg, echothiophate iodide) can be used to decrease accommodative convergence. These drugs act directly on the ciliary body, facilitating transmission at the myoneural junction. They reduce the central demand for accommodative innervation and thus reduce the amount of convergence induced by accommodation.

Fusional Vergence

Vergences move the 2 eyes in opposite directions. Fusional vergences are motor responses used to eliminate horizontal, vertical, or torsional image disparity. They can be grouped by the following functions:

- *Fusional convergence* eliminates bitemporal retinal disparity and controls an exophoria.
- *Fusional divergence* eliminates binasal retinal disparity and controls an esophoria.
- *Vertical fusional vergence* controls a hyperphoria or hypophoria.
- *Torsional fusional vergence* controls incyclophoria or excyclophoria.

Fusional vergences can be measured by using a haploscopic device (major amblyoscope), a rotary prism, or a bar prism, and gradually increasing the prism power until diplopia occurs. Accommodation must be controlled during fusional vergence testing. Fusional vergences can be changed by a number of mechanisms:

- *Involuntary by patient:* As a tendency to deviate evolves, the patient gradually develops a larger-than-normal fusional vergence for that deviation. Very large fusional vergences are common in compensated, long-standing vertical deviations and in exodeviations.
- *Visual acuity:* Improved acuity improves the fusional vergence mechanism. The treatment of reduced vision may change a symptomatic intermittent deviation to an asymptomatic phoria.
- *State of awareness:* Fatigue, illness, or drug and alcohol ingestion may decrease the fusional vergence mechanism, converting a phoria to a tropia.
- *Orthoptics:* The magnitude of the fusional vergence mechanism may be increased by exercises. This treatment works best for near fusional convergence, particularly for the relief of the syndrome of convergence insufficiency.
- *Optical stimulation of fusional vergence:* (1) In controlled accommodative esotropia, reducing the strength of the hyperopia or bifocal correction induces an esophoria that stimulates fusional divergence. (2) Prisms to control diplopia may be gradually reduced to stimulate a compensatory fusional vergence.

Special Motor Tests

Special motor tests include forced ductions, active force generation, and saccadic velocity. These are also discussed, with illustrations, in BCSC Section 5, *Neuro-Ophthalmology.*

- *Forced ductions* are performed by using forceps to move the eye into various positions, thus determining resistance to passive movement. This test is usually performed at the time of surgery but can sometimes be performed preoperatively with topical anesthesia in cooperative patients.
- *Active force generation* assesses the relative strength of a muscle. The patient is asked to move the eye in a given direction while the observer grasps the eye with an instrument. If the muscle tested is paretic, the examiner feels less than normal tension.
- *Saccadic velocity* can be recorded using a special instrument that graphically records the speed and direction of eye movement. This test is useful to differentiate paralysis from restriction. A paralyzed muscle generates a reduced saccadic velocity throughout the movement of the involved eye, whereas a restricted muscle produces an initially normal velocity that rapidly decelerates when the eye reaches the limit of its movement.

The field of single binocular vision may be tested on either a Goldmann perimeter or a tangent screen. These tests are useful for following the recovery of a paretic muscle or for measuring the outcome of surgery to alleviate diplopia. A small white test object is followed by both eyes in the various cardinal positions throughout the visual field. When the patient indicates that the test object is seen double, the point is plotted. The examiner then repeats the same procedure until the entire visual field has been plotted, noting the area in which the patient reported single vision and the area of double vision. The field of binocular fixation normally measures about 45°–50° from the fixation point except where it is blocked by the nose (Fig 6-7).

3-Step Test

Cyclovertical muscle palsies, especially those involving the superior oblique muscles, are often responsible for hyperdeviations. The 3-step test is an algorithm that can be used to help identify the paretic cyclovertically acting muscle. As helpful as this test is, however, it is not always diagnostic and can be misleading, especially in patients in whom more than one muscle is paretic, in patients who have undergone strabismus surgery, and in the presence of restrictions or dissociated vertical deviation (see Chapter 10).

The examiner must be familiar with the anatomy and motor physiology of the extraocular muscles in order to understand the test. There are 8 cyclovertically acting muscles: 4 work as depressors (2 in each eye), and 4 work as elevators (2 in each eye). The 2 *depressors* of each eye are the *inferior rectus* and *superior oblique muscles*; the 2 *elevators* of each eye are the *superior rectus* and the *inferior oblique muscles*. The 3-step test is performed as described in the following sections (Fig 6-8).

Step 1

Determine which eye is hypertropic by using the cover-uncover test (see Fig 6-1 and the discussion earlier in this chapter). Step 1 narrows the number of possible underacting muscles from 8 to 4. In the example shown in Figure 6-8, the right eye has been found to be hypertropic. This means that the paresis will be found in either the depressors of the right eye (RIR, RSO) or the elevators of the left eye (LIO, LSR). Draw an oval around these 2 muscle groups (Fig 6-8A).

Step 2

Determine whether the vertical deviation is greater in right gaze or in left gaze. In the example, the deviation is larger in left gaze. This implicates 1 of the 4 vertically acting

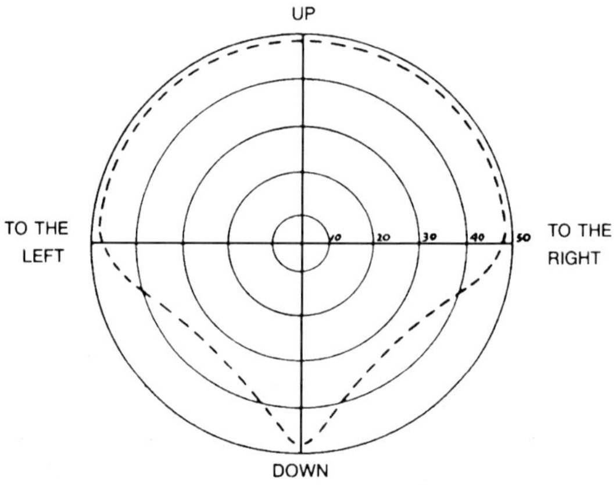

Figure 6-7 The normal field of single binocular vision.

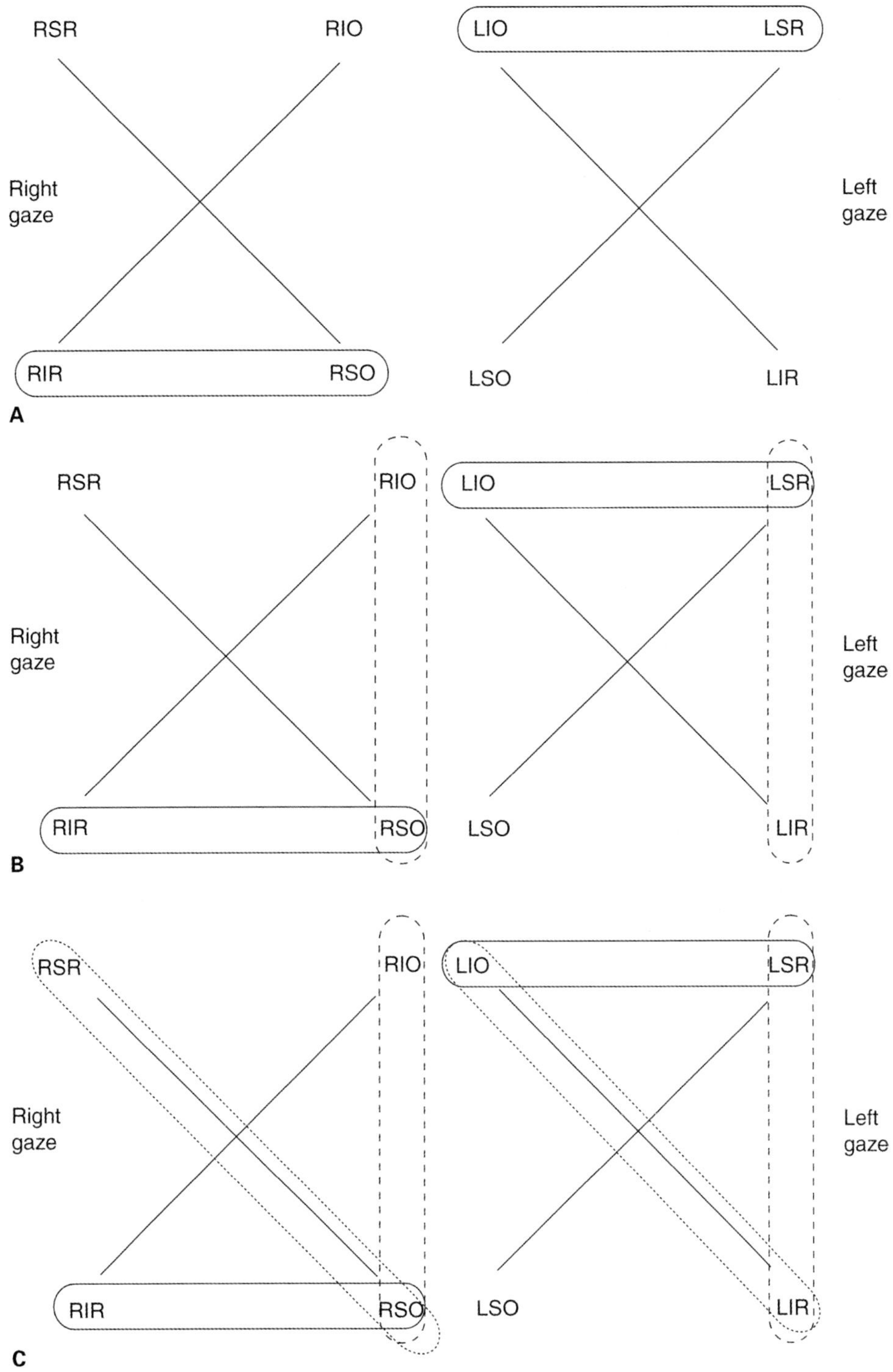

Figure 6-8 The 3-step test. **A,** Step 1: A right hypertropia suggests weakness in 1 of the 2 depressors of the right eye (RIR or RSO) or in 1 of the 2 elevators of the left eye (LIO or LSR). **B,** Step 2: Worsening of the right hypertropia on left gaze implicates either the RSO or the LSR. Note that, at the end of Step 2, 1 depressor and 1 elevator of opposite eyes will be the possible weak muscle. **C,** Step 3: The right head tilt causes intorsion (incycloduction) of the right eye. Because this rotation depends on activation of both the RSO (a depressor) and the RSR (an elevator), weakness of the RSO will cause the right hypertropia to increase.

muscles used in left gaze. Draw an oval around the 4 vertically acting muscles that are used in left gaze (Fig 6-8B). At the end of step 2, the 2 remaining possible muscles (1 in each eye) are both intortors or extortors and both superior or inferior muscles (1 rectus and 1 oblique). Note that in Figure 6-8B, the increased left-gaze deviation eliminates 2 inferior muscles and implicates 2 superior muscles.

Step 3

Known as the *Bielschowsky head-tilt test*, the final step involves tilting the head to the right and then to the left. Head tilt to the right stimulates intorsion of the right eye (RSR, RSO) and extorsion of the left eye (LIR, LIO). Head tilt to the left stimulates extorsion of the right eye (RIR, RIO) and intorsion of the left eye (LSR, LSO). Normally, the 2 intortors and the 2 extortors of each eye have *opposite* vertical actions that cancel each other. If 1 intortor or 1 extortor is paretic, it cannot act vertically, and the vertical action of the other ipsilateral torting muscle becomes manifest.

Figure 6-8C illustrates the results if step 2 had demonstrated that the deviation was greater in left gaze and the RSO was the paretic muscle. In this case, when the head is tilted to the right, in order to maintain fixation, the right eye must intort and the left eye must extort. Because the right superior oblique is paretic, the vertical action of the right superior rectus is unopposed. Contraction of this muscle in an attempt to incycloduct the eye results in an upward movement of the right eye, thus increasing the vertical deviation.

Parks MM. Isolated cyclovertical muscle palsy. *AMA Arch Ophthalmol.* 1958;60:1027–1035.

Prism Adaptation Test

In prism adaptation, the patient is fitted with prisms of sufficient magnitude to permit alignment of the visual axes. In many cases, this step provokes a restoration of sensory binocular cooperation in a form of fusion and even stereopsis. This technique simulates orthotropia and possibly offers some predictive value of whether fusion may be restored when the patient undergoes surgical alignment.

In some patients, however (especially those with acquired esotropia), placement of such prisms increases the deviation. In such cases, anomalous retinal correspondence based on the objective angle may drive the eyes to maintain this adaptive alignment even with prismatic correction. After wearing such prisms, the patient returns with a greater angle of deviation. Prism adaptation is used by some ophthalmologists in patients with acquired esotropia. The patient is reexamined every 1–2 weeks and given larger prism correction, if needed, until the deviation no longer increases. Surgery is then performed on the new, larger, prism-adapted angle. The Prism Adaptation Study demonstrated a smaller undercorrection rate when surgery was based on this deviation compared to standard surgery.

Repka MX, Connett JE, Scott WE. The one-year surgical outcome after prism adaptation for the management of acquired esotropia. *Ophthalmology.* 1996;103:922–928.

Tests of Binocular Sensory Cooperation

Assessment of the vergence system indicates the extent to which the 2 eyes can be directed at the same object. Sensory binocularity involves the use of both eyes together to form 1 perception. In general, normal sensory binocularity depends on normal fusional vergence. Ideally, testing should therefore be performed before binocularity is disrupted by occlusion of either eye. Two classes of tests are commonly used to assess sensory binocularity: Worth 4-dot testing (and its equivalents) and stereo acuity testing.

Worth 4-dot testing

The mechanics of *Worth 4-dot testing* are described in Chapter 4. Only patients who are using both eyes together can appreciate all 4 lights being projected (see Fig 4-11). If the right eye is suppressed, as often occurs if that eye is deviated, the patient will report seeing 3 green lights because the white light appears green. If the left eye is suppressed, the patient will report seeing 2 red lights because the white light appears red. If alternate eyes are suppressed, the patient may see 2 red and 3 green lights alternating. Patients with diplopia may report seeing 5 lights simultaneously.

Use of the Worth 4-dot test at distance illuminates a smaller, more central portion of the retina; testing at closer distances illuminates a progressively larger, more peripheral portion. Distance testing can reveal small suppression scotomata that may not be apparent on testing at near. Results of testing should be reported as fusion or suppression of 1 eye at distance and at near. Many cases of small-angle strabismus (eg, that associated with monofixation syndrome) may combine fusion at near with suppression of 1 eye at distance. A polarized version of the Worth 4-dot test is also available.

Stereo acuity testing

Worth 4-dot testing is best at detecting suppression, but *stereo acuity testing* assesses the use of the 2 eyes for binocular depth perception. Stereopsis occurs when the 2 retinal images, slightly disparate because of the normally different views provided by the horizontal separation of the 2 eyes, are cortically integrated. There are 2 types of stereopsis tests: *contour* and *random dot*. *Contour stereopsis tests* involve actual horizontal separation of the targets presented to each eye (with polarized or red-green glasses) such that monocular clues to depth are present at lower stereo acuity levels. *Random-dot stereopsis tests* circumvent the problem of monocular clues by embedding the stereo figures in a background of random dots.

In the *Stereo Fly test* (a contour stereopsis test), a card with superimposed images of a fly is shown to the patient. Ability to detect the elevation of the fly's wings above the plane of the card indicates stereopsis. Because the separation of the superimposed images is 3500 seconds of arc, this test is one of gross stereopsis. Other figures included on the same card contain less separated images. Thus, quantitation of finer stereo acuity may be possible in cooperative patients.

Several different types of random-dot stereopsis tests are clinically useful. The *Randot test*, in which polarized glasses are worn, can measure stereo acuity to 20 seconds of arc. The *Random-Dot E test* employs a preferential looking strategy to test stereopsis and is used in pediatric vision screening programs. Red-green glasses are used in the *TNO test* to provide separation of the images seen by each eye. The *Lang stereopsis tests* do not require glasses to produce a random-dot stereoscopic effect and therefore may be useful in young children who object to wearing glasses.

Stereopsis can also be measured at distance using the AO Project-O-Chart with Vectograph slide or the Smart System II PC Plus (M&S Technologies, Park Ridge, Illinois). Distance stereo acuity measurements may be helpful in monitoring control of intermittent exotropia.

Cycloplegic Refraction

One of the most important tests in the evaluation of any patient with complaints pertinent to binocular vision and ocular motility is refraction with cycloplegic agents. *Cyclopentolate* (1.0%) is the preferred drug for routine use in children, especially when combined with phenylephrine, which has no cycloplegic effect itself. Use of 0.5% strength is suggested in infants, and the clinician should be aware that some adverse psychological effects have been observed in children receiving cyclopentolate. *Homatropine* (5.0%) and *scopolamine* (0.25%) are occasionally used instead of cyclopentolate, but neither is as rapid acting or effective. *Tropicamide* (0.5% or 1.0%), which is used in conjunction with phenylephrine (2.5%) for routine dilation, is usually not strong enough for effective cycloplegia in children. Some ophthalmologists use a combination of cyclopentolate and tropicamide to achieve maximum dilation. Many ophthalmologists advocate *atropine* 1.0% drops or ointment, but this drug causes prolonged blurring and is more often associated with toxic or allergic side effects (see the following section). Nonetheless, 1% atropine drops (once per day to 1 eye only) are being used safely and with increasing frequency for the treatment of amblyopia (see Chapter 5).

Table 6-2 shows the schedule of administration and duration of action for commonly used cycloplegics. The duration of action varies greatly, and the pupillary effect occurs earlier and lasts longer than does the cycloplegic effect, so a dilated pupil does not necessarily indicate complete cycloplegia. For patients with accommodative esodeviations, frequent repeated cycloplegic examinations are essential when control is precarious, but not otherwise. Retinoscopic measurements should be made along the patient's visual axis.

Table 6-2 Administration and Duration of Cycloplegics

Medication	Administration Schedule	Duration of Mydriatic Action
Tropicamide	1 drop q 5 min × 2; wait 30 min	4–8 hr
Cyclopentolate	1 drop q 5 min × 2; wait 30 min	8–24 hr
Scopolamine	1 drop q 5 min × 2; wait 1 hr	1–3 d
Homatropine	1 drop q 5 min × 2; wait 1 hr	1–3 d
Atropine*	1 drop tid × 3 days; then 1 drop morning of appointment	1–2 wk

*Some physicians think that atropine ointment is a safer vehicle for delivery of the drug, given once a day × 3 days.

Side effects

Adverse reactions to cycloplegic agents include allergic (or hypersensitivity) reaction with conjunctivitis, edematous eyelids, and dermatitis. These reactions are more frequent with atropine than with any of the other agents. Hypnotic effect can be seen with scopolamine and occasionally with cyclopentolate or homatropine.

Systemic intoxication from atropine manifests in fever, dry mouth, flushing of the face, rapid pulse, nausea, dizziness, delirium, and erythema. Treatment is discontinuation of the medicine, with supportive measures as necessary. If the reaction is severe, physostigmine may be given. Remember, 1 drop of 1.0% atropine is 0.5 mg atropine.

CHAPTER 7

Esodeviations

An *esodeviation* is a latent or manifest convergent misalignment of the visual axes. Esodeviations are the most common type of strabismus, accounting for more than 50% of ocular deviations in the pediatric population. Three commonly recognized forms of esodeviation are grouped according to variations in fusional capabilities:

- *Esophoria* is a latent esodeviation that is controlled by fusional mechanisms so that the eyes remain properly aligned under normal binocular viewing conditions.
- *Intermittent esotropia* is an esodeviation that is intermittently controlled by fusional mechanisms but becomes manifest under certain conditions, such as fatigue, illness, stress, or tests that interfere with the maintenance of normal fusional abilities (such as covering 1 eye).
- *Esotropia* is an esodeviation that is not controlled by fusional mechanisms, so the deviation is constantly manifest.

Esodeviations can result from innervational, anatomical, mechanical, refractive, genetic, and accommodative causes. Table 7-1 lists the major types of esodeviation.

Pseudoesotropia

Pseudoesotropia is characterized by the false appearance of esotropia when the visual axes are actually aligned accurately. The appearance may be caused by a flat, broad nasal bridge; prominent epicanthal folds; or a narrow interpupillary distance. The observer sees less sclera nasally than would be expected, which creates the impression that the eye is turned in toward the nose, especially when the child gazes to either side. Because no real deviation exists, both corneal light reflex testing and cover testing results are normal. True esotropia can develop later in children with pseudoesotropia, so parents and pediatricians should be cautioned that reassessment is required if the apparent deviation does not improve.

Infantile (Congenital) Esotropia

Classic Congenital (Essential Infantile) Esotropia

Few children who are eventually diagnosed with classic congenital esotropia are actually born with an esotropia. Although the parents often describe the crossing as occurring at

Table 7-1 Types of Esodeviation

Pseudoesotropia

Infantile (congenital) esotropia
- Classic congenital (essential infantile) esotropia
- Nystagmus and esotropia
  - Ciancia syndrome
  - Manifest latent nystagmus
  - Nystagmus blockage syndrome

Accommodative esotropia
- Refractive (normal AC/A)
- Nonrefractive (high AC/A)
- Partially accommodative

Nonaccommodative acquired esotropia
- Basic
- Acute
- Cyclic
- Sensory deprivation
- Divergence insufficiency and divergence paralysis
- Spasm of the near synkinetic reflex
- Surgical (consecutive)

Incomitant esotropia
- Sixth nerve (abducens) paresis
- Medial rectus restriction
  - Thyroid-associated orbitopathy
  - Medial orbital wall fracture
- Duane syndrome and Möbius syndrome

birth, the exact date is not precisely established in most cases, and they rarely remember seeing the deviation in the newborn nursery. Documented presence of esotropia by age 6 months has been accepted as a defining element of congenital esotropia by most ophthalmologists. This criterion has been used in clinical studies. Some ophthalmologists prefer to describe this disorder as *infantile esotropia* to more accurately denote the timing of its development.

A family history of esotropia or strabismus is often present, but well-defined genetic patterns are unusual. Other than strabismus, children with congenital esotropia are usually normal. Esotropia, however, occurs in up to 30% of children with neurologic and developmental problems, including cerebral palsy and hydrocephalus.

Equal visual acuity associated with alternation of fixation from 1 eye to the other is common in children with congenital esotropia. Cross-fixation, in which a large-angle esotropia is associated with the use of the adducted eye for fixation of objects in the contralateral temporal field, is also frequent (Fig 7-1). Amblyopia may be present when a constant in-turning of only 1 eye occurs.

The misalignment is often readily apparent and the deviation is characteristically larger than 30Δ. There may be an apparent abduction deficit because of cross-fixation; children with equal vision have no need to abduct either eye on side gaze. If amblyopia is present, only the better-seeing eye will fixate in all fields of gaze, making the amblyopic eye appear to have an abduction weakness. The child's ability to abduct each eye may be

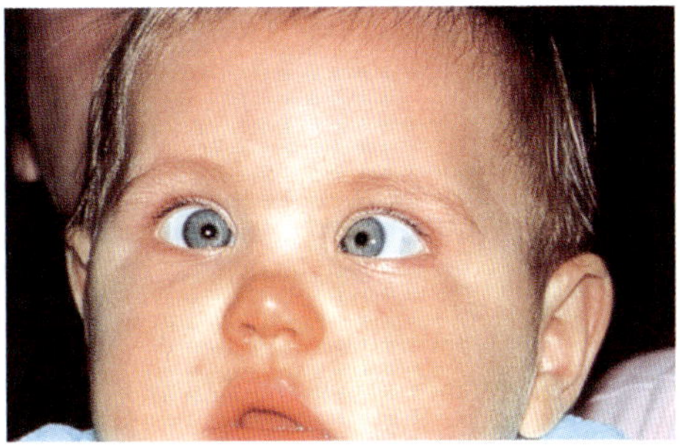

Figure 7-1 Classic congenital esotropia. *(Reproduced from Archer SM. Esotropia.* Focal Points: Clinical Modules for Ophthalmologists. *San Francisco: American Academy of Ophthalmology; 1994, module 12.)*

demonstrated with the doll's head maneuver, by rotating the child, or by observation with 1 eye patched. Inferior oblique muscle overaction and dissociated vertical deviation may occur in more than 50% of patients with congenital esotropia but are not commonly recognized until age 1 year or older.

Asymmetry of monocular horizontal smooth pursuit is normal in infants up to age 6 months, with nasal-to-temporal smooth pursuit less well developed than temporal-to-nasal smooth pursuit. Patients with congenital esotropia have persistent monocular smooth pursuit asymmetry that does not resolve.

Pathogenesis

The cause of congenital esotropia remains unknown. The debate regarding its etiology has focused on the implications of 2 conflicting theories. Worth's "sensory" concept was that congenital esotropia resulted from a deficit in a supposed fusion center in the brain. According to this theory, the goal of restoring binocularity was considered hopeless, because there was no way to provide this congenitally absent neural function. Chavasse disagreed with Worth's theory and believed the primary problem was mechanical and potentially curable if the deviation could be eliminated in infancy. Costenbader, Taylor, and Ing began to report favorable sensory results in some infants operated on between 6 months and 2 years of age. These encouraging results became the basis for the practice of early surgery for patients with congenital esotropia.

Management

Cycloplegic refraction characteristically reveals 1–2 D of hyperopia, which is the normal refractive error in young children. Significant astigmatism or myopia may be present and may require correction. Because accommodative esotropia can occur as early as age 4 months and often responds to hyperopic correction, significant refractive errors are corrected by prescribing the full cycloplegic retinoscopy findings. A small-angle esotropia that is variable or intermittent may be more likely to respond to hyperopic correction than a large-angle, constant esotropia. An atropine refraction may be useful in some hyperopic patients with esotropia to ensure that all the hyperopia has been identified.

Ocular alignment is rarely achieved without surgery in a child with early-onset esotropia. However, surgery should be undertaken only after correction of significant refractive errors and treatment of amblyopia. Failure to correct these problems may compromise stable surgical alignment of the eyes.

Most ophthalmologists agree that surgery should be undertaken early. The eyes should be aligned by age 24 months to optimize binocular cooperation. However, surgery can be performed in healthy children between ages 4 and 6 months to maximize binocular function such as stereopsis. The Congenital Esotropia Observational Study (CEOS) demonstrated that patients with a constant and stable esotropia of at least 40Δ who present between ages 2 and 4 months are unlikely to improve spontaneously. Based on this observation, some surgeons suggest even earlier surgery in hopes of achieving a superior sensory outcome. Smaller angles may be observed, as they may improve spontaneously.

The child's psychological and motor development may improve and accelerate after the eyes are straightened. Bonding is improved between infant and parents after surgical straightening of the eyes. Improved techniques have minimized the risk of general anesthesia such that anesthetic concerns need not dictate the age at which surgery is performed in healthy infants.

Various surgical approaches have been suggested for congenital esotropia. The most common procedure is recession of both medial rectus muscles. Recession of a medial rectus muscle combined with resection of the ipsilateral lateral rectus muscle is an acceptable alternative. Two-muscle surgery spares horizontal rectus muscles for subsequent surgery should it be needed; this is a common occurrence in patients with congenital esotropia. Some surgeons operate on 3 or even 4 horizontal rectus muscles at the time of the initial surgery if the deviation is larger than 50Δ. Associated overaction of the inferior oblique muscles is often treated at the time of the initial surgery using inferior oblique muscle-weakening procedures. Chapter 13 discusses surgical procedures in greater detail.

Botulinum toxin injections into the medial rectus muscles have been used by some ophthalmologists in the treatment of congenital esotropia. Multiple injections may be required and the long-term sensory and motor outcomes have not been shown to be superior to those from incisional surgery.

The goal of treatment in congenital esotropia is to reduce the deviation to orthotropia or as close to it as possible. Ideally, this results in normal sight in each eye and in the development of at least some degree of sensory fusion that will maintain motor alignment. However, approximately one third of children will require multiple surgeries. Alignment within 8Δ of orthotropia frequently results in the development of the monofixation syndrome, characterized by peripheral fusion, central suppression, and favorable appearance and is therefore considered a successful surgical result. This small-angle strabismus generally represents a stable, functional surgical outcome even though bifoveal fusion is not achieved.

Ing M, Costenbader FD, Parks MM, et al. Early surgery for congenital esotropia. *Am J Ophthalmol.* 1966;61:1419–1427.

Pediatric Eye Disease Investigator Group. The clinical spectrum of early-onset esotropia: experience of the Congenital Esotropia Observational Study. *Am J Ophthalmol.* 2002; 133:102–108.

von Noorden GK. A reassessment of infantile esotropia. XLIV Edward Jackson memorial lecture. *Am J Ophthalmol.* 1988;105:1–10.

Nystagmus and Esotropia

Nystagmus occurs in up to one third of patients with a history of early-onset esotropia. For a detailed discussion of nystagmus and esotropia, see Chapter 12 of this volume.

Accommodative Esotropia

Accommodative esotropia is defined as a convergent deviation of the eyes associated with activation of the accommodative reflex. All accommodative esodeviations are acquired, with the following characteristics:

- onset generally between 6 months and 7 years, averaging 2½ years of age (can be as early as age 4 months)
- usually intermittent at onset, becoming constant
- often hereditary
- sometimes precipitated by trauma or illness
- frequently associated with amblyopia
- diplopia may occur (especially in older children) but usually disappears as patient develops facultative suppression scotoma in the deviating eye

Types of accommodative esotropia are listed in Table 7-1 and discussed in the following sections.

Refractive Accommodative Esotropia

The mechanism of *refractive accommodative esotropia* involves 3 factors: (1) uncorrected hyperopia, (2) accommodative convergence, and (3) insufficient fusional divergence. The uncorrected hyperopia forces the patient to accommodate to sharpen the retinal image, thus inducing increased convergence. If the patient's fusional divergence mechanism is insufficient to compensate the increased convergence tonus, esotropia results. The angle of esotropia is generally between 20Δ and 30Δ and approximately equal at distance and near fixation. The amount of hyperopia averages +4 D.

Treatment of refractive accommodative esotropia consists of correction of the full amount of hyperopia, as determined under cycloplegia. Any concomitant amblyopia should be treated as well. Significant delay in the initiation of treatment following the onset of esotropia increases the likelihood that a portion of the esodeviation will fail to respond to antiaccommodative therapy. A gradual reduction of hyperopic correction may be possible over time if the patient can maintain control of the ensuing esophoria. This reduction stimulates the development of increased fusional divergence amplitudes, which in some patients may allow discontinuation of spectacle therapy in the future.

Parents must understand the importance of full-time wear of spectacle correction. The esodeviation, without glasses, may even increase initially after the correction is worn. Discussing this issue with parents at the time the prescription is first given is often more effective than the same explanation afterward. In addition, it is helpful to explain that the glasses help to control the strabismus, not cure it. This will help eliminate potential frustration when their child's eyes continue to cross when they are not wearing glasses.

Therapy with miotic agents (eg, echothiophate iodide) has been suggested as a substitute for glasses. However, because of potential ocular and systemic side effects from these medications, their use is usually confined to children who are uncooperative in wearing glasses at all or who spend long hours playing in the water when glasses may not be worn.

Surgical correction may be required when a patient with refractive accommodative esotropia fails to regain fusion with glasses or subsequently develops a nonaccommodative component to the deviation. However, the ophthalmologist must rule out latent uncorrected hyperopia before proceeding with surgery.

High Accommodative Convergence/Accommodative Esotropia

Patients with *high accommodative convergence/accommodation (AC/A)* have an abnormal relationship between accommodation and accommodative convergence. Excess convergence tonus results from accommodation, and esotropia develops in the setting of insufficient fusional divergence. Because more accommodation is required at near fixation than at distance, the angle of esotropia is greater at near. It can be reduced by +3.00 D bifocal lenses. Measurement of the angle of esotropia with fixation targets that require appropriate accommodation is critical to making the diagnosis of this type of esotropia.

High accommodative convergence/accommodative esotropia may occur in patients with large degrees of hyperopia or in patients with normal levels of hyperopia, emmetropia, or even myopia. In these latter groups of patients, the disorder is also referred to as *nonrefractive accommodative esotropia*. The refractive error in these patients averages +2.25 D.

No consensus exists on the best management of high AC/A esotropia. Several options are available:

- *Bifocals.* The most commonly used treatment option for nonrefractive accommodative esotropia is bifocal spectacles. If bifocals are employed, they should initially be prescribed in the executive or 35-mm flat-top style with a power of +2.50 or +3.00 D. The top of the segment should cross the pupil, and the vertical height of the bifocal should not exceed that of the distance portion of the lens. Detailed instructions concerning the bifocal should be given to the optician. Progressive bifocal lenses have been used successfully, but conventional bifocals are preferred. If progressive bifocals are used, they should be fitted higher than adult lenses (about 4 mm) and with a power up to +3.00 or the power needed to achieve alignment at near fixation. An ideal response to bifocal glasses is restoration of normal binocular function (fusion and stereopsis) at both distance and near fixation. An acceptable response is fusion at distance with less than 10Δ of residual esotropia through the bifocal at near fixation.
- *Long-acting cholinesterase inhibitors.* Ophthalmologists who use long-acting cholinesterase inhibitors suggest starting with maximum strength (0.125% echothiophate iodide drops) in both eyes once daily for 6 weeks. If such treatment is effective, strength or frequency should be decreased to the minimum effective dose.

Parents must be warned about the potentially serious side effects of these drugs, including deletion of pseudocholinesterase from the blood, which makes the patient highly susceptible to depolarizing muscle relaxants such as succinylcholine. Echothiophate iodide can also cause pupillary cysts to form; some ophthalmologists prescribe phenylephrine 2.5% drops twice daily concurrently to reduce the risk of cyst formation.

- *Surgery.* Some ophthalmologists advocate surgery for high AC/A esotropia. Surgery can normalize the AC/A ratio in these patients. It can be used in some patients, usually adolescents, to allow discontinuation of a bifocal and control of the esodeviation with single-vision glasses or contact lenses.
- *Observation.* Many patients will show a decrease in the near deviation with time and ultimately develop binocular vision at both distance and near fixation. Some ophthalmologists will observe the near deviation as long as the distance deviation allows for the development of fusion or if the patient is asymptomatic.

For the long-term management of both refractive and nonrefractive accommodative esotropia, it is important to remember that measured hyperopia usually increases until age 5–7 years. Therefore, if the esotropia with glasses increases, the cycloplegic refraction should be repeated and the full correction prescribed. After age 5–7 years, hyperopia may decrease, and the full cycloplegic refraction in place will thus blur vision and the prescription will need to be reduced.

If glasses or drugs correct all or nearly all of the esotropia and some degree of sensory binocular cooperation or fusion is present, the clinician may begin to reduce the strength of glasses or drugs to create a small esophoria when the patient reaches age 5 or 6. This reduction may stimulate the fusional divergence mechanism to redevelop normal magnitude. An increase in the fusional divergence combined with the natural decrease of both the hyperopia and the high AC/A ratio may enable the patient to maintain straight eyes without glasses, bifocals, or drugs. For example, in the case of a 5-year-old who has worn glasses since age 2 for esotropia and has a visual acuity of 20/25 in both eyes:

Hyperopia 4.00 D OU
  with +4.00 D OU: orthophoria at distance and near
  after 6–12 months of spectacle wear: with +3.00 D OU: $E = E' = 6\Delta$
Prescribe +3.00 OU

Further reductions may be possible if the child maintains good visual acuity, has control of the esophoria, and does not have asthenopic symptoms.

Another example is an 8-year-old child who had presented with new-onset esotropia at age 3 years:

Hyperopia 2.00 D OU
  with +2.00 D OU: $E = 4\Delta$; $E' = 24\Delta$
  +2.50 D bifocals prescribed: $E = E' = 4\Delta$
At age 6, hyperopia remains 2.00 D

with +2.00 D add: E = 4Δ; E′ = 8Δ
with +1.50 D add: E = 4Δ; E(T)′ = 12Δ
Prescribe +2.00 D sphere OU with +2.00 D add

Further bifocal reductions may be possible as long as the child maintains an asymptomatic esophoria. If the amount of hyperopia increases and is prescribed in new glasses, the bifocal add can sometimes be reduced by the same amount that the hyperopia increased without affecting the resultant lens power through the bifocal. This change increases the chance that the child will eventually be able to discontinue bifocal use.

Partially Accommodative Esotropia

Patients with partially accommodative esodeviations show a reduction in the angle of esotropia with glasses but have a residual esotropia despite treatment of amblyopia and provision of full hyperopic therapy. Sometimes, partially accommodative esotropia results from decompensation of a fully accommodative esotropia, but in other instances the child may have had an esotropia that subsequently developed an accommodative element. An interval of weeks to months between the onset of accommodative esotropia and the application of full cycloplegic refraction often results in some residual esotropia, even after the proper glasses are worn. Hence, prompt treatment of accommodative esotropia may offer substantial benefits. Patients with pure refractive accommodative esotropia who have been made orthotropic with glasses are less likely to develop a nonaccommodative component to their esodeviation than patients with the type of accommodative esotropia with a high AC/A ratio.

Treatment of partially accommodative esotropia consists of amblyopia management and prescription of the full hyperopic correction. Strabismus surgery may be warranted for the nonaccommodative portion depending on the size of the deviation and the wishes of the patient and family. It is important that the patient and parents understand before surgery that its purpose is to produce straight eyes with glassess—not to allow the child to discontinue wearing glasses altogether.

Mulvihill A, MacCann A, Flitcroft I, et al. Outcome in refractive accommodative esotropia. *Br J Ophthalmol.* 2000;84:746–749.

Nonaccommodative Acquired Esotropia

Basic (Acquired) Esotropia

Esotropia that develops after age 6 months and that is not associated with an accommodative component is called *basic,* or *acquired, esotropia.* As with infantile esotropia, an accommodative factor is usually absent, the amount of hyperopia is not significant, and the near deviation is the same as the distance deviation. Although most children with this form of esotropia are otherwise healthy, central nervous system lesions must be considered. Therapy consists of amblyopia treatment and surgical correction as soon as possible after the onset of the deviation.

When planning surgery for patients with acquired esotropia, some ophthalmologists advocate prism adaptation. Prism adaptation is a process of prescribing the full hyperopic correction if indicated and adding Press-On prisms to neutralize any residual esodeviation. The patient wears the glasses with the Press-On prisms for 1 or 2 weeks and is then reexamined. If the esodeviation increases with the prisms, new prisms are prescribed to neutralize the deviation. In some patients, the esodeviation increases as the patient "eats up" the prism—that is, the deviation continues to increase and more prism is required to correct it. Surgery is then planned for the full prism-adapted deviation. Prism adaptation may reduce the undercorrection rate associated with acquired or decompensated accommodative esotropia (see Prism Adaptation Test in Chapter 6).

Acute Esotropia

Occasionally, an acquired esotropia is acute in onset. In such cases, the patient immediately becomes aware of the deviation and frequently has diplopia. A careful motility evaluation is important to rule out an accommodative or paretic component. Artificial disruption of binocular vision, such as may follow treatment of an ocular injury or patching for amblyopia, is one of the known causes of acute esotropia. Because the onset of comitant esotropia in an older child may indicate an underlying neurologic disorder, neurologic evaluation may be indicated. Most patients with acute onset of esotropia have a history of normal binocular vision, and therefore the prognosis for restoration of single binocular vision with prisms and surgery is good. Prisms may be used during a period of observation before surgery is performed.

Cyclic Esotropia

Cyclic esotropia is rare, with an estimated incidence of 1:3000–1:5000 strabismus cases. Onset typically occurs during the preschool years, although a congenital case and several adult cases have been reported. The esotropia is present intermittently, usually every other day (48-hour cycle). Variable cycles and 24-hour cycles have also been documented.

Fusion and binocular vision are usually absent or defective on the strabismic day, with marked improvement on the straight day. Diplopia on strabismic days is unusual and has been a prominent symptom only in patients of a relatively older age who are unable to develop suppression.

Cyclic esotropia is noted for its unpredictable response to various forms of therapy, with the exception of surgery, which is usually curative. Occlusion therapy may convert the cyclic deviation into a constant one.

Helveston EM. Cyclic strabismus. *Am Orthopt J.* 1973;23:48–51.

Sensory Deprivation Esodeviation

Monocular vision loss from various causes, such as cataract, corneal scarring, optic atrophy, or prolonged blurred or distorted retinal images, may cause an esodeviation. Anisometropia with amblyopia is common in this type of esodeviation.

Obstacles preventing clear and focused retinal images and symmetric visual stimulation must be identified and remedied as soon as possible. Animal and clinical data indicate that restoration of normal, symmetric inputs must be accomplished at an early age if irreversible amblyopia is to be avoided. After all obstacles to balanced sensory inputs have been removed, any secondary amblyopia is treated, if possible. Surgery for residual esotropia may be indicated. The surgical management of these cases is similar to that of early-onset esotropia, except when good visual acuity cannot be restored as a result of irreversible amblyopia or organic defects. In such situations, strabismus surgery should generally be performed only on the abnormal eye.

Divergence Insufficiency

The characteristic finding of divergence insufficiency is an esodeviation, generally in adult patients, that is greater at distance than at near. The deviation does not change with vertical or horizontal gaze, and fusional divergence is reduced. Divergence paralysis may represent a more severe form of divergence insufficiency. Because true paralysis of divergence cannot generally be documented, the term *divergence insufficiency* is preferred. Divergence insufficiency can be divided into a primary isolated form and a secondary form associated with other neurologic abnormalities stemming from pontine tumors or severe head trauma. A thorough clinical evaluation can frequently distinguish between the 2 forms of divergence insufficiency. Primary isolated divergence insufficiency is frequently a benign condition: symptoms resolve in 40% of patients within several months. Patients with secondary divergence insufficiency may obtain relief from symptoms with treatment of the underlying neurologic disorder (eg, corticosteroids for temporal arteritis, treatment of intracranial hypertension). Management of diplopia consists of base-out prisms and, sometimes, surgery.

Jacobson DM. Divergence insufficiency revisited: natural history of idiopathic cases and neurologic associations. *Arch Ophthalmol.* 2000;118:1237–1241.

Spasm of the Near Synkinetic Reflex

Spasm of the near reflex is a spectrum of abnormalities of the near response. Thus, patients can present with varying combinations of excessive convergence, excessive accommodation, and miosis. The etiology is generally thought to be functional, related to psychological factors, but, rarely, it can be associated with organic disease. Patients may present with acute, persistent esotropia alternating at other times with orthotropia. The characteristic movement is the substitution of a convergence movement for a gaze movement on horizontal versions. Monocular abduction is normal in spite of marked abduction limitation on versions. Pseudomyopia may occur. Treatment, which may be problematic, has consisted of cycloplegic agents such as atropine or homatropine, plus lenses for patients with significant hyperopia and bifocals.

Surgical (Consecutive) Esodeviation

Esodeviation following surgery for exodeviation frequently improves spontaneously. Treatment includes base-out prisms, plus lenses or miotics (especially if the patient is hyperopic), alternate occlusion, and, finally, surgery. Unless the deviation is very large or symptomatic, surgery should be postponed for several months because of the possibility of spontaneous improvement.

A slipped or lost lateral rectus muscle produces varying amounts of esotropia, depending on the amount of slippage. A slipped muscle should be suspected in the case of consecutive esotropia with a large adduction deficit following surgery on a lateral rectus muscle. Surgical exploration and reattachment of the muscle to the globe is required. Transposition procedures may be necessary when lost muscles cannot be found. For slipped muscles, advancement of the muscle on the globe is required. (See Chapter 13, Fig 13-11, and the accompanying text discussion.)

Incomitant Esodeviation

The term *incomitant esodeviation* is used when esodeviation varies in different fields of gaze.

Sixth Nerve (Abducens) Paralysis

Paralysis of the lateral rectus muscle causes an incomitant esodeviation. Sixth nerve paralysis occurring at birth has been reported but is uncommon. Most cases of suspected congenital sixth nerve palsies represent infantile esotropia with cross-fixation. Congenital sixth nerve paralysis is thought to be caused by the increased intracranial pressure associated with the birth process and usually resolves spontaneously. Sixth nerve palsy occurs much more frequently in childhood than in infancy. Older patients may complain of double vision and often have a face turn toward the side of the paretic sixth nerve to avoid diplopia. Approximately one third of these cases are associated with intracranial lesions and may have associated neurologic findings. Other cases may be related to infectious or immunologic processes that involve cranial nerve VI. Spontaneous benign lesions usually resolve over several months.

The vision in both eyes is usually equal unless strabismic amblyopia or associated structural defects are found. The esotropia increases in gaze toward the paretic lateral rectus muscle. Saccadic velocities show slowing of the affected lateral rectus muscle, and active force generation tests document the weakness of that muscle. Versions show limited or no abduction of the affected eye.

A careful history should be taken to define antecedent infections, head trauma, or other possible inciting factors for sixth nerve palsy. Neurologic evaluation and computed tomography (CT) or magnetic resonance imaging (MRI) are indicated when neurologic signs or symptoms are present.

Patching may be required to maintain vision in the esotropic eye in children in the amblyopia age range, especially if the child has no face turn to maintain binocular fusion. Fresnel Press-On prisms are useful to correct the diplopia in primary position. Correction of a significant hyperopic refractive error may help to prevent the development of an accommodative esotropia. Spontaneous resolution may occur in more than half of patients with traumatic palsies, particularly if the paresis is unilateral. Injection of botulinum toxin into the antagonist medial rectus muscle may align the eye by temporarily paralyzing the medial rectus muscle. Botulinum treatment has not been shown to be helpful in preventing contracture of the medial rectus muscle or improving the rate of recovery.

Surgery is indicated when spontaneous resolution does not take place after 6 months or more of follow-up. In patients with some lateral rectus muscle function, a large recession of the antagonist medial rectus muscle with resection of the lateral rectus muscle is often a successful first operation. In cases of total paralysis, muscle transposition procedures may be required.

See additional discussions in Chapter 11, Special Forms of Strabismus, and Chapter 14, Chemodenervation Treatment of Strabismus and Blepharospasm Using Botulinum Toxin. See also BCSC Section 5, *Neuro-Ophthalmology.*

Foster RS. Vertical muscle transposition augmented with lateral fixation. *J AAPOS.* 1997;1: 20–30.

Holmes JM, Beck RW, Kip KE, et al. Botulinum toxin treatment versus conservative management in acute traumatic sixth nerve palsy or paresis. *J AAPOS.* 2000;4:145–149.

Other Forms of Incomitant Esodeviation

Medial rectus muscle restriction may result from thyroid myopathy, medial orbital wall fracture, or excessively resected medial rectus muscle (see Chapter 13).

For discussions of *Duane syndrome* and *Möbius syndrome*, see Chapter 11, Special Forms of Strabismus, and BCSC Section 5, *Neuro-Ophthalmology.*

Preferred Practice Patterns Committee, Pediatric Panel. *Esotropia and Exotropia.* San Francisco: American Academy of Ophthalmology; 2002.

CHAPTER 8

Exodeviations

An *exodeviation* is a divergent strabismus that can be latent (controlled by fusion) or manifest. Although the exact etiology of most exodeviations is unknown, proposed causes include anatomical and mechanical factors within the orbit as well as abnormalities of innervation such as excessive tonic divergence.

Pseudoexotropia

The term *pseudoexotropia* refers to an appearance of exodeviation when in fact the eyes are properly aligned. Pseudoexotropia may result from the following:

- wide interpupillary distance
- positive angle kappa without other ocular abnormalities (see the discussion of angle kappa in Chapter 6)
- positive angle kappa together with ocular abnormalities such as temporal dragging of the macula in retinopathy of prematurity

Exophoria

Exophoria is an exodeviation controlled by fusion under conditions of normal binocular vision. An exophoria is detected when binocular vision is interrupted, as during an alternate cover test. Exophoria may be asymptomatic if the angle of strabismus is small and fusional convergence amplitudes are adequate. Prolonged, detailed visual work or reading may bring about asthenopia. Treatment is usually not necessary unless an exophoria progresses to an intermittent exotropia.

Intermittent Exotropia

With the possible exception of exophoria at near, the most common type of exodeviation is *intermittent exotropia*, which is latent at times and manifest at others (Fig 8-1).

Clinical Characteristics

The onset of intermittent exotropia usually occurs early, before age 5, but it may be detected for the first time even later in childhood. Because proper eye alignment with

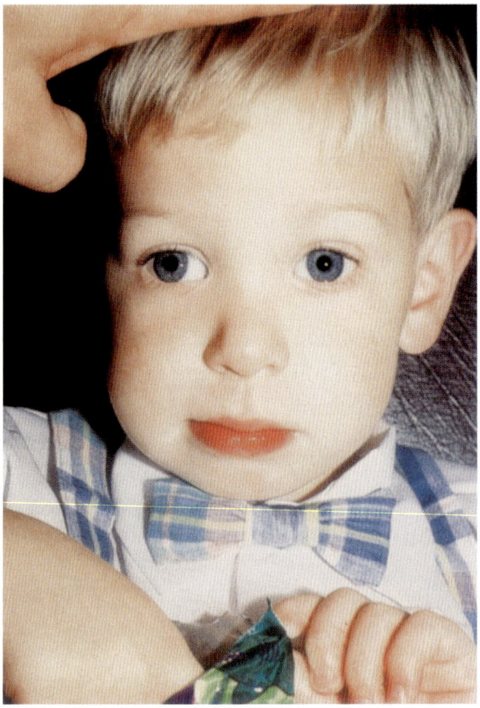

Figure 8-1 A 3-year-old boy with intermittent exotropia. *(Reproduced with permission from Wilson ME. Exotropia.* Focal Points: Clinical Modules for Ophthalmologists. *San Francisco: American Academy of Ophthalmology; 1995, module 11.)*

intermittent exotropia requires that compensatory fusional factors be active, the deviation often becomes manifest during times of visual inattention, fatigue, or stress. Parents of affected children often report that the exotropia occurs late in the day with fatigue or during illness, daydreaming, or drowsiness upon awakening. Exposure to bright light often causes a reflex closure of 1 eye.

During the early stages of the disorder, the deviation is usually larger for distance viewing than for near, and the exotropia is seen more frequently when the visual target is remote. Later, the near and distance exodeviations tend to be more equal in magnitude even if fusional control remains good. Intermittent exotropias can be associated with small hypertropias, A and V patterns, and oblique muscle dysfunction, all of which are discussed in Chapters 9 and 10.

In many patients, untreated intermittent exotropia progresses toward constant exotropia. During this progression, tropic episodes occur at lower levels of fatigue and last for longer periods of time. Children younger than 10 years of age may initially have diplopia but often develop the cortical adaptations of suppression and abnormal retinal correspondence with time. However, normal retinal correspondence and good binocular function remain when the eyes are straight. Amblyopia is uncommon unless the exotropia progresses to constant or nearly constant exotropia at an early age or unless another amblyogenic factor, such as anisometropia, is present.

Clinical Evaluation

The clinical evaluation begins with a history of the age of onset of the strabismus and a determination as to whether the exotropia is becoming more frequent. The clinician records how often and under what circumstances the deviation is manifest. A qualitative measurement of the control of the exodeviation exhibited throughout the examination is an important component of the evaluation and can be categorized as

- *Good control:* Exotropia manifests only after cover testing, and the patient resumes fusion rapidly without blinking or refixating.
- *Fair control:* Exotropia manifests after fusion is disrupted by cover testing, and the patient resumes fusion only after blinking or refixating.
- *Poor control:* Exotropia manifests spontaneously and may remain manifest for an extended time.

Prism and alternate cover testing should be used to evaluate the exodeviation at fixation distances of 20 feet and 14 inches. A far distance measurement at 100–200 feet (at the end of a long hallway or out a window) may more likely demonstrate a latent deviation or bring out an even larger one. The deviation at near fixation is often less than the deviation at distance fixation. This difference may be due to either a high accommodative convergence/accommodation (AC/A) ratio or to tenacious proximal fusion. The high AC/A ratio is a compensatory mechanism to help maintain alignment at near fixation. *Tenacious proximal fusion* is a proximal vergence aftereffect that occurs in some patients with intermittent exotropia; this aftereffect is due to a slow-to-dissipate fusion mechanism that prevents intermittent exotropia from manifesting at near fixation with a brief cover test. For patients with significantly more exodeviation in the distance than at near, a near prism and cover test after 1 hour of monocular occlusion to eliminate the effects of tenacious proximal fusion may help to distinguish between patients with a truly high AC/A ratio and those with a pseudo-high AC/A ratio. A patient with a pseudo-high AC/A ratio would have roughly equal distance and near measurements after occlusion; a patient with a truly high AC/A ratio would continue to have significantly less exodeviation at near. The abnormality of the AC/A ratio can be confirmed by testing with +3 D lenses at near or –2 D lenses at distance.

Kushner BJ, Morton GV. Distance/near differences in intermittent exotropia. *Arch Ophthalmol.* 1998;116:478–486.

Mohney BG, Huffaker RK. Common forms of childhood exotropia. *Ophthalmology.* 2003; 110:2093–2096.

Classification

Intermittent exotropia has traditionally been classified into several groups, based on the difference between alternating prism and cover test measurements at distance and at near and the change in near measurement produced by unilateral occlusion or +3 D lenses:

- *Basic* type exotropia is present when the exodeviation is approximately the same at distance and near fixation.

- *Divergence excess* type consists of an exodeviation that is greater at distance fixation than at near and can be divided into 2 subtypes.
  - *True divergence excess* type refers to those deviations that remain greater at distance than at near even after a period of monocular occlusion. Some of these patients prove to have a high gradient AC/A ratio when tested at near with +3 D lenses.
  - *Simulated divergence excess* type refers to a deviation that is initially greater at distance fixation than at near but that becomes about the same after 1 eye is occluded for 1 hour (to remove the effect of tenacious proximal fusion).
- The *convergence insufficiency* type is present when the exodeviation is greater at near than at distance. This type excludes isolated convergence insufficiency, which is discussed later in this chapter.

Sensory testing usually reveals excellent stereopsis with normal retinal correspondence when the exodeviation is latent and suppression with abnormal retinal correspondence when the exodeviation is manifest. However, if the deviation manifests rarely, diplopia may persist during those manifestations.

Treatment

Although many patients with intermittent exotropia will eventually require surgery, opinions vary widely regarding the timing of surgical intervention and the use of nonsurgical methods to delay or possibly to prevent the need for surgical intervention. Some ophthalmologists prefer to delay surgery in young children in whom good preoperative visual acuity and stereopsis could be exchanged for a small-angle esotropia, amblyopia, and decreased stereopsis. However, other ophthalmologists worry that delaying surgery too long could allow for the development of permanent suppression and loss of long-term stability following surgical correction.

Nonsurgical Management

Corrective lenses are prescribed for significant myopic, astigmatic, and hyperopic refractive errors. Correction of even mild myopia may improve control of the exodeviation. Mild to moderate degrees of hyperopia are not routinely corrected in children with intermittent exotropia for fear of worsening the deviation. However, some patients with more than 4.0 D of hyperopia (or more than 1.5 D of hyperopic anisometropia) may actually gain better control of the exodeviation after optical correction. Children with severe hyperopia may be unable to sustain the necessary accommodation for a clear image, and the lack of accommodative effort produces a blurred retinal image and manifest exotropia. Optical correction may improve retinal image clarity and help control the exodeviation.

Some ophthalmologists use additional minus lens power, usually 2–4 D beyond refractive error correction, to stimulate accommodative convergence to help control the exodeviation. This therapy may cause asthenopia in school-age children, but it can be effective as a temporizing measure to promote fusion and delay surgery during the visually immature years.

Part-time patching of the dominant (nondeviating) eye 4–6 hours per day, or alternate daily patching when no strong ocular preference is present, can be an effective treatment for small- to moderate-sized deviations, although the benefit produced is often temporary. The exact mechanism by which patching improves control of intermittent exotropia is not known; presumably, patching disrupts suppression and constitutes a passive orthoptic treatment.

Active orthoptic treatments, which consist of antisuppression therapy/diplopia awareness and fusional convergence training, can be used alone or in combination with patching, minus lenses, and surgery. For deviations of 20Δ or less, orthoptic treatment has been reported by some authors to have a long-term success rate comparable to that of surgery. Others have found no benefit and recommend surgery for any poorly controlled deviation.

Base-in prisms can be used to promote fusion in intermittent exotropia, but this treatment option is seldom chosen for long-term management because it can cause a reduction in fusional vergence amplitudes.

Surgical Treatment

Many patients with intermittent exotropia ultimately require surgery, which is customarily performed when progression toward constant exotropia is documented. No consensus exists regarding specific indications; however, the best sensory outcomes are probably achieved with motor alignment before age 7 or before 5 years of strabismus duration, or while the deviation is still intermittent. Many surgeons use manifestation of the deviation more than 50% of the time as criterion for surgery.

Abroms AD, Mohney BG, Rush DP, et al. Timely surgery in intermittent and constant exotropia for superior sensory outcome. *Am J Ophthalmol.* 2001;131:111–116.

Symmetric recession of both lateral rectus muscles is the most common surgical procedure for intermittent exotropia. Recession of 1 lateral rectus muscle combined with resection of the ipsilateral medial rectus muscle is an acceptable alternative and may be preferred for patients with basic type intermittent exotropia. Some strabismus surgeons perform unilateral lateral rectus muscle recession for patients with smaller exodeviations.

Kushner BJ. Selective surgery for intermittent exotropia based on distance/near differences. *Arch Ophthalmol.* 1998;116:324–328.

Olitsky SE. Early and late postoperative alignment following unilateral lateral rectus recession for intermittent exotropia. *J Pediatr Ophthalmol Strabismus.* 1998;35:146–148.

Management of surgical overcorrection

A temporary overcorrection of up to 10Δ–15Δ is desirable after bilateral lateral rectus muscle recessions. Persistent overcorrection (beyond 3–4 weeks) may require treatment with base-out prisms (usually Fresnel Press-On prisms) or alternate patching to prevent amblyopia or relieve diplopia. Corrective lenses or miotics should be considered if hyperopia is significant. Bifocals can be used for a high AC/A ratio. Unless deficient ductions suggest a slipped or lost muscle, a delay of several months is recommended before reoperation because spontaneous improvement is common. Following a bilateral lateral rectus muscle recession, a medial rectus muscle recession in 1 or both eyes can be performed, provided abduction is normal in both eyes. Unilateral lateral rectus muscle recession/medial rectus muscle resection surgery can be followed by medial rectus muscle recession/lateral rectus muscle resection surgery on the other eye. Botulinum toxin injection into 1 medial rectus muscle may be effective in the management of consecutive esotropia, particularly when fusion is present.

Raab EL, Parks MM. Recession of the lateral recti: early and late postoperative alignments. *Arch Ophthalmol.* 1969;82:203–208.

Management of surgical undercorrection

Mild to moderate residual exodeviation is often treated by observation alone if fusional control is good. However, manifest exotropia commonly returns in time. Therefore, some surgeons recommend aggressive base-in prism management for undercorrections, with a gradual weaning of the prism dosage. Postoperative patching and orthoptic treatment can also be applied. In small doses, botulinum toxin injection has also been used to treat surgical undercorrections, but supportive data are limited. Indications for reoperation in undercorrected patients are the same as for initial surgery. If lateral rectus muscle recessions have been performed bilaterally, a unilateral or bilateral medial rectus muscle resection may be chosen when reoperation is needed. Unilateral lateral rectus muscle recession/medial rectus muscle resection is often followed by a similar recess/resect procedure on the other eye. The surgical dose–response curve appears to be similar to that for the initial surgery. Therefore, the surgical dosage, for previously unoperated muscles, can often be selected as though the surgery were a primary operation.

Constant Exotropia

Constant exotropia is encountered more often in older patients manifesting sensory exotropia or decompensated intermittent exotropia.

Surgical treatment for constant exotropia consists of appropriate bilateral recessions of the lateral rectus muscles or unilateral lateral rectus recession combined with a medial rectus resection. In some cases, patients with an enlarged field of peripheral vision because of rapid alternation of fixation may notice a field constriction when the eyes are straight.

Congenital Exotropia

Congenital exotropia presents before age 6 months with a large-angle constant deviation. It is uncommon in otherwise healthy infants, and many children with congenital exotropia have associated neurologic impairment or craniofacial disorders (Fig 8-2). Patients with constant congenital exotropia are operated on early in life in the same manner as are patients with congenital esotropia. As with patients with congenital esotropia, early surgery can lead to gross binocular vision but perfect binocular function is rare. These patients also tend to develop dissociated vertical deviation and inferior oblique muscle overaction and should be followed closely for the development of these associated motility disturbances.

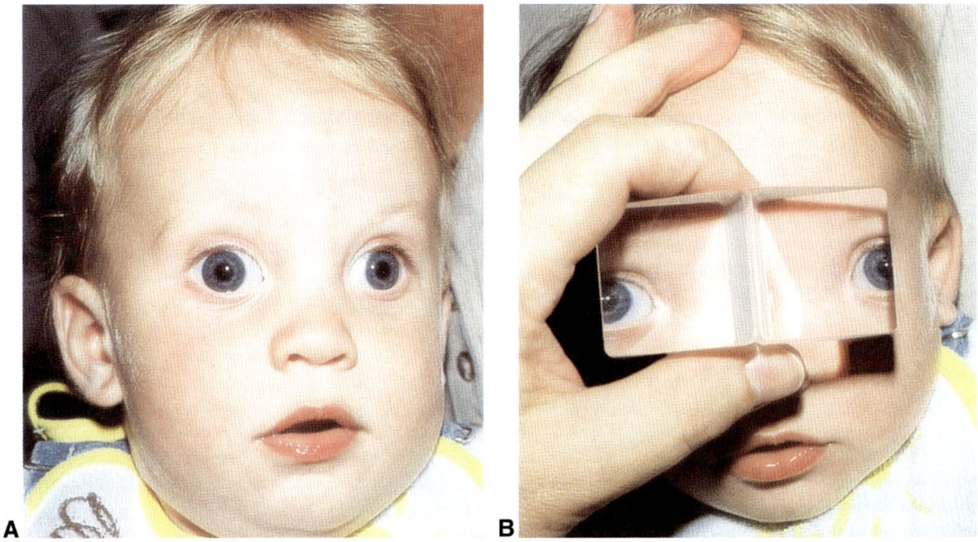

Figure 8-2 **A,** This 10-month-old infant with congenital exotropia also shows moderate motor developmental delay. **B,** Krimsky testing uses two 45Δ prisms placed base-to-base in the frontal plane to measure 90Δ of exotropia. *(Reproduced with permission from Wilson ME. Exotropia.* Focal Points: Clinical Modules for Ophthalmologists. *San Francisco: American Academy of Ophthalmology; 1995, module 11.)*

Hunter DG, Ellis FJ. Prevalence of systemic and ocular disease in infantile exotropia: comparison with infantile esotropia. *Ophthalmology.* 1999;106:1951–1956.

Sensory Exotropia

Any condition that reduces visual acuity in 1 eye can cause sensory exotropia. The causes include anisometropia, corneal or lens opacities, optic atrophy or hypoplasia, macular lesions, and amblyopia. It is not known why some persons become esotropic after unilateral visual loss and others become exotropic. Both sensory esotropia and sensory exotropia are common in children, but exotropia predominates in older children and adults.

If the eye with sensory exotropia can be visually rehabilitated, peripheral fusion may sometimes be reestablished after surgical realignment, provided the sensory exotropia has not been present for an extended period. Loss of fusional abilities, known as *central fusional disruption*, or *horror fusionis*, can lead to constant and permanent diplopia when adult-onset sensory exotropia has been present for several years prior to visual rehabilitation and realignment. In these patients, intractable diplopia may persist, even with well-aligned eyes.

Consecutive Exotropia

Consecutive exotropia is defined as exotropia that follows previous surgery for esotropia. Treatment of consecutive exotropia depends on many factors, including the size of the deviation, the type and amount of surgery that preceded its development, the presence of duction limitations, lateral incomitance, and the level of visual acuity in each eye. The planning of strabismus surgery is discussed in Chapter 13.

Exotropic Duane (Retraction) Syndrome

Duane syndrome can present with exotropia, usually accompanied by a face turn away from the affected eye. Adduction is most often markedly deficient; other signs include eyelid narrowing, globe retraction, and characteristic upshoots and downshoots. See Chapter 11 for further discussion of Duane syndrome.

Neuromuscular Abnormalities

A constant exotropia may result from third nerve palsy, internuclear ophthalmoplegia, or myasthenia gravis. These conditions are discussed in detail in BCSC Section 5, *Neuro-Ophthalmology*.

Dissociated Horizontal Deviation

Dissociated strabismus may contain vertical, horizontal, and torsional components. When the dissociated abduction movement is predominant, it is called *dissociated horizontal deviation*. Although not a true exotropia, dissociated horizontal deviation can be confused with a constant or intermittent exotropia. Dissociated vertical deviation and latent nystagmus often coexist with dissociated horizontal deviation (Fig 8-3). Treatment usually consists of unilateral or occasionally bilateral lateral rectus recession in addition to any necessary oblique or vertical muscle surgery.

Wilson ME, Hutchinson AK, Saunders RA. Outcomes from surgical treatment for dissociated horizontal deviation. *J AAPOS*. 2000;4:94–101.

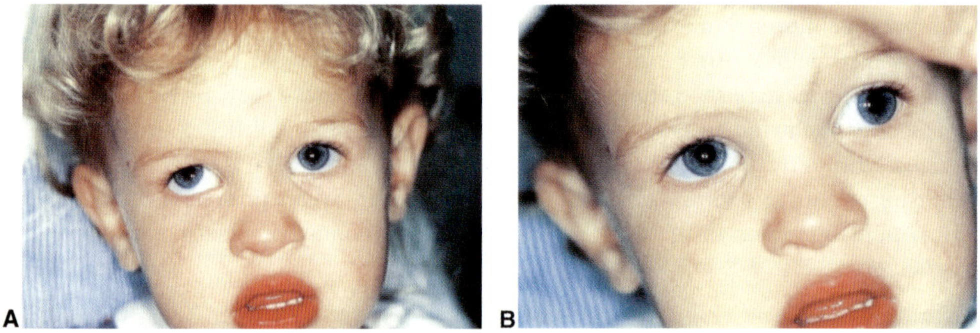

Figure 8-3 Dissociated strabismus complex. **A,** When the patient fixates with the left eye, a prominent dissociated vertical deviation is shown in the right eye. **B,** However, when the patient fixates with the right eye, a prominent dissociated horizontal deviation (DHD) is shown in the left eye. *(Reproduced with permission from Wilson ME. Exotropia.* Focal Points: Clinical Modules for Ophthalmologists. *San Francisco: American Academy of Ophthalmology; 1995, module 11.)*

Convergence Insufficiency

Characteristics of convergence insufficiency include asthenopia, blurred near vision, and reading problems in the presence of poor near fusional convergence amplitudes and a remote near point of convergence. The patient, typically an older child or adult, may have an exophoria at near but, by definition, should not have an exotropia. Rarely, accommodative spasms may occur if accommodation and convergence are stimulated in an effort to overcome the convergence insufficiency. Convergence insufficiency, as discussed here, should not be confused with the convergence insufficiency type of intermittent exotropia discussed previously.

Treatment of convergence insufficiency usually involves orthoptic exercises. Base-out prisms can be used to stimulate fusional convergence during reading. Stereograms, "pencil pushups," and other near point exercises are often used. If these exercises fail, base-in prism reading glasses may be needed. Medial rectus muscle resection, unilateral or bilateral, has been used in rare cases when nonsurgical treatments have been unsatisfactory, but this surgery carries a substantial risk of diplopia in distance viewing. Patients with combined convergence and accommodative insufficiency may benefit from plus lenses and base-in prisms for reading.

Choi DG, Rosenbaum AL. Medial rectus resection(s) with adjustable suture for intermittent exotropia of the convergence insufficiency type. *J AAPOS.* 2001;5:13–17.

Convergence Paralysis

Convergence paralysis, a condition distinct from convergence insufficiency and usually secondary to an intracranial lesion, is characterized by normal adduction and accommodation with exotropia and diplopia on attempted near fixation only. Convergence paralysis differs from convergence insufficiency in its relatively acute onset and the patient's inability to overcome any base-out prism. Convergence paralysis usually results from a lesion in the corpora quadrigemina or the nucleus of cranial nerve III and may be associated with Parinaud syndrome.

Treatment is limited to providing base-in prisms at near to alleviate the diplopia. Occasionally, accommodation also is weakened, particularly in a chronically ill patient, and plus lenses may also be required at near. These patients have little if any fusional vergence amplitudes at near, and it may not be possible to restore comfortable single binocular vision. Occlusion of one eye at near is indicated in such cases, and eye muscle surgery is contraindicated.

Kushner BJ. Exotropic deviations: a functional classification and approach to treatment. 18th Richard G. Scobee Memorial Lecture. *Am Orthopt J.* 1988;38:81–93.

CHAPTER 9

A- and V-Pattern Horizontal Strabismus

Some horizontal deviations change in magnitude in upgaze and downgaze. An A pattern is present when a horizontal deviation shows a more convergent (less divergent) alignment in upgaze compared with downgaze. V pattern describes a horizontal deviation that is more convergent (less divergent) in downgaze compared with upgaze. Other, less common variations of pattern horizontal strabismus that will not be discussed include Y, λ, and X patterns. An A or V pattern is found in 15%–25% of horizontal strabismus cases.

Each of the following conditions has been considered a cause of A and V patterns:

- *Bilateral oblique muscle dysfunction.* Inferior oblique muscle overaction is associated with V patterns (Figs 9-1, 9-2), and superior oblique muscle overaction is associated with A patterns (Figs 9-3, 9-4). These associations reflect the ancillary abducting action in upgaze and downgaze, respectively, of these muscles.
- *Horizontal rectus muscle dysfunction.* Increased lateral rectus muscle action in upgaze or increased medial rectus muscle action in downgaze produces a V pattern. Decreased horizontal rectus muscle action in these respective gazes produces an A pattern.
- *Vertical rectus muscle dysfunction.* For example, if the superior rectus muscles are underacting, their tertiary adducting effect in upgaze will decrease, resulting in a V pattern. Similarly, underaction of the inferior rectus muscle results in an A pattern.

Patients with upward- or downward-slanting palpebral fissures (Fig 9-5) may also show A and V patterns. In these cases, the pattern is most likely due to altered force vectors of the extraocular muscles; the alteration is caused by an underlying variation in orbital configuration, reflected in the orientation of the fissures.

Similarly, patients with Apert or Crouzon syndrome (see Chapter 28) frequently show a V-pattern exotropia or esotropia with marked elevation of the adducting eye, resembling the pattern caused by overacting inferior oblique muscles. The cause of this unusual motility disorder may be a combination of mechanical factors (eg, excyclorotation of the entire bony orbit) and structural abnormalities (eg, abnormal size, number,

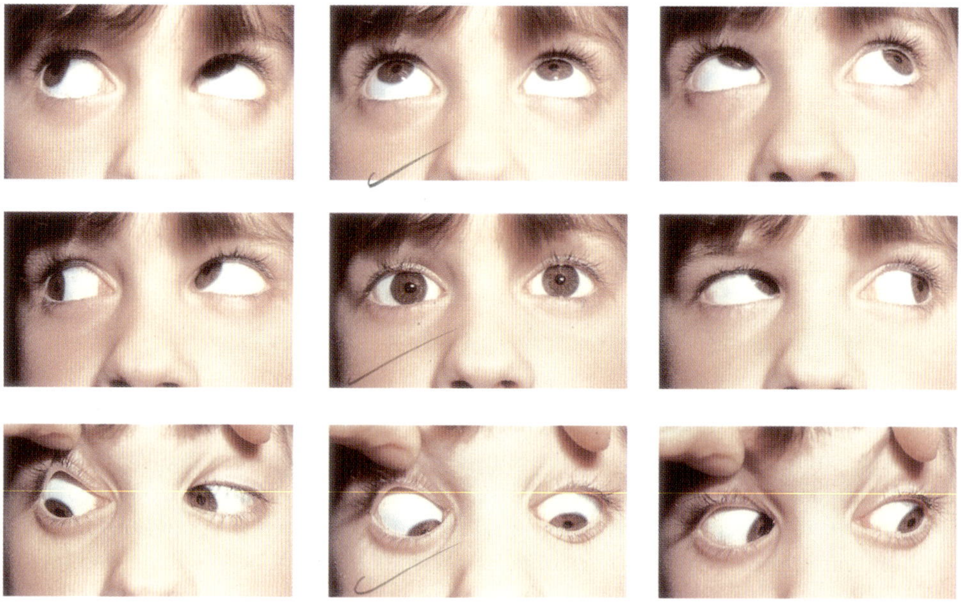

Figure 9-1 V-pattern esotropia. Note overelevation (overaction of the inferior oblique muscles) and limitation of depression (underaction of the superior oblique muscles) of each eye when in adduction.

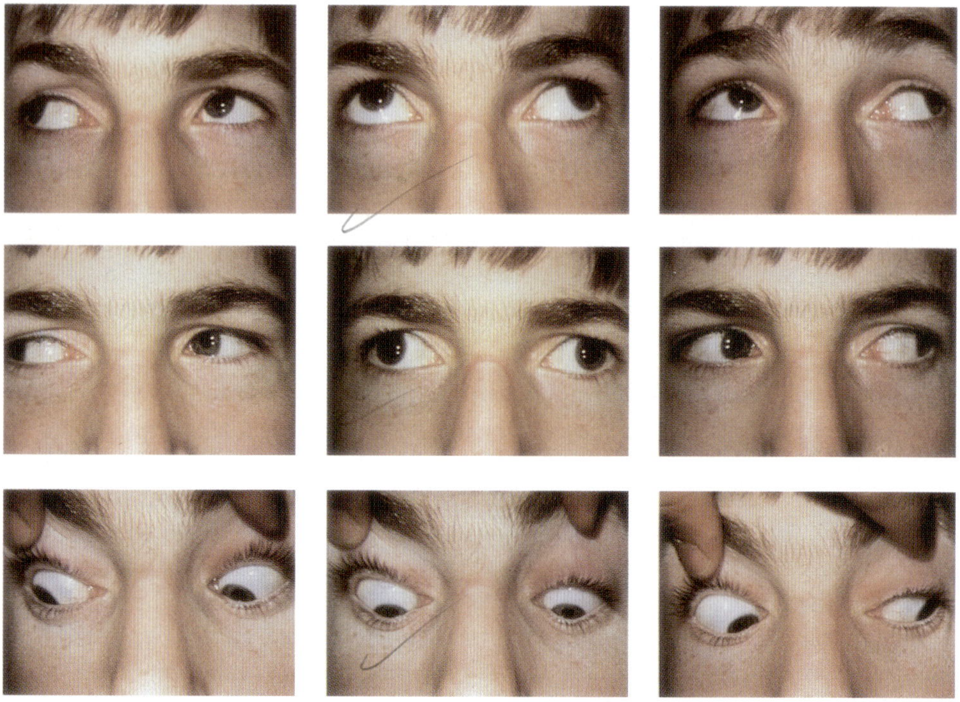

Figure 9-2 V-pattern exotropia with moderate overaction of the inferior oblique muscles OU. There is no apparent underaction of either superior oblique muscle.

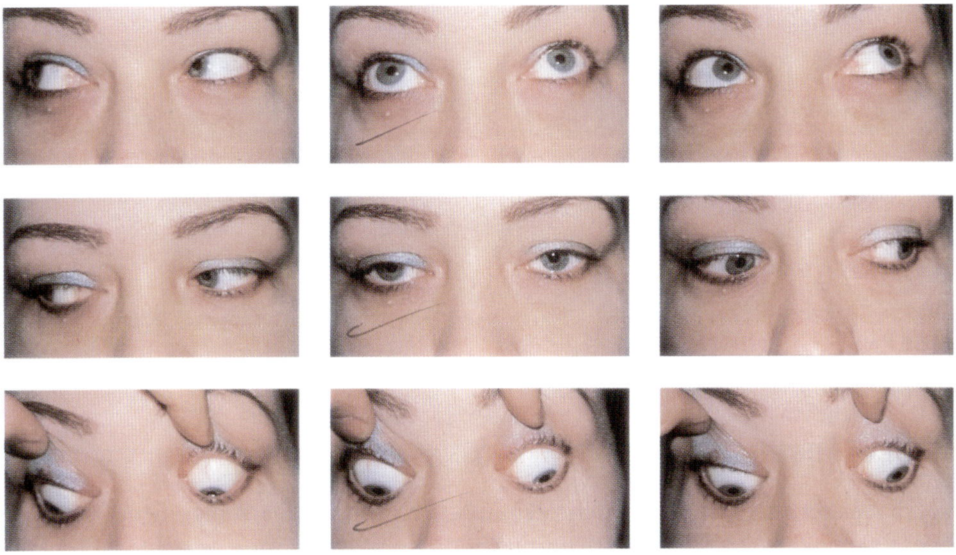

Figure 9-3 A-pattern exotropia with overaction of the superior oblique muscles and slight underaction of only the right inferior oblique muscle, with depression of the adducted right eye. Asymmetry of oblique muscle over- and underactions is not uncommon and usually is ignored in correcting A or V patterns when the discrepancy is minimal.

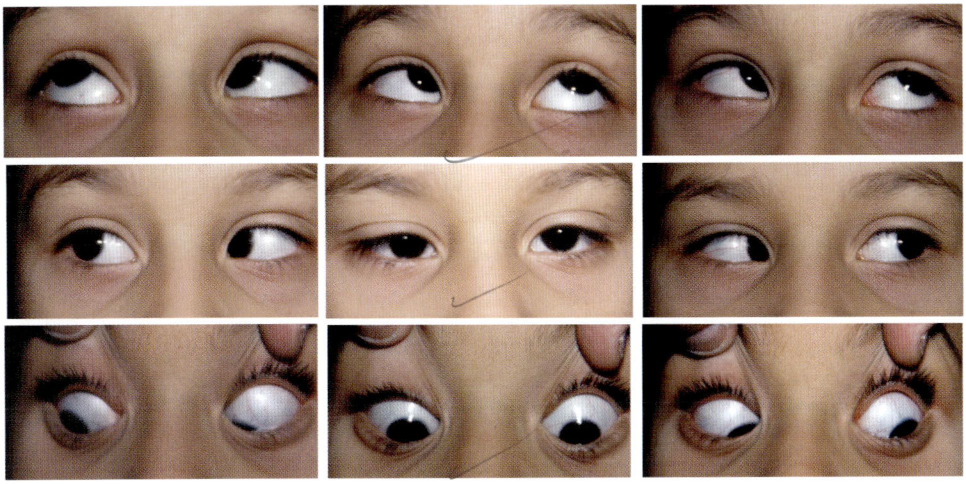

Figure 9-4 A-pattern esotropia with bilateral superior oblique muscle overaction and inferior oblique muscle underaction. *(Photographs courtesy of Edward L. Raab, MD.)*

or insertion of muscles). Surgical correction can be difficult. In addition, facial surgery for these conditions may produce a large ocular alignment shift, usually in an esotropic direction.

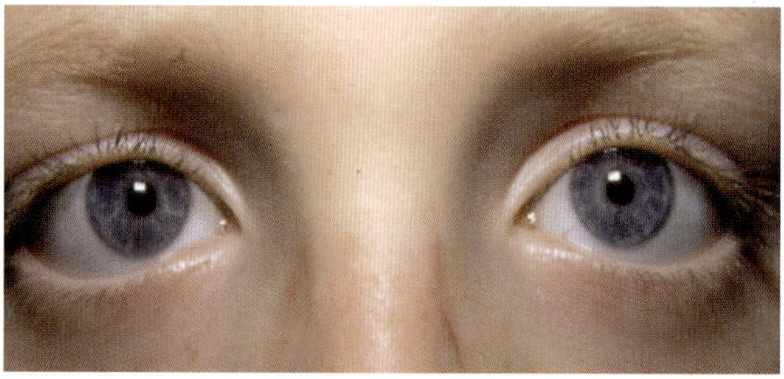

Figure 9-5 Downward slant of the palpebral fissures, often associated with a V-pattern horizontal deviation. *(Photograph courtesy of Edward L. Raab, MD.)*

Clinical Features

A and V patterns are determined by measurement of the patient's alignment while he or she is fixating on an accommodative target at distance, with fusion prevented. Proper refractive correction is necessary during measurement. Underactions and overactions of the oblique muscles are detected by study of the versions. Any compensatory head position (chin up or chin down) must be noted.

According to the traditional (and somewhat arbitrary) definition, an A pattern is considered clinically significant only when the difference in measurement between upgaze and downgaze, each approximately 25° from the primary position, is at least 10Δ. To be a clinically significant V pattern, the difference must be at least 15Δ. Accordingly, we encounter V-pattern esotropia, V-pattern exotropia, A-pattern esotropia, and A-pattern exotropia.

Management

Clinically significant patterns (defined earlier in the chapter) typically are treated surgically, most often in combination with correction of the underlying horizontal deviation. The following are guidelines for planning surgical correction of A- and V-pattern deviations:

- Primary and reading positions are functionally the most important positions of gaze.
- Appropriate surgery to eliminate the horizontal deviation in primary position should be independently selected.
- Patients with large A or V patterns usually also have significant corresponding oblique muscle dysfunction.
- Most surgeons use the presence or absence of significant oblique dysfunction to determine their surgical approach. If the pattern is related to overaction of the oblique muscles, these are weakened as part of the surgical plan. Weakening the inferior oblique muscles or tightening the superior oblique tendons corrects up to 15Δ–20Δ of V pattern.

- Bilateral superior oblique tenotomies correct up to 35Δ–45Δ of A pattern (ie, they produce 35Δ–45Δ of esotropic shift in downgaze).
- Displacing the horizontal rectus muscle insertions (see the following discussion) is indicated when there is no oblique dysfunction, but this is not an effective substitute for oblique muscle surgery when overaction is present.

When horizontal rectus muscles are vertically displaced to correct A- or V-pattern strabismus, the amount of displacement usually is one half to a full tendon width. The medial rectus muscles are always moved toward the direction of vertical gaze where *convergence is greater* or *divergence is less* (ie, upward in A patterns and downward in V patterns). The lateral rectus muscles are moved toward the direction of vertical gaze in which the *divergence is greater* or *convergence is less* (ie, upward in V patterns and downward in A patterns). These rules apply whether the horizontal recti are weakened or tightened.

When recession-resection surgery is indicated for an A pattern, displacement of the medial rectus muscle upward and the lateral rectus muscle downward has no net vertical or torsional effect in the primary position, but in upgaze the medial rectus muscle will be relaxed and the lateral rectus muscle tightened, thereby decreasing the A pattern. Similarly, for V patterns, the medial rectus muscle is displaced downward and the lateral rectus muscle upward. In downgaze, the medial rectus muscle will be relaxed and the lateral rectus muscle will be tightened, thereby decreasing the V pattern without a vertical or torsional effect.

A useful mnemonic for these procedures is MALE: *m*edial rectus muscles to the *a*pex of the pattern, *l*ateral rectus muscles to the *e*mpty space (Fig 9-6). For more precise consideration of the applicable mechanics, observe that the muscle is moved in the direction in which the muscle's horizontal effect is to be least (eg, medial rectus muscles downward for a V pattern).

Some surgeons vertically displace the tendon without keeping its reattachment parallel to the limbal tangent; this increases the effect on the pattern. Others have described a procedure in which, instead of displacing the reattached horizontal rectus muscles, one corner (upper or lower) of the insertion is placed farther from the limbus than the other

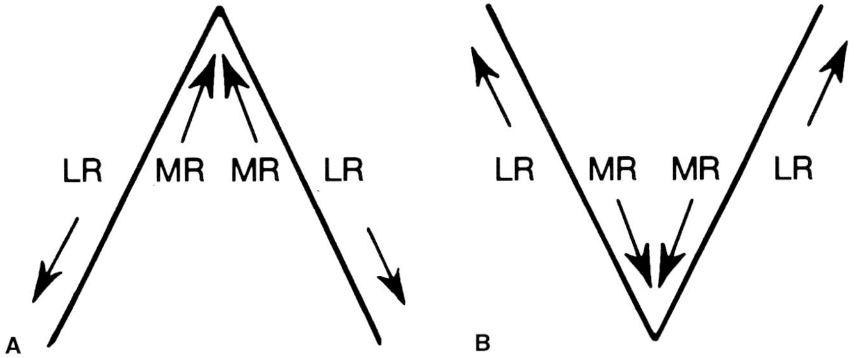

Figure 9-6 Direction of displacement of medial rectus (MR) and lateral rectus (LR) muscles in operations to treat A-pattern deviations **(A)** and V-pattern deviations **(B)**. *(Reprinted from von Noorden GK.* Binocular Vision and Ocular Motility*. 5th ed. St Louis: Mosby; 1996:388.)*

(slanted insertion), giving an effect similar to that of displacement in the direction of the farther corner.

Ohba M, Nakagawa T. Treatment for "A" and "V" exotropia by slanting muscle insertions. *Jpn J Ophthalmol.* 2000;44:433–438.

When A- and V-pattern horizontal strabismus was initially described, anomalous function of the vertical rectus muscles was proposed as a possible causative factor, to be remedied by shifting the muscles' insertions (eg, temporal displacement of the superior rectus muscles for A-pattern esotropia, temporal displacement of the inferior rectus muscles for V-pattern esotropia). Although such procedures are theoretically appealing, especially when the oblique muscles are not found to be dysfunctional, they are rarely used because the horizontal rectus muscle operations required for the underlying eso- or exotropia can correct the pattern when appropriate displacements of the latter muscles are utilized.

Sample Treatment Plans for the Various Patterns

V-Pattern Esotropia

If inferior oblique muscle overaction is present, the inferior oblique muscles should be weakened, and the deviation in primary position should be corrected with the appropriate horizontal rectus muscle procedure. This procedure has a negligible effect on primary position alignment (see Chapter 10). If inferior oblique muscle overaction is not present, the preferred choices are bilateral medial rectus muscle recession with downward displacement, bilateral resection of the lateral rectus muscles with upward displacement, or a recession-resection operation moving the medial rectus muscle downward and the lateral rectus muscle upward, depending on other pertinent factors in the case (eg, prior surgery, unimprovable vision in 1 eye).

Caldeira JA. V-pattern esotropia: a review; and a study of the outcome after bilateral recession of the inferior oblique muscle: a retrospective study of 78 consecutive patients. *Binocul Vis Strabismus Q.* 2003;18:35–48.

V-Pattern Exotropia

The same scheme as is used for V-pattern esotropia should be followed for V-pattern exotropia, except that the opposite horizontal deviation is present and horizontal surgery is chosen accordingly.

Caldeira JA. Some clinical characteristics of V-pattern exotropia and surgical outcome after bilateral recession of the inferior oblique muscle: a retrospective study of 22 consecutive patients and a comparison with V-pattern esotropia. *Binocul Vis Strabismus Q.* 2004;19:139–150.

A-Pattern Esotropia

If superior oblique muscle overaction is present (more likely in exotropia than in esotropia), these muscles can be weakened by bilateral tenotomies or tendon-lengthening procedures. Weakening of superior oblique muscle action can correct up to 35Δ–45Δ of excess divergence in downgaze, if present. There is a risk of induced torsional imbalance, especially in patients with fusion capacity. An alternative treatment, with or without superior oblique muscle overaction, is horizontal rectus muscle surgery with the appropriate displacement.

The effect of bilateral superior oblique muscle weakening on primary position horizontal alignment remains somewhat controversial. Some surgeons think the loss of abducting force after bilateral superior oblique muscle weakening increases convergence in primary position by 10Δ–15Δ. These surgeons suggest adjusting horizontal surgery to compensate for this expected change. Other surgeons think superior oblique tenotomy or other weakening procedures have no significant effect on primary position alignment, and thus no adjustment of horizontal surgery is warranted. Because the amount of horizontal rectus surgery required is difficult to predict when superior oblique tenotomies are completed, adjustable sutures on the horizontal muscles may be helpful in a suitable patient.

Biglan AW. Pattern strabismus. In: Rosenbaum AL, Santiago AP, eds. *Clinical Strabismus Management: Principles and Surgical Techniques*. Philadelphia: Saunders; 1999:202–215.

von Noorden GK. *Binocular Vision and Ocular Motility: Theory and Management of Strabismus*. 6th ed. St Louis: Mosby; 2002.

A-Pattern Exotropia

The appropriate plan, depending on whether the superior oblique muscles are overacting, can be inferred by extension of the schemes outlined in the previous section.

CHAPTER 10

Vertical Deviations

A vertical deviation (vertical misalignment of the visual axes) may be comitant or incomitant (noncomitant). Either form of vertical deviation can occur alone or be associated with a horizontal deviation. Such an association is the more typical setting for comitant vertical deviations, which usually are small.

The majority of vertical deviations are incomitant. They are associated with so-called dysfunctional overactions or underactions of the superior and inferior oblique muscles, paralysis (paresis or palsy) or contracture of one or more of these cyclovertical muscles, or restriction of vertical movement. Although nearly every vertical paralytic deviation is incomitant at onset, it may with time approach comitance unless there are associated restrictions, as might occur with an orbital blowout fracture or thyroid-associated orbitopathy.

A vertical deviation is described according to the direction of the vertically deviating nonfixating eye. If the right eye is higher than the left and the left eye is fixating, this is called a *right hypertropia.* If the nonfixating right eye is lower than the fixating left eye, this is called a *right hypotropia.* If the ability to alternately fixate is present, the deviation is named for the usually hyperdeviating eye in ordinary visual circumstances (ie, not during cover testing).

The following references are excellent sources of in-depth information on the entities discussed in this chapter, as well as on other topics in strabismus:

Rosenbaum AL, Santiago AP. *Clinical Strabismus Management: Principles and Surgical Techniques.* Philadelphia: Saunders; 1999.

Spector RH. Vertical diplopia. *Surv Ophthalmol.* 1993;38:31–62.

von Noorden GK, Campos EC. *Binocular Vision and Ocular Motility: Theory and Management of Strabismus.* 6th ed. St Louis: Mosby; 2002.

Inferior Oblique Muscle Overaction

Overaction of the inferior oblique muscle is termed *primary* when it is not associated with superior oblique muscle paralysis. It is called *secondary* when it accompanies paresis or palsy of its antagonist superior oblique muscle or yoke inferior rectus muscle.

The cause of primary overaction is not well understood. One explanation involves vestibular influences governing postural tonus of the extraocular muscles. Some observers have questioned the concept of a true inferior oblique overaction, preferring to describe the movement as *overelevation in adduction*. Magnetic resonance imaging (MRI) studies have demonstrated a connective tissue pulley where the inferior oblique muscle's path crosses that of the inferior rectus muscle, the latter also having a pulley. This arrangement is said to lead to a dynamic interaction of these structures during vertical rotation that could give the appearance of overaction.

Demer JL, Oh SY, Clark RA, et al. Evidence for a pulley of the inferior oblique muscle. *Invest Ophthalmol Vis Sci.* 2003;44:3856–3865.

Stager DR. Costenbader Lecture. Anatomy and surgery of the inferior oblique muscle: recent findings. *J AAPOS.* 2001;5:203–208.

Clinical Features

Primary inferior oblique muscle overaction has been reported to develop between ages 1 and 6 years in up to two thirds of patients with congenital esotropia. The entity also occurs, less frequently, in association with acquired esotropia or exotropia and occasionally in patients with no other form of strabismus. A bilateral overaction can be asymmetric, because of either different times of onset or different degrees of severity.

In adduction, the eye is elevated; this is apparent with the eyes in lateral gaze and the abducting eye fixating, as well as with the eyes in lateral upgaze (Fig 10-1). Alternate cover testing under these conditions shows that the higher eye refixates with a downward movement and that the lower eye does so with an upward movement. When inferior oblique overaction is bilateral, the higher and lower eyes reverse in the opposite lateral gaze. These features differentiate inferior oblique overaction from dissociated vertical deviation (DVD; see the discussion later in the chapter), in which neither eye refixates with an upward movement whether adducted, abducted, or in primary position. In addition, a V-pattern horizontal deviation is common with overacting inferior oblique muscles but not with DVD.

Management

In all but the mildest cases, a weakening procedure on the inferior oblique muscle (recession, disinsertion, myectomy, or anterior transposition) is indicated (see also Chapter 13). Structural variations in this muscle or its path may affect the surgical result. Weakening the inferior oblique muscles has an insignificant effect on primary position horizontal alignment. An associated horizontal deviation requiring surgical correction is treated at the same operative session.

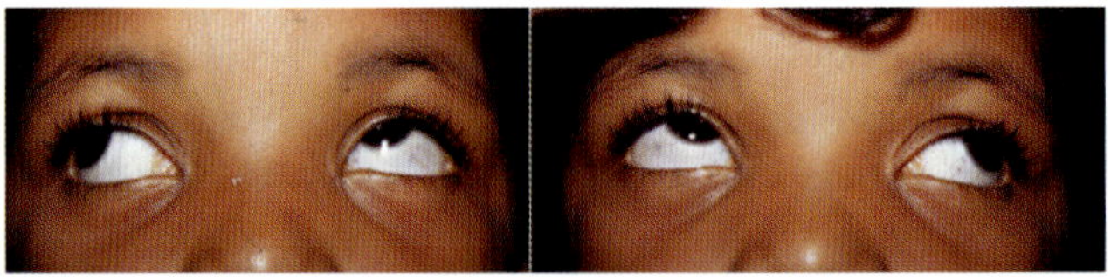

Figure 10-1 Bilateral inferior oblique overaction. Overelevation in adduction, seen best in the upper fields. *(Photographs courtesy of Edward L. Raab, MD.)*

Anterior transposition is another effective weakening procedure that can correct marked overaction of the inferior oblique muscles and DVD, particularly when both are present simultaneously. Excessive excyclotorsion due to the overaction can also be improved by this procedure. Actual results vary according to the new location of the anterior and posterior fibers of the reinserted inferior oblique muscle. Caution is advisable because excessively anterior and spread-out reattachment can restrict elevation, especially when the eye is abducted (anti-elevation syndrome).

De Angelis D, Makar I, Kraft SP. Anatomic variations of the inferior oblique muscle: a potential cause of failed inferior oblique weakening surgery. *Am J Ophthalmol.* 1999;128:485–488.

Elliott RL, Nankin SJ. Anterior transposition of the inferior oblique. *J Pediatr Ophthalmol Strabismus.* 1981;18:35–38.

Santiago AP, Isenberg SJ, Apt L, et al. The effect of anterior transposition of the inferior oblique muscle on ocular torsion. *J AAPOS.* 1997;1:191–196.

Superior Oblique Muscle Overaction

For clinical purposes, and unlike with inferior oblique muscle overaction, almost all cases of bilateral superior oblique muscle overaction can be considered primary, because paralysis of the inferior rectus and inferior oblique muscles is uncommon.

Clinical Features

A vertical deviation in primary position often occurs with unilateral or asymmetric bilateral overaction of the superior oblique muscles. The lower eye contains the unilaterally, or more prominent bilaterally, overacting superior oblique muscle. An associated horizontal deviation, most often exotropia, may be present. The overacting superior oblique muscle also causes depression, with resulting hypotropia of the adducting eye in lateral gaze, which is accentuated in lateral downgaze (Fig 10-2). An alternative term for this finding is *overdepression in adduction.*

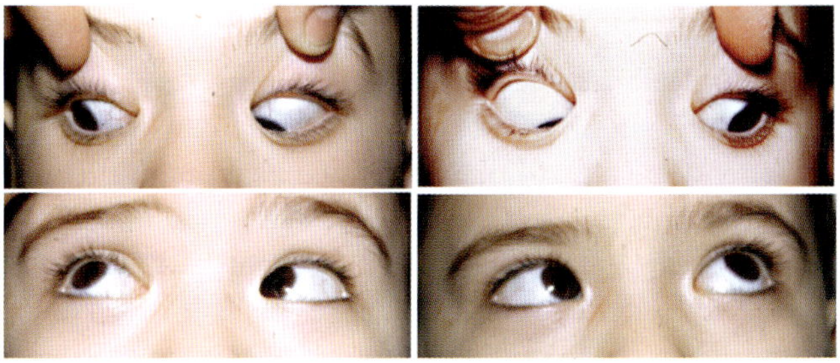

Figure 10-2 Top row, Bilateral superior oblique overaction. Overdepression in adduction, seen best in the lower fields. **Bottom row,** Associated bilateral inferior oblique underaction. *(Photographs courtesy of Edward L. Raab, MD.)*

Management

In a patient with a clinically significant hyper- or hypotropia or an A pattern, a bilateral superior oblique tendon–weakening procedure (recession, tenotomy, tenectomy, or lengthening by insertion of a silicone expander or nonabsorbable suture or by Z-splitting) may be indicated (see also Chapter 13). However, many surgeons are reluctant to perform superior oblique weakening in patients with normal stereopsis, in whom the resulting sometimes asymmetric torsional and/or vertical effects can cause diplopia or secondary superior oblique palsy with a head tilt. As with inferior oblique muscle overaction, the associated horizontal deviation is corrected at the same operative session. Some surgeons, anticipating a convergent effect, adjust their surgical amounts for horizontal rectus muscles modestly when simultaneously weakening the superior oblique muscles.

Bardorf CM, Baker JD. The efficacy of superior oblique split Z-tendon lengthening for superior oblique overaction. *J AAPOS.* 2003;7:96–102.

Lee SY, Rosenbaum AL. Surgical results in patients with A-pattern horizontal strabismus. *J AAPOS.* 2003;7:251–255.

Dissociated Vertical Deviation

Dissociated vertical deviation (DVD) is a common innervational disorder, found in 50%–90% of patients with congenital esotropia and in other forms of strabismus. The cause is unknown, but DVD appears to be associated with early disruption of binocular development. Recent work has suggested that DVD may be the result of compensating mechanisms for latent nystagmus, with the oblique muscles having the principal role.

Brodsky MC. Dissociated vertical divergence: a righting reflex gone wrong. *Arch Ophthalmol.* 1999;117:1216–1222.

Brodsky MC. DVD remains a moving target. *J AAPOS* [editorial]. 1999;3:325–327.

Guyton DL. Costenbader Lecture. Dissociated vertical deviation: etiology, mechanism, and associated phenomena. *J AAPOS.* 2000;4:131–134.

Clinical Features

DVD usually presents after age 2 years, whether or not the horizontal deviation it accompanies has been surgically corrected. Either eye may spontaneously and slowly drift upward and outward, with simultaneous extorsion, when an eye is occluded or during periods of visual inattention (Fig 10-3). Some patients attempt to compensate by tilting the head, for reasons that still have not been conclusively identified.

As the vertically deviated eye moves down (and intorts) to fixate when the previously fixating fellow eye is occluded, the latter makes no downward movement. Note that with true hypertropia, when the hypertropic eye refixates, the occluded fellow eye moves downward into a hypotropic position of equal magnitude. In contrast, as noted, eyes with DVD have no corresponding hypotropia of the fellow eye when the hypertropic eye refixates. In this respect, Hering's law of equal innervation appears not to apply to DVD.

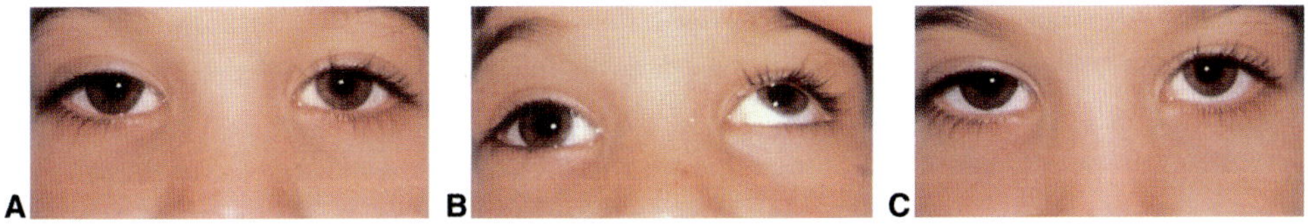

Figure 10-3 Dissociated vertical deviation, left eye. **A,** Straight eyes when binocular vision allowed. **B,** Large left hyperdeviation immediately after the eye is uncovered. **C,** Left eye drifts back down toward horizontal.

The vertical movement usually predominates, but sometimes the principal dissociated movement is one of abduction *(dissociated horizontal deviation).*

The condition is usually bilateral although frequently asymmetric. DVD may occur spontaneously (manifest DVD) or only when 1 eye is occluded (latent DVD). In addition to dissociated horizontal deviation, latent nystagmus (see Chapter 12) and horizontal strabismus are often associated with DVD. A prior history of congenital esotropia is particularly common. A coexisting vertical deviation subject to Hering's law can also occur.

Santiago AP, Rosenbaum AL. Dissociated vertical deviation and head tilts. *J AAPOS.* 1998;2: 5–11.

Measurement of DVD is difficult and imprecise. One method uses base-down prism in front of the upwardly deviating eye while it is behind an occluder. The occluder is then switched to the fixating lower eye. The base-down prism power is adjusted until the deviating eye shows no downward movement to refixate. Results are similar when a red Maddox rod is used to generate a horizontal stripe viewed by the dissociated higher eye while the other eye fixates on a small light; vertical prism power is used to eliminate the separation of the light and the line. Each eye is tested separately in cases of bilateral DVD.

Another method, using a modified form of the Krimsky test, is particularly useful in evaluating patients who cannot fixate with the deviating eye. The deviation can also simply be graded on a 1+ (least) to 4+ (most) scale. The earlier discussion of inferior oblique muscle overaction describes the features that distinguish that condition from DVD.

Management

Treatment for DVD is indicated if the vertical deviation occurs spontaneously, is frequent, and is cosmetically significant. Changing the fixation preference by patching or by penalization is effective mostly in unilateral or highly asymmetric bilateral DVD. Surgical treatment often improves the condition but rarely eliminates it. Distinguishing DVD from overaction of the inferior oblique muscles is important because the surgical approaches to these 2 conditions are different in most cases, although inferior oblique muscle anterior transposition can be suitable in either entity (see also Chapter 13).

Engman JH, Egbert JE, Summers CG, et al. Efficacy of inferior oblique anterior transposition placement grading for dissociated vertical deviation. *Ophthalmology.* 2001;108:2045–2050.

Quinn AG, Kraft SP, Day C, et al. A prospective evaluation of anterior transposition of the inferior oblique muscle, with and without resection, in the treatment of dissociated vertical deviation. *J AAPOS.* 2000;4:348–353.

Superior Oblique Muscle Paralysis (Palsy or Paresis)

The most common single cyclovertical muscle paralysis encountered by the ophthalmologist is the fourth cranial (trochlear) nerve palsy, involving the superior oblique muscle. It can be congenital or acquired, the latter usually as a result of closed head trauma or, less commonly, central nervous system vascular problems, diabetes, or brain tumors. The same clinical features can result from a congenitally lax, attenuated, or even absent superior oblique tendon, a developmental rather than a neurologic feature, or from unusual pathways of the muscle or functional consequences of orbital pulleys. Superior oblique muscle underaction can also occur in several craniofacial abnormalities (see Chapter 28).

Kono R, Demer JL. Magnetic resonance imaging of the functional anatomy of the inferior oblique muscle in superior oblique palsy. *Ophthalmology.* 2003;110:1219–1229.

To differentiate congenital from acquired superior oblique muscle palsy, it is helpful to examine old family photographs to detect a compensatory head tilt extending back to childhood. Facial asymmetry from long-standing head tilting and large vertical fusional amplitudes also indicate chronicity. Congenital cases are usually unilateral, and acquired cases are more often bilateral. The distinction is important because acquired palsies that cannot be reasonably attributed to known instances of trauma suggest the possibility of serious intracranial lesions and the need for often extensive neurologic investigation.

Markedly asymmetric bilateral palsies that initially appear to be unilateral have prompted the term *masked bilateral.* Direct trauma to the tendon or the trochlear area is an unusual cause of unilateral superior oblique muscle palsy.

Clinical Features

Examination of versions usually reveals underaction of the involved superior oblique muscle and overaction of its antagonist inferior oblique muscle. The diagnosis of superior oblique muscle palsy is supported by results of the 3-step determination and double Maddox rod testing (see Chapter 6) to measure torsional imbalance. However, 3-step test results can be abnormal in some cases of DVD or entities involving restriction and therefore can be misleading. Furthermore, some cases of skew deviation show results on the 3-step test that mimic a superior oblique muscle palsy. Intorsion—instead of the expected extorsion—determined by double Maddox rod testing and by ophthalmoscopy, identifies such cases, especially when there are associated neurologic findings.

Assessment of the ocular deviation in the diagnostic gaze positions, as well as with right and left head tilt, is important in diagnosing and planning treatment for superior oblique muscle palsy (Fig 10-4). Some ophthalmologists document serial changes in the deviation by means of the Hess screen or Lancaster red-green test, or plot the field of binocular single vision, to follow patients with superior oblique muscle palsy (see Chapter 6).

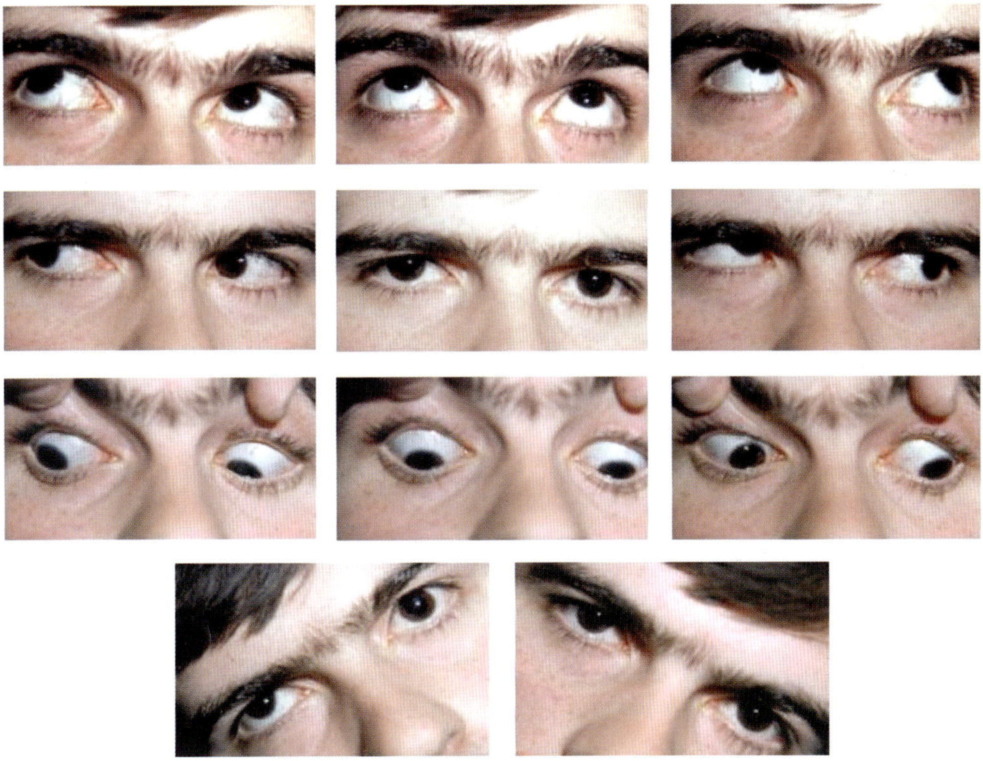

Figure 10-4 Right superior oblique palsy. There is a right hypertropia in primary position that increases on left gaze and with head tilted to the right. Note accompanying overaction of the right inferior oblique muscle. *(Photographs courtesy of Edward L. Raab, MD.)*

The possibility of bilateral paralysis should always be considered. To differentiate bilateral from unilateral superior oblique muscle paresis or palsy, the following criteria are used:

- *Unilateral cases* usually show little if any V pattern (see Chapter 9) and less than 5° of excyclotorsion. The patient may present with hypertropia in primary position. The 3-step test yields positive results for the involved side only. The action of the superior oblique muscle may appear normal or diminished. Either the normal or the affected eye can be preferred for fixation. Abnormal head positions are common, usually a head tilt toward the shoulder opposite the side of the weakness. Amblyopia is uncommon in acquired palsies but may be present in congenital ones. A complaint of apparent tilting of objects is common in acquired bilateral cases.
- *Bilateral cases* usually show a V pattern. Excyclotorsion usually is at least 5° and is highly diagnostic when 10° or more. The Bielschowsky head-tilt test (see Chapter 6) yields positive results on tilt to each side—that is, right head tilt shows a right hypertropia and left head tilt a left hypertropia. The ductions attributable to both superior oblique muscles usually are diminished. Signs of bilaterality in cases initially thought to be unilateral include bilateral objective fundus excyclotorsion,

esotropia in downgaze, and even the mildest degree of inferior oblique overaction (see earlier in the chapter) on the presumed uninvolved side.

Management

Indications for treatment are abnormal head position, significant vertical deviation, diplopia, or asthenopia. Surgery is indicated in most cases. Prisms may be used to overcome diplopia in small, symptomatic, nearly comitant deviations that lack a prominent torsional component. Common operative strategies are discussed in the following sections and in Chapter 13.

Unilateral superior oblique paralysis

The first approach to *unilateral superior oblique paralysis* is usually weakening of the antagonist inferior oblique muscle when it is overacting and the deviation in primary position is no greater than 15Δ. The amount of deviation in primary position that is corrected by any weakening technique is proportional to the degree of overaction of the inferior oblique muscle. Correcting mild overaction may yield only 5Δ–8Δ of primary gaze vertical correction. Weakening a moderate to severely overacting muscle often can achieve 10Δ–15Δ of correction. It is important to determine that the case is not one of skew deviation, as inferior oblique muscle weakening would aggravate the incyclotorsion of the higher eye. In the minority of cases in which the antagonist inferior oblique muscle does not appear to be overacting, most ophthalmologists nevertheless consider inferior oblique muscle weakening to be a reasonable choice.

If the deviation is greater than 15Δ, one should consider adding a second muscle to the procedure. The usually favored choices are recession of the contralateral (yoke) inferior rectus muscle, which has the additional advantage of facilitating use of an adjustable suture, or tucking the tendon of the weak superior oblique muscle if it is significantly lax. As a basic guideline, each millimeter of recession of a vertical rectus muscle results in approximately 3Δ of vertical correction. The ability to determine the quantity of tuck for a superior oblique tendon comes with experience. The goal is to tuck the tendon until forced ductions of both superior oblique muscles are comparable. Excessive tucking risks the possibility of Brown syndrome (see Chapter 11).

The surgical plan should include recession of the ipsilateral superior rectus muscle if a forced duction test shows limited depression on the side of the hypertropia. This finding is more common in long-standing superior oblique palsy, due to ipsilateral superior rectus muscle contracture. For example, with right superior oblique muscle weakness, the hypertropia is usually greatest in left gaze. In cases with contracture of the ipsilateral superior rectus muscle, the deficient depression and the deviation in right gaze are more like those of the deviation in primary position and left gaze, a so-called *spread of comitance.* On version testing, Hering's law may cause this to appear to represent superior oblique muscle overaction in the normal left eye. If the surgeon is misled and performs superior oblique tenotomy on the normal eye, thereby converting a unilateral superior oblique palsy to a bilateral one, disabling torsional diplopia can result.

In the unusually severe case with a vertical deviation greater than 35Δ in primary position, 3-muscle surgery usually is required. In this situation, most surgeons would favor recession of the overacting antagonist inferior oblique muscle, superior oblique tendon tuck, and either ipsilateral superior rectus recession or contralateral inferior rectus recession, as dictated by forced duction test results.

Whatever the approach, it is important to avoid overcorrection of a long-standing unilateral superior oblique muscle paralysis in an adult patient: overcorrection will be aggravated with time and often causes disabling diplopia resembling the original problem.

Bilateral superior oblique paralysis

In the case of *bilateral superior oblique paralysis,* surgery is performed on both eyes, graded for unequal severity if necessary. Bilateral inferior oblique muscle weakening is appropriate but may not be completely effective. Other options, as for unilateral palsy, are inferior rectus muscle recession, tucking of the superior oblique tendon, and the Harada-Ito procedure.

As noted earlier, inferior rectus muscle recession can be adjusted and is easily graded; care is required to avoid postoperative recession of the lower eyelid margin. The Harada-Ito procedure is preferred in bilateral cases with predominantly torsional complaints. This operation involves anterior and temporal displacement of the anterior portions of the superior oblique tendons to a location adjacent to the upper edge of the lateral rectus muscle, about 8 mm posterior to that muscle's insertion. The procedure, which can be done with adjustable sutures, corrects the deficient intorsion but not the vertical deviation in primary position. The effect tends to lessen with time.

Helveston EM, Mora JS, Lipsky SN, et al. Surgical treatment of superior oblique palsy. *Trans Am Ophthalmol Soc.* 1996;94:315–334.

Nishimura JK, Rosenbaum AL. The long-term effect of the adjustable Harada-Ito procedure. *J AAPOS.* 2002;6:141–144.

Siatkowski RM. Third, fourth, and sixth nerve palsies. *Focal Points: Clinical Modules for Ophthalmologists.* San Francisco: American Academy of Ophthalmology; 1996, module 8.

Brown Syndrome

Although included in most listings of vertical deviations, Brown syndrome is best considered as a special form of strabismus; it is discussed in Chapter 11.

Inferior Oblique Muscle Palsy

Damage to the inferior division of cranial nerve III and especially to the branch that supplies the inferior oblique muscle has been proposed as the cause of inferior oblique muscle palsy. However, it is difficult to understand how such a lesion might occur; thus, whether this rare condition actually exists is controversial. It has been suggested recently that at least some cases, especially those with an associated history of head trauma or with additional neurologic findings, are a form of skew deviation. The descriptive term *underelevation in adduction* may be preferable.

Clinical Features

As with Brown syndrome (see Chapter 11), elevation is deficient in the adducted position of the eye. Forced ductions are free when the adducted eye is elevated. An A pattern and overaction of the ipsilateral superior oblique muscle are usually present (Table 10-1).

Even if the diagnosis of inferior oblique muscle palsy is supported by findings of the 3-step test (Fig 10-5), the same results have been observed in some cases thought to represent skew deviation. In inferior oblique muscle palsy, the hypotropic eye should be incyclotorted; in skew deviation, the hypotropic eye is seen to be excyclotorted, a finding incompatible with the former diagnosis. These phenomena are analogous to those described for superior oblique palsy (see earlier in this chapter). When the 3-step results are not clear, such cases may represent asymmetric or unilateral primary superior oblique muscle overaction with secondary underaction of the inferior oblique muscle.

Donahue SP, Lavin PJM, Mohney B, et al. Skew deviation and inferior oblique palsy. *Am J Ophthalmol.* 2001;132:751–756.

Management

Indications for treatment of "true" inferior oblique muscle palsy are abnormal head position, vertical deviation in primary gaze, and diplopia. Management consists of either ipsilateral superior oblique muscle weakening or contralateral superior rectus muscle recession. The former procedure will aggravate the excyclotorsion of the hypotropic eye that is already present if skew deviation is the underlying cause.

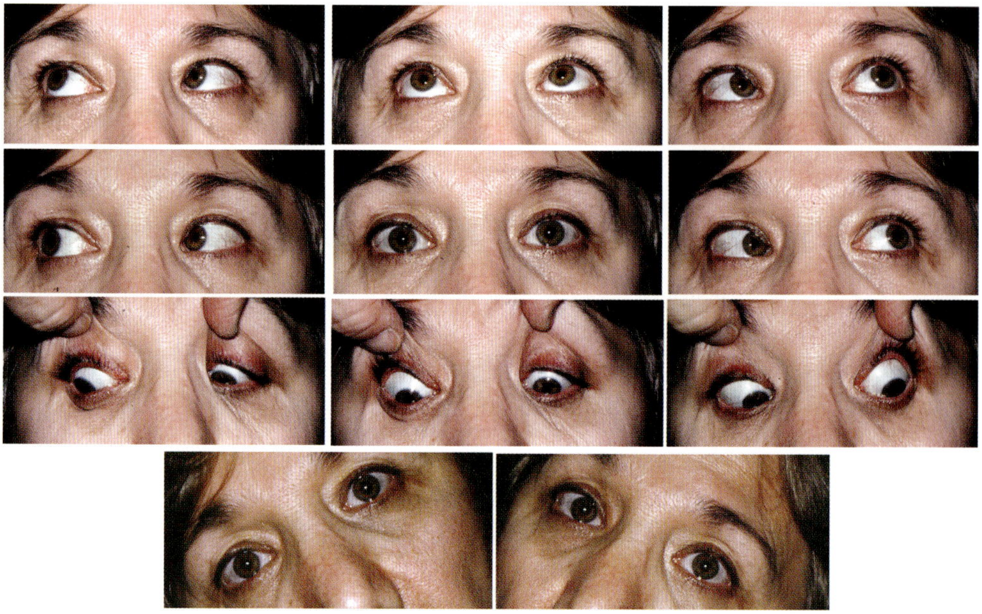

Figure 10-5 Right inferior oblique muscle palsy. Small left hypertropia in primary position, increasing in left gaze and in left head tilt. This patient had no abnormal neurologic findings. Note convergence in straight upgaze, a point of differentiation from Brown syndrome. *(Photographs courtesy of Edward L. Raab, MD.)*

Table 10-1 Comparison of Inferior Oblique Muscle Palsy With Brown Syndrome

	Inferior Oblique Muscle Palsy	Brown Syndrome
Forced ductions	Negative	Positive
Strabismus pattern	A pattern	V pattern
Superior oblique muscle overaction	Usually present	None or minimal

Monocular Elevation Deficiency (Double Elevator Palsy)

The term *double elevator palsy* implies a paralysis of the inferior oblique and superior rectus muscles of the same eye. However, *double elevator palsy* has become an umbrella term for any strabismus manifesting deficient elevation in all horizontal orientations of the eye. Because this motility pattern is well known to be caused by inferior rectus muscle restriction as well as by weakness of one or both elevator muscles, "double elevator muscle palsy" is a misnomer and has been replaced by *monocular elevation deficiency.*

Clinical Features

Monocular elevation deficiency is characterized by limitation of elevation in adduction as well as in abduction and in straight upgaze. There is hypotropia of the involved eye that increases in upgaze, a chin-up position with fusion in downgaze, and ptosis or pseudoptosis (Fig 10-6). An element of true ptosis is present in 50% of patients, some with the Marcus Gunn jaw-winking phenomenon.

Three types of monocular elevation deficiency are found:

1. with inferior rectus restriction
    - positive forced duction for elevation
    - normal elevation force generation and elevation saccadic velocity (no muscle paralysis)
    - often an extra or deeper lower eyelid fold on the affected side
    - poor or absent Bell's phenomenon
2. with elevator weakness
    - free forced ductions
    - reduced elevation force generation and saccadic velocity
    - Bell's phenomenon often preserved (indicating a supranuclear cause)
3. combination (inferior rectus restriction and weak muscles of elevation)
    - positive forced duction for elevation
    - reduced force generation and saccadic velocity for elevation

Management

Indications for treatment include a large vertical deviation in primary position, with or without ptosis, and an abnormal head position, usually chin-up. If inferior rectus muscle

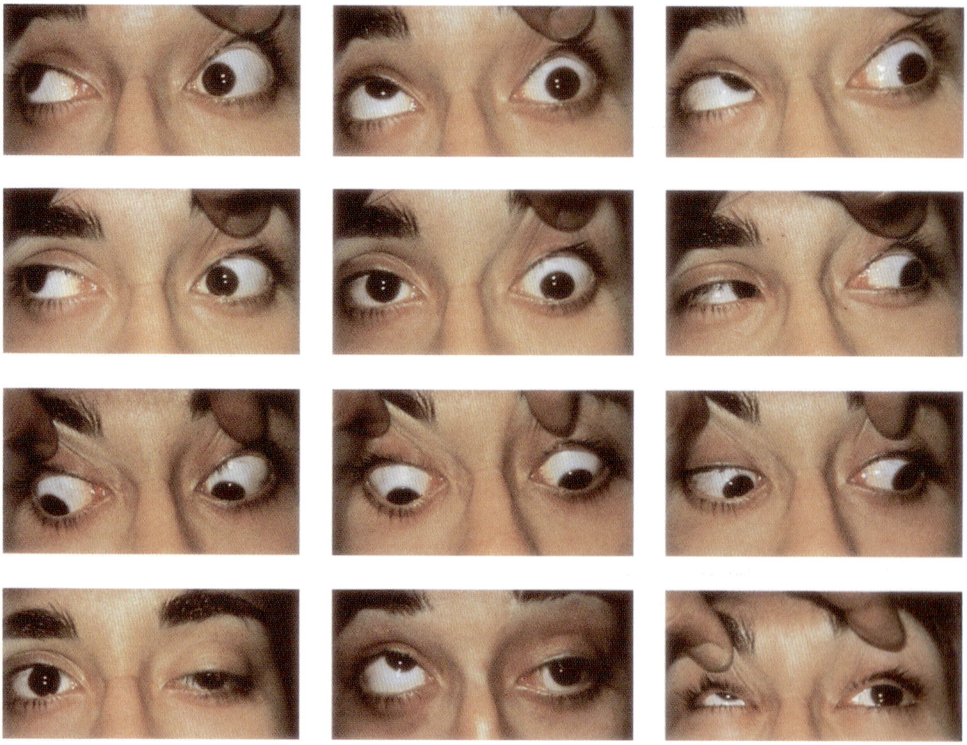

Figure 10-6 Monocular elevation deficiency of the left eye. **Top row,** No voluntary elevation of the left eye above horizontal. **Second row,** Hypotropia of the left eye. **Third row,** Depression of the left eye is unaffected. **Bottom left,** Ptosis (true and pseudo-) of the left upper eyelid when fixating with the right eye, persisting when fixating with the left eye **(bottom center).** [In the top 3 rows, the left upper lid is elevated manually.] **Bottom center,** Also shows the marked secondary overelevation of the right eye when fixating with the left eye. **Bottom right,** A partial Bell's phenomenon, with the left eye elevating above the horizontal on forced eyelid closure.

restriction is present, this muscle should be recessed. If there is no restriction, the medial rectus and the lateral rectus muscles should be transposed toward the superior rectus muscle *(Knapp procedure).* Upper eyelid surgery for ptosis should be deferred until after the vertical deviation has been corrected.

Raab EL. Double elevator palsy. In: Roy FH, ed. *Master Techniques in Ophthalmic Surgery.* Baltimore: Williams & Wilkins; 1995:267–274.

Orbital Floor Fractures

Blunt facial trauma is the usual cause of orbital floor fractures; auto accidents account for most of these. The injury is considered to be caused by an acute increase in intraorbital pressure from a direct impact that closes the orbital entrance, with or without injury to its rim. In the latter instance, this is termed *blowout fracture.*

Fracture of the orbital floor can be part of more extensive fractures of the midface, including the orbital rim or the zygomatic complex. Damage to the inferior rectus muscle with resulting weakness may be caused by hemorrhage or ischemia from direct trauma to the muscle or injury to its nerve; it can occur either at the time of injury or at the time the orbital floor fracture is repaired.

Clinical Features

The clinical features of orbital floor fractures are as follows:

- ecchymosis of the involved eye
- diplopia in some or all positions of gaze, often immediately following injury
- paresthesia or hypoesthesia of the infraorbital area secondary to damage of the infraorbital nerve, a sign more meaningful if present after the initial swelling subsides
- crepitus of the lower eyelid
- enophthalmos, either early or late
- evidence on imaging studies of entrapment of the inferior rectus muscle, inferior oblique muscle, or surrounding tissues
- hypotropia in the primary position that increases with upgaze and may decrease or become a hypertropia in downgaze. The latter suggests combined restriction to elevation and inferior rectus weakness from the injury (Fig 10-7)
- if inferior rectus muscle paralysis without entrapment (rare), hypertropia usually seen in primary position
- if associated medial orbital wall fracture, resulting in entrapment of the medial rectus muscle, limited horizontal rotations usually seen, especially abduction
- decreased vision, abnormal color vision, and an afferent pupillary defect (indications of optic neuropathy)

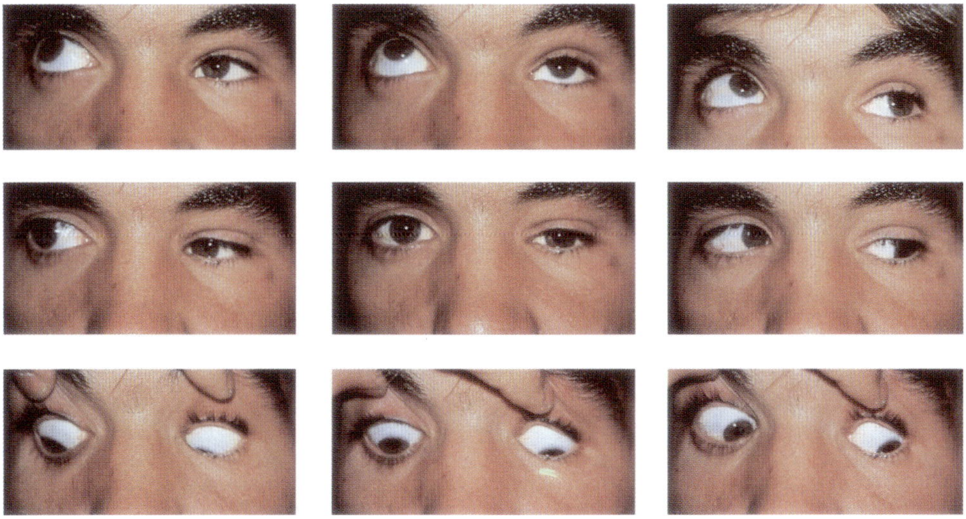

Figure 10-7 Left orbital fracture with inferior rectus muscle entrapment. Note limitation of elevation of the left eye and pseudoptosis from enophthalmos.

In the presence of limited elevation or depression, a positive forced duction test indicates the presence of restriction. Saccadic velocity and force generation testing help determine whether the eye is further limited in movement because of a paralytic process. Orbital CT and MRI studies of the involved soft tissues are useful to indicate the extent of the fracture and the degree of damage. In some cases, bradycardia, heart block, nausea, or syncope occurs as a vagal response to entrapment. *A complete eye examination should be done to detect associated ocular injury.*

Management

Surgical management of orbital floor fractures is controversial. Some clinicians advocate immediate exploration once the diagnosis is made, irrespective of forced duction test results. The justification for this approach, especially when supported by serial exophthalmometry, is that with large floor fractures, orbital contents can progressively herniate into the adjacent maxillary sinus, resulting in disfiguring enophthalmos. Others recommend waiting, from a few days to 2 weeks, for orbital edema and hematoma to subside before considering surgery; these surgeons will operate only when there is evidence of restriction, in which case exploration of the fracture and release of the inferior rectus muscle and surrounding tissues may limit the subsequent damage. A few ophthalmologists do not attempt repair of the fracture and deal only with any subsequent strabismus.

The initial management of inferior rectus muscle weakness without entrapment is observation, because the weakness may reverse with time. If recovery does not take place within 6 months of the injury, resection of the affected muscle combined with recession of the ipsilateral superior rectus muscle can be performed. Alternatively, a recession of the contralateral inferior rectus muscle with or without the addition of a posterior fixation suture can be used to limit downgaze and match the duction deficiency of the injured eye. This approach is known as *fixation duress* and is particularly useful when diplopia occurs in the reading position but no deviation is present in primary position (see also BCSC Section 7, *Orbit, Eyelids, and Lacrimal System*). Transposition of the ipsilateral medial and lateral rectus muscles to the inferior rectus muscle (inverse Knapp procedure) can be performed for complete inferior rectus muscle palsy.

Bansagi ZC, Meyer DR. Internal orbital fractures in the pediatric age group: characterization and management. *Ophthalmology.* 2000;107:829–836.

Burnstine MA. Clinical recommendations for repair of isolated orbital floor fractures: an evidence-based analysis. *Ophthalmology.* 2002;109:1207–1211.

CHAPTER 11

Special Forms of Strabismus

The following general reference is a valuable summary of current knowledge concerning many eye movement disorders in children.

Cassidy L, Taylor D, Harris C. Abnormal supranuclear eye movements in the child: a practical guide to examination and interpretation. *Surv Ophthalmol.* 2000;44:479–506.

Duane Syndrome

Duane syndrome is a spectrum of motility disturbances, all of which are characterized by retraction of the globe in actual or attempted adduction. Horizontal eye movement is usually somewhat limited in both directions. Upshoot or downshoot *(leash phenomenon)* of the affected eye in attempted adduction is common in more severe cases; it has been attributed to co-contraction of the medial and lateral rectus muscles and, alternatively, to slipping of the lateral rectus muscle over the outer aspect of the eye.

A defect in development occurring in the fourth week of gestation appears to be the cause of Duane syndrome, according to studies of patients prenatally exposed to thalidomide. Although most affected patients have Duane syndrome alone, many associated systemic defects have been observed, including Goldenhar syndrome (hemifacial microsomia, ocular dermoids, ear anomalies, preauricular skin tags, and upper eyelid colobomas) and Wildervanck syndrome (sensorineural hearing loss, Klippel-Feil anomaly with fused cervical vertebrae).

Most cases of Duane syndrome are sporadic, but about 5%–10% show autosomal dominant inheritance. A higher prevalence in females is reported in most series. Discordance in monozygotic twins raises the possibility that the intrauterine environment may be important. The many nonfamilial cases and the predilection for the left eye also suggest nongenetic factors.

In most anatomical and imaging studies, the nucleus of the sixth cranial nerve is absent, and an aberrant branch of the third cranial nerve has innervated the lateral rectus muscle. Electromyographic studies have shown paradoxical innervation of the lateral rectus muscle (innervation on attempted adduction and reduced innervation on attempted abduction). Anomalous synergistic innervation of the medial, inferior, and superior rectus muscles and the oblique muscles has been demonstrated as well. Although considered an innervational anomaly, tight and broadly inserted medial rectus muscles and fibrotic lateral rectus muscles, with corresponding forced duction abnormalities, are often encountered at surgery.

Ozkurt H, Basak M, Oral Y, et al. Magnetic resonance imaging in Duane's syndrome. *J Pediatr Ophthalmol Strabismus.* 2003;40:19–22.

Clinical Features

The most widely used classification of Duane syndrome defines 3 groups (although these may represent differences only in severity of the limited horizontal rotations): type 1 consists of poor abduction, frequently with primary position esotropia (Fig 11-1); type 2 consists of poor adduction and exotropia (Fig 11-2); and type 3 consists of poor abduction and adduction, with esotropia, exotropia, or no primary position deviation (Fig 11-3). About 15% of cases are bilateral; the type and severity need not be the same in each eye. For designing management strategies, consideration of the direction of the strabismus in primary gaze is more useful than identifying the type.

Type 1 Duane syndrome with esotropia and deficient abduction is the most common form (50%–80% in several series). Parents often incorrectly believe that what is actually the normal eye is turning in excessively, not realizing that the involved eye is not abducting. Careful observation for globe retraction on adduction, particularly viewing from the side of the patient, obviates a neurologic investigation for a sixth nerve palsy, although retraction can be hard to appreciate in an infant. Another indicator pointing away from

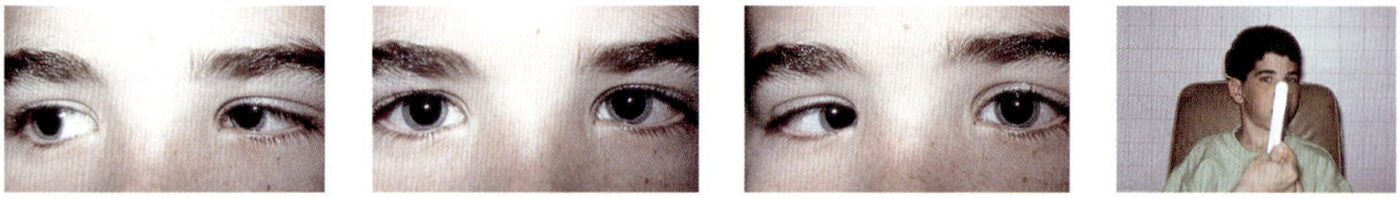

Figure 11-1 Type 1 Duane syndrome with esotropia, left eye, showing limitation of abduction and almost full adduction. Retraction of the globe on adduction. **Extreme right,** Compensatory left face turn. *(Photographs courtesy of Edward L. Raab, MD.)*

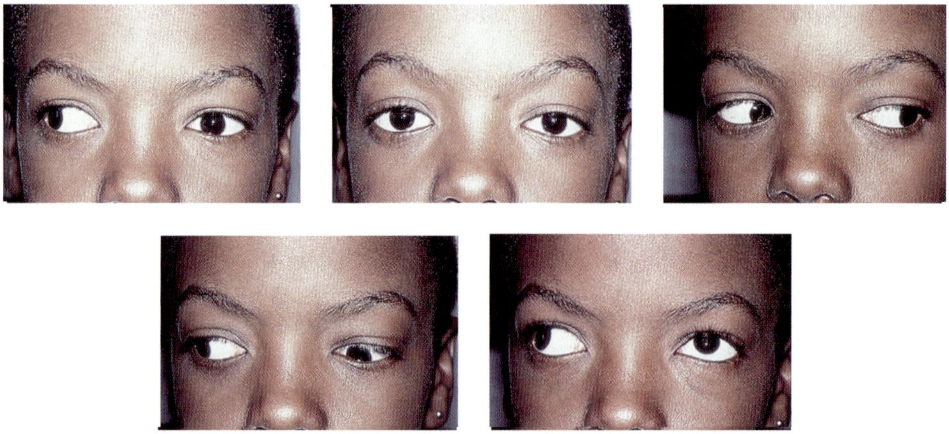

Figure 11-2 Type 2 Duane syndrome, left eye. **Top row,** Full abduction and marked limitation of adduction. **Bottom row,** Variable up- or downshoot of the left eye with extreme right gaze effort. The typical primary position exotropia is not present in this patient. *(Photographs courtesy of Edward L. Raab, MD.)*

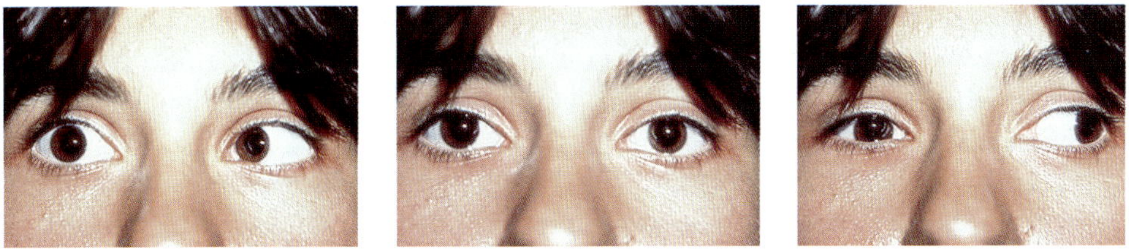

Figure 11-3 Type 3 Duane syndrome, right eye. Severe limitation of abduction and adduction, with palpebral fissure narrowing even though adduction cannot be accomplished. No deviation in primary position. *(Photographs courtesy of Edward L. Raab, MD.)*

sixth cranial nerve palsy is the lack of correspondence between the absent or typically modest primary position esotropia and the usually profound abduction deficit (a comparison useful in ruling out paralysis in other entities as well). A further point of differentiation is that, even in esotropic Duane syndrome, a small-angle exotropia frequently is present in gaze to the side opposite the affected eye, a finding not present in lateral rectus muscle paralysis.

Alexandrakis G, Saunders RA. Duane retraction syndrome. *Ophthalmol Clin North Am.* 2001;14:407–417.

Management

Because any surgical approach results in partial improvement at best, surgery is reserved primarily for cases with primary position deviations, an abnormal head position, marked globe retraction, or large upshoots or downshoots. Many patients with Duane syndrome have some position of gaze in which the eyes are properly aligned, allowing the development of binocular vision. One goal of surgery is to centralize and expand the field of single binocular vision.

For Duane syndrome with esotropia, recession of the medial rectus muscle on the involved side has been the most often used procedure to correct primary position deviation and eliminate the head turn. Abduction is not improved by this operation. Adding recession of the opposite medial rectus has been recommended for deviations over 20Δ in primary position. Although primary position overcorrection by medial rectus recession is not a significant risk, when the involved eye is adducted, postoperative exotropia is possible. Recession of the lateral rectus muscle of the uninvolved eye can offset this effect.

Resection of the lateral rectus muscle for Duane syndrome with esotropia is not favored because of the likelihood that globe retraction will worsen, although one study reported favorable results with unilateral recession-resection procedures. Partial or full transposition of the vertical rectus muscles has been advocated to improve abduction but may exaggerate the effects of co-contraction. Posterior scleral fixation of the transposed portions of the vertical rectus muscles, as described by Foster, has been found helpful, not only in Duane syndrome but in several types of paralytic strabismus as well. The value of botulinum injection into the medial rectus muscle to improve abduction is controversial.

The recommended surgery for Duane syndrome with exotropia and deficient adduction (type 2) is comparable to that for esotropic Duane syndrome: recession of the lateral rectus on the involved side for small deviations and of both lateral recti for large deviations, with avoidance of resection of the medial rectus. The latter aspect is especially important when an up- or downshoot is present on attempted adduction, because this finding indicates severe co-contraction.

Patients with type 3 Duane syndrome who have poor abduction and adduction often have straight eyes in or near the primary position and little, if any, head turn. Severe globe retraction may be helped by recession of both the medial and the lateral rectus muscles, which also may benefit the induced anomalous vertical excursion. Additional suggested procedures for the up- or downshoot are splitting the lateral rectus muscle in a Y configuration or a posterior fixation procedure on this muscle. Disinsertion of the lateral rectus muscle and reattachment to the lateral wall of the orbit is the most recent procedure to be tried.

Foster RS. Vertical muscle transposition augmented with lateral fixation. *J AAPOS.* 1997;1: 20–30.

Jampolsky A. Duane syndrome. In: Rosenbaum AL, Santiago AP, eds. *Clinical Strabismus Management: Principles and Surgical Techniques.* Philadelphia: Saunders; 1999:325–346.

Morad Y, Kraft SP, Mims JL 3rd. Unilateral recession and resection in Duane syndrome. *J AAPOS.* 2001;5:158–163.

Paysse EA, McCreery KMB, Ross A, et al. Use of augmented rectus muscle transposition surgery for complex strabismus. *Ophthalmology.* 2002;109:1309–1314.

Rao VB, Helveston EM, Sahare P. Treatment of upshoot and downshoot in Duane syndrome by recession and Y-splitting of the lateral rectus muscle. *J AAPOS.* 2003;7:389–395.

Rosenbaum AL. Costenbader Lecture. The efficacy of rectus muscle transposition surgery in esotropic Duane syndrome and VI nerve palsy. *J AAPOS.* 2004;8:409–419.

Brown Syndrome

Brown syndrome was described by Harold W. Brown in 1950 as the *superior oblique tendon sheath syndrome.* The characteristic restriction of elevation in adduction was originally thought to be caused by shortening of the anterior sheath of the superior oblique tendon. Brown and others later abandoned this theory in favor of an explanation implicating restriction of the superior oblique tendon at the trochlear pulley.

Brown syndrome occurs in congenital or acquired form. Prominent causes of acquired Brown syndrome include trauma in the region of the trochlea and systemic inflammatory conditions. The latter often result in intermittent Brown syndrome, which may resolve spontaneously. Resolution of congenital Brown syndrome is unusual but possible. This condition is bilateral in approximately 10% of cases.

Clinical Features

Well-recognized clinical features of Brown syndrome include deficient elevation in adduction that improves in abduction but often not completely (Fig 11-4). Several findings, along with positive forced duction testing results, differentiate Brown syndrome from inferior oblique muscle palsy (discussed in Chapter 10).

Attempts at straight-ahead elevation usually cause divergence (V pattern). This finding is an important difference from inferior oblique muscle palsy. In adduction, the

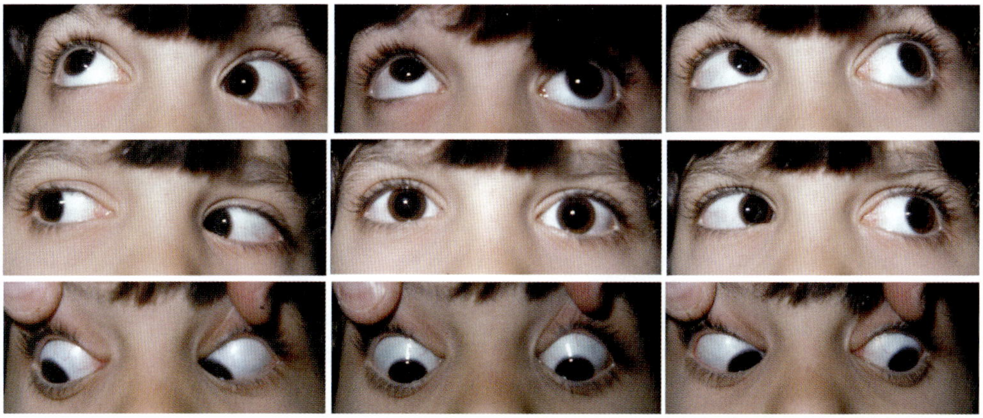

Figure 11-4 Brown syndrome, left eye. No elevation of the left eye when adducted. Left eye is depressed instead. Elevation is also severely limited in straight-up gaze and moderately so even in up-and-left gaze. The characteristic divergence in straight-up gaze should be noted. *(Photographs courtesy of Edward L. Raab, MD.)*

palpebral fissure widens and a downshoot of the involved eye is often seen; it can be distinguished from superior oblique muscle overaction because downshoot in the latter condition occurs less abruptly as adduction is increased.

Brown syndrome can be graded as mild, moderate, or severe. In the mild form, no hypotropia is present in primary position and no downshoot of the eye occurs in adduction. Moderate cases may have a downshoot in adduction but still no primary gaze hypotropia. Severe Brown syndrome cases have both a downshoot in adduction and a primary gaze hypotropia, often accompanied by a chin-up head posture and sometimes by a face turn-away from the affected eye. Absence of an abnormal head position in a severe case could be an indication of amblyopia.

An unequivocally positive forced duction test demonstrating restricted passive elevation in adduction is essential for the diagnosis of Brown syndrome. Retropulsion of the globe during this determination stretches the superior oblique tendon and accentuates the restriction. When inferior rectus muscle fibrosis or inferior orbital blowout fracture (the principal entities to be differentiated) produces a restrictive elevation deficiency, the limitation to passive elevation is accentuated by forceps-induced proptosis of the eye rather than by retropulsion. In addition, the elevation deficiency produced by inferior rectus muscle fibrosis or blowout fracture is usually more marked in abduction than in adduction.

Management

Observation alone remains the most common form of management for the mild and moderate forms that make up about two thirds of all Brown syndrome cases. When associated with rheumatoid arthritis or other systemic inflammatory diseases, resolution may occur as systemic treatment brings the underlying disease into remission or by corticosteroids injected near the trochlea. Sinusitis has also led to Brown syndrome, and it has been recommended that patients with an acute-onset presentation of Brown syndrome of undetermined cause undergo CT of the orbits and paranasal sinuses to investigate this possibility.

Surgical treatment is indicated for the most severe cases—those having primary position hypotropia, anomalous head posture, or both. Brown's original advocacy of sheathectomy has been abandoned in favor of ipsilateral superior oblique tenotomy. However, iatrogenic superior oblique muscle palsy may occur postoperatively. Although the occurrence rate of this sequel has been reported to be 44%–82%, it is reduced by careful preservation of the intermuscular septum during tenotomy. This modification often produces an early undercorrection that gradually improves with time.

To further reduce the consequences of superior oblique muscle palsy after tenotomy, some surgeons perform simultaneous ipsilateral inferior oblique muscle weakening. Others have advocated a guarded tenotomy using an inert spacer sewn to the cut ends of the superior oblique tendon or controlling the gap between the cut ends with an adjustable suture. These procedures eliminate the need for simultaneous inferior oblique muscle weakening but sometimes result in a downgaze restriction due to adhesions to the nasal border of the superior rectus muscle. Care must be taken to avoid contact of the spacer to nearby structures by preserving the intermuscular septum.

Helveston EM. The influence of superior oblique anatomy on function and treatment. The 1998 Bielschowsky Lecture. *Binocul Vis Strabismus Q.* 1999;14:16–26.

Wright KW. Brown's syndrome: diagnosis and management. *Trans Am Ophthalmol Soc.* 1999;97:1023–1109.

Third Cranial (Oculomotor) Nerve Palsy

The causes of *third cranial nerve palsy* in children include congenital disorders (40%–50%), trauma, inflammation, viral infection, migraine, and (infrequently) neoplastic lesions. In adults, third cranial nerve palsy may be caused by intracranial aneurysm, diabetes, neuritis, trauma, infection, or, rarely, tumor. Diabetic third cranial nerve palsy generally resolves spontaneously within 3–4 months. The majority of adults referred for surgical treatment have palsy due to trauma.

Clinical Features

Third cranial nerve palsy results in limited adduction, elevation, and depression of the eye, causing exotropia and often hypotropia. These findings would be expected because the remaining unopposed muscles are the lateral rectus (abductor) and the superior oblique (abductor and depressor). Upper lid ptosis usually is present, often with a pseudoptosis component due to the depressed position of the involved eye (Fig 11-5).

In congenital and traumatic cases, the clinical findings and treatment may be complicated by aberrant regeneration (misdirection) of the damaged nerve, presenting as anomalous eyelid elevation, pupil constriction, or depression of the globe on attempted adduction (see also BCSC Section 5, *Neuro-Ophthalmology*).

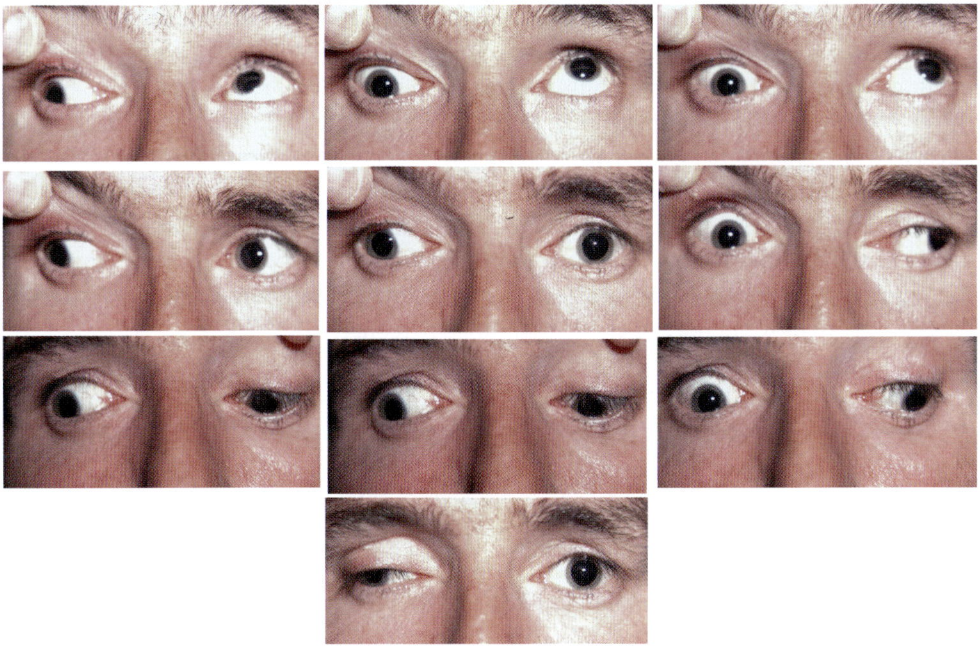

Figure 11-5 Third cranial nerve palsy, right eye, with ptosis and limited adduction, elevation, and depression. *(Photographs courtesy of Edward L. Raab, MD.)*

Management

Except in congenital cases of third cranial nerve palsy, it is advisable to wait 6–12 months for any spontaneous recovery before surgical correction is planned. Patients with at least partial recovery are much better candidates for good functional, as well as cosmetic, results. Because the visual system is still developing in pediatric patients, amblyopia is a common finding that must be treated aggressively.

Third cranial nerve palsies present difficult surgical challenges because multiple extraocular muscles as well as the levator may be involved. Replacing all of the lost rotational forces on the globe is impossible; therefore, the goals of surgery must be thoroughly discussed with patients so their expectations are realistic. Adequate alignment for binocular function in primary position and in slight downgaze for reading may be all that can be expected.

Although good primary position alignment can be achieved in most patients, surgery should be undertaken cautiously in patients with complete palsy and previously good binocular visual function, because elevation of the eyelid and incomplete realignment without useful single binocular fields may produce incapacitating diplopia. Prism adaptation testing has shown that adult patients who can achieve single binocular vision with prisms of any power before surgery are most likely to do well with surgical therapy. The occurrence rate of diplopia in patients under age 8 years is small because of the ability of the young binocular visual system to suppress conflicting visual information, resulting in amblyopia.

Planning for the appropriate surgical procedure is dictated by the number and condition of the involved muscles and the presence of noticeable paradoxical rotations. Frequently, a large recession-resection procedure on the horizontal rectus muscles to correct the exodeviation, with supraplacement of both to correct the hypotropia, is effective, especially with incomplete paralysis. Most surgeons reserve correction of ptosis for a subsequent procedure, which allows for a more accurate assessment.

Some surgeons use superior oblique tenotomy instead of supraplacement of the horizontal rectus muscles for hypotropia correction when the palsy is complete. Transfer of the tendon to the upper nasal quadrant of the globe also has been employed; however, anomalous eye movements can result from this procedure.

Aoki K, Sakaue T, Kubota N, et al. Outcome of surgery for bilateral third nerve palsy. *Jpn J Ophthalmol.* 2002;46:540–547.

Mudgil AV, Repka MX. Ophthalmologic outcome after third cranial nerve palsy or paresis in childhood. *J AAPOS.* 1999;3:2–8.

Schumacher-Feero LA, Yoo KW, Solari FM, et al. Third cranial nerve palsy in children. *Am J Ophthalmol.* 1999;128:216–221.

Siatkowski RM. Third, fourth, and sixth nerve palsies. *Focal Points: Clinical Modules for Ophthalmologists.* San Francisco: American Academy of Ophthalmology; 1996, module 8.

Sixth Cranial (Abducens) Nerve Palsy

The causes, features, and treatment of sixth cranial nerve palsy are discussed in Chapter 7. Features distinguishing sixth cranial nerve palsy from Duane syndrome include the absence of up- or downshoots and of retraction of the globe on adduction and, especially in sixth cranial nerve palsy, the presence of esotropia in primary position that is commensurate with the usually severe limitation of abduction (Fig 11-6).

Graves Eye Disease

Graves eye disease is also discussed in several other volumes of the BCSC as *thyroid ophthalmopathy* or *thyroid-associated orbitopathy* (consult the *Master Index*). Additional terms used elsewhere in the literature include *thyroid orbitopathy* and *thyroid-related immune orbitopathy.* European literature uses the eponym *von Basedow* rather than *Graves.* With this condition, the eye and the orbit can be affected in a variety of ways that are discussed in BCSC Section 7, *Orbit, Eyelids, and Lacrimal System.* Only motility disturbances are covered in this volume.

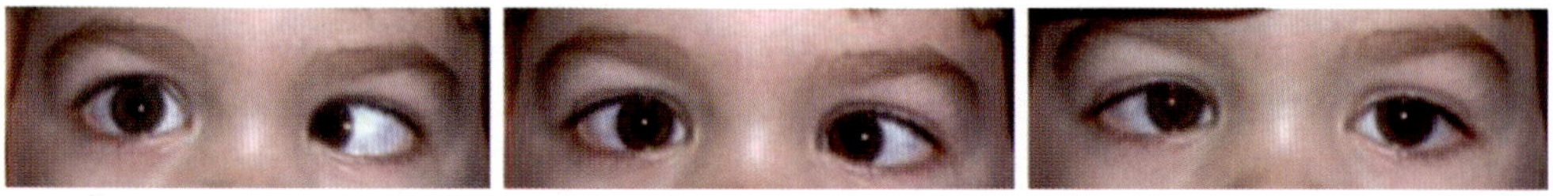

Figure 11-6 Sixth cranial nerve palsy, right eye. **Left,** No abduction in gaze to the right. Esotropia in primary position greater with fixation by palsied right eye **(center)** than by left eye **(right),** consistent with Hering's law (see Chapter 3). *(Photographs courtesy of Edward L. Raab, MD.)*

Edema, inflammation, and fibrosis are present in this disease because of lymphocytic infiltration. These conditions result in massive enlargement of affected extraocular muscles and may not only restrict motility but also cause compressive optic neuropathy. Detection of this muscle enlargement by orbital ultrasound, CT, or MRI helps confirm the diagnosis of Graves eye disease.

The myopathy is not caused by thyroid dysfunction. Rather, both conditions probably result from a common autoimmune disease. Therefore, patients may be euthyroid, hyperthyroid, or hypothyroid at the time of diagnosis. Some patients with Graves disease also have myasthenia gravis (discussed later in the chapter), complicating the clinical findings. It is mostly a disease of adults but can occur in children.

Clinical Features

Severe restrictive myopathy may occur with Graves disease. The muscles affected, in decreasing order of severity and frequency, are the inferior rectus, medial rectus, superior rectus, and lateral rectus. The condition most often is bilateral and asymmetric. Forced duction test results are almost always positive in 1 or more directions.

The patient presents most often with some degree of proptosis, hypotropia, or esotropia (Fig 11-7). Upper eyelid retraction often is present. Graves eye disease is a common cause of acquired vertical deviation in adults, especially females, but is rare in children.

Management

Indications for strabismus surgery include diplopia and abnormal head position. Surgery may eliminate diplopia in primary gaze but rarely restores normal motility because of

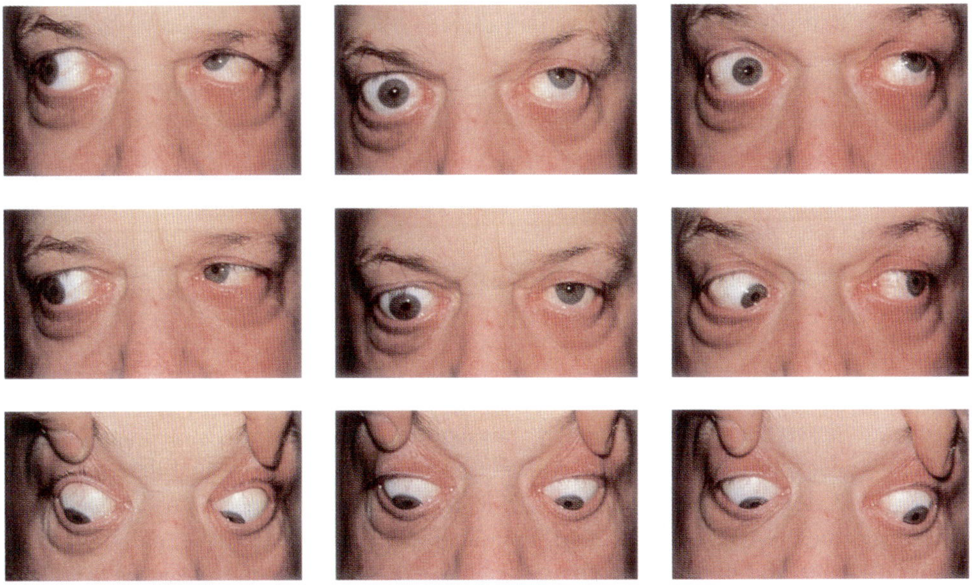

Figure 11-7 Graves disease (thyroid ophthalmopathy), right eye. Note upper eyelid retraction and restrictive right hypotropia with very limited elevation. Other rotations are not affected.

the restrictive myopathy, the need for very large recessions to allow the eye to be in primary position, and the replacement of muscle tissue by fibrous scar because of the underlying disease.

It is important to establish stability of the strabismus measurements before surgery is performed; waiting for at least 6 months is recommended. In the meantime, prisms may alleviate diplopia in primary position or for reading, but they are not necessarily effective in other positions of gaze. One recent study investigated performance of surgery prior to the achievement of stability but beyond the period of acute inflammation. The results were favorable, although half of the patients required repeat operation.

Recession of the affected muscles is the preferred surgical treatment. Strengthening procedures are rarely performed because they usually worsen restriction. Adjustable sutures are helpful in these difficult cases. Slight initial undercorrection is desirable, because late progressive overcorrection is common, especially with large inferior rectus recessions. Nonabsorbable sutures may decrease the likelihood of overcorrection. Limited depression of the eyes after inferior rectus muscle recessions can interfere with bifocal use by patients after surgery. Proptosis can become worse after extraocular muscle recessions.

If the need for orbital decompression is foreseeable, it is usually preferable to postpone strabismus surgery until that has been accomplished. Likewise, eyelid surgery usually is performed at a later time because upper eyelid retraction may be improved when the patient no longer strains to elevate the eye.

Large recessions of very tight inferior rectus muscles can cause lower eyelid retraction severe enough to require subsequent eyelid surgery. Severing the lower eyelid retractors as part of the strabismus surgery has led to some success at preventing this complication. If necessary, a spacer of banked sclera or synthetic material can be placed to vertically lengthen the lower lid tarsus (see also Chapter 13).

Coats DK, Paysse EA, Plager DA, et al. Early strabismus surgery for thyroid ophthalmopathy. *Ophthalmology;* 1999;106:324–329.

Cockerham KP, Kennerdel JS. Thyroid-associated orbitopathy. *Focal Points: Clinical Modules for Ophthalmologists.* San Francisco: American Academy of Ophthalmology; 1997, module 1.

Mills MD, Coats DK, Donahue SP, et al. Strabismus surgery for adults: a report by the American Academy of Ophthalmology. *Ophthalmology.* 2004;111:1255–1262.

Chronic Progressive External Ophthalmoplegia

Clinical Features

Chronic progressive external ophthalmoplegia (CPEO) usually begins in childhood with ptosis and slowly progresses to total paralysis of the eyelids and extraocular muscles. CPEO may be sporadic or familial. Although a true pigmentary retinal dystrophy usually is absent, constricted fields and electrodiagnostic abnormalities can occur. Defects in mitochondrial DNA have been found in some patients. The triad of retinal pigmentary changes, CPEO, and cardiomyopathy (especially heart block) is called *Kearns-Sayre syndrome.* BCSC Section 2, *Fundamentals and Principles of Ophthalmology*, discusses this condition in greater detail.

Management

Treatment options are limited. Cautious surgical elevation (suspension) of the upper eyelids is indicated to lessen a severe chin-up head position.

Myasthenia Gravis

Onset of *myasthenia gravis* may occur at any age but is uncommon in children. A transient neonatal form, caused by the placental transfer of acetylcholine receptor antibodies of mothers with myasthenia gravis, usually subsides rapidly. Another variety is not immune-mediated and exhibits a familial incidence.

The disease may be purely ocular but, in the most severe form, frequently (30%–50%) occurs as part of a major systemic disorder, with other skeletal muscles involved as well. Childhood myasthenia gravis is more common in females. BCSC Section 5, *Neuro-Ophthalmology*, discusses both the ocular and the systemic aspects of myasthenia gravis in depth.

Clinical Features

The principal ocular manifestation is extraocular muscle weakness, including weakness of the levator muscle. The majority of cases (90%) have both ptosis and limited ocular rotations. Affected muscles fatigue rapidly, so ptosis typically increases when the patient is required to look upward for 30 seconds. In the sleep test, ptosis often resolves after 20–30 minutes in a dark room with the eyelids closed. The presence of *Cogan twitch*, an overshoot of the eyelid when the patient looks straight ahead after looking down for several minutes, also is highly suggestive.

In the Tensilon test, a preliminary dose of 2 mg edrophonium chloride is injected intravenously. The patient's eyelids and eye movements are observed. If function improves obviously (Fig 11-8), no additional drug is needed. If no adverse reaction or improvement occurs, 2-mg increments are injected intravenously to a total of 10 mg. Atropine for IV administration is kept available as an antidote should a severe adverse cholinergic reaction occur. A similar test using neostigmine (Prostigmine), administered intramuscularly following pretreatment with atropine, has been described for use in children because the effect begins later and is prolonged, allowing more time for

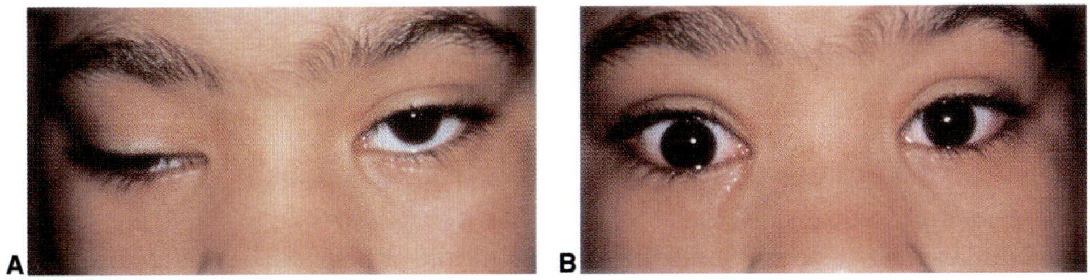

Figure 11-8 Myasthenia gravis. **A,** Bilateral ptosis with right hypotropia and exotropia. **B,** Following Tensilon injection, the eyes show orthophoria, normal eyelid position, and the lacrimation that frequently accompanies Tensilon injection.

measurement of changes in alignment, which is difficult with edrophonium because of the latter's brief action.

External application of ice for 2–5 minutes improves function of the levator and other affected extraocular muscles, giving a rapid and reliable method of establishing this diagnosis without the need for drug administration.

Electromyography shows decreased electrical activity of involved muscles after prolonged voluntary innervation and increased activity (including saccadic velocity) after the administration of edrophonium or neostigmine. Documentation of abnormalities in single-fiber electromyography or the presence of circulating antiacetylcholine receptor antibodies is confirmatory, although a negative result does not rule out the presence of this disease.

Ellis FD, Hoyt CS, Ellis FJ, et al. Extraocular muscle responses to orbital cooling (ice test) for ocular myasthenia gravis diagnosis. *J AAPOS.* 2000;4:271–281.

Mullaney P, Vajsar J, Smith R, et al. The natural history and ophthalmic involvement in childhood myasthenia gravis at the Hospital for Sick Children. *Ophthalmology.* 2000;107:504–510.

Table 11-1 compares the features of Graves disease with CPEO and myasthenia gravis.

Management

A full discussion of treatment of the various forms of myasthenia gravis is beyond the scope of this chapter. The ocular manifestations frequently are resistant to the usual systemic myasthenia treatment. If and when the ocular deviation has stabilized, standard eye muscle surgery can be helpful in restoring binocular function in at least some gaze positions.

Congenital Fibrosis Syndrome

Congenital fibrosis syndrome is a group of rare congenital disorders characterized by restriction of the extraocular muscles and replacement of the muscles by fibrous tissue. The spectrum ranges from isolated fibrosis of a single muscle to bilateral involvement of all extraocular muscles. The cause of congenital fibrosis syndrome is unknown. Some forms have been noted to be inherited and involve developmental defects of cranial nerve nuclei.

Engle EC. Applications of molecular genetics to the understanding of congenital ocular motility disorders. *Ann N Y Acad Sci.* 2002;956:55–63.

Clinical Features

Generalized fibrosis is the most severe form of the disease, involving all the extraocular muscles of both eyes, including the levator palpebrae superioris. This disorder is usually transmitted as an autosomal dominant but may be inherited as an autosomal recessive.

Congenital unilateral fibrosis with enophthalmos and ptosis is nonfamilial, with fibrosis of all the extraocular muscles and the levator on 1 side.

Table 11-1 Differentiation of Conditions Producing Ptosis and Extraocular Muscular Involvement

	Graves Disease (Thyroid-Associated Orbitopathy)	Chronic Progressive External Ophthalmoplegia (CPEO)	Myasthenia Gravis
Age	Any age	Any age	Any age
Muscle preferentially involved	Inferior rectus, medial rectus muscles	Levator, extraocular muscles	Levator, extraocular muscles
Fatiguability	No, unless coexistent myasthenia gravis	No	Yes
Response to Tensilon	No, unless coexistent myasthenia gravis	No	Yes
Other eye signs	External eye signs	Pigmentary retinopathy, optic neuropathy	No
Forced ductions	Restriction	Restriction if long-standing	Normal
Clinical course	May resolve or progress	Slowly progressive	Fluctuation; may have generalized weakness
Eyelids	Retraction	Ptosis	Ptosis
Diplopia	Yes	No	Yes
Other signs and symptoms	Tachycardia, arrhythmia, tremor, weight loss, diarrhea, heat intolerance	Heart block (manifestation of Kearns-Sayre syndrome)	Dysphagia, jaw weakness, limb weakness, dyspnea

Congenital fibrosis of the inferior rectus muscle alone may be unilateral or bilateral and sporadic or familial. This condition is commonly inherited as an autosomal dominant trait.

Strabismus fixus involves the horizontal recti, usually the medial rectus muscles, causing severe esotropia. Occasionally, the lateral recti are affected. The condition usually is sporadic and can be acquired late.

Vertical retraction syndrome involves the superior rectus muscle, with inability to depress the eye.

Diagnosis depends on finding limited voluntary motion, with restriction confirmed by forced duction testing. The congenital origin is an important distinction from thyroid-associated orbitopathy.

Management

Surgery is difficult and requires release of the restricted muscles (ie, weakening procedures). Fibrosis of the adjacent tissues may be present as well. A good surgical result aligns the eyes in primary position, but full ocular rotations cannot be restored and the outcome is unpredictable.

Yazdani A, Traboulsi EI. Classification and surgical management of patients with familial and sporadic forms of congenital fibrosis of the extraocular muscles. *Ophthalmology.* 2004;111:1035–1042.

Möbius Syndrome

Clinical Features

Möbius syndrome (or "sequence"; see Chapter 15) is a rare condition characterized by the association of both sixth and seventh cranial nerve palsies, the latter causing masklike facies. Patients may also manifest gaze palsies that can be attributed to abnormalities in the pontine paramedian reticular formation, indicating that the lesion is not only nuclear (see also BCSC Section 5, *Neuro-Ophthalmology*). Many patients also show limb, chest, and tongue defects, and some geneticists think that Möbius syndrome is one of a family of syndromes in which hypoplastic limb anomalies are associated with orofacial and cranial nerve defects. Poland syndrome (absent pectoralis muscle) is another variant.

The patient may have an esotropia or straight eyes in primary position. Both abduction and adduction may be limited (Fig 11-9); in some patients, adduction is better with convergence than with versions, similar to a gaze paralysis. Some patients appear to have palpebral fissure changes on adduction, and a few have vertical extraocular muscle involvement.

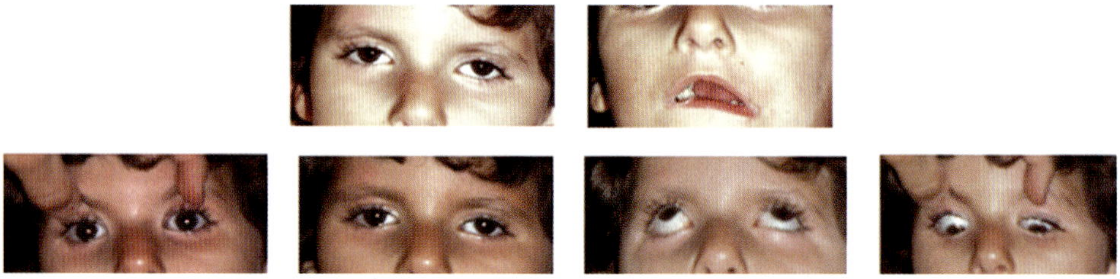

Figure 11-9 Möbius syndrome (sequence). **Top row, left,** Straight eyes in primary position; **right,** the patient cannot smile because of bilateral seventh cranial nerve palsy. **Bottom row,** Bilaterally absent adduction and severely limited abduction. Vertical movements are not affected. *(Photographs courtesy of Edward L. Raab, MD.)*

Management

Medial rectus muscle recession has been advocated, but caution should be exercised in the presence of a significant limitation of adduction. Some surgeons have undertaken to improve abduction by vertical rectus muscle transposition procedures after medial rectus muscle restriction has been relieved.

Miller MT, Stromland K. The Möbius sequence: a relook. *J AAPOS.* 1999;3:199–208.

Esotropia Associated With High Myopia

In highly myopic patients, the posterior portion of the eye can herniate out of the muscle cone after stretching and slippage of the lateral rectus pulley and other supporting tissues. Treatment includes measures to reinforce the defect by stabilizing the position of the lateral rectus muscle.

Internuclear Ophthalmoplegia

A prominent group of fibers called the *median longitudinal fasciculus (MLF)* is located dorsally on either side of the brain stem midline and passes between the sixth cranial nerve nuclei, below and lateral to the fourth and third cranial nerve nuclei. This group of fibers integrates the nuclei of the cranial nerves governing ocular motility and has major connections with the vestibular nuclei. An intact median longitudinal fasciculus is essential for the production of conjugate eye movements.

Bilateral internuclear ophthalmoplegia is an abnormality of the eye movement system in patients with demyelinating disease, but it may also occur in patients who have had a cerebrovascular accident or brain tumor.

Clinical Features

Injury to the median longitudinal fasciculus results in a typical pattern of disconjugate movement called internuclear ophthalmoplegia. In this condition, the eye ipsilateral to the lesion adducts slowly and incompletely or not at all, whereas the abducting eye exhibits a characteristic horizontal nystagmus. Both eyes adduct normally on convergence. Some degree of skew deviation may be present. (See also BCSC Section 5, *Neuro-Ophthalmology*.)

Management

If a large horizontal deviation persists after 6 months, medial rectus muscle resection and contralateral lateral rectus muscle recession (to limit exotropia in lateral gaze) can be helpful in eliminating diplopia, particularly in bilateral cases.

Congenital Ocular Motor Apraxia

Congenital ocular motor apraxia is a rare disorder of ocular motility, sometimes associated with strabismus. It is more common in males than in females and may be familial. At least some variants are inherited autosomal recessively.

This condition has been associated with premature birth and developmental delay. Central nervous system abnormalities, including bilateral lesions of the frontoparietal cortex, agenesis of the corpus callosum, hydrocephalus, and Joubert syndrome (abnormal eye movements, developmental delay, microcephaly, and retinal dysplasia, among several anomalies) also have been associated, as have kidney abnormalities. Several case reports have identified mass lesions of the cerebellum that compress the rostral part of the brain stem. Assessment of children with ocular motor apraxia by neuroimaging of the skull, as well as a complete systemic and developmental evaluation, is prudent.

Clinical Features

This condition is characterized by an inability to generate normal voluntary horizontal saccades. Instead, changes in horizontal fixation are made by a head thrust that overshoots the target, followed by a rotation of the head back in the opposite direction once fixation is established. The initial thrust serves to break fixation and may be associated with a blink that serves the same purpose. Vertical saccades and random eye movements are intact, but vestibular and optokinetic nystagmus are impaired. Reading can be difficult. The head thrust may improve in later childhood.

The differential diagnosis of acquired ocular motor apraxia subsumes conditions that affect the generation of voluntary saccades, including metabolic and degenerative diseases such as Huntington chorea. (See also BCSC Section 5, *Neuro-Ophthalmology*.)

Le Ber I, Moreira MC. Rivaud-Pechoux S, et al. Cerebellar ataxia with oculomotor apraxia type 1: clinical and genetic studies. *Brain.* 2003;126:2761–2772.

Tusa RJ, Hove MT. Ocular and oculomotor signs in Joubert syndrome. *J Child Neurol.* 1999;14:621–627.

Superior Oblique Myokymia

Superior oblique myokymia is a rare entity whose cause is poorly understood. There is some evidence that it is caused by aberrant regeneration of fourth cranial nerve fibers after minor damage. Another suggested etiology is vascular compression of the nerve, which can be confirmed by MRI.

Clinical Features

The condition is unilateral and consists of episodic rapid, low-amplitude torsional movements of the eye that cause diplopia and monocular oscillopsia. Patients are usually otherwise neurologically normal. The recurring symptoms may persist indefinitely, but the disorder is considered benign.

Management

Treatment is not necessary if the patient is not disturbed by the visual symptoms. Various medications have given inconsistent results. For surgical treatment to be effective, the superior oblique muscle must be permanently disconnected from the globe, usually by generous tenectomy. This can be expected to result in palsy, requiring further surgical management. (See also BCSC Section 5, *Neuro-Ophthalmology*.)

Plager DA. Superior oblique palsy and superior oblique myokymia. In: Rosenbaum AL, Santiago AP, eds. *Clinical Strabismus Management: Principles and Surgical Techniques.* Philadelphia: Saunders;1999:219–229.

Special Settings for Strabismus

In addition to the unique varieties of ocular motility disturbance just discussed, there are several familiar clinical settings in which strabismus is one of the consequences. These are mentioned briefly here.

Refractive surgery that creates monovision in adults in the presbyopic age range to facilitate visual clarity at distance and near without spectacles or contact lenses can result in dissimilar sensory input to the 2 eyes sufficient to cause loss of motor control of the extraocular muscles and disruption of fusion in predisposed patients.

Surgery for retinal detachment can lead to scarring of the fascial tissues covering the globe, with restricted rotations. Corrective surgery can be extremely difficult, especially if it is deemed necessary to remove the elements attached to the globe as part of the repair of the detachment. The presence of a retinal surgeon for guidance during the strabismus correction is valuable. The recently introduced modality of macular translocation surgery can cause torsional diplopia and other binocular sensory disturbances.

Aqueous drainage devices are another source of scarring and interference with ocular rotations. Treatment may require removal of the device and relocation or substitution of another size or type, a dilemma if it has been functioning well.

The extraocular muscles can be damaged after retrobulbar injection of anesthetic agents. Such damage may result from direct injury of the muscle or from a toxic effect of the injected material. Rotation deficiency should be managed according to the principles outlined for extraocular muscle paralysis, including the allowance of several months to permit spontaneous recovery. Because of the usual placement of these injections, the vertical rectus and inferior oblique muscles are the most vulnerable.

Laceration of the medial rectus muscle has been described as one of several serious ocular and orbital complications of pterygium removal or endoscopic sinus surgery. In the most severe form, an entire section of the muscle can be excised inadvertently. Restoration of function can be an extremely difficult surgical challenge.

Bhatti MT, Stankiewicz JA. Ophthalmic complications of endoscopic sinus surgery. *Surv Ophthalmol.* 2003;48:389–402.

Suh DW. Acquired esotropia in children and adults. *Focal Points: Clinical Modules for Ophthalmologists.* San Francisco: American Academy of Ophthalmology; 2003, module 10.

CHAPTER 12

Childhood Nystagmus

The child with nystagmus presents a difficult diagnostic challenge. The primary goal of the ophthalmic evaluation is to determine whether the nystagmus is a sign of a significant neurologic abnormality necessitating immediate intervention (Table 12-1), an ocular abnormality that may affect visual development, or a motor defect compatible with good visual function. In many children with nystagmus, the condition has an ophthalmic cause that can be determined by standard office examination techniques. BCSC Section 5, *Neuro-Ophthalmology*, discusses the neurologic implications of nystagmus.

Abadi RV, Bjerre A. Motor and sensory characteristics of infantile nystagmus. *Br J Ophthalmol.* 2002;86:1152–1160.

Nomenclature

Nystagmus is an involuntary, rhythmic to-and-fro oscillation of the eyes. In *pendular nystagmus*, the eyes oscillate with equal velocity in each direction. *Jerk nystagmus* denotes a movement of unequal speed; by convention, the fast component defines the direction of the nystagmus—for example, a right jerk nystagmus has a slow movement to the left and a fast movement (jerk) to the right.

Table 12-1 Common Intracranial Tumors in Childhood

Type	Location
Glial tumors	
Astrocytoma	Cerebellum Brain stem Hypothalamus Optic nerve/chiasm
Ependymoma	Fourth ventricle
Neural tumors	
Medulloblastoma	Cerebellum
Neuroblastoma	
Congenital tumors	
Germinomas	
Craniopharyngioma	Suprasellar, chiasmal
Arachnoid cysts	

The nystagmus movement can be further classified according to the frequency (number of oscillations per unit of time) and the amplitude (the angular distance traveled during the movement). The movements may be horizontal, vertical, rotary, oblique, or circular. Characteristics of the eye movements may change with different gaze direction. A pendular nystagmus can become jerk on extreme gaze.

Certain gaze positions can affect the amplitude and frequency. This is especially true of jerk nystagmus, which typically has a *null point* (the gaze location where the nystagmus is minimal) located in the gaze opposite the fast-phase component *(Alexander's law)*. Thus, a right jerk nystagmus becomes much worse on right gaze and improves significantly on left gaze. A patient with a right jerk nystagmus would therefore develop a right head turn and left gaze preference (Fig 12-1).

Hertle RW, Zhu X. Oculographic and clinical characterization of thirty-seven children with anomalous head postures, nystagmus, and strabismus: the basis of a clinical algorithm. *J AAPOS.* 2000;4:25–32.

Evaluation

History

Many forms of nystagmus are inherited, either as a direct genetic abnormality or because of an association with other ocular diseases (Table 12-2). A thorough family history is important in the initial evaluation. Questions should be asked about other types of inherited ocular diseases, systemic diseases, or syndromes known to affect visual development. Congenital motor nystagmus may be inherited as an autosomal dominant, recessive, or X-linked trait. Examination of family members with nystagmus can provide valuable prognostic information about the anticipated visual function in affected children.

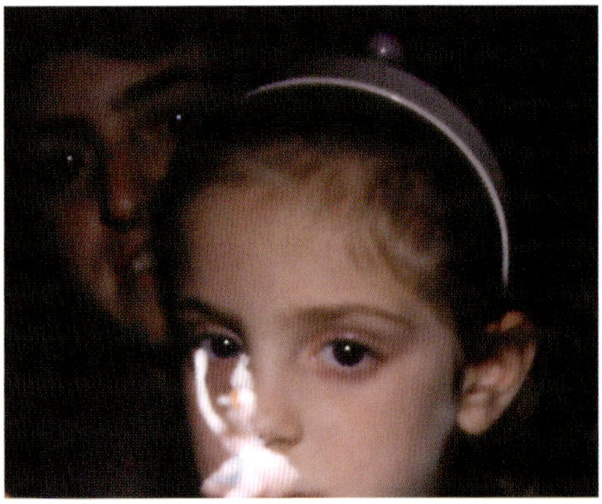

Figure 12-1 Patient with a right face turn, left gaze preference due to a right-beating jerk nystagmus. *(Photograph courtesy of Edward L. Raab, MD.)*

Table 12-2 Ocular Conditions Associated With Nystagmus

- Ocular coloboma
  - Optic nerve
  - Retinal
- Congenital cataract
- Congenital glaucoma
- Retinoblastoma
- Cicatricial retinopathy of prematurity
- Iridocorneal dysgenesis
- Aniridia
- Retinal dysplasia
- Congenital toxoplasmosis
- Congenital "macular coloboma"
- Leber congenital amaurosis
- Bilateral optic nerve hypoplasia/atrophy
- Albinism
  - Ocular albinism
  - Oculocutaneous albinism
- Achromatopsia
- Congenital stationary night blindness
- Congenital retinoschisis

Events at the time of delivery can significantly affect the developing visual system and, if severe enough, can result in nystagmus. Inquiries as to whether there were problems with labor and delivery, maternal infections, and prematurity can illuminate the cause of nystagmus. In children older than 3 months, parental observations about head tilts, head movements, gaze preference, and viewing distances can aid in diagnosis.

Ocular Examination

The ophthalmic evaluation should concentrate on visual acuity testing, pupillary responses, ocular motility, and funduscopic examination.

Visual acuity testing

The level of visual function can be helpful in determining the cause of nystagmus. Patients with nystagmus and nearly normal visual acuity usually have congenital motor nystagmus, which is a benign entity. Markedly decreased visual acuity usually implies either retinal or optic nerve abnormalities. Visual acuity should be measured at distance and near as well as under binocular conditions, allowing children to use whatever head position or movement they choose. This last measurement is crucial in establishing the true functional visual performance.

Near visual acuity is usually better than at distance and can indicate the difficulty the child is likely to experience in a school setting. Many children with 20/400 or worse distance acuity can read at the 20/40 to 20/60 level by viewing the material at close range. Glasses or other devices can enable these children to master the school curriculum. In preverbal children, if a vertical *optokinetic nystagmus (OKN)* response can be superimposed on the child's underlying nystagmus, the visual function is usually 20/400 or better.

Preferential looking also can be used, but the response can be more easily observed with the card held vertically in patients with a horizontal nystagmus.

Pupils

Pupils should be assessed for asymmetry, direct reaction to light, afferent defect, reaction to darkness, and anatomical structure.

Sluggish or absent response to light or an afferent defect indicates severe anterior visual pathway abnormalities, such as optic nerve or retinal dysfunction. Responses can be normal in mild abnormalities, such as macular hypoplasia, rod monochromatism, and primary motor nystagmus. The normal response to darkness is the immediate dilation of the pupil. If, instead of dilating, the pupils paradoxically constrict, optic nerve or retinal disease is present (Table 12-3).

In addition to pupillary responses, iris structure should be assessed. Defects such as colobomas suggest similar optic nerve or retinal defects. Excess iris transillumination is a hallmark of albinism. Aniridia and albinism are associated with macular hypoplasia, poor vision, and nystagmus.

Ocular motility

Patients with nystagmus often have strabismus, either as a result of poor vision or as an attempt to damp the nystagmus by converging. Children with motor nystagmus usually fixate with the preferred eye in adduction and turn their heads to look across their noses (Fig 12-2). They use this maneuver at distance or near to improve visual acuity.

Fundus

Optic nerve or macular hypoplasia is common in children with nystagmus. Although many of the retinal disorders are associated with visible abnormalities, in some, the fundus appears normal or there are subtle retinal pigmentary changes (Table 12-4). In patients with nystagmus and normal-appearing posterior poles, electrophysiologic testing may be necessary to identify the cause.

Buckley EG. The clinical approach to the pediatric patient with nystagmus. *Int Pediatr.* 1990; 5:225–231.

Childhood Nystagmus Types

Some authors have described a transient nystagmus in children occurring prior to 2 months of age and subsiding after about 6 months. In the absence of other causes, the nystagmus was attributed to as-yet immature and unstable motor control.

Good WV, Hou C, Carden SM. Transient, idiopathic nystagmus in infants. *Dev Med Child Neurol.* 2003;45:304–307.

Congenital Nystagmus

Congenital motor nystagmus

Congenital motor nystagmus is a binocular conjugate nystagmus that is usually horizontal and commonly remains so on up- and downgaze. Congenital motor nystagmus can be

Table 12-3 Differential Diagnosis of Paradoxical Pupillary Phenomena

Congenital stationary night blindness
Congenital achromatopsia
Optic nerve hypoplasia
Leber congenital amaurosis
Best disease
Albinism
Retinitis pigmentosa

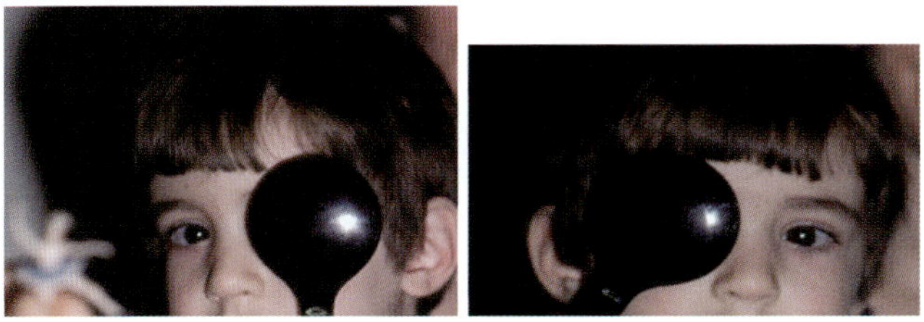

Figure 12-2 Congenital motor nystagmus. There is a right face turn when fixating with the right eye. The head turn reverses when fixating with the left eye. In children with good vision in each eye, the nystagmus null point is almost always with the fixating eye in adduction. *(Photographs courtesy of Edward L. Raab, MD)*

Table 12-4 Conditions Associated With Decreased Vision and Minimal Fundus Changes

Leber congenital amaurosis
Rod monochromacy
Blue-cone monochromacy
Hereditary optic atrophy
Optic nerve hypoplasia
Ocular albinism
Congenital stationary night blindness

pendular, jerk, circular, or elliptical, and more than 1 type may exist in the same individual. The characteristic waveform of congenital motor jerk nystagmus is a slow phase with an exponential increase in velocity. A null point, or *neutral zone*, may be present; this is a gaze position in which the intensity of oscillations is diminished and the visual acuity improves. If the null point is not in primary position, anomalous head postures may be adopted to damp the nystagmus and provide the best visual acuity. Head bobbing or movement may also be present at first, although this usually decreases with age. Oscillopsia is rare. See Table 12-5.

Table 12-5 Characteristics of Congenital Nystagmus

Bilateral
Conjugate
Horizontal
Worsens with attempted fixation
Improves with convergence
Null point often present with head position
Two thirds of patients have "inverted" OKN response
Oscillopsia usually not present

Congenital motor nystagmus is damped by convergence and therefore is often associated with esotropia. This combination of nystagmus and esotropia has been termed *nystagmus blockage syndrome*, a distinction from those in which esotropia and nystagmus happen to coexist. Nystagmus blockage syndrome presents characteristically as an esotropia that "eats up prism" on attempted measurement and exhibits an increased jerk nystagmus on attempted lateral gaze.

Purely congenital motor nystagmus is not associated with other central nervous system abnormalities. Visual function can be near normal. Patients develop a preferred gaze position to utilize a null location, thereby increasing foveation time, during which their acquisition of visual information occurs. This head position becomes more obvious as the child reaches school age.

Approximately two thirds of these patients exhibit a paradoxical inversion of the OKN response. Normally, if a patient with right jerk nystagmus views an OKN drum rotating to the patient's left (eliciting a pursuit left, jerk right response), the right jerk nystagmus will increase. However, patients with congenital motor nystagmus exhibit either a damped right jerk nystagmus or possibly even a left jerk nystagmus. This paradoxical response occurs only in congenital motor nystagmus.

Stevens DJ, Hertle RW. Relationship between visual acuity and anomalous head posture in patients with congenital nystagmus. *J Pediatr Ophthalmol Strabismus.* 2003;40:259–264.

Sensory defect nystagmus

Sensory defect nystagmus, another form of congenital nystagmus, is secondary to an abnormality in the afferent visual pathway and is the most common cause of nystagmus in the pediatric population. Inadequate image formation results in failure of development of the normal fixation reflex. If this is present at birth, the resulting nystagmus begins in the first 3 months of life. Its severity depends on that of the visual loss. All waveforms may be present, but pendular nystagmus is most common. On lateral gaze, the nystagmus may become jerk.

Searching, slow, wandering, or conjugate eye movements may also be observed. Searching nystagmus, defined as a roving or drifting, typically horizontal, movement of the eyes without fixation, is usually observed in children whose vision is worse than 20/200. Pendular nystagmus occurs when the visual acuity is better than 20/200 in at least 1 eye. Jerk nystagmus is often associated with visual acuity between 20/60 and 20/100. (See Table 12-2 for the ocular conditions that can give rise to sensory nystagmus.)

Periodic alternating nystagmus

Periodic alternating nystagmus (PAN) is an unusual form of congenital motor jerk nystagmus that periodically changes direction. The motion typically starts with a jerk nystagmus in 1 direction that lasts for 60–90 seconds and then slowly begins to damp, until it reaches a period of no nystagmus that lasts from 10 to 20 seconds, followed by nystagmus that jerks in the opposite direction in a repeating process. Some children adopt an alternating head position to take advantage of the changing null position. The cause of congenital PAN is unknown, but it has been associated with oculocutaneous albinism.

Latent nystagmus

Latent nystagmus is a congenital conjugate horizontal jerk nystagmus that occurs under conditions of monocular fixation. When 1 eye is occluded, a jerk nystagmus develops in both eyes with the fast phase directed toward the uncovered eye. Thus, a left jerk nystagmus of both eyes occurs when the right eye is covered. This nystagmus is the only form that reverses direction as driven by a change in fixation. Asymmetries in amplitude, frequency, and velocity of the nystagmus also can be present, depending on which eye is covered.

Latent nystagmus usually is noted in early childhood, especially in patients with congenital esotropia and dissociated vertical deviation. The cause is unknown but may be related to the mechanism of vestibular nystagmus. Because a nystagmus is induced when an eye is covered, binocular visual acuity is better than monocular, and occlusion must be avoided during monocular tests of vision. Use of polarizing lenses and a polarized chart, blurring of the nontested eye with a +5.00 D sphere, or repositioning of the occluder several inches in front of the eye not being tested can be effective.

Latent nystagmus may become manifest (manifest latent nystagmus) when both eyes are open but only 1 eye is being used for vision (ie, the other eye is suppressed or amblyopic). Just as with motor nystagmus, on which it often is superimposed, occlusion of the preferred eye results in a change in the direction of the jerk nystagmus. Electronystagmographic evaluation of latent and manifest latent nystagmus reveals a similar waveform with an exponential decrease in velocity of the slow phase. This pattern is the opposite of congenital motor nystagmus, which shows an exponential increase in slow-phase velocity (Fig 12-3).

Brodsky MC, Tusa RJ. Latent nystagmus: vestibular nystagmus with a twist. *Arch Ophthalmol.* 2004;122:202–209.

Gottlob I. Nystagmus. *Curr Opin Ophthalmol.* 2001;12:378–383.

Acquired Nystagmus

Spasmus nutans

Spasmus nutans is an acquired nystagmus that occurs in children in the first 2 years of life, presenting as a triad of nystagmus, head nodding, and torticollis. The nystagmus generally is bilateral and of small amplitude and high frequency (shimmering); however, it can be monocular, asymmetric, and variable in different gaze positions. It can be horizontal, vertical, or rotary and is occasionally intermittent.

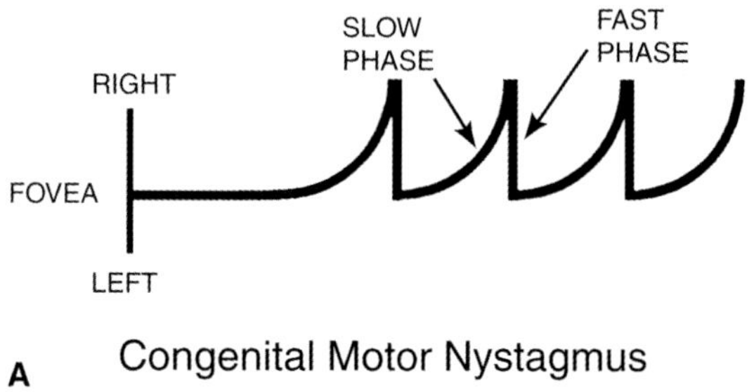

A

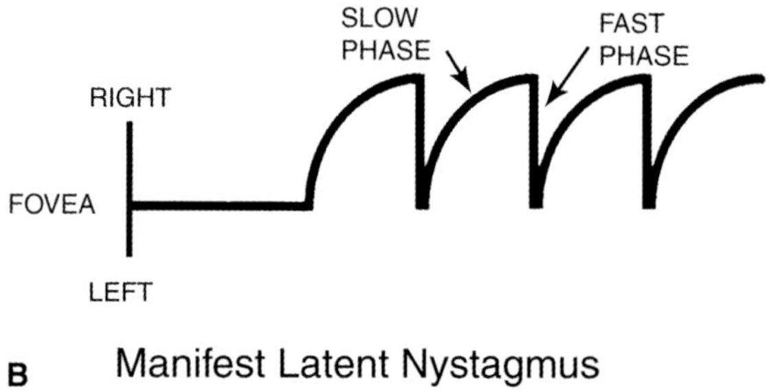

B

Figure 12-3 Left jerk nystagmus. **A,** Electronystagmographic evaluation of congenital motor nystagmus shows an exponential increase in velocity of the slow phase. **B,** Manifest latent nystagmus shows a waveform with a new exponential decrease in velocity of the slow phase.

Spasmus nutans occasionally can be familial and has been present in monozygotic twins. It usually disappears by age 3–4 years. It is a benign disorder in most cases, but nystagmus characteristic of spasmus nutans has been associated with chiasmal or suprachiasmal tumors in children who have other central nervous system abnormalities. When doubt persists about the cause of presumed spasmus nutans, neuroradiologic investigation is warranted.

Gottlob I, Wizov SS, Reinecke RD. Spasmus nutans. A long-term follow-up. *Invest Ophthalmol Vis Sci.* 1995;36:2768–2771.

Shaw FS, Kriss A, Russel-Eggitt I, et al. Diagnosing children presenting with asymmetric pendular nystagmus. *Dev Med Child Neurol.* 2001;43:622–627.

Unsold R, Ostertag C. Nystagmus in suprasellar tumors: recent advances in diagnosis and therapy. *Strabismus.* 2002;10:173–177.

See-saw nystagmus

See-saw nystagmus, an unusual but dramatic type of nystagmus, has both vertical and torsional components. The name derives from the action of the familiar playground device. If 2 eyes were placed on a see-saw, one at either end, they would “roll down the plank” as the see-saw rose, with the high eye intorting and the low eye extorting. As the direction of the see-saw changed, so would that of the eye movement. Thus, the eyes make alternating movements of elevation and intorsion followed by depression and extorsion.

This type of nystagmus is often associated with a lesion in the rostral midbrain or the suprasellar area. In children, the most likely associated intracranial tumor is a craniopharyngioma. Confrontation visual fields may elicit a bitemporal defect. Neuroradiologic evaluation is necessary. The treatment for see-saw nystagmus is removal of the inciting cause.

Nystagmus retractorius

Nystagmus retractorius, or *convergence-retraction nystagmus*, is part of the dorsal midbrain syndrome associated with paralysis of upward gaze, defective convergence, and pupillary light–near dissociation. In the pediatric age group, nystagmus retractorius is most commonly secondary to congenital aqueductal stenosis or a pinealoma. Unlike other types of childhood nystagmus, this form may be noticed only under particular circumstances. It is best elicited on attempted fast upgaze, when co-contraction of all the horizontal extraocular muscles occurs and the eyes are pulled into the orbit (hence the term *retractorius*). The eyes often converge on attempted upgaze as well. However, voluntary convergence is minimal.

Opsoclonus

Opsoclonus, an extremely rare eye movement disorder, is not a true nystagmus but a bizarre rapid and involuntary ocular oscillation. It can be present intermittently and often has a very-high-frequency, low-amplitude movement. The movements are so fast and chaotic that they are not easily confused with other forms of infantile nystagmus.

The most common cause of opsoclonus is an acute cerebellar ataxia of childhood. Opsoclonus can also be a sign of occult neuroblastoma, a consequence of epidemic encephalitis of viral origin, or an effect of hydrocephalus.

Downbeat nystagmus

Downbeat nystagmus is a jerk nystagmus with the fast component downward. It obeys Alexander's law (see Nomenclature, near the beginning of this chapter) and is maximum in downgaze and down to the left and right. Downbeat nystagmus often has a null position in upgaze. When congenital, this condition is associated with good vision and normal neurologic findings, although a hereditary form of downbeat nystagmus may precede spinocerebellar degeneration.

More commonly, downbeat nystagmus is acquired, secondary to structural abnormalities such as the Arnold-Chiari malformation. In this condition, the cerebellar tonsils herniate through the foramen magnum, compressing the brain stem and resulting in downbeat nystagmus. Decompression of this area often results in complete resolution. Pharmacologic agents such as codeine, lithium, tranquilizers, and anticonvulsants may also cause this condition.

Monocular nystagmus

Monocular nystagmus has been reported to occur in severely amblyopic and blind eyes. The oscillations are pendular, chiefly vertical, slow, small in amplitude, and irregular in frequency.

Dissociated nystagmus

Nystagmus only in the abducting eye *(dissociated nystagmus)* occurs in several conditions, the most familiar being internuclear ophthalmoplegia. Myasthenia gravis may simulate an internuclear ophthalmoplegia. Surgical weakening of the medial rectus muscle has been reported to cause a nystagmus of the contralateral abducting eye similar to that seen with internuclear ophthalmoplegia but without the slowing of saccades in the adducting eye that occurs in the latter condition.

Differential Diagnosis

Figure 12-4 lists the signs and symptoms of various forms of horizontal nystagmus in children, along with guidelines for testing and systemic associations.

Treatment

Prisms

Prisms can optically improve head positions by shifting the image into the null zone or can improve visual acuity by inducing convergence. They can be used as the sole treatment or as a trial to predict surgical success. Fresnel Press-On prisms are useful for this because powers of 10Δ–20Δ are often necessary.

To correct head positions, each prism is mounted with the apex pointing to the direction of the null zone. For example, with a left head turn and a null zone in right gaze, prisms before the right eye should be oriented base-in and prisms before the left eye should be oriented base-out. This shifts the image to the right and decreases the amount of turn the patient requires to gain the same visual benefit. If this technique improves the head position, strabismus surgery is also likely to be effective. A limitation of prism treatment is that, unlike surgery, it does not bring the eyes out of the gaze position necessary to achieve the null zone.

Prism spectacles improve visual acuity by stimulating fusional convergence, which damps the nystagmus. In this situation, base-out prisms are placed in front of both eyes in amounts determined by trial and error.

Nystagmus Surgery

Extraocular muscle surgery for nystagmus is indicated to correct a head turn by shifting the null point closer to the primary position. Surgery can also improve visual acuity by decreasing nystagmus intensity. The types of surgery typically recommended are a recession-resection procedure performed on both eyes *(Kestenbaum-Anderson)* or a 4-horizontal-muscle recession.

In the Kestenbaum-Anderson procedure, the eyes are surgically rotated toward the direction of the head turn and away from the null zone or preferred position of gaze. Each eye undergoes a recession-resection procedure to move the eyes in the same direction. For example, if a patient with congenital nystagmus has a left face turn and null zone in right gaze, the eyes are surgically rotated to the left by recession of the right lateral and left medial rectus muscles and by resection of the right medial and left lateral

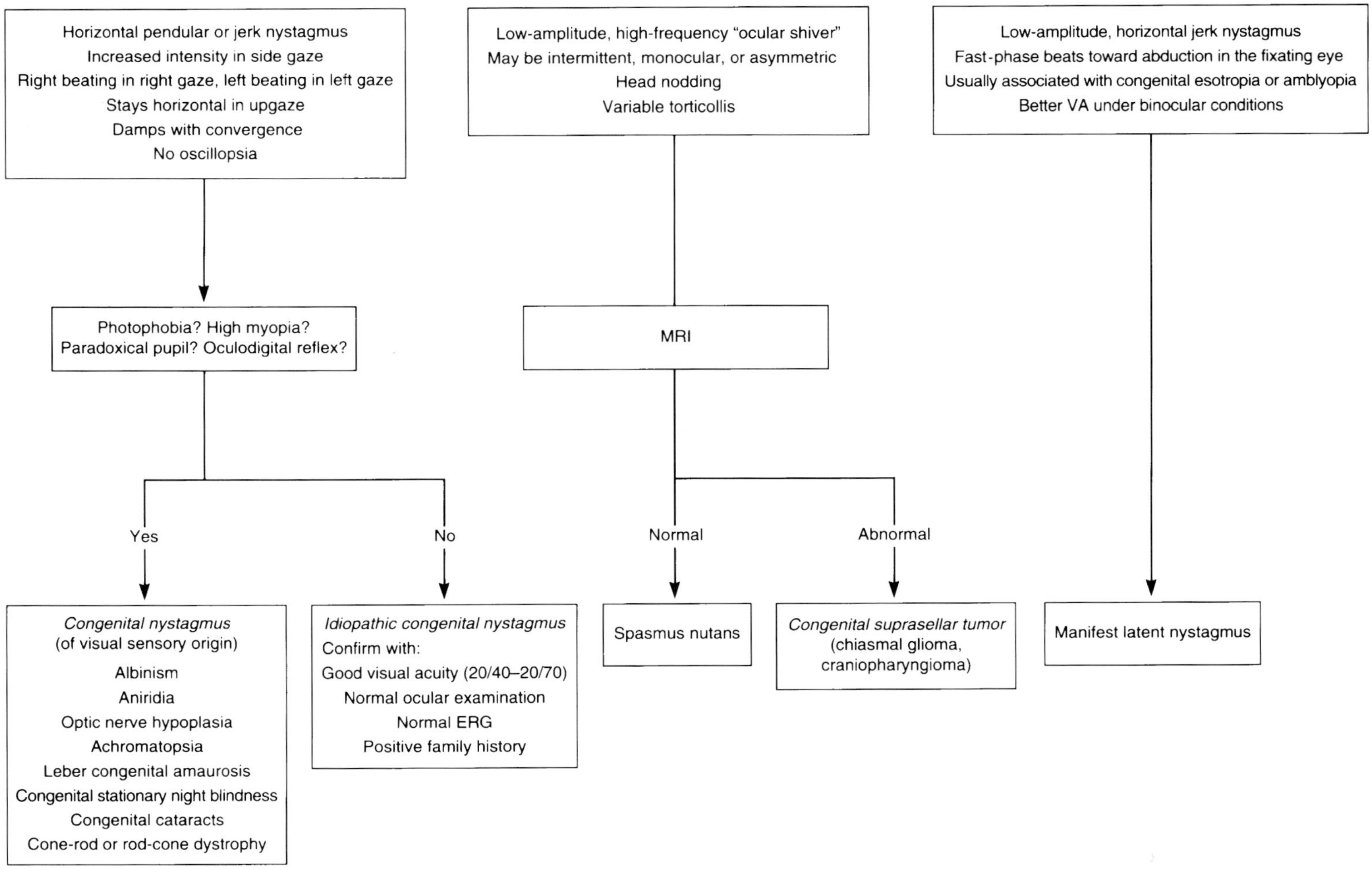

Figure 12-4 Differential diagnosis of horizontal nystagmus in children. *(Modified from Brodsky MC, Baker RS, Hamed LM.* Pediatric Neuro-Ophthalmology. *New York: Springer-Verlag; 1995:339.)*

rectus muscles. This makes it more difficult for the patient to look into right gaze, thereby damping the nystagmus more toward the primary position (Fig 12-5).

The amount of recession-resection performed in the Kestenbaum-Anderson procedure has been modified through experience. Table 12-6 describes the original operation plus 2 modifications in which the amount of surgery is increased by 40% or 60%. The resulting amounts are rounded off to the nearest 0.5 mm. The total amount of surgery for each eye (as measured in millimeters) is equal in order to rotate each globe an equal amount. For face turns of 30°, the 40% augmented procedure is recommended; for turns of 45°, the 60% augmentation procedure is employed. The augmented procedures may cause restriction of motility, which is usually necessary to achieve a satisfactory result.

If vertical torticollis is present with congenital nystagmus, chin-up or -down posturing may be ameliorated in some cases by vertical prism (again, apex toward the null zone) or by surgery on the vertical rectus muscles. As with horizontal nystagmus, the eyes are rotated away from the null point. Thus, if a chin-up, eyes-down posture is

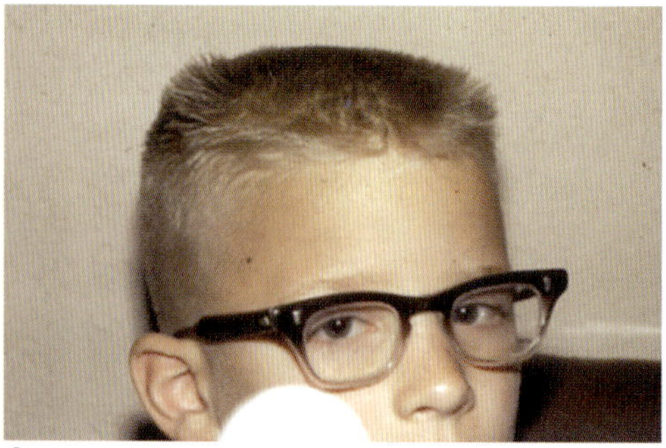

A

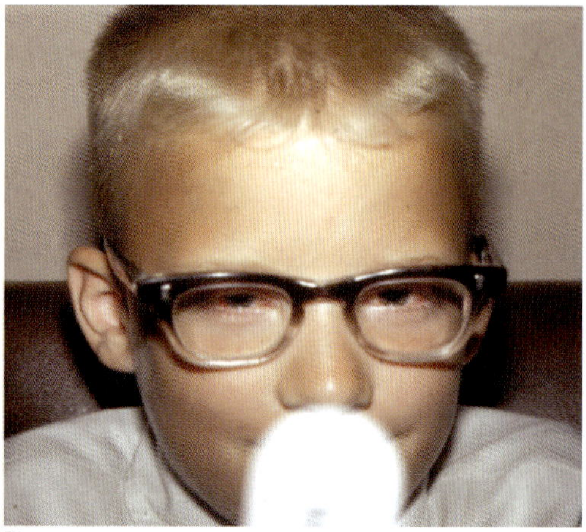

B

Figure 12-5 **A,** Congenital motor nystagmus with the null point in right gaze. **B,** Null point shifted by the Kestenbaum-Anderson procedure, eliminating the necessity for a head turn. *(Photographs courtesy of Edward L. Raab, MD.)*

Table 12-6 **Kestenbaum-Anderson Procedure and Modifications**

Procedure	Kestenbaum	40% Augmented	60% Augmented
Recess medial rectus	5.0 mm	7.0 mm	8.0 mm
Resect medial rectus	6.0 mm	8.4 mm	9.6 mm
Recess lateral rectus	7.0 mm	9.8 mm	11.2 mm
Resect lateral rectus	8.0 mm	11.2 mm	12.8 mm
Total surgery	13.0 mm	18.2 mm	20.8 mm
R + R	(5 + 8) = (6 + 7)	(7 + 11.2) = (8.4 + 9.8)	(8 + 12.8) = (9.6 + 11.2)

present, the inferior rectus muscles are recessed and the superior rectus muscles are resected. The amount of surgery is usually 5–7 mm of recession and resection on each eye.

Recession of all the horizontal rectus muscles to a position posterior to the equator is an alternative to the Kestenbaum-Anderson procedure. It usually requires 8–10 mm of recession of both medial rectus muscles and 10–12 mm of recession of both lateral rectus muscles. This approach may be especially beneficial for improving visual function when the head position is not a problem, but a newly generated deviation is possible. Further, recent studies have found that merely disinserting and reattaching the horizontal rectus muscles, without recession or resection, may be beneficial to damp the nystagmus and improve visual acuity. Nystagmus surgery in the absence of abnormal head posture is controversial.

Surgery for nystagmus blockage syndrome involves recession of the medial rectus muscles, usually with amounts that are slightly larger than normal. This can be combined with posterior fixation sutures to enhance the effect.

For nystagmus patients with strabismus, the surgery must be performed on the dominant fixating eye; surgery on the nondominant eye is adjusted to account for the strabismus. For example, a patient who is right-eye dominant and has a right head turn and left gaze null zone would undergo a right medial rectus recession and right lateral rectus resection in the amounts indicated in Table 12-6. This procedure could lessen or eliminate a coexisting esotropia and would increase an exotropia. Surgery on the nonpreferred eye is tailored to these possibilities.

Hertle RW, Dell'Osso LF, FitzGibbon EJ, et al. Horizontal rectus tenotomy in patients with congenital nystagmus: results in 10 adults. *Ophthalmology*. 2003;110:2097–2105.

Reinecke RD. Costenbader Lecture. Idiopathic infantile nystagmus: diagnosis and treatment. *J AAPOS*. 1997;1:67–82.

Roberts EL, Saunders RA, Wilson ME. Surgery for vertical head position in null point nystagmus. *J Pediatr Ophthalmol Strabismus*. 1996;33:219–224.

Zubcov AA, Stark N, Weber A, et al. Improvement of visual acuity after surgery for nystagmus. *Ophthalmology*. 1993;100:1488–1497.

CHAPTER 13

Surgery of the Extraocular Muscles

Both the experienced and the beginning strabismus surgeon should become familiar with the basic references and surgical atlases given in the following list. The discussion in this chapter does not specifically refer to these works, but the reader should turn to them when additional information is needed. See also Chapters 2 and 3 of this volume.

Burian HM, von Noorden GK. *Burian-von Noorden's Binocular Vision and Ocular Motility: Theory and Management of Strabismus.* 5th ed. St Louis: Mosby; 1996.

Rosenbaum AL, Santiago AP. *Clinical Strabismus Management: Principles and Surgical Techniques.* Philadelphia: Saunders; 1999.

Wright KW. *Color Atlas of Strabismus Surgery: Strabismus.* Irvine, CA: Wright; 2000.

A thorough knowledge of the anatomy of the extraocular muscles and surrounding fascia, along with an understanding of their motor physiology, is essential to planning and executing strabismus surgery. Guided by this knowledge and the use of appropriate surgical technique, the surgeon can help prevent lifelong problems for the patient. The surgeon should also become familiar with the appropriate types of surgical instruments, sutures, and needles used in strabismus surgery. The preceding references are excellent resources for this information.

The history and a detailed motility evaluation (often repeated at a subsequent visit to corroborate the initial findings), in conjunction with a complete ocular examination, provide the information necessary to plan the correct surgery. Evaluation may include sensory testing, forced duction testing, active force generation testing, saccadic velocities, and diplopia visual fields. Preoperative planning must address the patient's and family's expectations, as well as those of the surgeon; risks and complications must be discussed. Such communication is the basis of informed patient consent.

Indications for Surgery

Surgery is performed to improve function, appearance, and well-being. The indications for surgery may be subtle or obvious. Asthenopia, a vague but real sense of ocular fatigue, is common in patients with phorias or intermittent tropias. Occasionally, subconjunctival scar tissue or restricted muscles from prior muscle surgery may warrant additional surgical revision to improve appearance or to relieve mechanical restriction.

Double vision in one or all fields of gaze is often the complaint of patients with adult-onset strabismus, and eliminating diplopia is one of the goals of strabismus surgery.

If some degree of fusion can be achieved, postsurgical ocular alignment will be improved. Alignment of the visual axes can restore stereopsis in some patients or allow the development of a certain amount of stereopsis in others, especially if the preoperative deviation is intermittent or of recent onset.

Some patients assume an abnormal head position to relieve diplopia (eg, with superior oblique or lateral rectus muscle weakness) or to improve vision (eg, with nystagmus and an eccentric null point). Surgical treatment may not only increase the field of useful vision but reduce habitual head posturing. Correcting an abnormal head position or eliminating an ocular deviation can, in turn, improve the patient's self-image and sense of well-being. Strabismus is not a variation of normal; therefore, correcting it is reconstructive rather than cosmetic surgery, even if enhanced fusion is not feasible.

Coats DK, Paysse EA, Towler AJ, et al. Impact of large angle horizontal strabismus on ability to obtain employment. *Ophthalmology.* 2000;107:402–405.

Costello PA, Simon JW, Jia Y, et al. Acquired esotropia: subjective and objective outcomes. *J AAPOS.* 2001;5:193–197.

Satterfield D, Keltner JL, Morrison TL. Psychosocial aspects of strabismus study. *Arch Ophthalmol.* 1993;111:1100–1105.

Surgical Techniques for the Muscles and Tendons

Weakening Procedures

Table 13-1 defines various weakening procedures and describes when each is used.

Strengthening Procedures

To strengthen or enhance the effect of a rectus muscle, surgeons usually use the resection technique:

1. Absorbable sutures are placed at a predetermined distance posterior to the muscle insertion.
2. The muscle anterior to the position of the sutures is excised (resected).
3. The shortened muscle is reattached to the globe at or near the original insertion.

This technique is commonly used on any of the rectus muscles but rarely used to strengthen either of the oblique muscles. For detailed descriptions of the techniques, see the basic references listed at the beginning of the chapter.

A rectus muscle can also be strengthened by *advancing* the insertion nearer the limbus, a technique especially useful if the muscle has been previously recessed. Advancement of a muscle to a position anterior to its original anatomical insertion is rarely performed because the muscle may become visible under the conjunctiva. The anterior half of the superior oblique tendon may be advanced temporally and toward the limbus, in the Harada-Ito procedure, to reduce excyclotorsion in patients with superior oblique muscle paresis.

The *tucking procedure* can be performed on the superior oblique tendon to enhance its effect, especially for superior oblique muscle paresis. However, tucking the superior

Table 13-1 Weakening Procedures Used in Strabismus Surgery

Procedure	Used For
Myotomy: cutting across a muscle *Myectomy:* removing a portion of muscle	Used by some surgeons to weaken the inferior oblique muscles
Marginal myotomy: cutting partway across a muscle, usually following a maximal recession	To weaken a rectus muscle further
Tenotomy: cutting across a tendon *Tenectomy:* removing a portion of tendon	Both used routinely to weaken the superior oblique muscle; recently, silicone spacers have been interposed by some surgeons to control the weakening effect
Recession: removal and reattachment of a muscle (rectus or oblique) so that its insertion is closer to its origin	The standard weakening procedure for rectus muscles
Denervation and extirpation: the ablation of the entire portion of the muscle, along with its nerve supply, within Tenon's capsule	Used only on severely or recurrently overacting inferior oblique muscles
Recession and anteriorization: movement of the muscle's insertion anterior to its original position	Also used only on the inferior oblique muscle, to change its elevation function; particularly useful when an inferior oblique muscle overaction and dissociated vertical deviation (DVD) both exist
Posterior fixation suture (fadenoperation): attachment of a rectus muscle to the sclera 11–18 mm posterior to the insertion using a nonabsorbable suture; this procedure is difficult to perform	Used to weaken a muscle in its field of action by decreasing its mechanical advantage; often used in conjunction with recession; sometimes used in DVD, nystagmus, high AC/A esotropia, and noncomitant strabismus

oblique tendon may produce an iatrogenic Brown syndrome. For step-by-step techniques, see the basic references listed at the beginning of the chapter.

Adjustable Suture Techniques

Adjustable strabismus sutures have been used for many years to improve the outcome of strabismus surgery. Their intended purpose is to increase the likelihood of reaching the desired surgical alignment with 1 operation, thereby decreasing the need for staged operations and reoperations. Adjustable suture techniques do not solve the problem of long-term alignment (or permanence of the surgical results), which depends on the potential for fusion, the establishment of focused and comparable retinal images in both eyes, and the effect of tonic and innervational forces acting on the extraocular muscles. Various types of adjustable suture techniques have been described; several are discussed in the following sections.

Postoperative (2-stage) adjustment

Strabismus surgery is completed in the operating room using externalized sutures and knots so that the position of the muscle can be altered during the postoperative period as needed to obtain alignment.

Operation/reoperation

Strabismus surgery is completed using only short-acting or reversible anesthetic agents and externalized sutures and knots. The patient is examined a short time after surgery and reanesthetized for the final tying or adjustment of the sutures, as indicated by the postoperative evaluation. This method has been used successfully in children. However, because a second general anesthesia is required, the technique offers little advantage over standard nonadjustable surgery with possible reoperation.

Topical anesthesia

The surgery is completed with the patient awake. Drugs that might affect ocular motility are avoided, and the patient's dynamic ocular motility and ocular alignment are observed and adjusted at the time of surgery. This technique requires a cooperative patient and is not appropriate for most patients with significant scarring who need a reoperation, persons with thyroid ophthalmopathy, and almost all children. (Anesthesia is discussed later, under Anesthesia for Extraocular Muscle Surgery.)

Pull-over (stay) sutures

A temporary suture is attached to the limbus and secured to periocular skin to fix the eye in a selected position during postoperative healing. This technique is particularly useful in cases with severely restricted rotations.

Transposition Procedures

Transposition procedures involve moving the extraocular muscles out of their original planes of action. These procedures are generally reserved for treatment of paralytic strabismus, small vertical and horizontal deviations, and A and V patterns. The usual indications for transposition procedures include paralysis of cranial nerves III and VI, as well as monocular elevation deficiency. In specific circumstances, nonabsorbable sutures that secure transposed tendons to the sclera have been particularly useful in augmenting the surgical effect.

Foster RS. Vertical muscle transposition augmented with lateral fixation. *J AAPOS.* 1997;1:20–30.

Rosenbaum AL. Costenbader Lecture. The efficacy of rectus muscle transposition surgery in esotropic Duane syndrome and VI nerve palsy. *J AAPOS.* 2004;8:409–419.

Considerations in Planning Surgery for Strabismus

Incomitance

Deviations that vary in different gaze positions require special alterations in technique to make the postoperative alignment more nearly comitant.

Vertical incomitance

If a horizontal deviation in the primary position is significantly different in upgaze and downgaze, an A or a V pattern is present. Surgical treatment may include surgery on the oblique muscles or displacement (upward or downward) of the horizontal rectus muscles. (See Other Rectus Muscle Surgery later in the chapter.)

Horizontal incomitance

If the deviation in left and right gaze is significantly different from the deviation in primary gaze, a paresis or restriction is likely. In general, restrictive forces must be relieved for surgery to be effective. If there is no restriction, surgical correction, as illustrated in the following example, might be considered:

XT = 20Δ	XT = 30Δ	XT = 40Δ
right gaze	primary position	left gaze

The surgeon might do one of the following:

- Perform a recession of each lateral rectus muscle, the left more than the right, to achieve greater reduction of the exotropia in the field of action of the left lateral rectus (ie, left gaze).
- Perform a greater recession of the left lateral rectus muscle and lesser resection of the left medial rectus muscle than the standard amount to achieve greater effect in left gaze.

Lateral incomitance

Standard amounts of surgery for intermittent exotropia may result in overcorrection if measurements in side gaze are substantially less than in primary position. Consider the following:

XT = 15Δ	XT = 30Δ	XT = 15Δ
right gaze	primary position	left gaze

Some surgeons recommend reducing the amount of recession of each lateral rectus slightly in these patients.

Moore S. The prognostic value of lateral gaze measurements in intermittent exotropia. *Am Orthopt J.* 1969;19:69–71.

Prior Surgery

It is technically easier and therefore preferable to operate on muscles that have not undergone prior surgery. However, each case must be considered individually. In cases of mechanical restriction from excessive resection/scarring, the restrictive forces must be relieved by reoperation on the involved muscle to obtain optimal surgical results. Previous operative reports may be helpful in surgical planning. If retinal detachment surgery has been performed in the past, consultation with the retinal surgeon is advisable. In some cases, it may be preferable to operate on the other eye.

Cyclovertical Strabismus

In many patients with vertical strabismus, the deviation is different in right and left gaze. In some patients, the vertical deviation is different between upgaze to one side and downgaze to that side. In general, surgery should be performed on those muscles whose field of action is in the same field as the greatest vertical deviation. For example, in a patient with a right hypertropia that is greatest down and to the patient's left, the surgeon should strongly consider either strengthening the right superior oblique muscle or weakening the left inferior rectus muscle. If the right hypertropia is the same in left upgaze, straight left, and left downgaze, then any of the four muscles whose greatest vertical action is in left gaze may be chosen for surgery. In this example, the left superior rectus muscle or right superior oblique muscle could be strengthened, or the left inferior rectus muscle or right inferior oblique muscle could be weakened. Larger deviations may require surgery on more than 1 muscle.

Visual Acuity

Most surgeons prefer to avoid surgery on the good eye whenever possible in patients with severe visual loss in the other eye. Surgery is normally delayed until the vision has been made equal or nearly so by whatever means are appropriate, including spectacles and amblyopia therapy.

Simon JW, Dannemann AF, Hampton GR, et al. "Which eye will you be straightening, Doctor?" *J Pediatr Ophthalmol Strabismus.* 1989;26:55.

Guidelines for Strabismus Surgery

Two surgeons are unlikely to perform a specific surgical procedure in exactly the same way. Thus, the amount of dissection, the measurement and placement of sutures in the muscle and sclera, and the placement of the conjunctival incision will vary slightly between surgeons, even when both are following the same surgical table. Nonetheless, the beginning surgeon will find the following guidelines a useful starting point for routine strabismus surgery. Each surgeon must standardize his or her approach by continually reviewing the results and adjusting the amount of surgery to achieve the best possible outcomes. Thus, the surgery should be planned according to the surgeon's own ocular motility measurements and judgment. In addition, each patient's expectations and sensory status should be considered.

Esodeviation

Symmetric surgery

The amounts of medial rectus recession often performed in each eye of patients with specified deviations are given in Table 13-2. Some surgeons advocate medial rectus muscle recessions of 6.5–7.0 mm for 60Δ–80Δ of esotropia; others avoid these very large recessions and favor operating on 3 or 4 muscles for large angles.

Monocular recess-resect procedures

The same figures given in Table 13-2 may be used in monocular recess-resect procedures, with the surgeon selecting the appropriate number of millimeters for each muscle, as shown in Table 13-3. For example, for an esotropia of 30Δ, the surgeon would recess the medial rectus muscle 4.5 mm and resect the lateral rectus muscle 7.0 mm.

Exodeviation

Symmetric surgery

The surgical guidelines for exodeviation are listed in Table 13-4. Some surgeons advocate bilateral lateral rectus muscle recessions of 9.0 mm or greater for deviations larger than 45Δ. Others advocate surgery on a third muscle for large-angle exotropias.

Monocular recess-resect procedures

As with esodeviations, the surgical table can be used for monocular procedures as well as for symmetric surgery, with the surgeon reading across according to the angle of deviation (Table 13-5). For example, for an exodeviation of 15Δ, the surgeon would recess the lateral rectus muscle 4.0 mm and resect the antagonist medial rectus muscle 3.0 mm. Monocular surgery of large-angle exotropia is likely to result in a limitation of abduction.

Value of immediate overcorrection in exodeviation

The surgical dosages listed in Table 13-4 for bilateral lateral rectus recessions tend to produce a small overcorrection of exotropia in the early postoperative period. Available evidence suggests that a small temporary esotropia during the first few days or weeks

Table 13-2 Symmetric Surgery for Esodeviation

Angle of Esotropia	Recess MR OU	or	Resect LR OU
15Δ	3.0 mm		4.0 mm
20Δ	3.5 mm		5.0 mm
25Δ	4.0 mm		6.0 mm
30Δ	4.5 mm		7.0 mm
35Δ	5.0 mm		8.0 mm
40Δ	5.5 mm		9.0 mm
50Δ	6.0 mm		9.0 mm

Table 13-3 Monocular Recess-Resect Procedures for Esodeviation

Angle of Esotropia	Recess MR	and	Resect LR
15Δ	3.0 mm		4.0 mm
20Δ	3.5 mm		5.0 mm
25Δ	4.0 mm		6.0 mm
30Δ	4.5 mm		7.0 mm
35Δ	5.0 mm		8.0 mm
40Δ	5.5 mm		9.0 mm
50Δ	6.0 mm		9.0 mm

Table 13-4 Symmetric Surgery for Exodeviation

Angle of Exotropia	Recess LR OU	or	Resect MR OU
15Δ	4.0 mm		3.0 mm
20Δ	5.0 mm		4.0 mm
25Δ	6.0 mm		5.0 mm
30Δ	7.0 mm		6.0 mm
40Δ	8.0 mm		6.0 mm

after surgery may yield the most favorable long-term result. Many patients have diplopia during the time they are esotropic, and they should be advised of this possibility.

Raab EL, Parks MM. Recession of the lateral recti. Early and late postoperative alignments. *Arch Ophthalmol.* 1969;82:203–208.

Oblique Muscle-Weakening Procedures

Weakening the inferior oblique muscle

In cases that show a marked asymmetry of the overactions of the inferior oblique muscles with no superior oblique muscle paresis, unilateral surgery on the muscle with the most marked overaction is often followed by a significant degree of overaction in the fellow eye. Therefore, some surgeons recommend bilateral inferior oblique–weakening procedures for asymmetric cases. A good symmetric result is the rule, and overcorrections are rare. Inferior oblique muscles that are not overacting should not undergo a surgical weakening procedure.

Secondary overaction of the inferior oblique muscle occurs in some patients who have superior oblique muscle paresis. In this situation, the greatest vertical deviation appears in the field of action of the ipsilateral inferior oblique muscle. A weakening of that inferior oblique muscle could be expected to correct up to 15Δ of vertical deviation in primary position. The amount of vertical correction is roughly proportional to the degree of preoperative overaction (see Chapter 10). Frequently, a weakening procedure is performed on each inferior oblique muscle for V-pattern strabismus. Such surgery can be expected to cause 15Δ or more of eso shift in upgaze (decrease of an exodeviation or increase of an esodeviation), but it has almost no effect on primary position or downgaze.

Goldchmit M, Felberg S, Souza-Dias C. Unilateral anterior transposition of the inferior oblique muscle for correction of hypertropia in primary position. *J AAPOS.* 2003;7:241–243.

Stager DR. Costenbader Lecture. Anatomy and surgery of the inferior oblique muscle: recent findings. *J AAPOS.* 2001;5:203–208.

Stager DR Jr, Wang X, Stager DR Sr, et al. Nasal myectomy of the inferior oblique muscles for recurrent elevation in adduction. *J AAPOS.* 2004;8:462–465.

Weakening the superior oblique muscle

Procedures to weaken the superior oblique include tenotomy, tenectomy, z-lengthening, insertion of silicone spacers or nonabsorbable sutures, and recession. Unilateral weakening of a superior oblique muscle is not commonly performed except as part of the treatment

Table 13-5 Monocular Recess-Resect Procedures for Exodeviation

Angle of Exotropia	Recess LR	and	Resect MR
15Δ	4.0 mm		3.0 mm
20Δ	5.0 mm		4.0 mm
25Δ	6.0 mm		5.0 mm
30Δ	7.0 mm		6.0 mm
40Δ	8.0 mm		6.0 mm
50Δ	9.0 mm		7.0 mm
60Δ	10.0 mm		8.0 mm
70Δ	10.0 mm		9.0 mm
80Δ	10.0 mm		10.0 mm

for Brown syndrome (see also the discussion of Brown syndrome in Chapter 10). This procedure may also be performed for an isolated inferior oblique muscle weakness, which is rare.

Bilateral weakening of the superior oblique muscle is often performed, with or without horizontal muscle surgery, for A-pattern deviations. This surgery can be expected to cause an eso shift of up to 30Δ–40Δ in downgaze, little change in primary position, and almost no change in upgaze. In surgery on patients with normal binocularity, the possibility of creating diplopia from vertical or torsional strabismus must be considered.

Vertical Rectus Muscle Surgery for Hypotropia and Hypertropia

Because vertical deviations have many causes (eg, cyclovertical muscle palsy, mechanical restriction), no single approach for surgical correction can be recommended for all situations. Surgical planning must be individualized according to suspected cause and size of deviation. For comitant vertical deviations, recession and resection of vertical rectus muscles is frequently advocated. Recession of the inferior rectus in the hypotropic eye with recession of the superior rectus in the hypertropic eye has the advantage of changing the alignment symmetrically on up- and downgaze, as well as on left and right gaze. The atlases cited at the beginning of the chapter offer more specific guidance concerning selection of muscles and determination of the size of the recession or resection.

Dissociated vertical deviation

When treatment of dissociated vertical deviation is indicated, one of several surgical methods can be used. A recession of the superior rectus muscle, possibly on a "hang-back" suture of 6–10 mm, is considered effective. Bilateral, perhaps asymmetric, superior rectus muscle recession may be indicated whenever either eye can fixate. If only one eye can fixate, unilateral surgery is possible. Resection of the inferior rectus muscle for dissociated vertical deviation ranges from 4 mm for small-angle deviations to 8 mm for large-angle deviations. This technique may advance the lower eyelid, especially if careful dissection is not performed. Some surgeons favor the fadenoperation, or posterior fixation suture on the superior rectus muscle(s), often combined with recession.

Recessing the inferior oblique muscle and moving its insertion anteriorly to a point adjacent to the lateral border of the inferior rectus has been found effective in reducing or eliminating dissociated vertical deviation; the mechanical tethering/depressing effect is important. This procedure is especially useful when a patient has both dissociated vertical deviation and a component of inferior oblique overaction.

Elliott RL, Nankin SJ. Anterior transposition of the inferior oblique. *J Pediatr Ophthalmol Strabismus.* 1981;18:35–38.

Other Rectus Muscle Surgery

Vertical displacement of the horizontal rectus muscles for A and V patterns

Vertical displacement of 2 horizontal rectus muscles (one-half tendon width) produces about 15Δ of additional weakening of those muscles in the direction of gaze at which they are displaced. The muscles should thus be displaced in the direction of the desired additional weakening effect, whether the muscles were weakened or strengthened. The medial rectus muscle should be moved toward the apex of the A or V pattern (up in A pattern, down in V pattern). The lateral rectus muscle should be moved toward the open end of the A (down) or V (up). This guideline applies whether surgery is performed on 1 or both eyes. For example, a patient with a V-pattern exotropia might undergo recession of both lateral recti with upward transposition or a recession of 1 lateral rectus with upward transposition, along with a resection of the ipsilateral medial rectus with downward transposition.

Knapp P. A and V patterns. In: Burian HM, ed. *Symposium on Strabismus: transactions of the New Orleans Academy of Ophthalmology.* St Louis: Mosby; 1971:242–254.

Metz HS, Schwartz L. The treatment of A and V patterns by monocular surgery. *Arch Ophthalmol.* 1977;95:251–253.

Lateral rectus muscle paralysis

The treatment of lateral rectus muscle paralysis varies according to the degree of weakness of the lateral rectus muscle and the degree of contracture of the antagonist ipsilateral medial rectus muscle. Apart from the use of botulinum toxin, there are basically 2 treatment options:

1. resection of the lateral rectus muscle with recession of the ipsilateral medial rectus muscle (recess-resect procedure)
2. transposition of the vertical recti, perhaps with recession of the ipsilateral medial rectus muscle

Transposition procedures are more effective than recess-resect surgery in cases with severe paralysis, but anterior segment ischemia may be a risk, especially if medial rectus recession is added (see Anterior Segment Ischemia later in this chapter). Some surgeons prefer to isolate and preserve the ciliary vessels; others avoid simultaneous surgery on the medial rectus. Options to be considered include augmenting the effect of the transposition by resecting the transposed muscles or attaching them to the sclera along the border of the lateral rectus muscle, 16 mm posterior to the limbus. Another option is botulinum injection of the medial rectus.

Brooks SE. Transposition procedures. *Focal Points: Clinical Modules for Ophthalmologists.* San Francisco: American Academy of Ophthalmology; 2001, module 10.

Brooks SE, Olitsky SE, deB Ribeiro G. Augmented Hummelsheim procedure for paralytic strabismus. *J Pediatr Ophthalmol Strabismus.* 2000;37:189–195.

Foster RS. Vertical muscle transposition augmented with lateral fixation. *J AAPOS.* 1997;1:20–30.

McKeown CA, Lambert HM, Shore JW. Preservation of the anterior ciliary vessels during extraocular muscle surgery. *Ophthalmology.* 1989;96:498–506.

Anesthesia for Extraocular Muscle Surgery

Topical anesthetic drops alone (eg, tetracaine 0.5%, proparacaine 0.5%, cocaine 4%) can be used effectively in cooperative patients for certain procedures. Lid blocks are not necessary if the eyelid speculum is not spread to the point of causing pain. Topical anesthesia is effective for making incisions in the conjunctiva and Tenon's capsule, placing sutures into the muscle, and disinserting the muscle from the globe. Such anesthesia is not effective in controlling the pain produced by pulling on or against a muscle. Topical anesthesia is effective for simple recession procedures but is not as effective for resection procedures or for recession procedures involving restricted muscles or difficult exposure.

Both local infiltration (peribulbar) and retrobulbar anesthesia make most extraocular muscle procedures pain-free. Such anesthesia should be considered in adults for whom general anesthesia may pose an undue hazard. The administration of a short-acting hypnotic by an anesthesiologist just before retrobulbar injection greatly improves patient comfort. Because injected anesthesia may influence alignment during the first few hours after surgery, suture adjustment is best delayed for at least half a day following the surgery.

General anesthesia is necessary for children and is frequently used for adults as well, particularly those requiring bilateral surgery. Neuromuscular blocking agents such as succinylcholine, which are often administered to facilitate intubation for general anesthesia, can temporarily affect the results of a traction test. Today, laryngeal mask airways are often used, avoiding the need for intubation.

France NK, France TD, Woodburn JD Jr, et al. Succinylcholine alteration of the forced duction test. *Ophthalmology.* 1980;87:1282–1287.

Conjunctival Incisions

Fornix Incision

The fornix incision is made in either the superior or (more frequently) the inferior oblique quadrants. The incision is located on bulbar conjunctiva, not actually in the fornix, 1–2 mm to the limbal side of the cul-de-sac. The incision is parallel to the fornix and approximately 8 mm in length. It begins from an imaginary line dropped into the cul-de-sac from the mid-cornea and extends either nasally or temporally. It is usually possible to avoid making 2 contiguous incisions, which tend to become connected. All 6 extraocular muscles can be approached, if necessary, through an inferotemporal and a superonasal conjunctival incision.

Bare sclera is exposed by incising Tenon's capsule perpendicular to the conjunctival incision in its midportion. The muscle is engaged from this bare scleral exposure using a succession of muscle hooks. The conjunctival incision is pulled or stretched over the point of the hook that has passed under the muscle belly.

When properly placed, the 2-plane incision can be self-closed by gently massaging the conjunctiva into the fornix. Some surgeons prefer to close the incision with conjunctival sutures.

Parks MM. Fornix incision for horizontal rectus muscle surgery. *Am J Ophthalmol.* 1968;65: 907–915.

Limbal or Peritomy Incision

The initial incision through conjunctiva and Tenon's capsule to the sclera is made in an oblique quadrant, close to and radial to the limbus, on the side of the eye nearest the muscle. The combined layer of conjunctiva and Tenon's capsule is then cleanly severed from the limbus. A second, short radial incision is made at the other end of the peritomy so that the combined conjunctiva/Tenon's capsule flap can be retracted to expose the muscle for surgery. At the completion of surgery, the flap is reattached to its original position with a single suture in each corner. If the conjunctiva is tight, contributing to a restriction of motility, it can be recessed at the end of surgery.

von Noorden GK. The limbal approach to surgery of the rectus muscles. *Arch Ophthalmol.* 1968;80:94–97.

Complications of Strabismus Surgery

Unsatisfactory Alignment

The most common complication of surgery for strabismus is unsatisfactory postoperative alignment. With the guidelines in the preceding sections, undercorrections are more common than overcorrections. In some cases, it is apparent to both the patient and the surgeon in the immediate postoperative period that the alignment is not satisfactory. Even satisfactory initial alignment may not be permanent, however. Among the reasons for this unpredictability are poor fusion, poor vision, altered accommodation, and contracture of scar tissue. In many patients, the cause of the unstable alignment is unknown. Reoperations are often necessary.

Refractive Changes

Changes in refractive error are most common when strabismus surgery is performed on 2 rectus muscles of 1 eye. An induced with-the-rule astigmatism of low magnitude usually resolves within several months.

Thompson WE, Reinecke RD. The changes in refractive status following routine strabismus surgery. *J Pediatr Ophthalmol Strabismus.* 1980;17:372–374.

Diplopia

Diplopia occasionally occurs following strabismus surgery in older children and, especially, in adults. The surgery can move the image of the object of regard in the deviating eye out of a suppression scotoma. In the hours to several months following surgery, various responses are possible:

- Fusion of the 2 images can occur, obviating the need for a suppression scotoma.
- A new suppression scotoma may form, which corresponds to the new angle of alignment.
- Diplopia may persist.

If the initial strabismus was acquired before age 10, the ability to suppress is generally well developed, and a new suppression scotoma can usually be established to match the postoperative alignment, especially on the same side of the midline. Prolonged postoperative diplopia is, therefore, uncommon unless the patient's strabismus is overcorrected. If strabismus was first acquired in adulthood, however, the diplopia that was symptomatic before surgery is likely to persist unless fusion is regained. Prisms may be helpful in preoperatively assessing the fusion potential and the risk of bothersome postoperative diplopia.

Further treatment is indicated for patients, mainly adults, whose symptomatic diplopia persists more than 3–4 weeks following surgery, especially if it is severe and in the primary position. Patients with unequal visual acuities can frequently be taught to ignore the dimmer, fuzzier, nondominant image by closing the nondominant eye intermittently. If vision is equal or nearly so, temporary prisms should be tried, generally with the full correction in a single prism over the nonpreferred eye, tilted to correct both vertical and horizontal deviations. If diplopia is eliminated, gradually decreasing the prisms or replacing them with permanent ground-in prism split between both eyes may provide long-term relief. If this approach fails, additional surgery or botulinum toxin injection may be needed (see Chapter 14).

Perforation of the Sclera

A needle may perforate into the suprachoroidal space or through the choroid and retina. In most cases, this perforation creates no problem other than a chorioretinal scar. Indeed, most perforations are probably unrecognized. However, perforation can lead to vitreous hemorrhage, retinal detachment, or endophthalmitis (Fig 13-1). Presumably, perforation of the sclera with a suture pass provides access for infection within the globe. Periodic fundus examination is advised, with further treatment as indicated. Prophylactic topical antibiotics are generally used during the immediate postoperative period.

Awad AH, Mullaney PB, Al-Hazmi A, et al. Recognized globe perforation during strabismus surgery: incidence, risk factors, and sequelae. *J AAPOS.* 2000;4:150–153.

Dang Y, Racu C, Isenberg SJ. Scleral penetrations and perforations in strabismus surgery and associated risk factors. *J AAPOS.* 2004;8:325–332.

Postoperative Infections

Serious infection is uncommon following strabismus surgery. Some patients develop mild conjunctivitis, which may be caused by allergy to suture material or postoperative medications, as well as by infectious agents. Preseptal or orbital cellulitis with proptosis, eyelid swelling, chemosis, and fever are also rare complications of strabismus surgery (Fig 13-2).

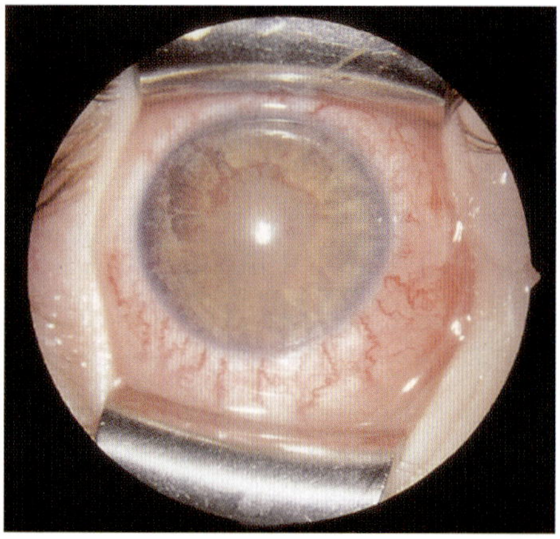

Figure 13-1 Endophthalmitis following muscle surgery of the right eye. Although rare, this complication can occur following scleral perforation.

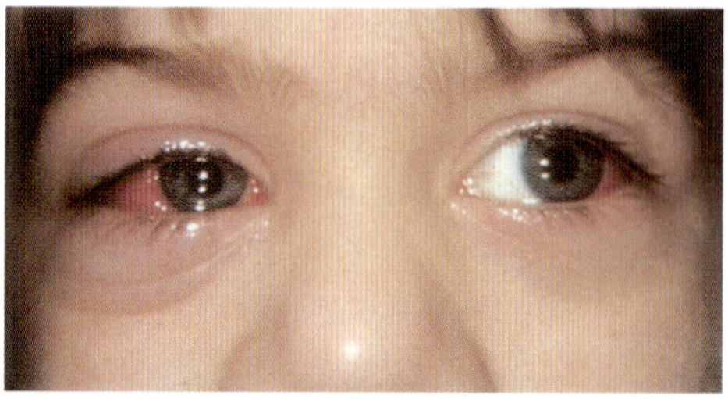

Figure 13-2 Orbital cellulitis, right eye, 2 days after bilateral recession of lateral rectus muscles. Typically noted 2 or 3 days postoperatively, the infection usually responds quickly to antibiotics, especially if given parenterally.

These conditions usually develop 2–3 days after surgery and generally respond well to systemic (especially parenteral) antibiotics. As noted earlier, frank endophthalmitis has also been reported after strabismus surgery, which is identical to endophthalmitis following other types of ophthalmic surgery in its presentation, diagnosis, and treatment. Patients should be warned of the signs and symptoms of orbital cellulitis and endophthalmitis prior to discharge so they will seek emergency consultation if those signs or symptoms develop.

Kivlin JD, Wilson ME Jr. Periocular infection after strabismus surgery. Periocular Infection Study Group. *J Pediatr Ophthalmol Strabismus.* 1995;32:42–49.

Recchia FM, Baumal CR, Sivalingam A, et al. Endophthalmitis after pediatric strabismus surgery. *Arch Ophthalmol.* 2000;118:939–944.

Foreign-Body Granuloma and Allergic Reaction

Occasionally, a foreign-body granuloma develops several weeks after surgery, often at the suture site. The granuloma is characterized by a localized, elevated, slightly hyperemic, slightly tender mass, usually less than 1 cm in diameter. The granuloma may respond to topical corticosteroids. Surgical excision may be necessary if the granuloma persists (Fig 13-3). Some suture materials may incite a vigorous allergic reaction, but such reactions are rare today because gut suture has largely been replaced in strabismus surgery (Fig 13-4).

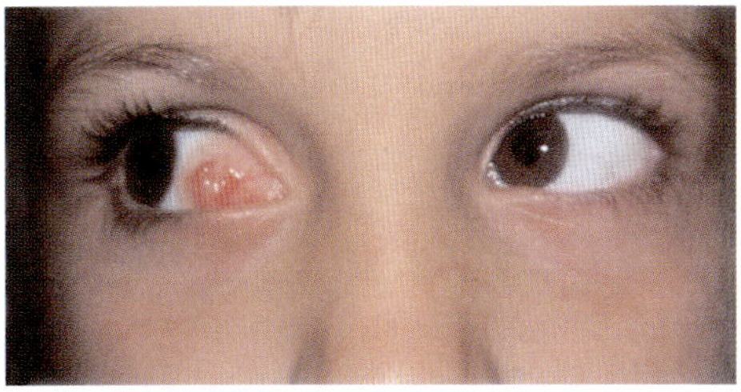

Figure 13-3 Severe postoperative granuloma over the right medial rectus persists 1 year after medial rectus recessions OU.

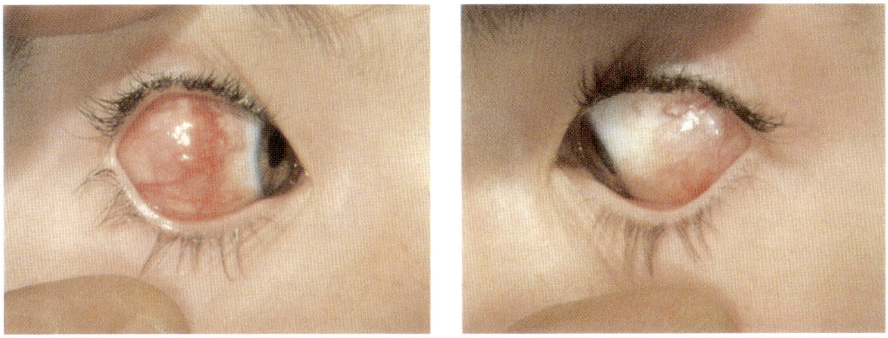

Figure 13-4 Chromic gut was used in the right eye *(left)* and polyglycolic acid suture in the left eye *(right)*. Right eye shows a severe allergic reaction 3 weeks postoperatively.

Conjunctival Inclusion Cyst

If any conjunctival epithelium is buried during muscle reattachment or closure of the incision, a conjunctival cyst may appear (Fig 13-5). This noninflamed translucent mass under the conjunctiva appears several days to several years after surgery. Topical steroids may be helpful, although persistent cases may require surgical excision.

Conjunctival Scarring

Improved alignment may occasionally be overshadowed by unsightly scarring of the conjunctiva and Tenon's capsule. The tissues may remain hyperemic or salmon pink instead of returning to their usual whiteness. This complication may result from the following factors:

- *Advancement of thickened Tenon's capsule too close to the limbus.* In resection procedures, pulling the muscle forward may advance into view the thicker Tenon's capsule that normally lies over and between the muscles. This situation is especially likely in reoperations, when the Tenon's capsule around and anterior to the insertion may be hypertrophied.
- *Advancement of the plica semilunaris onto bulbar conjunctiva.* In surgery on the medial rectus muscle using the limbal approach, the surgeon sometimes mistakes the plica semilunaris for a conjunctival edge and incorporates it or a portion of it into the closure. Although not strictly a conjunctival scar, the plica semilunaris,

now pulled forward over bulbar conjunctiva, retains its normal fleshy color long after the remainder of the conjunctiva has returned to its normal color (Fig 13-6). A restrictive esotropia is also likely.

Adherence Syndrome

Violation of Tenon's capsule with prolapse of orbital fat into the sub–Tenon's space can cause formation of a pink fibrofatty scar of the muscle and globe, which may restrict motility. If an inadvertent rent in Tenon's capsule is recognized at the time of surgery, the prolapsed fat can be excised and the rent can be closed with absorbable sutures. Otherwise, the prognosis for normal motility is poor. Meticulous surgical technique usually prevents this serious complication.

Dellen

The term *dellen* (*delle*, singular), derived from the German word for "dents," refers to shallow depressions or corneal thinning just anterior to the limbus. Dellen occur when raised abnormal tissue on the bulbar conjunctiva prevents the eyelid from adequately resurfacing the cornea with tears during blinking (Fig 13-7). Fluorescein pools in these depressions but does not stain the stroma. Dellen occasionally occur when the limbal

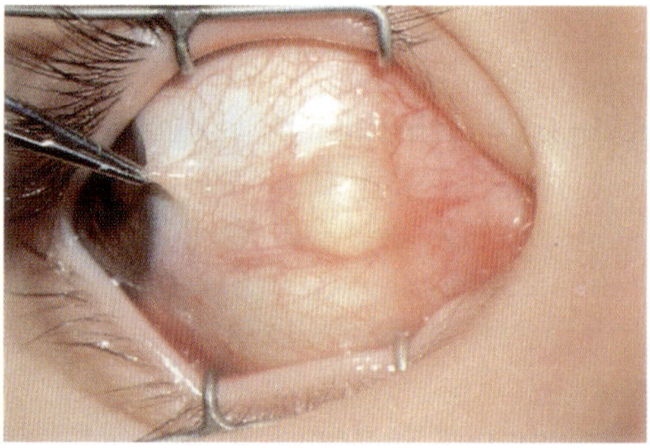

Figure 13-5 Postoperative conjunctival epithelial inclusion cyst following right medial rectus recession using fornix incision technique.

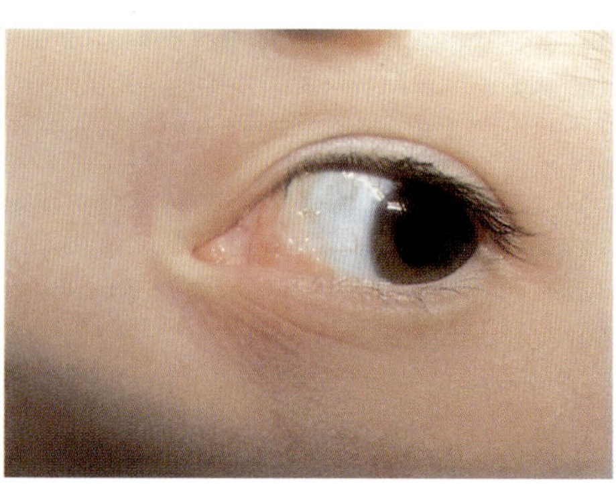

Figure 13-6 Involvement of plica semilunaris incision.

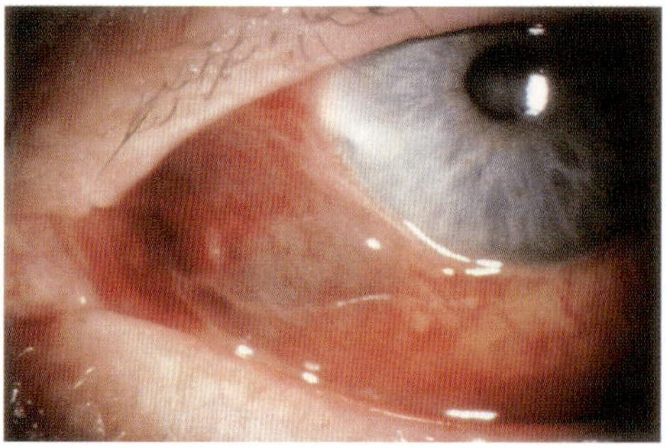

Figure 13-7 Corneal delle subsequent to postoperative subconjunctival hemorrhage.

approach to muscle surgery is used. They cause mild discomfort and should be followed carefully. Artificial tears or lubricants may be needed until the chemosis and conjunctival hemorrhage subside. Patching of the eye may be helpful.

Anterior Segment Ischemia

Most of the blood supply to the anterior segment of the eye comes through the anterior ciliary arteries that travel in the 4 rectus muscles. Simultaneous surgery on 3 of these rectus muscles, or even 2 of them in patients with poor blood flow, may lead to anterior segment ischemia. The earliest sign of this complication is cell and flare in the anterior chamber. More severe cases are characterized by corneal epithelial edema, folds in Descemet's membrane, and other signs of anterior uveitis (Fig 13-8). If severe, the complication may lead to anterior segment necrosis and phthisis bulbi. Treatment is directed at the anterior uveitis, which often responds to frequent administration of topical, subconjunctival, or systemic steroids.

It may be possible to recess or resect a rectus muscle while sparing its anterior ciliary vessels by using an operating microscope and vitrectomy microinstruments. Although difficult and time-consuming, this technique may be indicated in high-risk cases. Staging surgeries, with surgery on the third muscle performed several months after the first procedure, may also be helpful.

Saunders RA, Bluestein EC, Wilson ME, et al. Anterior segment ischemia after strabismus surgery. *Surv Ophthalmol.* 1994;38:456–466.

Change in Eyelid Position

Change in the position of the eyelids is most likely with surgery on the vertical rectus muscles. Pulling the inferior rectus muscle forward, as in a resection, pulls the lower eyelid up over the lower limbus; recessing the muscle pulls the lower eyelid down, exposing bare sclera below the lower limbus (Figs 13-9, 13-10). Surgery on the superior rectus muscle is somewhat less likely to affect the upper eyelid position.

Eyelid position changes can be obviated somewhat by careful dissection. In general, all intermuscular septum and fascial connections of the operated vertical rectus muscle must be severed at least 12–15 mm posterior to the muscle insertion (to the point at which the muscle disappears through Tenon's capsule). Some surgeons have advocated

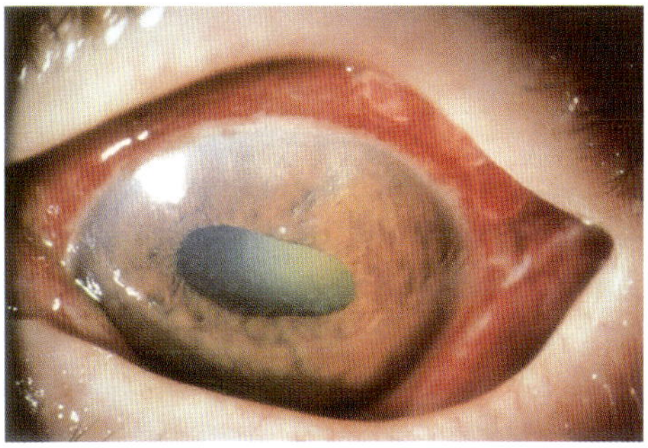

Figure 13-8 Superotemporal segmental anterior segment ischemia after simultaneous superior rectus muscle and lateral rectus muscle surgery following scleral buckling procedure.

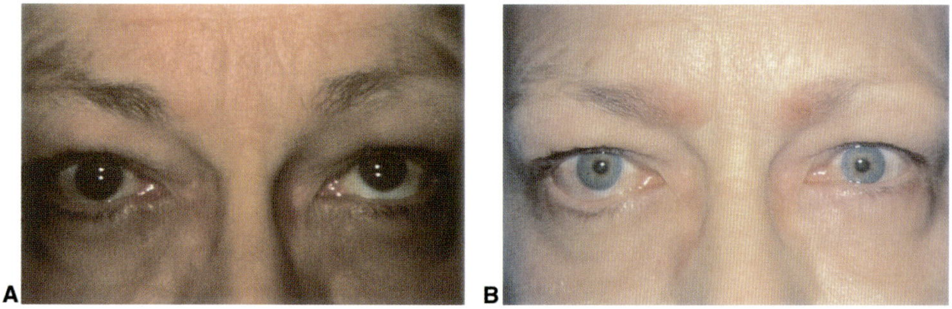

Figure 13-9 **A,** Preoperative photograph of patient who underwent recession of the right inferior rectus muscle, which pulled the right lower eyelid down, and a resection of the left inferior rectus muscle, which pulled the left lower eyelid up, causing postoperative asymmetry. **B,** Postoperative photograph.

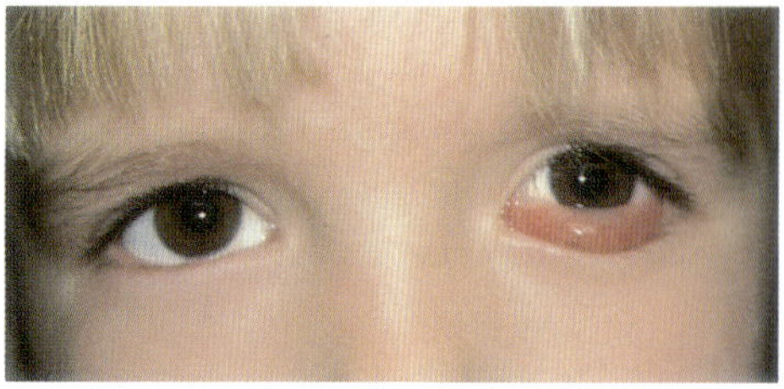

Figure 13-10 One year after resection of the left inferior rectus muscle, which caused the left lower eyelid to be pulled up and the conjunctiva to prolapse.

release of the lower eyelid retractors or advancement of the capsulopalpebral head to prevent lower eyelid retraction after inferior rectus muscle recession.

Kim DB, Meyer DR, Simon JW. Retractor lysis as prophylaxis for lower lid retraction following inferior rectus recession. *J Pediatr Ophthalmol Strabismus.* 2002;39:198–202.

Lost Muscle

After a muscle is freed from its insertion, it sometimes slips out of the sutures or surgical instruments and is lost posteriorly in the orbit. The problem is most severe with the medial rectus, especially after a resection. The surgeon should immediately make every attempt to find the lost muscle. It is important to realize that a lost or retracted muscle usually does not remain next to the globe posterior to the equator but instead retracts into Tenon's capsule along the orbital wall. Generally, pulling Tenon's capsule forward in a "hand-over-hand" fashion brings the muscle into view. Malleable retractors and a headlight may be helpful. Care must be taken not to violate Tenon's capsule, in which case fibrofatty proliferation can occur (see the earlier discussion, Adherence Syndrome). When the diagnosis is made in the immediate postoperative period, the patient should be promptly returned to surgery for exploration and attempted retrieval of the lost muscle by a surgeon experienced with this potentially complex surgery. Muscle transposition surgery may be required if the lost muscle is not found, although anterior segment ischemia may be a risk.

Slipped Muscle

Occasionally, an inadequately sutured muscle slips posteriorly within the muscle capsule during the postoperative period. Clinically, the patient manifests a weakness of that muscle, with limited rotations and decreased saccades in its field of action. Surgery should be performed as soon as possible in order to replace the slipped muscle before further retraction and contracture take place. This problem can be prevented by adequately securing the muscle prior to tenotomy with full-thickness lock bites to include muscle tissue and not just capsule (Fig 13-11).

Plager DA, Parks MM. Recognition and repair of the "lost" rectus muscle. A report of 25 cases. *Ophthalmology.* 1990;97:131–137.

Plager DA, Parks MM. Recognition and repair of the slipped rectus muscle. *J Pediatr Ophthalmol Strabismus.* 1988;25:270–274.

Postoperative Nausea and Vomiting

Nausea and vomiting are common following eye muscle surgery. The incidence and severity can be reduced using newer anesthetic agents and antiemetics.

Oculocardiac Reflex

The oculocardiac reflex is a slowing of the heart rate caused by traction on the extraocular muscles. In its most severe form, the reflex can produce asystole. The surgeon should be aware of the possibility of inducing the oculocardiac reflex when manipulating a muscle and should be prepared to release tension if the heart rate drops excessively. Intravenous atropine and other agents can protect against this reflex.

Malignant Hyperthermia

Malignant hyperthermia (MH) is an acute metabolic disorder that can be fatal if diagnosis and treatment are delayed. In its fully developed form, MH is characterized by extreme heat production. MH may be triggered by many inhalational anesthetics, by the muscle relaxant succinylcholine, and by local anesthetics of the amide type. MH is a disorder of calcium binding by the sarcoplasmic reticulum of skeletal muscle. In the presence of an anesthetic triggering agent, unbound intracellular calcium increases, stimulating muscle contracture. As this increased metabolism outstrips oxygen delivery, anaerobic metabolism develops with lactate production and massive acidosis. Hyperthermia results from

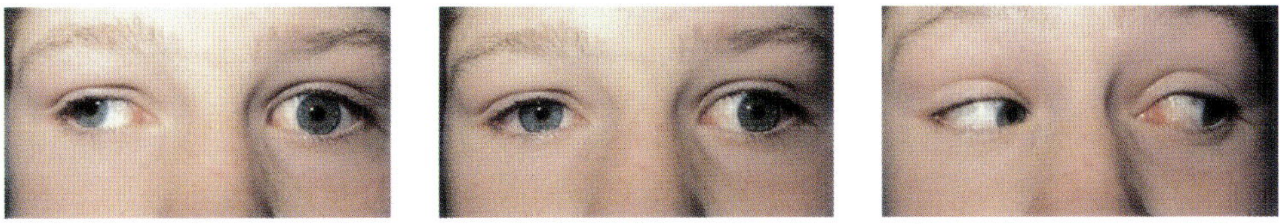

Figure 13-11 Slipped left medial rectus muscle. **Left,** Gaze right shows widening of palpebral fissure of left eye and inability to adduct. **Middle,** Exotropia in primary position with widened palpebral fissure. **Right,** Gaze left shows full abduction with normal width of fissure.

the hypermetabolic state. As cells are depleted of adenosine triphosphate, cell breakdown occurs with loss of potassium and myoglobin. MH can occur as an isolated case or as a dominantly inherited disorder with incomplete penetrance. Other disorders associated with MH include strabismus, myopathies, ptosis, and other musculoskeletal abnormalities. The incidence is variously reported as between 1:6000 and 1:60,000 and is thought to be higher in children. MH occurs in all age groups. Although the mortality rate used to be as high as 70%, today, with modern treatment, it is probably lower than 10%.

Diagnosis

The diagnosis of MH is based on clinical signs and may be confirmed by laboratory studies. Muscle biopsy with in vitro halothane and caffeine contraction testing is the most specific method to confirm the clinical diagnosis. When the diagnosis is unconfirmed but the personal or family history is suspicious for MH, susceptibility testing may be warranted. If testing is not available, non-triggering anesthetic agents should be used and the patient treated as if MH is possible.

Clinical picture

Frequently, the earliest sign of MH is tachycardia that is greater than expected for the patient's anesthetic and surgical status. If the patient is being monitored with capnography, elevated end-tidal carbon dioxide may be the presenting sign. Other arrhythmias may also occur, as can unstable blood pressure. Other early signs include tachypnea, sweating, muscle rigidity, blotchy discoloration of the skin, cyanosis, and dark urine. Onset may be manifested during the induction of anesthesia by trismus caused by masseter muscle spasm, although the significance of masseter spasm is controversial. Most of these patients do not develop MH, but they should be observed closely. A later sign is a rise in temperature, which may reach extremely high levels. Other later signs include respiratory and metabolic acidosis, hyperkalemia, hypercalcemia, myoglobinuria and renal failure, skeletal muscle swelling, heart failure, disseminated intravascular coagulation, and cardiac arrest. Ideally, MH should be diagnosed and treated before the temperature rises significantly. Survival is greatly improved when treatment begins early.

Treatment

Early treatment of unexpected cases of MH cannot be overemphasized. Table 13-6 gives the protocol for this treatment. Once the condition is recognized, anesthetic agents should be discontinued, hyperventilation with oxygen started, and treatment with intravenous dantrolene begun. Dantrolene works to prevent release of calcium from the sarcoplasmic reticulum, preventing the excessive contractile response of muscle. Surgery should be terminated as soon as possible, even if incomplete. Temperature monitoring should be established, along with an intra-arterial catheter for the monitoring of blood pressure and arterial blood gases. Electrolytes, electrocardiograms, urine output, prothrombin time, partial thromboplastin time, fibrinogen, and pulse oximetry should also be monitored. Central venous or pulmonary artery pressure may be monitored if indicated by the patient's condition.

Table 13-6 Malignant Hyperthermia Protocol

1. Stop the triggering agents immediately and conclude surgery as soon as possible.
2. Hyperventilate with 100% oxygen at high flow rates.
3. Administer
   a. Dantrolene: 2–3 mg/kg initial bolus with increments up to 10 mg/kg total. Continue to administer dantrolene until symptoms are controlled. Occasionally, a dose greater than 10 mg/kg may be needed.
   b. Sodium bicarbonate: 1–2 mEq/kg increments guided by arterial pH and pCO_2. Bicarbonate will combat hyperkalemia by driving potassium into cells.
4. Actively cool patient:
   a. If needed, IV iced saline (not Ringer's lactate) 15 mL/kg q 10 minutes × 3. Monitor closely.
   b. Lavage stomach, bladder, rectum, and peritoneal and thoracic cavities with iced saline.
   c. Surface cool with ice and hypothermia blanket.
5. Maintain urine output. If needed, administer mannitol 0.25 gm/kg IV, furosemide 1 mg/kg IV (up to 4 doses each). Urine output greater than 2 mL/kg/hr may help prevent subsequent renal failure.
6. Calcium channel blockers *should not* be given when dantrolene is administered because hyperkalemia and myocardial depression may occur.
7. Insulin for hyperkalemia. Add 10 units of regular insulin to 50 mL of 50% glucose and titrate to control hyperkalemia. Monitor blood glucose and potassium levels.
8. Postoperatively: Continue dantrolene 1 mg/kg IV q6h × 72 hours to prevent recurrence. Lethal recurrences of MH may occur. Observe in an intensive care unit.
9. For expert medical advice and further medical evaluation, call the MHAUS MH Hotline consultant at (800) 644-9737. For nonemergency professional or patient information, call (800) 986-4287. E-mail address is info@mhaus.org; Internet address is mhaus.org.

CHAPTER 14

Chemodenervation Treatment of Strabismus and Blepharospasm Using Botulinum Toxin

Pharmacology and Mechanism of Action

Botox (purified botulinum toxin A) is a protein drug produced by the bacterium *Clostridium botulinum*. For patients with strabismus or blepharospasm, the toxin is injected directly into selected extraocular muscles or into the orbicularis muscle, localized with a portable electromyographic device. Following injection, botulinum toxin is bound and internalized in 24–48 hours within local motor nerve terminals, where it remains for many weeks to interfere with the release of acetylcholine. Paralysis of the injected muscle begins within 2–4 days after injection and lasts clinically for at least 5–8 weeks in the extraocular muscle and for 3 or more months in the orbicularis muscle. An extraocular muscle lengthens while it is paralyzed by botulinum, and its antagonist contracts. These changes may produce long-term improvement in the alignment of the eyes.

Indications, Techniques, and Results

Clinical trials have shown botulinum to be most effective when used in the following conditions:

- small- to moderate-angle esotropia and exotropia (<40Δ)
- postoperative residual strabismus (2–8 weeks following surgery or later)
- acute paralytic strabismus (especially sixth nerve palsy) to eliminate diplopia while the palsy recovers
- cyclic esotropia
- active thyroid ophthalmopathy (Graves disease) or inflamed or prephthisical eyes, when surgery is inappropriate

Studies have shown this treatment to be disappointing in patients with large deviations, restrictive or mechanical strabismus (trauma, chronic Graves disease, or multiple reoperations), or secondary strabismus wherein a muscle has been overrecessed. Injection is ineffective in A and V patterns, dissociated vertical deviations, oblique muscle disorders, and chronic paralytic strabismus. Multiple injections are frequently required. As with surgical treatment, results are best when there is fusion to stabilize the alignment.

The percentage of patients achieving a deviation of 10Δ or less at least 6 months after the last injection has ranged from 33% for large-angle exotropia to 72% for small-angle esotropia. Overcorrections are rare, and adults and children have responded similarly. The increased potency of surgical correction may be important, especially in larger-angle strabismus cases. The long-term recovery rate for patients with acute sixth nerve palsy who were treated with observation alone is similar to that of patients who received botulinum.

Complications

The most common side effects of botulinum use have been temporary ptosis, lasting from 3 weeks to 3 months (16% of adults and 25% of children) and induced vertical strabismus (17% of all patients). In rare cases, these effects have persisted beyond 6 months (0.16% with slight residual ptosis and 2% with residual vertical strabismus of 2Δ or more). Other reported rare complications include scleral perforation (0.13%), retrobulbar hemorrhage (0.2%), pupillary dilation (0.6%), and permanent diplopia in 1 patient as a result of loss of suppression. Systemic botulism has been reported in animals and humans following massive injections of large muscle groups, but this has not been encountered in ophthalmology.

Cobb DB, Watson WA, Fernandez MC. Botulism-like syndrome after injections of botulinum toxin. *Vet Hum Toxicol.* 2000;42:163.

Cohen DA, Savino PJ, Stern MB, et al. Botulinum injection therapy for blepharospasm: a review and report of 75 patients. *Clin Neuropharmacol.* 1986;9:415–429.

Holmes JM, Beck RW, Kip KE, et al. Botulinum toxin treatment versus conservative management in acute traumatic sixth nerve palsy or paresis. *J AAPOS.* 2000;4:145–149.

McNeer KW, Tucker MG, Spencer RF. Management of essential infantile esotropia with botulinum toxin A: review and recommendations. *J Pediatr Ophthalmol Strabismus.* 2000;37:63–67.

Scott AB, Magoon EH, NcNeer KW, et al. Botulinum treatment of strabismus in children. *Trans Am Ophthalmol Soc.* 1989;87:174–184.

PART II

Pediatric Ophthalmology

INTRODUCTION TO PART II

Growth and Development of the Eye

The human eye undergoes dramatic anatomical and physiologic development throughout infancy and early childhood (Table II-1). Ophthalmologists caring for children should be familiar with the normal growth and development of the pediatric eye, since departures from the norm may indicate pathology.

Dimensions of the Eye

Most of the growth of the eye takes place in the first year of life. The change in the axial length of the eye occurs in 3 phases (Fig II-1). The first phase is a rapid period of growth in the first 6 months of life during which the axial length increases by about 4 mm. During the second (age 2–5 years) and third (age 5–13 years) phases, growth slows; only about 1 mm of growth is added during each of these phases.

Similarly, the cornea grows rapidly over the first several months of life (Fig II-2). Keratometry values change markedly in the first year of life, starting at approximately 52 D at birth, flattening to 46 D by 6 months, and reaching their adult power of 42–44 D by age 12. The average corneal horizontal diameter is 9.5–10.5 mm in newborns, increasing to 12 mm in adulthood; most of this change occurs in the first year of life. Mild corneal clouding can be normal in newborns and is expected in premature infants; it resolves as the cornea gradually thins from an average central thickness of 0.96 mm at birth to 0.52 mm at 6 months.

The power of the infant lens decreases dramatically over the first several years of life, an important fact to consider when implanting intraocular lenses (IOLs) in children undergoing cataract extraction in infancy and early childhood. Figure II-3 shows the theoretical power of the pediatric lens at a given age, based on modified SRK IOL power calculations using pediatric keratometry and axial length values.

Refractive Errors

The refractive state of the eye changes as the axial length of the eye increases and the cornea and lens flatten. In general, infants are hyperopic at birth, become slightly more hyperopic until age 7, and then experience a myopic shift until the eye reaches its adult

Table II-1 Dimensions of Newborn and Adult Eyes

	Newborn	Adult
Anterioposterior length (mm)	17	24
Corneal horizontal diameter (mm)	9.5–10.5	12
Radius of corneal curvature (mm)	6.6–7.4	7.4–8.4

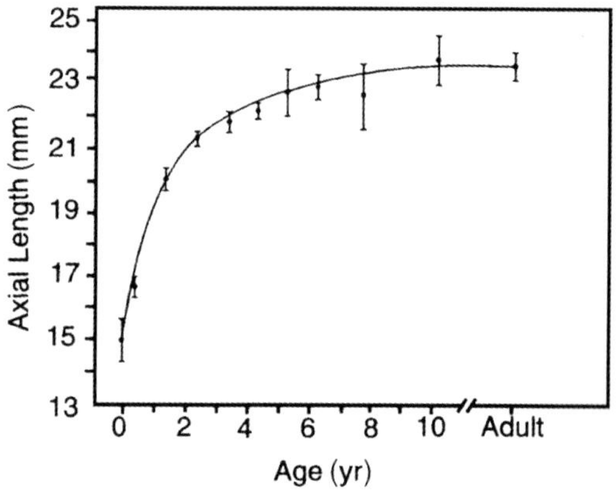

Figure II-1 Axial length plotted with respect to age. *Dots* represent mean values for age group indicated; *bars* represent standard deviations. *(Figures II-1 to II-3 reproduced by permission from Gordon RA, Donzis PB. Refractive development of of the human eye.* Arch Ophthalmol. *1985;103:785–789. © 1985, American Medical Association.)*

size, usually by about age 16 (Fig II-4). Changes in refractive error vary widely, but if myopia presents before age 10, there is a higher risk of eventual progression to myopia of 6 D or greater. Oblique astigmatism is common in infants and often regresses.

Orbit and Ocular Adnexa

During infancy and childhood, orbital volume increases, the shape of the orbital opening becomes less circular and more like a horizontal oval, the lacrimal fossa becomes more superficial, and the inner angle of the orbit becomes more convergent.

The palpebral fissure measures about 18 mm horizontally and 8 mm vertically at birth and changes very little during the first year of life, but a rapid increase in palpebral fissure length occurs during the first decade, causing the round infant eye to acquire an elliptical adult shape.

Although the development of the nasolacrimal duct is complete in most infants, a substantial number of infants show clinical evidence of nasolacrimal duct (NLD) obstruction. Spontaneous resolution of NLD obstruction is seen in 75%–90% of cases.

Iris, Pupil, and Anterior Chamber

Most iris color changes occur over the first 6 to 12 months of life, as pigment accumulates in the iris stroma and melanocytes, but the iris may continue to pigment until later in life. The infant pupil is relatively small compared to adults', but a pupil size smaller than

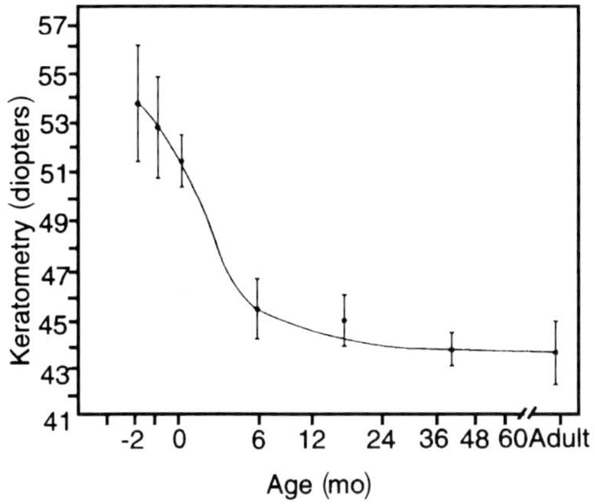

Figure II-2 Keratometry values plotted with respect to age on a logarithmic scale. The negative number represents months of prematurity; *dots*, mean value for age group indicated; and *bars*, standard deviations.

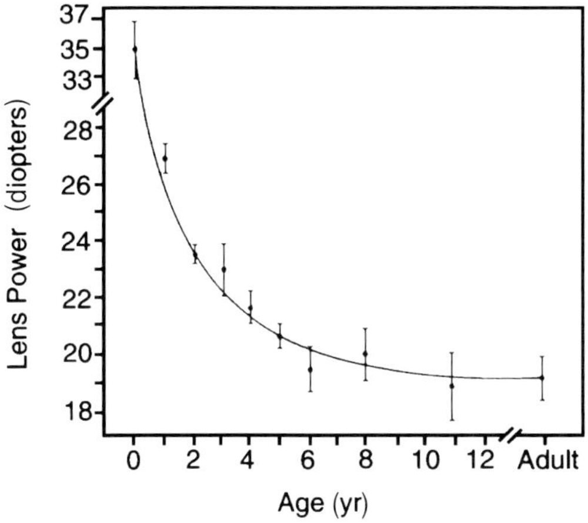

Figure II-3 Mean values *(dots)* and standard deviations *(bars)* for calculated lens power as determined by modified SRK formula, plotted with respect to age.

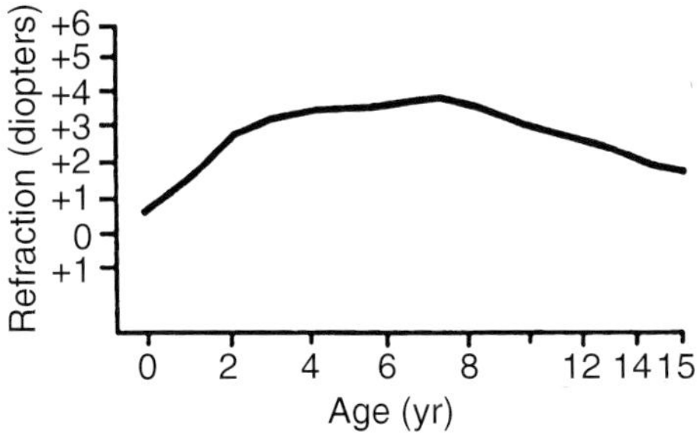

Figure II-4 Change in mean refractive error as a function of age. *(Reproduced with permission from Wright KE, Spiegel PH, eds.* Pediatric Ophthalmology and Strabismus. *2nd ed. New York: Springer-Verlag; 2003:49.*

1.8 mm or greater than 5.4 mm is suggestive of an abnormality. A pupillary light response is expected to be present in infants of 31 or more weeks' gestational age. At birth, the iris insertion is near the level of the sclcral spur, but during the first year of life, the lens and ciliary body migrate posteriorly, resulting in the formation of the angle recess.

Intraocular Pressure

Intraocular pressure determination in infants can be difficult, and normal pressures vary depending on the method used to obtain them. Nevertheless, normal intraocular pressure is lower in infants than in adults, and a pressure of greater than 21 mm Hg should be considered abnormal. Axial length, gonioscopy, corneal diameter, and clarity are helpful when assessing an infant for suspected glaucoma. As has also been observed in adults, central corneal thickness is greater in children with ocular hypertension than in control subjects or those with glaucoma; therefore, pressure readings could be falsely raised.

Extraocular Muscle Anatomy and Physiology

Infant rectus muscles are smaller than those of adults; muscle insertions on average are 2.3 mm to 3 mm narrower than in adults; and the tendons are thinner and more easily disinserted. In infants, the distance from the rectus muscle insertion to the limbus is roughly 2 mm less than in adults; by age 6 months, it is 1 mm less; and at 20 months, it is similar to that of adults. Posteriorly, the topographic anatomy of neonates differs substantially from that of adults and older children; enlargement of the posterior segment occurs during the first 2 years of life, resulting in a separation between the superior and inferior oblique insertions of 4–5 mm and migration of the inferior oblique insertion temporally.

Development of extraocular muscle function continues after birth. Vestibular-driven eye movements are present as early as 34 weeks' gestational age. Conjugate horizontal gaze is present at birth, but vertical gaze may not be fully functional until 6 months of age. About two thirds of infants are exotropic in infancy, but most will have straight eyes by 2–3 months of age. Accommodation and fusional convergence are usually present by 3 months.

Retina

The macula is poorly developed at birth but changes rapidly until about age 4. Most notable are changes in macular pigmentation, annular ring, foveal light reflex, and cone photoreceptor differentiation. Improvement in visual acuity with growth is attributed to 3 processes: differentiation of cone photoreceptors, reduction in the diameter of the rod-free zone, and an increase in foveal cone density. Retinal vascularization proceeds in a centrifugal manner, starting at the optic disc and reaching the temporal ora serrata by 40 weeks' gestational age.

Visual Acuity and Stereoacuity

Two major methods are used to determine visual acuity in preverbal infants and toddlers: *visual evoked potentials (VEP)* and *preferential looking (PL)*. VEP shows improvement of vision from about 20/400 in infancy to 20/20 by age 6–7 months. However, PL studies estimate the vision of a newborn infant to be about 20/600, improving to 20/120 by 3 months and to 20/60 by 6 months. Acuity of 20/20 is not reached with PL testing until age 3–5 years. The discrepancy between these 2 methods may relate to the higher cortical processing required for PL compared to VEP. Stereoacuity reaches 60 sec arc by about 5–6 months.

Eustis HS, Guthrie ME. Postnatal development. In: Wright KE and Spiegel PH, eds. *Pediatric Ophthalmology and Strabismus.* 2nd ed. New York: Springer-Verlag; 2003:39–53.

CHAPTER 15

Congenital Anomalies

Many details and definitions pertaining to genetics, chromosomal anomalies, and developmental embryology are discussed and illustrated in BCSC Section 2, *Fundamentals and Principles of Ophthalmology.* See the glossary in this chapter for terms frequently associated with dysmorphology and congenital anomalies.

Major congenital anomalies occur in 2%–3% of live births. Causes include single genes, chromosomal anomalies, multifactorial disorders, environmental agents, and unknown causes. The last category, unknown causes, accounts for 50% or more of these malformations. Regardless of etiology, from a developmental point of view, congenital anomalies may be organized into the following categories (examples are given in parentheses):

- *agenesis:* developmental failure (anophthalmos)
- *hypoplasia:* developmental arrest (optic nerve hypoplasia)
- *hyperplasia:* developmental excess (distichiasis)
- abnormal development (cryptophthalmos)
- failure to divide or canalize (congenital nasolacrimal duct obstruction)
- *dysraphia:* failure to fuse (choroidal coloboma)
- persistence of vestigial structures (persistent fetal vasculature)

A *malformation* implies a morphologic defect present from the onset of development or from a very early stage. A disturbance to a group of cells in a single developmental field may cause multiple malformations. Multiple causes may result in similar field defects and patterns of malformation. A single structural defect or factor can lead to a cascade, or domino effect, of secondary anomalies called a *sequence.* However, "sequence" does not always imply a single causative factor. The Pierre Robin group of anomalies (cleft palate, glossoptosis, micrognathia, respiratory problems) may represent a sequence caused by abnormal descent of the tongue and is seen in many syndromes (such as Stickler and fetal alcohol) and chromosomal anomalies. A *syndrome* is a recognizable and consistent pattern of multiple malformations known to have a specific cause, which is usually a mutation of a single gene, a chromosome alteration, or an environmental agent. An *association* represents defects known to occur together in a statistically significant number of patients, such as the CHARGE association (ocular *c*oloboma, *h*eart defects, choanal *a*tresia, mental *r*etardation, and *g*enitourinary and *e*ar anomalies). An association may represent a variety of yet-unidentified causes. Two or more minor anomalies in combination significantly increase the chance of an associated major malformation.

Cohen MM Jr. *The Child With Multiple Birth Defects.* 2nd ed. New York: Oxford University Press; 1997.

Jones KL. *Smith's Recognizable Patterns of Human Malformation.* 6th ed. Philadelphia: Elsevier Saunders; 2005.

Wyllie AH. The genetic regulation of apoptosis. *Curr Opin Genet Dev.* 1995;5:97–104.

Glossary

The following additional terms are frequently used in discussions of congenital anomalies and dysmorphology:

Apoptosis An orderly sequence of events in which cells shut down and self-destruct without causing injury to neighboring cells that are necessary for the development of the embryo. Persistent fetal vasculature is a likely example of a defect in apoptosis in the eye's development. Also called *programmed cell death.*

Congenital anomalies All forms of developmental defects present at birth, whether due to genetic, chromosomal, or environmental causes.

Deformation Abnormal form, shape, or position of a part of the body caused by a mechanical process such as intrauterine compression.

Developmental field A group of cells that respond as a coordinated unit to embryonic interaction defects in development, resulting in multiple malformations.

Disruption A morphologic defect resulting from the extrinsic breakdown of, or interference with, an originally normal developmental process.

Dysplasia Abnormal organization of cells into tissue(s) and its morphologic result; the process (and consequence) of abnormality of histogenesis (eg, collagen formation in the joints and zonular fibers of a patient with Marfan syndrome).

Neurocristopathy A constellation of malformations or a craniofacial syndrome involving structures that are primarily derived from neural crest cells (eg, Goldenhar syndrome).

Teratogen Any agent that can produce a permanent morphologic or functional abnormality. This category includes not only drugs and environmental agents such as ionizing radiation but also viruses and other pathogenic organisms (eg, rubella virus, *Toxoplasma gondii*) and metabolic abnormalities (eg, diabetes).

CHAPTER 16

Orbital Dysmorphology and Eyelid Disorders

Orbital and eyelid malformations can be isolated conditions or features of a syndrome; therefore, systematic evaluation of the orbit is an essential part of the clinical evaluation of a dysmorphic infant. Morphologic measurements of the orbit can be performed with transparent rulers or calipers and compared to normal reference measures (Fig 16-1). Alternatively, indices such as the Farcas canthal index, defined by the inner to outer intercanthal ratio $\times$ 10, can be used. Hypotelorism and hypertelorism are defined as having a canthal index greater than 42 and less than 38, respectively. It is important to consider ethnic variations.

Terminology and Associations of Abnormal Interocular Distance

Hypotelorism

Hypotelorism is characterized by a reduced distance between the medial walls of orbits with reduced inner and outer canthal distances. The finding is associated with over 60 syndromes. Hypotelorism can be the result of skull malformation or a failure in brain development.

Hypertelorism

Orbital hypertelorism refers to lateralization of the entire orbit. *Ocular hypertelorism* is defined as an increase in both the inner and outer intercanthal distances. Clinically, interpupillary distance is the best parameter of this anomaly. Hypertelorism occurs in over 550 disorders and is thought to be caused by early ossification of the lesser wing of the sphenoid, which fixes the orbits in the fetal position; by failure of development of the nasal capsule, which allows the primitive brain to protrude, as in frontal encephalocele; or by a disturbance in the development of the skull base, as in craniosynostosis syndromes.

Exorbitism

Some clinicians define *exorbitism* as prominent eyes due to shallow orbits; others define it as an increased angle of divergence of the orbital walls.

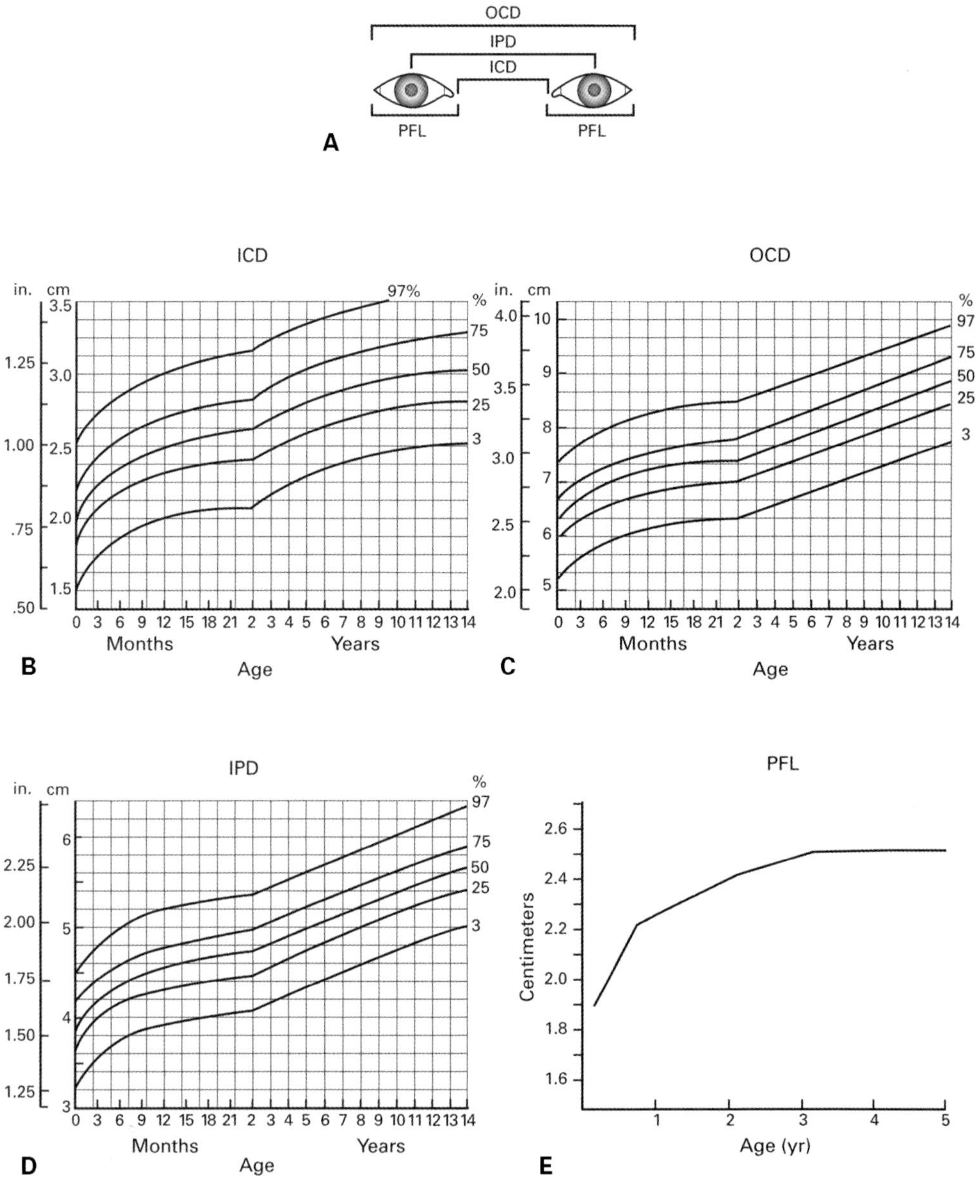

Figure 16-1 **A,** Schematic representation of measurements involved in the evaluation of the orbital region. *OCD* = outer canthal distance; *ICD* = inner canthal distance; *IPD* = interpupillary distance; *PFL* = palpebral fissure length. **B,** ICD measurements according to age. **C,** OCD measurements according to age. **D,** IPD measurements according to age. **E,** Normal PFL measurements according to age. *(Reproduced with permission from Dollfus H, Verloes A. Dysmorphology and the orbital region: a practical clinical approach.* Surv Ophthalmol. *2004;49:549).*

Telecanthus

Telecanthus is a condition characterized by an increased distance between the inner canthi. It is considered primary if the interpupillary measurement is normal and secondary if it is greater than normal. Telecanthus is common in many syndromes.

Dystopia Canthorum

Dystopia canthorum is specific for Waardenberg syndrome type 1. It is described as lateral displacement of both the inner canthi and the lacrimal puncta such that an imaginary vertical line drawn connecting the upper and lower puncta crosses the cornea (Fig 16-2).

Dollfus H, Verloes A. Dysmorphology and the orbital region: a practical clinical approach. *Surv Ophthalmol.* 2004;49:547–561.

Eyelid Disorders

Congenital eyelid disorders can result from abnormal differentiation of the eyelids and adnexa, developmental arrest, intrauterine environmental insults, and other unknown factors. Examples of these groups are discussed below. See also BCSC Section 2, *Fundamentals and Principles of Ophthalmology*, and Section 7, *Orbit, Eyelids, and Lacrimal System.*

Cryptophthalmos

Cryptophthalmos, a rare condition, results from failure of differentiation of eyelid structures. The skin passes uninterrupted from the forehead over the eye to the cheek and blends in with the cornea of the eye, which is usually malformed (Fig 16-3). Fraser syndrome is an autosomal recessive disorder that is characterized by partial syndactyly and genitourinary anomalies; it may include cryptophthalmos and other ocular malformations.

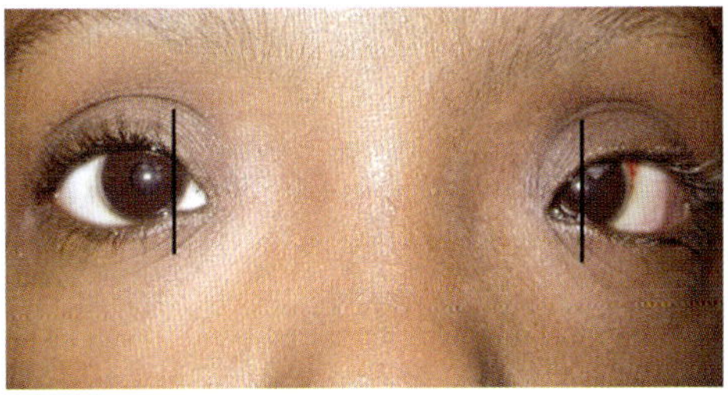

Figure 16-2 Dystopia canthorum in a patient with Waardenberg syndrome. Notice that the imaginary vertical lines drawn through the puncta intersect the cornea. *(Photograph courtesy of Amy Hutchinson, MD.)*

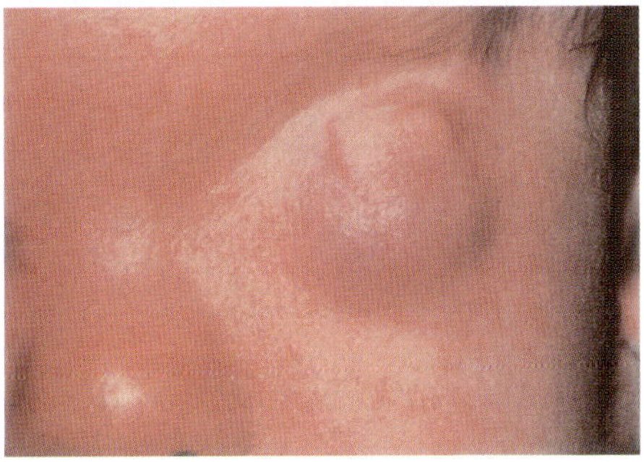

Figure 16-3 Cryptophthalmos, left eye.

Congenital Coloboma of the Eyelid

Congenital coloboma of the eyelid usually involves the upper eyelid and can range from a small notch to the absence of the entire length of the eyelid, which can be fused to the globe (Fig 16-4). Eyelid colobomas are commonly associated with Goldenhar syndrome. The eye of an infant with a congenital coloboma should be observed for exposure keratopathy, which is uncommon. Surgical closure of the eyelid defect is eventually required in most cases.

Ankyloblepharon

Fusion of part or all of the eyelid margins is known as *ankyloblepharon.* This condition may be dominantly inherited. A variant is *ankyloblepharon filiforme adnatum,* in which the eyelid margins are connected by fine strands (Fig 16-5). Treatment is surgical.

Congenital Ectropion

Congenital ectropion is a disorder characterized by eversion of the eyelid margin that usually involves the lower eyelid secondary to a vertical deficiency of the skin. A lateral tarsorrhaphy may be needed for mild cases. More severe cases may require a skin flap or graft.

Congenital Entropion

Congenital entropion of the lower eyelid is uncommon and often asymptomatic; it should be differentiated from epiblepharon (see the following section). Surgery should be reserved for persistent cases that threaten the cornea. Congenital entropion of the upper eyelid usually results from congenital horizontal tarsal kink (see later in the chapter) or microphthalmos.

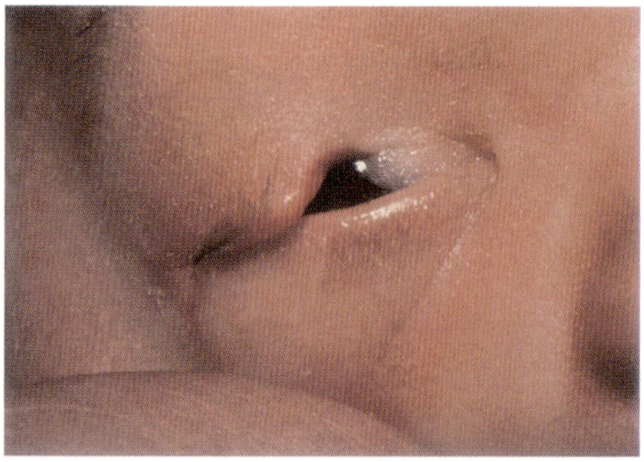

Figure 16-4 Congenital eyelid coloboma, right eye. The eyelid is fused to the globe.

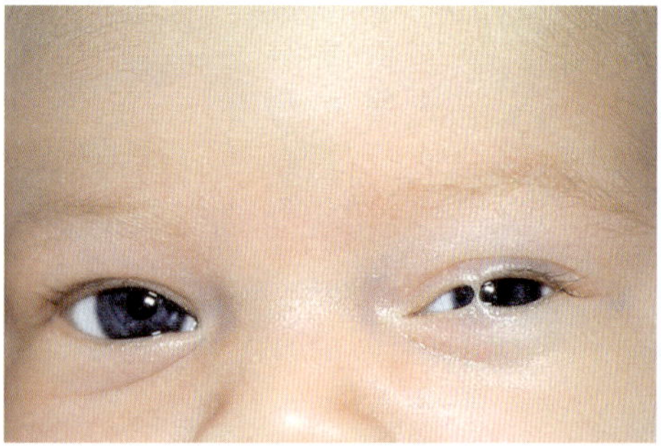

Figure 16-5 Ankyloblepharon. The eyelid margins are fused by a fine strand. The eyelids were easily separated with blunt Wescott scissors in the office without anesthesia. *(Photograph courtesy of Amy Hutchinson, MD.)*

Epiblepharon

Epiblepharon is a congenital anomaly characterized by a horizontal fold of skin adjacent to either the upper or lower eyelid—most commonly, the lower eyelid—that may turn the lashes against the cornea. The cornea often tolerates this condition surprisingly well, and in the first several years of life, epiblepharon usually resolves spontaneously. Severe cases require surgical repair.

Congenital Tarsal Kink

The origin of congenital tarsal kink is unknown, but a child with this condition is born with the upper eyelid bent back and open. The upper tarsal plate often has an actual 180° fold. As with large congenital colobomas, the cornea may be exposed and traumatized by the bent edge, resulting in ulceration. Minor defects can be managed by manually unfolding the tarsus and taping the eyelid shut with a pressure dressing for 1–2 days. More severe cases require surgical incision of the tarsal plate or even excision of a V-shaped wedge from the inner surface to permit unfolding (Fig 16-6).

Distichiasis

A partial or complete accessory row of eyelashes growing out of or slightly posterior to the meibomian gland orifices is known as *distichiasis*. The abnormal lashes tend to be thinner, shorter, softer, and less pigmented than normal cilia and are therefore often well tolerated. Treatment is indicated if the patient is symptomatic or if corneal irritation is evident (Fig 16-7).

Euryblepharon

Enlargement of the lateral part of the palpebral aperture with downward displacement of the temporal half of the lower eyelid is known as *euryblepharon*. This condition gives the appearance of a very wide palpebral fissure or a droopy lower eyelid.

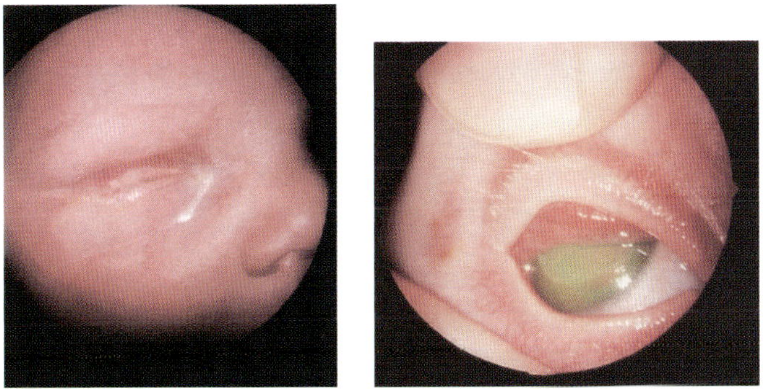

Figure 16-6 Congenital tarsal kink. Note the large corneal epithelial defect.

Epicanthus

Epicanthus, a crescent-shaped fold of skin running vertically between the eyelids and overlying the inner canthus, is shown in Figure 16-8. There are 4 types of epicanthus:

1. *epicanthus tarsalis:* fold is most prominent in the upper eyelid
2. *epicanthus inversus:* fold is most prominent in the lower eyelid
3. *epicanthus palpebralis:* fold is equally distributed in the upper and lower eyelids
4. *epicanthus supraciliaris:* fold arises from the brow and terminates over the lacrimal sac

Epicanthus may be associated with blepharophimosis or ptosis, or it may be an isolated finding. Surgical correction is only occasionally required.

Palpebral Fissure Slants

In the normal eye, the lids are generally positioned so that the lateral canthus is about 1 mm higher than the medial canthus. Slight upward or downward slanting of palpebral

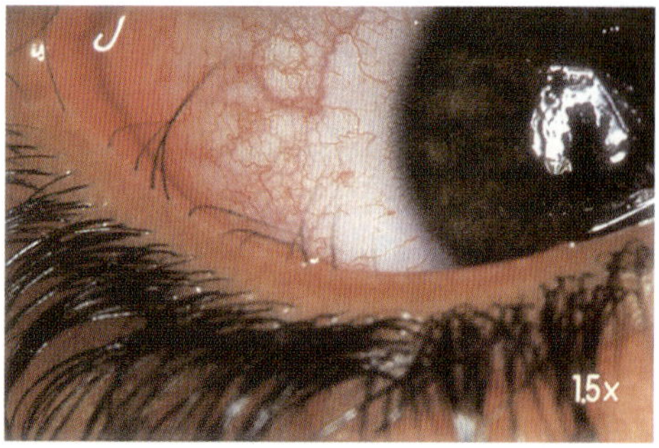

Figure 16-7 Distichiasis. An accessory row of eyelashes exits from the meibomian gland orifices. *(Reproduced by permission from Byrnes GA, Wilson ME. Congenital distichiasis.* Arch Ophthalmol. *1991;109:1752–1753. ©1991, American Medical Association.)*

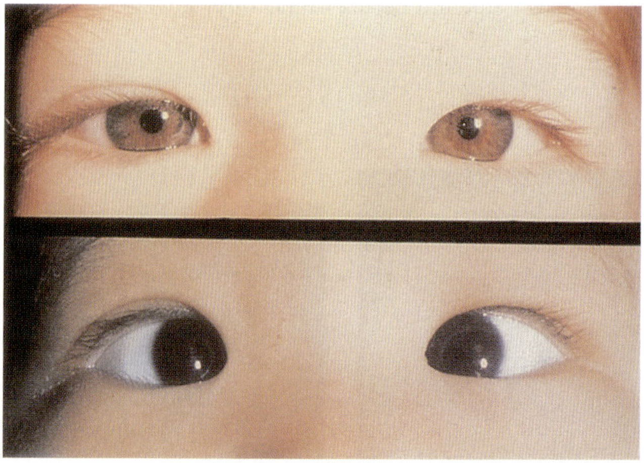

Figure 16-8 Epicanthus, bilateral. **Top,** Epicanthus tarsalis. **Bottom,** Epicanthus palpebralis. *(Reproduced by permission from Crouch E.* The Child's Eye: Strabismus and Amblyopia. *Slide script. San Francisco: American Academy of Ophthalmology; 1982.)*

fissures normally occurs on a familial basis or in groups such as people of Asian descent. However, certain craniofacial syndromes frequently cause palpebral fissures to have a characteristic upward (eg, Down syndrome) or downward (eg, Treacher Collins syndrome) slant (see Fig 28-10).

Blepharophimosis Syndrome

Blepharophimosis syndrome consists of blepharophimosis, epicanthus inversus, telecanthus, and ptosis; it may occur as an isolated or autosomal dominant disorder. The palpebral fissures are shortened horizontally and vertically *(blepharophimosis)* with poor levator function and no eyelid fold (Fig 16-9). The horizontal palpebral fissure length, normally 25–30 mm, is reduced to 18–22 mm in these patients. Repair of the ptosis, usually with frontalis suspension procedures, is often needed early in life. Because the epicanthus and telecanthus may improve with age, repair of these defects is often delayed.

Ptosis

Ptosis (blepharoptosis) describes eyelid droop; the condition can be congenital or acquired. Acquired ptosis has been classified according to its various causes (Table 16-1). Evaluation of ptosis involves a thorough history that includes the date of onset and reviews any ocular disorders in the family. A complete examination, including slit-lamp examination and refraction, should be performed. Astigmatic errors may be associated with ptosis and are the most common cause of amblyopia in these patients; total occlusion of the

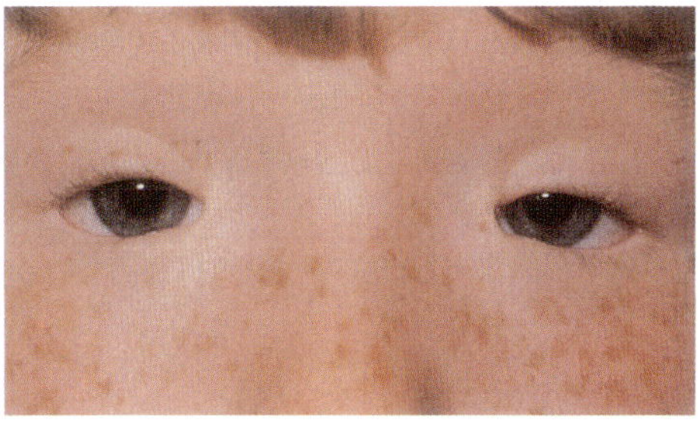

Figure 16-9 Blepharophimosis syndrome: blepharophimosis, epicanthus inversus, telecanthus, and ptosis.

Table 16-1 Classification of Ptosis

Pseudoptosis

Congenital ptosis

Acquired ptosis
- *Myogenic*
  - Myasthenia gravis
  - Progressive external ophthalmoplegia
- *Neurogenic*
  - Horner syndrome
  - Third nerve palsy
- *Mechanical*

visual axis is uncommon. Astigmatism often persists after eyelid surgery. The eyelid is evaluated by description of the upper fold, and the amount of ptosis is documented by measuring the height of the palpebral fissure. Levator function is measured while the effect of the frontalis muscle is blocked. Both tear function and corneal sensitivity should be evaluated because exposure and drying will be compounded by surgical repair. If Bell's phenomenon is poor, the cornea can decompensate quickly after ptosis repair. A documentary photograph of the patient is desirable.

Correction of ptosis in a child can often be delayed until the patient is several years old, although consistent chin-up head posturing may justify earlier surgery. Although rarely encountered, a completely closed eyelid must be elevated early in infancy to avoid occlusion amblyopia. Surgical techniques include levator resection, tucking of the levator aponeurosis, and eyelid suspension anchored into the frontalis muscle. When levator function is less than 4 mm, frontalis suspension surgery is usually performed. Some surgeons prefer autogenous fascia lata for frontalis suspension surgery. However, others report good results with silicone rods or human donor fascia lata. Autogenous fascia cannot be obtained until the patient is 3 or 4 years old. One study reported a 50% recurrence rate by 8–10 postoperative years when human donor fascia lata was used.

Marcus Gunn Jaw Winking

In the typical Marcus Gunn jaw-winking syndrome, there is a congenital trigemino-oculomotor synkinesis. This results in ptosis, and the ptotic eyelid is elevated with jaw movement. Discussion with the family regarding their concerns about the ptosis versus the eyelid excursion is important. The eyelid excursion is the greater concern in some patients, and they may elect to dennervate the levator(s) and use a sling to elevate one or both eyelids. Many children learn to control eyelid movement, so surgery can be avoided.

Meyer DR. Congenital ptosis. *Focal Points: Clinical Modules for Ophthalmologists.* San Francisco: American Academy of Ophthalmology; 2001, module 2.

Wilson ME, Johnson RW. Congenital ptosis. Long-term results of treatment using lyophilized fascia lata for frontalis suspensions. *Ophthalmology.* 1991;98:1234–1237.

CHAPTER 17

Infectious and Allergic Ocular Diseases

Intrauterine and Perinatal Infections of the Eye

Maternally transmitted congenital infections cause ocular damage in 3 ways:

1. through direct action of the infecting agent, which damages tissue
2. through a teratogenic effect resulting in malformation
3. through a delayed reactivation of the agent after birth, with inflammation that damages developed tissue

These infections can cause ongoing tissue damage; therefore, long-term evaluation is required to determine their full impact. Most perinatal disorders have an exceedingly broad spectrum of clinical presentation, ranging from silent disease to life-threatening tissue and organ damage. Only the common types of congenital infections are included in this chapter. They can be remembered by the acronym *TORCHES: to*xoplasmosis; *r*ubella; *c*ytomegalic inclusion disease; *h*erpesviruses, including *E*pstein-Barr; *s*yphilis. Other well-known causes of in utero infections include the CLAP diseases—*c*hickenpox, *L*yme disease *(Borrelia burgdorferi)*, *A*IDS (human immunodeficiency), and *p*arvovirus B19.

Stamos JK, Rowley AH. Timely diagnosis of congenital infections. *Pediatr Clin North Am.* 1994;41:1017–1033.

Toxoplasmosis

The etiologic agent of *toxoplasmosis, Toxoplasma gondii*, is an obligate intracellular parasite. Cats are the definitive host, wherein the parasite resides in the intestinal mucosa in the form of an oocyst. Once secreted into the environment, the oocyst can be ingested by many animals, including humans. Humans can also acquire the disease secondarily by ingesting undercooked infected meat such as pork, lamb, or even chicken.

The ingested cyst has a predilection for muscle, including the heart, and neural tissue, including the retinas. Encysted organisms can remain dormant indefinitely or the cyst can rupture, releasing hundreds of thousands of *tachyzoites*, the proliferative phase of the protozoan. The stimulus for local reactivation of an infected cyst is unknown.

Systemic infection in humans is common and usually goes undiagnosed. Symptoms may include fever, lymphadenopathy, and sore throat. The proportion of antibody titer–positive persons in North America increases with age from less than 10% in early childhood to greater than 80% in octogenarians.

Toxoplasmosis can be acquired congenitally via transplacental transmission from an infected mother to the fetus. Congenital infection can result in varying degrees of retinitis, hepatosplenomegaly, intracranial calcifications, microcephaly, and developmental delay.

Ocular manifestations include retinitis, sometimes with associated choroiditis, iritis, and anterior uveitis (Fig 17-1). The active area of retinal inflammation is usually thickened and cream-colored with an overlying vitritis. The area may be at the edge of an old flat atrophic scar, frequently in the macular area, or adjacent to the scar (a so-called satellite lesion). Most cases of apparently acquired *Toxoplasma* retinitis probably represent reactivation of a congenital infection.

Diagnosis

Diagnosis is primarily clinical, based on the characteristic retinal lesions. It can be supported by a positive enzyme-linked immunosorbent assay (ELISA) for *Toxoplasma* antibody. Any positivity, even undiluted, is significant, but the rate of false-positive results is very high. Lack of antibody essentially rules out the diagnosis. In the infant, maternal IgM does not cross the placenta, so finding IgM in the infant serum is evidence of congenital infection in the infant. (See Chapter 4 of BCSC Section 4, *Ophthalmic Pathology and Intraocular Tumors*, and Chapter 9 of BCSC Section 9, *Intraocular Inflammation and Uveitis*.)

Dodds EM. Ocular toxoplasmosis: clinical presentations, diagnosis, and therapy. *Focal Points: Clinical Modules for Ophthalmologists.* San Francisco: American Academy of Ophthalmology; 1999, module 10.

Montoya JG, Parmley S, Liesenfeld O, et al. Use of the polymerase chain reaction for diagnosis of ocular toxoplasmosis. *Ophthalmology.* 1999;106:1554–1563.

Treatment

Ocular inflammation from reactivated toxoplasmosis does not require treatment unless it threatens vision. Vision can be compromised by the location of the reactivation adjacent to the macula or optic nerve or by significant vitritis. If the lesion is in the periphery of the eye and does not affect vision, it will likely quiet on its own in 1–2 months. If the macula or optic nerve is involved or if massive vitritis threatens vision, treatment may be indicated. Systemic treatment involves use of oral corticosteroids to quiet the inflammation in combination with 1 or more antimicrobial drugs aimed at the proliferating organisms. Steroids should never be used alone without antimicrobial coverage. Depot injection of steroid should not be used to treat ocular toxoplasmosis.

The commonly used antimicrobials are

- *pyrimethamine:* can cause bone marrow suppression, so its use is always accompanied by concomitant therapy with folinic acid. Patients should undergo weekly blood and platelet counts while on this drug. Pyrimethamine is usually used in combination with 1 of the following 2 agents:
  - *sulfadiazine*—a sulfa drug long used in treatment of toxoplasmosis
  - *clindamycin*—also effective against *Toxoplasma*; patients should be monitored for development of severe diarrhea from pseudomembranous colitis

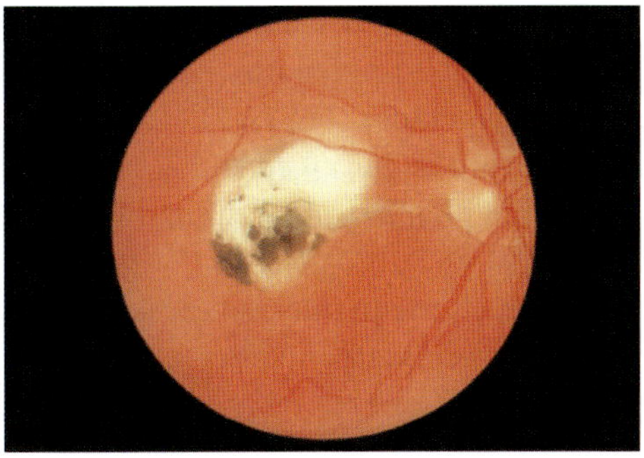

Figure 17-1 Toxoplasmosis, right eye.

- *trimethoprim-sulfamethoxazole:* combination can be used if the other drugs are not available or not tolerated
- *atovaquone:* newer antimicrobial that has been shown to be effective against *Toxoplasma* but is not a first-line therapy and is not effective unless used in combination with other drugs, such as pyrimethamine

Oral prednisone can be used judiciously to combat inflammation only while the patient is taking appropriate antimicrobial therapy.

Classic triple-drug therapy refers to pyrimethamine, sulfadiazine, and prednisone. Quadruple drug therapy includes the addition of clindamycin.

Additional details of drug therapy for toxoplasmosis is contained in BCSC Section 9, *Intraocular Inflammation and Uveitis.*

Dodds EM. Ocular toxoplasmosis: clinical presentations, diagnosis, and therapy. *Focal Points: Clinical Modules for Ophthalmologists.* San Francisco: American Academy of Ophthalmology; 1999, module 12.

Mets MB, Holfels E, Boyer KM, et al. Eye manifestations of congenital toxoplasmosis. *Am J Ophthalmol.* 1996;122:309–324.

Remington JS, McLeod R, Thulliez P, et al. Toxoplasmosis. In: Remington JS, Klein JO, eds. *Infectious Diseases of the Fetus and Newborn Infant.* 6th ed. Philadelphia: Elsevier Saunders; 2006.

Rubella

Congenital rubella (German measles) syndrome is a well-defined combination of ocular, otologic, and cardiac abnormalities, along with microcephaly and variable mental deficiency. The syndrome is caused by transplacental transmission of the rubella virus from an infected mother. The incidence of congenital rubella syndrome has decreased markedly in North America since widespread vaccination of children was instituted in the late 1960s, although rubella remains a cause of infant morbidity and mortality in less-developed countries. The number of cases in the United States has decreased from 58,000 in 1969, when mass immunization began, to 200–400 cases/year in 1998 to less than 25 cases/year between 2001 and 2004. Humans are the only known host.

Ocular abnormalities from rubella include a peculiar nuclear cataract that is sometimes floating in a liquefied lens cortex, microphthalmos, and retinopathy varying from a subtle salt-and-pepper appearance to pseudoretinitis pigmentosa (Fig 17-2).

Diagnosis is based on the characteristic clinical picture as described and is supported by serologic testing. The virus itself can be isolated from pharyngeal swabs and from the lens contents at the time of cataract surgery.

Lensectomy can be performed in the usual manner, although infected eyes are prone to excessive postoperative inflammation and subsequent secondary membrane formation. Topical steroids and mydriatics should be used aggressively.

Cooper LZ, Alford CA. Rubella. In: Remington JS, Klein JO, eds. *Infectious Diseases of the Fetus and Newborn Infant.* 6th ed. Philadelphia: Elsevier Saunders; 2006.

Wolff SM. The ocular manifestations of congenital rubella. *Trans Am Ophthalmol Soc.* 1972;70: 577–614.

Zimmerman LE. Histopathologic basis for ocular manifestations of congenital rubella syndrome. *Am J Ophthalmol.* 1968;65:837–862.

Cytomegalovirus

Cytomegalovirus (CMV) is a member of the herpesvirus family. CMV can cause a variety of human disease manifestations, both congenital and acquired, although symptomatic acquired infections occur almost exclusively in immunocompromised persons. Over 80% of adults in developed countries have antibodies to the virus.

Congenital infection with CMV, or *cytomegalic inclusion disease,* is the most common congenital infection in humans, occurring in approximately 1% of infants, although over 90% of these remain asymptomatic. Transmission to the newborn can occur transplacentally, from contact with an infected birth canal during delivery, or perhaps from infected breast milk or maternal secretions. Congenital CMV disease is characterized by fever, jaundice, hematologic abnormalities, deafness, microcephaly, and periventricular calcifications.

Ophthalmic manifestations of congenital infection include retinochoroiditis, optic nerve anomalies, microphthalmos, cataract, and uveitis (Fig 17-3). The retinochoroiditis usually presents with bilateral focal involvement consisting of areas of retinal pigment epithelium atrophy and whitish opacities mixed with retinal hemorrhages. The retinitis can be progressive.

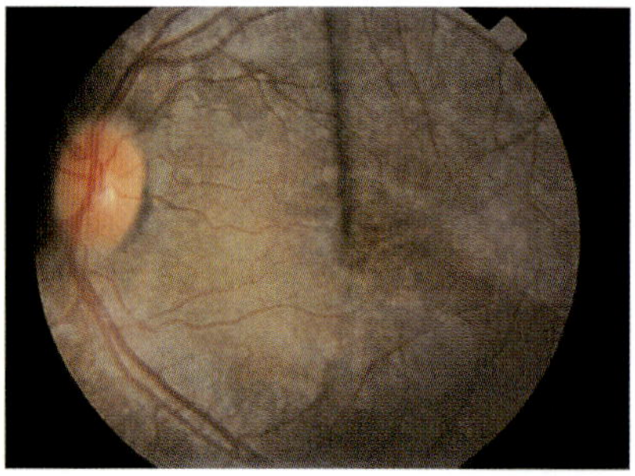

Figure 17-2 Fundus photograph of a 6-year-old with rubella syndrome (ERG normal).

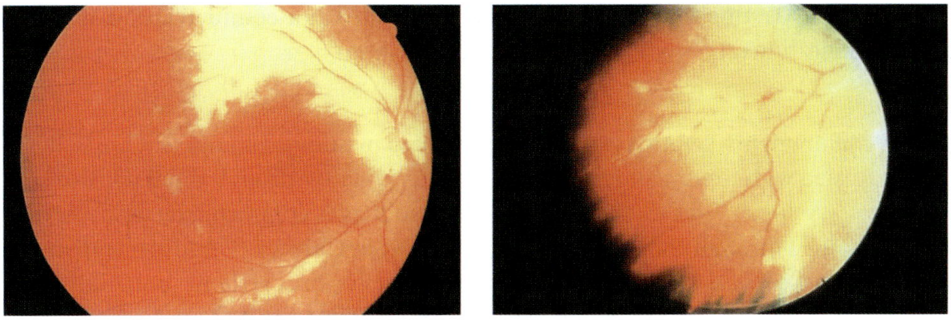

Figure 17-3 Active CMV retinochoroiditis in a premature infant, right eye.

CMV retinitis can be acquired in children who are immunocompromised (most frequently by AIDS) or iatrogenically following organ transplantation or chemotherapy. The retinitis is a diffuse retinal necrosis with areas of retinal thickening and whitening, hemorrhages, and venous sheathing. Vitritis may also be present.

Diagnosis is based on the clinical presentation in acquired disease and supplemented by serologic testing for antibodies to CMV in congenital infection. The virus can be recovered from bodily secretions in infected infants through cell culture techniques.

Currently, 5 drugs are available for treatment: ganciclovir, valganciclovir, foscarnet, cidofovir, and fomivirsen.

Coats DK, Demmler GJ, Paysse EA, et al. Ophthalmologic findings in children with congenital cytomegalovirus infection. *J AAPOS.* 2000;4:110–116.

Stagno S, Britt W. Cytomegalovirus infections. In: Remington JS, Klein JO, eds. *Infectious Diseases of the Fetus and Newborn Infant.* 6th ed. Philadelphia: Elsevier Saunders; 2006.

Herpes Simplex

Herpes simplex virus (HSV) is a member of the herpesvirus family that includes 2 types of simplex virus (HSV-1 and HSV-2), herpes zoster, Epstein-Barr virus, and CMV. HSV-1 typically affects the eyes, skin, and mouth region and is transmitted by close personal contact. HSV-2 is typically associated with genital infection through venereal transmission and is responsible for most neonatal infections.

Congenital infection is usually acquired during passage through an infected birth canal. The neonatal infection is confined to the central nervous system, skin, oral cavity, and eyes in one third of cases. It commonly manifests with vesicular skin lesions, ulcerative mouth sores, and keratoconjunctivitis. Disseminated disease occurs in two thirds of cases and can involve the liver, adrenal glands, and lungs. The mortality rate from disseminated disease is significant, and survivors usually have permanent impairment.

Eye involvement in congenital infection can include conjunctivitis, keratitis, retinochoroiditis, and cataracts. Keratitis can be epithelial or stromal. Retinal involvement can be severe, including massive exudates and retinal necrosis.

Diagnosis is based on the clinical presentation, confirmed with viral cultures taken from vesicular fluid, conjunctival or corneal swabs, or nasal secretions. Polymerase chain reaction (PCR) testing detects viral nucleic acids but is not commercially available for clinical applications.

Treatment

Herpes conjunctivitis/keratitis is usually self-limited in immunocompetent hosts, but it is usually treated with topical antivirals such as trifluridine 1% drops 9 times daily or sometimes oral acyclovir. Vidarabine 3% ointment is no longer commercially available, but it can be obtained through compounding pharmacies. See Chapter 19 for further discussion of treatment of corneal disease. Disseminated disease requires systemic antivirals such as acyclovir given under the direction of a specialist in pediatric infectious disease.

Diagnosis and treatment of acquired herpes simplex keratoconjunctivitis in children is similar to that in adults. See BCSC Section 8, *External Disease and Cornea.*

Arvin AM, Whitley RJ, Gutierrez KM. Herpes simplex virus infections. In: Remington JS, Klein JO, eds. *Infectious Diseases of the Fetus and Newborn Infant.* 6th ed. Philadelphia: Elsevier Saunders; 2006.

Overall JC. Herpes simplex virus infection of the fetus and newborn. *Pediatr Ann.* 1994; 23:131–136.

Parrish CM. Herpes simplex virus eye disease. *Focal Points: Clinical Modules for Ophthalmologists.* San Francisco: American Academy of Ophthalmology; 1997, module 2.

Schwartz GS, Holland EJ. Oral acyclovir for the management of herpes simplex virus keratitis in children. *Ophthalmology.* 2000;107:278–282.

Syphilis

Syphilis is caused by the spirochete *Treponema pallidum*, and sexual contact is the usual route of transmission. Fetal infection occurs following maternal spirochetemia. The longer the mother has had syphilis, the lower the risk of transmitting the disease to her child. If the mother has contracted primary or secondary disease, about half of her offspring will be infected. In cases of untreated late maternal syphilis (the most common form), about 70% of infants are healthy.

Congenital syphilis should be considered in premature births of unexplained cause, large placenta, persistent rhinitis, intractable rash, unexplained jaundice, hepatosplenomegaly, pneumonia, anemia, generalized lymphadenopathy, and metaphyseal abnormalities or periostitis on radiograph. Congenitally acquired infection can lead to neonatal death or premature delivery. Early eye involvement in congenital syphilis is rare.

Chorioretinitis appears as a salt-and-pepper granularity of the fundus in some infants. An appearance of pseudoretinitis pigmentosa may ensue; rarely, anterior uveitis, glaucoma, or both may develop. In other cases, symptoms may not appear until late childhood or adolescence. Widely spaced, peg-shaped teeth; eighth nerve deafness; and interstitial keratitis constitute *Hutchinson triad.* Other manifestations include saddle nose, short maxilla, and linear scars around body orifices. Bilateral interstitial keratitis is the classic ophthalmic finding in older children and adults, occurring in approximately 10% of patients.

Diagnosis

The Centers for Disease Control and Prevention define confirmed congenital syphilis by identification of *T pallidum* by dark-field microscopy. Congenital syphilis can be presumptively diagnosed by the combination of a positive result with the Venereal Disease Research Laboratory (VDRL) test and 1 or more of the following:

- evidence of congenital syphilis on physical examination
- long-bone radiographic evidence
- a positive result on VDRL testing of cerebrospinal fluid
- otherwise unexplained elevation of cerebrospinal fluid protein or cell count
- quantitative nontreponemal serologic titer 4 times greater than the mother's
- a positive FTA-ABS

Treatment

Treatment for congenital syphilis in neonates younger than 1 month includes aqueous crystalline penicillin G, 50,000 units/kg IV every 12 hours for 1 week, then every 8 hours, for a total of 10 days. Infants older than 1 month receive aqueous crystalline penicillin G every 6 hours for 10 days. Serologic tests should be repeated at 2 to 4, 6, and 12 months after conclusion of treatment or until results become nonreactive or the titer has decreased fourfold. Persistent positive titers or a positive cerebrospinal fluid VDRL test result at 6 months should prompt retreatment.

Ingall D, Sanchez P, Baker CJ. Syphilis. In: Remington JS, Klein JO, eds. *Infectious Diseases of the Fetus and Newborn Infant.* 6th ed. Philadelphia: Elsevier Saunders; 2006.

Ophthalmia Neonatorum

Ophthalmia neonatorum refers to conjunctivitis occurring in the first month of life caused by a number of different agents, including bacterial, viral, and chemical agents. Widespread effective prophylaxis has diminished the morbidity of this problem to very low levels in industrialized countries, but ophthalmia neonatorum remains a significant source of ocular morbidity, blindness, and even death in medically underserved areas around the world.

Etiology

Worldwide, the incidence of ophthalmia neonatorum is high in areas with high rates of sexually transmitted disease. Incidence ranges from 0.1% in highly developed countries with effective prenatal care to 10% in areas such as East Arica.

The organism usually infects the infant through direct contact during passage through the birth canal. Infections are known to ascend to the uterus so that even infants delivered via cesarean section can be infected. This possibility is enhanced by prolonged rupture of membranes at the time of delivery.

Most Important Agents

Neisseria

The most serious form of ophthalmia neonatorum is caused by *Neisseria gonorrhoeae.* Onset is typically in the first 3–4 days of life but may be delayed for up to 3 weeks. Though some cases may present with mild conjunctival hyperemia and discharge, severe cases have marked chemosis, copious discharge, and possibly rapid corneal ulceration and perforation of the eye (Fig 17-4). Systemic infection can cause sepsis, meningitis, and arthritis.

Diagnosis Gram stain of the conjunctival exudate showing gram-negative intracellular diplococci allows a presumptive diagnosis of *N gonorrhoeae* infection, and treatment should be started immediately. Ophthalmia neonatorum from *Neisseria meningitidis* has also been reported. The 2 *Neisseria* organisms cannot be differentiated by Gram stain. Definitive diagnosis is based on culture of the conjunctival discharge. The specimen should be cultured on both selective (Thayer-Martin) and nonselective (chocolate agar) media and incubated at 37°C.

Treatment Treatment must be systemic. Increasing resistance to traditionally effective antibiotics such as penicillin, tetracycline, and erythromycin has made treatment more difficult, but effective medications are available. Ceftriaxone given intravenously or intramuscularly 50 mg/kg daily for 1 week is highly effective. Penicillin (aqueous crystalline penicillin G) is effective for many strains.

Topical irrigation of the eyes can be helpful to mechanically debride large amounts of conjunctival discharge, but topical antibiotics, in the absence of corneal ulcer, provide no added benefit.

Chlamydia

The agent responsible for *Chlamydia trachomatis* (called *trachoma-inclusion conjunctivitis,* or *TRIC*) is an obligate intracellular organism. The infant comes into contact with the organism during passage through the birth canal of an infected mother, but like other organisms, the TRIC agent can also ascend to the uterus and infect an infant delivered by cesarean section.

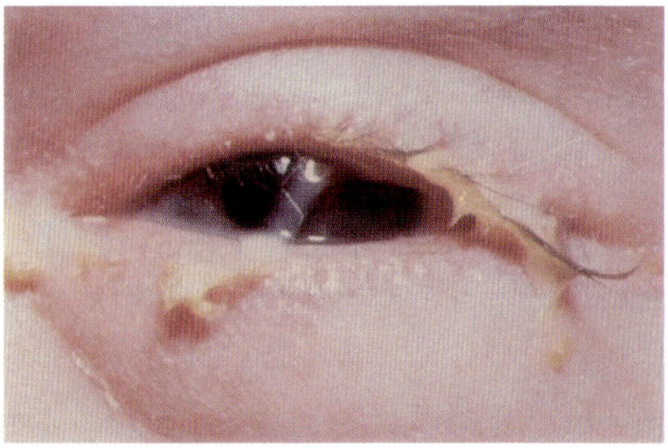

Figure 17-4 *Neisseria gonorrhoeae* conjunctivitis.

Onset of conjunctivitis in the infant usually occurs around 1 week of age, although onset may be earlier, especially in cases with premature rupture of membranes. Eye infection is characterized by usually mild swelling, hyperemia, and a papillary reaction with minimal to moderate discharge. Rare severe cases can be accompanied by more copious discharge and pseudomembrane formation. A follicular conjunctival reaction typical of adult inclusion conjunctivitis can occur after about 1 month of age.

Diagnosis The gold standard for diagnosis is culture from conjunctival scrapings; however, improper handling of specimens can reduce sensitivity. Several more-rapid indirect laboratory tests are available, including enzyme-linked immunoassays (eg, Chlamydiazyme, Abbott Diagnostics, Chicago, and MicroTrak EIA, Genetic Systems, Seattle), direct fluorescent antibody tests (eg, Syva MicroTrak, Genetics Systems, and Pathfinder, Sanofi-Pasteur, Chaska, Minnesota), and DNA probes.

Treatment Chlamydial conjunctivitis is a self-limited disease, although it can last for a year or more in untreated cases. However, treatment is mandated in part because of the associated systemic involvement that can result in pneumonia or gastrointestinal infection. Treatment of the eye disease must be systemic; topical erythromycin ointment can be applied but is probably superfluous when systemic erythromycin is used.

The treatment of choice is oral erythromycin, 50 mg/kg per day in 4 divided doses for 14 days. As with other venereally transmitted diseases, public health authorities should be contacted to initiate evaluation and treatment of other maternal contacts.

Herpes simplex

Infection with herpes simplex virus (HSV) is a rarer form of ophthalmia neonatorum. It typically presents later than infection with *N gonorrhoeae* or *C trachomatis*, frequently in the second week of life. See the discussion of herpes simplex conjunctivitis later in this chapter.

Chemical conjunctivitis

Chemical conjunctivitis refers to a mild, self-limited irritation and redness of the conjunctiva occurring in the first 24 hours after instillation of silver nitrate, a preparation used for prophylaxis of ophthalmia neonatorum. These symptoms can suggest the onset of conjunctivitis in the newborn, but the condition will improve spontaneously by the second day.

Prophylaxis for Ophthalmia Neonatorum

In 1880, Crede introduced the concept of widespread prophylaxis for gonorrheal ophthalmia neonatorum with 2% silver nitrate. It significantly reduced the incidence of gonorrheal conjunctivitis and is still used in many places today. This method is not effective against TRIC and therefore has been supplanted by agents effective against *Gonococcus* and TRIC, such as erythromycin and tetracycline ointments.

Povidone-iodine drops have been shown effective and less toxic when compared to erythromycin or silver nitrate ointment in a clinical trial in Kenya. This agent may be particularly useful in developing countries due to its low cost and ease of application.

Holland GN. Infectious diseases. In: Isenberg SJ, ed. *The Eye in Infancy.* 2nd ed. St Louis: Mosby; 1994:493–504.

Isenberg SJ, Apt L, Wood M. A controlled trial of povidone-iodine as prophylaxis against ophthalmia neonatorum. *N Engl J Med.* 1995;332:562–566.

Conjunctivitis

Common causes of conjunctival inflammation, or red eye, in infants and children are listed in Table 17-1. The majority of cases of acute conjunctivitis in children are bacterial; a viral etiology has been found in 20%–40% of cases in children. BCSC Section 8, *External Disease and Cornea*, discusses conjunctivitis in detail.

Common clinical findings in children with infectious conjunctivitis are burning, stinging, foreign-body sensation, ocular discharge, and matting of the eyelids. Symptoms and signs may present unilaterally or bilaterally. The character of the discharge, which can provide some diagnostic help, may be serous, mucopurulent, or purulent. Purulent discharge suggests a polymorphonuclear response to a bacterial infection, mucopurulence suggests a viral or chlamydial infection, and a serous or watery discharge suggests a viral or allergic reaction.

Bacterial Conjunctivitis

The most common causes of bacterial conjunctivitis in school-age children are *Streptococcus pneumoniae*, some *Haemophilus* species, and *Moraxella*. The relative incidence of infection from *Haemophilus* has dropped in recent years because immunization for this genus has become widespread, but *Haemophilus influenzae* remains an important cause of bacterial conjunctivitis in children. In older children, cases present with unilateral or bilateral signs of conjunctival hyperemia, discharge, morning lid sealing, and perhaps foreign-body sensation. In clinical practice, culture to identify the offending agent usually is not necessary. If untreated, symptoms will be self-limited but may last up to 2 weeks. A broad-spectrum topical ophthalmic drop or ointment should shorten the course to a

Table 17-1 Causes of Conjunctival Inflammation in Children

Infectious conjunctivitis
Bacterial
Viral
Chlamydial
Blepharoconjunctivitis
Allergic conjunctivitis
Trauma
Foreign body
Drug, toxin, or chemical reaction
Nasolacrimal duct obstruction
Iritis
Episcleritis or scleritis

few days. Usually effective medications include sulfacetamide, trimethoprim-polymyxin B, gentamicin or tobramycin, erythromycin ointment, third-generation fluoroquinolones such as ciprofloxacin, and newer, fourth-generation fluoroquinolones such as moxifloxacin and gatifloxicin.

More severe forms of bacterial conjunctivitis accompanied by copious discharge suggest infection with more virulent organisms, including *N gonorrhoeae, N meningitidis*, or various *Streptococcus, Staphylococcus*, or *Haemophilus* species. In such cases, calcium alginate swabs of the conjunctival surface should be obtained for a Gram stain and culture.

Although infection with *N gonorrhoeae* in children usually is associated with ophthalmia neonatorum from passage through an infected birth canal, older children who are sexually active or victims of sexual abuse can contract this infection.

For further discussion of diagnosis and treatment of gonorrheal conjunctivitis, see BCSC Section 8, *External Disease and Cornea.*

Viral Conjunctivitis

Most viral conjunctivitis is caused by adenovirus, a DNA virus that can cause a range of human diseases, including upper respiratory infection, gastroenteritis, and conjunctivitis. Some serotypes (types 18, 19, and 37) are associated with epidemic keratoconjunctivitis, others with pharyngoconjunctival fever (types 3 and 7), acute hemorrhagic conjunctivitis (types 11 and 21), or an acute follicular conjunctivitis (types 1, 2, 3, 4, 7, and 10).

Epidemic keratoconjunctivitis

Epidemic keratoconjunctivitis is a highly contagious conjunctivitis that tends to occur in epidemic outbreaks. This infection is an acute follicular conjunctivitis that is usually unilateral at onset and associated with preauricular lymphadenopathy. Initial complaints are foreign-body sensation and periorbital pain. A diffuse superficial keratitis is followed by focal epithelial lesions that stain. After 11–15 days, subepithelial opacities begin to form under the focal epithelial infiltrates. The epithelial component fades by day 30, but the subepithelial opacities may linger for up to 2 years. In severe infections, particularly in infants, a conjunctival membrane and marked swelling of the eyelids occur and must be differentiated from orbital or preseptal cellulitis (discussed later under Orbital and Adnexal Infections).

The infection is easily transmitted and occurs in epidemic outbreaks. Infected children may need to be kept out of school or child care for up to 2 weeks. Medical personnel who become infected should be excluded from ophthalmic examination areas for at least 2 weeks, and isolation areas should be designated for examination of patients known to have adenoviral infections.

Diagnosis is usually made on clinical grounds but can be confirmed by isolation of the agent or increased antibody titer to the specific adenovirus type. The organism can be recovered from the eyes and throat for 2 weeks after onset, demonstrating that patients are infectious during this period. Complications include persistent subepithelial opacities and conjunctival scar formation. Treatment is supportive. Topical steroids administered 3 to 4 times daily may be used judiciously in severe cases causing visual compromise, but such agents may prolong the time to full recovery. Steroid use in adenovirus infections is seldom indicated in children. Artificial tears and cold compresses can provide symptomatic relief.

Pharyngoconjunctival fever

Pharyngoconjunctival fever presents with conjunctival hyperemia and frequently with subconjunctival hemorrhage, edema, epiphora, and even lid swelling. It is accompanied by sore throat and fever. Within a few days, a follicular conjunctival reaction and preauricular adenopathy develop. Pharyngoconjunctival fever is caused by an adenovirus, usually type 3 or 7. Symptoms may last for 2 weeks or more. No topical or systemic treatment alters the course of the disease.

Herpes simplex conjunctivitis

Herpes simplex virus (HSV) conjunctivitis can occur as a primary or secondary infection and typically presents with ocular redness, discomfort, foreign-body sensation, or a combination of these; a watery discharge; and preauricular adenopathy. HSV conjunctivitis is more commonly unilateral. Typical herpetic eyelid vesicles help identify the cause of the conjunctivitis, but they are not always present. Bulbar conjunctival ulceration, although rare, is highly suggestive of HSV infection.

Most cases of primary eye involvement are caused by HSV-1 and are associated with gingivostomatitis or recurrent orolabial infection. HSV-2 is associated with genital infection and is the more common cause of neonatal eye infections. Recurrent disease is characterized by dendritiform or geographic keratitis (Fig 17-5).

Diagnosis is usually made based on characteristic clinical findings. Epithelial disease is marked by epithelial vesicles and dendritic ulcers. Atypical or questionable cases can be confirmed with ELISA testing.

Treatment of pure conjunctival disease does not seem to alter the course of disease, although treatment is definitely indicated when the cornea is involved. Treatment includes topical drops of trifluridine 1%, 9 drops per day. Oral acyclovir has been shown to be effective for treatment of herpetic epithelial keratitis and for reducing the rate of recurrences when used prophylactically.

Corneal involvement can be treated with debridement of the infected area, in addition to topical drops. See BCSC Section 8, *External Disease and Cornea*, for more discussion of the various forms of corneal disease and their treatment.

Varicella and zoster

Varicella (chickenpox) is a contagious viral exanthem of childhood that causes fever and vesicular eruptions of skin and mucous membranes. The cause is varicella-zoster (VZV), a herpes family virus. Clinical manifestations of the primary infection with VZV include fever and characteristic skin lesions. Ocular involvement is usually mild and self-limited. Conjunctival vesicles or ulcerations and internal ophthalmoplegia can occur. The cornea may be involved with a dendritic ulcer, opacification, punctate epithelial keratitis, or interstitial keratitis. Anterior uveitis can be seen but is usually mild and resolves without treatment.

Treatment of the conjunctivitis is symptomatic. Topical steroids are contraindicated except for late nonulcerative interstitial keratitis. Topical antibiotics may prevent second-

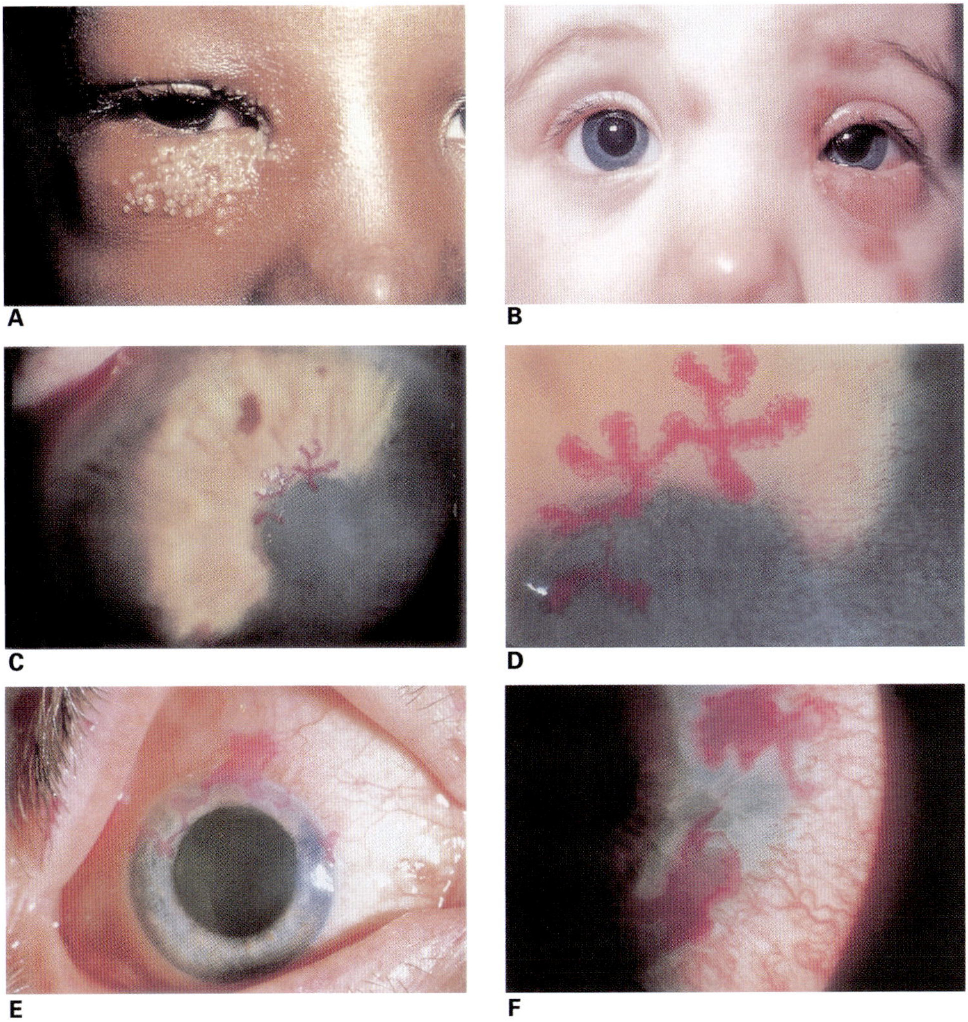

Figure 17-5 Herpes simplex. **A,** Vesicular lesions, right lower eyelid. **B,** Medial canthal distribution, left eye. **C** and **D,** Dendritic keratitis demonstrated by stain with rose bengal solution. **E** and **F,** Dendritic keratoconjunctivitis.

ary infection. Intravenous or oral acyclovir may be considered in the treatment of immunocompromised children with chickenpox but should be administered under the direction of an expert in pediatric infectious diseases.

Reactivation of latent VZV from dorsal root and cranial nerve ganglia results in zoster. When it does, vesicular lesions may erupt on the periorbital skin with subsequent ocular involvement (Fig 17-6). Ocular involvement is most likely if the nasociliary branch of V1 is affected. Keratitis and anterior uveitis can result.

Treatment of herpes zoster includes steroids for the inflammation and for iritis, if present. Systemic antivirals (famciclovir, valacyclovir, acyclovir) can be used in infants and children with herpes zoster infection.

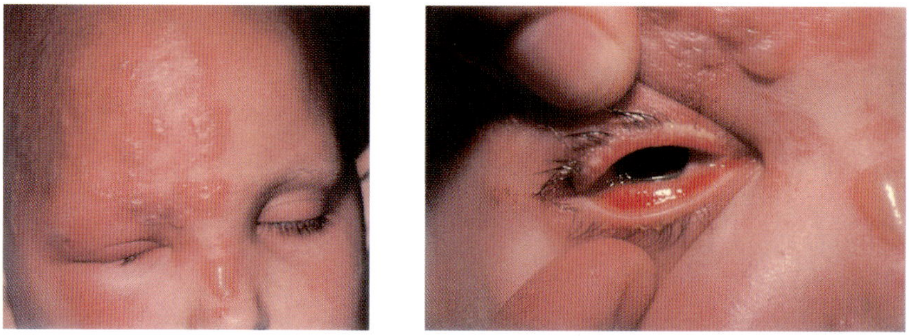

Figure 17-6 Herpes zoster.

Infectious mononucleosis

Infectious mononucleosis is caused by Epstein-Barr virus. The disease usually occurs between ages 15 and 30 years and is benign and self-limited. Findings include fever, widespread lymphadenopathy, pharyngitis, hepatic involvement, and the presence of atypical lymphocytes and heterophil antibodies in the circulating blood. Conjunctivitis occurs in a very high percentage of cases. Treatment is supportive, including bed rest, antipyretics, analgesics, and cool compresses to the eyes.

Influenza virus

Acute conjunctivitis with superficial punctate or interstitial keratitis, chemosis, and secondary bacterial infection may be caused by influenza virus type A, B, or C. The clinical manifestations include headache, fever, malaise, myalgias, nasal congestion, nausea, cough, and pharyngitis. Treatment is supportive, with topical antibiotics to prevent secondary infection.

Mumps virus

Acute viremia may lead to ocular involvement. The conjunctival manifestations are chemosis, follicular or papillary conjunctivitis, hyperemia, and subconjunctival hemorrhages. Treatment is supportive, with topical antibiotics to prevent secondary bacterial infection.

Rubeola

Rubeola, an acute contagious febrile illness, primarily affects school-age children and is caused by a paramyxovirus. Clinical manifestations include maculopapular rash, keratoconjunctivitis, and inflammation of the respiratory tract. Treatment includes antipyretics, analgesics, and cool compresses on the eyelids.

Molluscum contagiosum

Molluscum contagiosum is caused by a DNA pox virus and presents most commonly as numerous umbilicated skin lesions in the periocular region (Fig 17-7). Lesions on or near the lid margin can release viral particles onto the conjunctival surface, resulting in a follicular conjunctivitis. The lesions tend to be self-limited, but those causing conjunc-

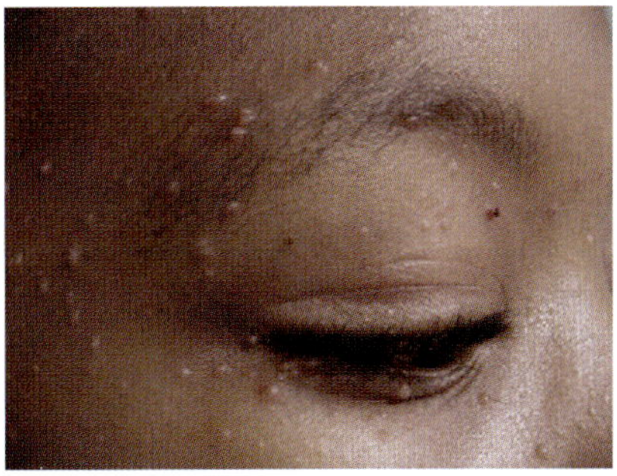

Figure 17-7 Molluscum contagiosum lesions on lid. *(Photograph courtesy of David A. Plager, MD.)*

tivitis, in particular, should be treated by incising and debriding the central core from each lesion. For young children, this usually requires general anesthesia.

Other Types of Conjunctivitis

Parinaud oculoglandular syndrome

Parinaud oculoglandular syndrome (POS) manifests as a unilateral granulomatous conjunctivitis associated with preauricular and submandibular adenopathy. The adenopathy can be very marked (Fig 17-8). Cat-scratch disease is the most common cause of POS.

Cat-scratch disease is usually associated with a scratch from a young kitten, although a cat bite and perhaps even touching the eye with a hand that has been licked by an infected kitten can cause the disease. The etiologic agent, which is endemic in cats, has been identified as *Bartonella henselae*, a pleomorphic gram-negative bacillus.

Diagnosis is made on clinical grounds and supported by a compatible history of exposure to cats. An immunofluorescent assay directed at *B henselae* is available.

Treatment can be supportive in mild cases because the disease is self-limited and is not known to cause corneal complications. In more severe cases, oral agents including azythromycin, ciprofloxacin, rifampin, trimethoprim-sulfamethoxazole, and erythromycin have been reported to be successful, although there is no generally accepted first-line choice of medication.

Other organisms that can cause POS include *Mycobacterium tuberculosis, Mycobacterium leprae, Francisella tularensis, Yersinia pseudotuberculosis, Treponema pallidum*, and *C trachomatis.*

Grando D, Sullivan LJ, Flexman JP, et al. Bartonella henselae associated with Parinaud's oculoglandular syndrome. *Clin Infect Dis.* 1999;28:1156–1158.

Trachoma

Except in areas of the South and on Native American reservations, trachoma is uncommon in the United States. Most cases are mild. Clinical manifestations include acute purulent conjunctivitis, follicles, papillary hypertrophy, vascularization of the cornea, and progressive cicatricial changes of the cornea and conjunctiva. Diagnosis is made from corneal scrapings, which reveal cytoplasmic inclusion bodies. Expressed follicle material demonstrates large macrophages and lymphoblasts. Treatment includes topical or systemic sulfonamides (or both), erythromycin, and tetracyclines.

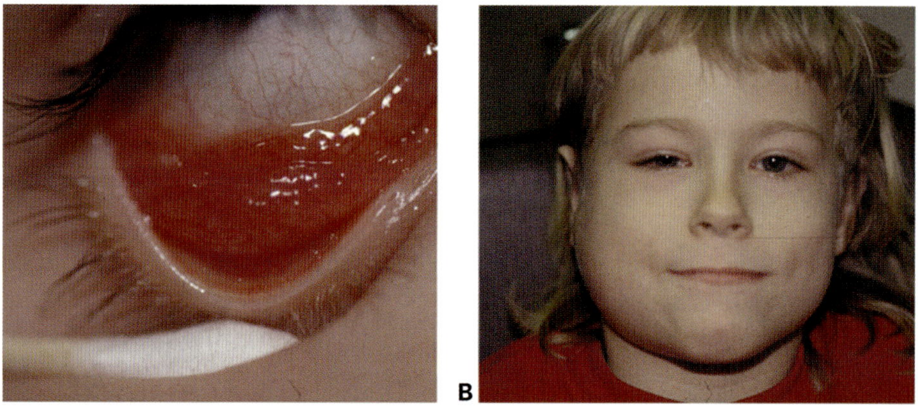

Figure 17-8 Parinaud oculoglandular syndrome. **A,** Marked follicular reaction in lower fornix. **B,** Massive submandibular lymph node enlargement on affected right side. *(Photographs courtesy of David A. Plager, MD.)*

Orbital and Adnexal Infections

Orbital cellulitis and preseptal cellulitis are both usually more rapidly progressive and more severe in children than in adults. See also BCSC Section 7, *Orbit, Eyelids, and Lacrimal System.*

Preseptal Cellulitis

Preseptal cellulitis, a common infection in children, is an inflammatory process involving the tissues anterior to the orbital septum. Eyelid edema may extend into the eyebrow and forehead. The periorbital skin becomes taut and inflamed, and edema may appear on the contralateral eyelids. Proptosis is not a feature of preseptal cellulitis, and the globe remains uninflamed. Full ocular motility and absence of pain on eye movement help distinguish preseptal from orbital cellulitis.

Preseptal cellulitis can occur in 1 of 3 ways. Posttraumatic cellulitis occurs following puncture, laceration, or abrasion of the eyelid skin. In these cases, organisms found in the skin, such as *Staphylococcus aureus* or *Streptococcus pyogenes*, are most commonly responsible for the infection.

The second cause of preseptal cellulitis is severe conjunctivitis such as epidemic keratoconjunctivitis or skin infection such as impetigo or herpes zoster infection.

The third mechanism for preseptal cellulitis tends to occur in young children and is secondary to upper respiratory or sinus infection or to unknown cause. Until the 1990s, *H influenzae* was the most common causative agent. It could be recognized by a typical deep violaceous hue of the infected lids. *Haemophilus* preseptal cellulitis may still be seen in medically underserved regions, but the incidence has dropped markedly since widespread use of Hib vaccine began in the early 1990s. More recently, *S pneumoniae* and other streptococcal infections and *S aureus* are the most common causes.

Children with nonsevere preseptal infections who are not systemically ill can be treated on an outpatient basis with oral antibiotics. Broad-spectrum drugs effective against the most common pathogens, such as cephalosporins or ampicillin-clavulanic acid combination, are usually effective.

If the child is younger than 1 year or has signs of systemic illness such as sepsis or meningeal involvement, hospitalization (for appropriate cultures, imaging of the sinuses and orbits, and intravenous antibiotics) is appropriate.

Orbital Cellulitis

Orbital cellulitis is an infection of the orbit that involves the tissues posterior to the orbital septum. Orbital cellulitis is commonly associated with ethmoid or frontal sinusitis and subperiosteal abscess and can follow penetrating injuries of the orbit. A retained foreign body can trigger orbital cellulitis months after the initial injury.

The etiologic agents most commonly responsible for orbital cellulitis vary with age. In general, children younger than 9 years have infections caused by a single aerobic pathogen. Children older than 9 years may have complex infections with multiple pathogens, both aerobic and anaerobic. *S aureus* and gram-negative bacilli are most common in the neonate. In older children and adults, *S aureus, S pyogenes, S pneumoniae*, and various anaerobic species are common pathogens. Gram-negative organisms are found primarily in immunosuppressed patients.

Diagnosis

Early signs and symptoms of orbital cellulitis include lethargy, fever, eyelid edema, rhinorrhea, headache, orbital pain, and tenderness on palpation. The nasal mucosa becomes hyperemic, with a purulent nasal discharge. Increased venous congestion may cause elevated intraocular pressure. Proptosis and limited ocular movement suggest orbital involvement. In general, children with orbital cellulitis present with more systemic manifestations than children of similar age with preseptal involvement only. It is crucial to distinguish orbital cellulitis from preseptal cellulitis because the former requires hospitalization with IV antibiotics. Paranasal sinusitis is the most common cause of bacterial orbital cellulitis (Fig 17-9). In children younger than 10 years, the ethmoid sinuses are most frequently involved. If orbital cellulitis is suspected, computed tomography (CT) is indicated to confirm orbital involvement, to document the presence and extent of sinusitis and subperiosteal abscess, and to rule out a foreign body in a patient with a history of trauma (Fig 17-10).

The differential diagnosis of orbital cellulitis includes inflammatory pseudotumor, benign orbital tumors such as lymphangioma and hemangioma, rhabdomyosarcoma or other malignant tumors, metastatic disease, and leukemia.

Complications of orbital cellulitis include cavernous sinus thrombosis or intracranial extension (subdural or brain abscesses, meningitis, periosteal abscess), which may result in death. Cavernous sinus thrombosis can be difficult to distinguish from simple orbital cellulitis. Paralysis of eye movement in cavernous sinus thrombosis is often out of proportion to the degree of proptosis. Pain on motion and tenderness to palpation are absent. Decreased sensation along the maxillary division of cranial nerve V (trigeminal) supports the diagnosis. Bilateral involvement is virtually diagnostic of cavernous sinus thrombosis.

Other complications of orbital cellulitis include corneal exposure with secondary ulcerative keratitis, neurotropic keratitis, secondary glaucoma, septic uveitis or retinitis,

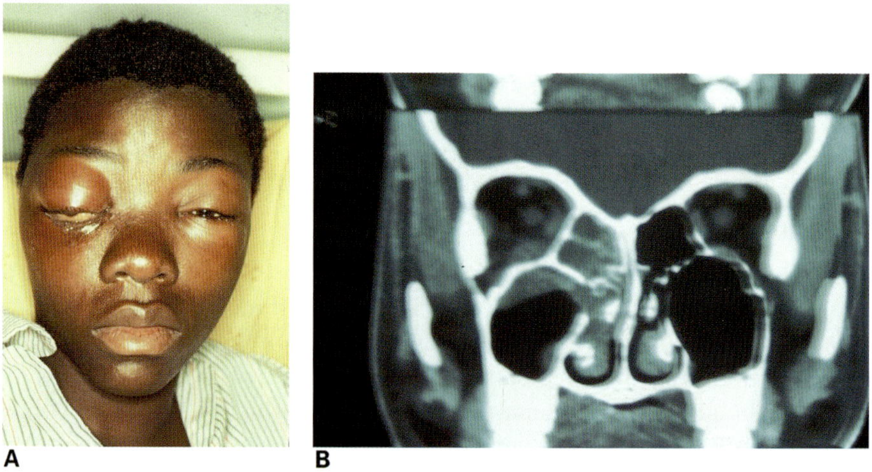

Figure 17-9 Orbital cellulitis with proptosis **(A)** secondary to sinusitis **(B)**. *(Photographs courtesy of Jane Edmond, MD.)*

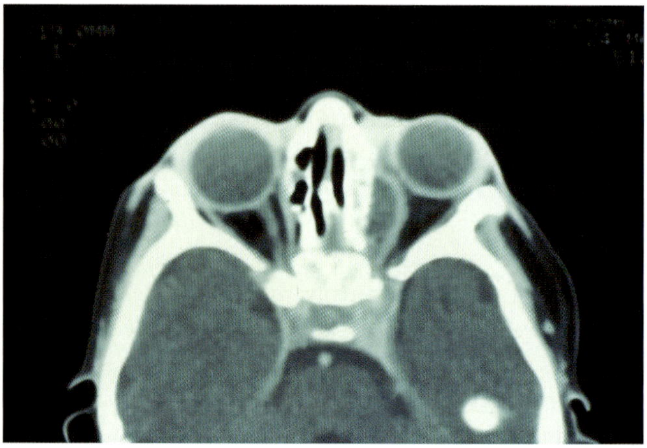

Figure 17-10 Axial CT showing a medial subperiosteal abscess of the right orbit associated with ethmoid sinusitis. *(Image courtesy of Jane Edmond, MD.)*

exudative retinal detachment, optic nerve edema, inflammatory neuritis, infectious neuritis, central retinal artery occlusion, and panophthalmitis.

Treatment

Orbital cellulitis in children is a serious disease that requires hospitalization and treatment with intravenous broad-spectrum antibiotics. Orbital imaging with CT or MR should be performed. If associated sinusitis or subperiosteal abscess is present, other specialists should be consulted. The patient should be followed closely for signs of visual compromise.

Choice of intravenous antibiotic should be based on the most likely pathogens until results from nasal, nasopharyngeal, or blood cultures are known. Most subperiosteal abscesses in children will resolve without medical management; however, emergency drainage of a subperiosteal abscess is indicated for a patient of any age with evidence of optic nerve compromise (decreasing vision, relative afferent pupillary defect) and an enlarging subperiosteal abscess. Even in the absence of optic nerve dysfunction, surgical drainage may be required for clinical deterioration despite 48 hours of intravenous antibiotics or to relieve significant discomfort.

Harris GJ. Subperiosteal abscess of the orbit: age as a factor in bacteriology and response to treatment. *Ophthalmology.* 1994;101:585–595.

Harris GJ. Subperiosteal abscess of the orbit: computed tomography and the clinical course. *Ophthal Plast Reconstr Surg.*1996;12:1–8.

Related conditions

Maxillary osteomyelitis is a rare condition of early infancy. Infection spreads from the nose into the tooth buds with unilateral erythema and edema of the eyelids, cheek, and nose. Infection may spread and cause orbital cellulitis.

Fungal orbital cellulitis (mucormycosis) occurs most frequently in patients with ketoacidosis or severe immunosuppression. The infection causes thrombosing vasculitis with ischemic necrosis of involved tissue (Fig 17-11). Cranial nerves often are involved, and extension into the central nervous system is common. Smears and biopsy of the involved tissues reveal the fungal organisms. Treatment includes debridement of necrotic and infected tissue plus administration of amphotericin. Predisposing factors such as metabolic acidosis should be controlled.

Ocular Allergy

Allergic ocular disease is a common problem in children, often associated with asthma, allergic rhinitis, and atopic dermatitis. Marked itching and bilateral conjunctival inflammation of a chronic, recurrent, and possibly seasonal nature are hallmarks of external ocular disease of allergic origin. Other signs and symptoms may be nonspecific and include tearing, stinging, burning, and photophobia.

Three specific types of ocular allergy are discussed in this section: seasonal allergic conjunctivitis, vernal keratoconjunctivitis, and atopic keratoconjunctivitis. All have some element of type I hypersensitivity reaction caused by the interaction between an allergen

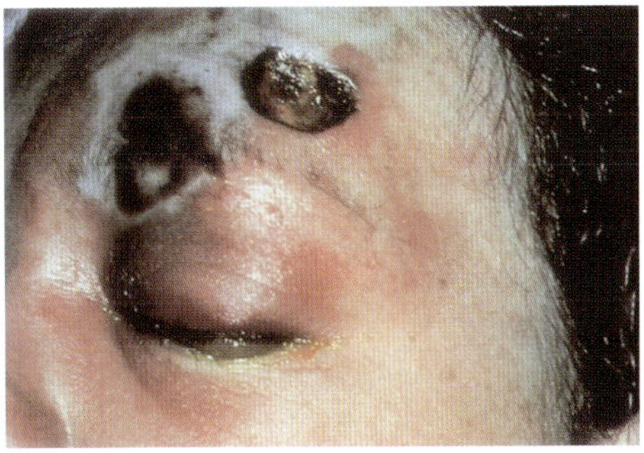

Figure 17-11 Mucormycosis, left orbit.

and specific IgE antibodies on the surface of mast cells in the conjunctiva. This interaction results in the initiation of a cascade of biochemical events involved in mediation of the allergic response and includes prostaglandins and leukotrienes. Among the mediators released as a result of these interactions is histamine. Histamine is known to cause much of the itching, vasodilation, and edema that are so characteristic of the ocular allergic response.

Seasonal Allergic Conjunctivitis

Seasonal allergic conjunctivitis is a common clinical entity, affecting approximately 40 million people living in the United States, including many children. As the name implies, it is a seasonal affliction, occurring in the spring and fall and triggered by environmental contact with specific airborne allergens such as pollens from grasses, flowers, weeds, and trees. Conjunctival scrapings reveal eosinophils, a finding that is almost diagnostic of an allergic response. Patients typically present with reddened, watery eyes, boggy-appearing conjunctiva, and complaints of itchy eyes. Lower-lid ecchymoses termed *allergic shiners* are common.

Perennial allergic conjunctivitis is a related, though usually milder and less seasonal, form of type I hypersensitivity reaction to more ubiquitous household allergens, such as dust mites and dander from domestic pets.

Vernal Keratoconjunctivitis

Vernal keratoconjunctivitis shows evidence of a mast cell/lymphocyte–mediated allergic response. This condition most commonly affects males in the first 2 decades of life and, like seasonal allergic conjunctivitis, usually occurs in the spring and fall. It occurs in 2 forms—palpebral and bulbar—depending on which conjunctival surface is most affected.

The chief pathological findings include overgrowth of the subconjunctival tissues in the substantia propria. The tissue is infiltrated with lymphocytes, plasma cells, and eosinophils. With progression, large numbers of cells accumulate, forming nodules of tissue that project from the tarsal plate. New blood vessels are formed, producing giant papillae, the hallmark of this entity.

Clinically, the palpebral form of vernal keratoconjunctivitis preferentially affects the tarsal conjunctiva of the upper eyelid (Fig 17-12). Changes in the lower eyelid are rare and slight. In the early stages, the eye may be diffusely injected, with little discharge, and the conjunctiva appears milky. The most prominent features are photophobia and intense itching. There may be no progression beyond this stage. However, papillae may multiply, covering the tarsal area with a mosaic of flat papules. The conjunctiva is then covered with a milky veil.

The discharge is characteristically thick, ropy, and dirty white. It contains epithelial cells, leukocytes, and large numbers of eosinophils. Itching can be intense and accompanied by blepharospasm, foreign-body sensation, and photophobia.

The limbal, or bulbar, form of vernal keratoconjunctivitis is also bilateral and seasonal, etiologically and pathogenically similar to the palpebral disease. Intense itching is the most constant clinical feature. The earliest changes are thickening and opacification of the conjunctiva at the limbus, usually most marked at the upper margin of the cornea.

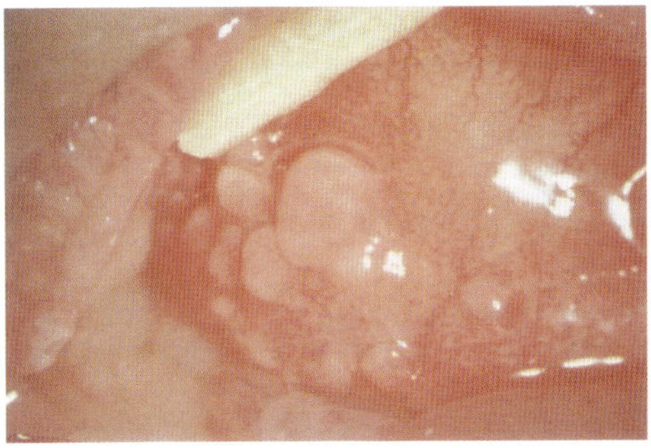

Figure 17-12 Palpebral vernal keratoconjunctivitis, upper eyelid.

The discrete limbal nodules that appear in this thickened conjunctiva are gray, jellylike, elevated lumps with vascular cores. They may increase in number and become confluent. These nodules persist as long as the seasonal exacerbation of the disease lasts. A whitish center may occur in the raised lesion filled with eosinophils and epithelioid cells. The complex is called a *Trantas* or *Horner-Trantas dot.*

The cornea can become involved with punctate epithelial erosions, especially superiorly. Corneal involvement can progress to a large confluent area of epithelial defect, typically in the upper half of the cornea, called a *shield ulcer.* The ulcer is sterile and clinically looks like an ovoid corneal abrasion.

Atopic Keratoconjunctivitis

Atopic keratoconjunctivitis has elements of a variety of immune responses, including type I and cell-mediated response. This condition is relatively rare in children and tends to present in males from the late teens to the sixth decade of life. Atopic keratoconjunctivitis is not seasonal and occurs in atopic persons with a tendency to develop hypersensitivity reactions such as atopic dermatitis, eczema, and asthma. Chronic inflammation of the eyelids is usually apparent. Unlike the case with vernal keratoconjunctivitis, the inferior palpebral conjunctiva is usually involved with papillae and scarring.

Other ocular involvement is common, including punctate corneal erosions and cataracts.

Treatment

Treatment of all allergic eye disorders is fundamentally similar to treatment of other allergy-related disorders. The most effective treatment is to remove the offending allergens from the patient's environment. Unfortunately, such attempts at removal frequently fall short of what is required to adequately alleviate the patient's symptoms.

Medical treatment can be systemic or topical. In general, oral medications—specifically, antihistamines aimed at ameliorating itching, swelling, and redness—are not very effective for ocular symptoms. The sedating effect of most drugs outweighs their therapeutic benefit for ocular allergy, although some recently introduced antihistamines induce less drowsiness than previous generations of these medications (Table 17-2).

Eyedrops are the preferred therapy for most patients. Therapeutic strategies are to stabilize mast cells, block H_1 receptors, or both. Available topical drops are listed in Table 17-3.

Table 17-2 Oral Antihistamines

Cetirizine hydrochloride (Zyrtec)
Fexofenadine hydrochloride (Allegra)
Loratidine (Claritin, Alavert)

Table 17-3 Topical Drops for Treatment of Allergic Eye Disorders

Mast cell stabilizers
Cromolyn sodium 4% (Crolom, Opticrom)
Lodoxamide tromethamine 0.1% (Alomide)
H_1-receptor antagonists
Emedastine difumarate 0.05% (Emadine)
Levocabastine hydrochloride 0.05% (Livostin)
Drops with both mast cell stabilizer and H_1-blocking activity
Ketotifen fumarate 0.025% (Zaditor)
Olopatidine hydrochloride 0.1% (Patanol)
Nedocromil sodium 2% (Alocril)
Pemirolast potassium 0.1% (Alamast)
Azelastine hydrochloride (Optivar)
Steroids
Fluoromethalone 1%/0.25% (FML/FML-F)
Prednisolone acetate 1%/0.12% (Pred Fort/Pred Mild)
Rimexolone 1% (Vexol)
Loteprednol etabonate 0.5%/0.2% (Lotemax, Alrex)
Medrysone 1% (HMS)

Cromolyn sodium, derived from khellin, a substance found in a Mediterranean plant, is the prototype mast cell stabilizer. Cromolyn acts by decreasing the release of granules containing inflammatory mediators from allergen-stimulated mast cells.

H_1-blocking antihistamines act by competitive inhibition of the H_1 sites responsible for the itching response and for some of the vascular permeability and vasodilation reactions.

A topical nonsteroidal anti-inflammatory medication, ketorolac tromethamine (Acular), is also available.

Topical steroid drops used in pulsed doses can be effective in reducing allergic ocular symptoms, but patients using topical steroids, unlike those using other nonsteroidal drops, must be closely monitored for steroid side effects, including glaucoma and cataracts.

Bouchard C. The ocular immune response. In: Krachmer JH, Mannis MJ, Holland EJ, eds. *Cornea.* St Louis: Mosby; 1997.

Dinowitz M, Rescigno R, Bielory L. Ocular allergic diseases: differential diagnosis, examination techniques, and testing. *Clin Allergy Immunol.* 2000;15:127–150.

Heidemann DG. Atopic and vernal keratoconjunctivitis. *Focal Points: Clinical Modules for Ophthalmologists.* San Francisco: American Academy of Ophthalmology; 2001, module 1.

Mets MB, Noffke AS. Ocular infections of the external eye and cornea in children. *Focal Points: Clinical Modules for Ophthalmologists.* San Francisco: American Academy of Ophthalmology; 2002, module 2.

Stevens-Johnson Syndrome

Stevens-Johnson syndrome (erythema multiforme) is an acute inflammatory polymorphic disease affecting skin and mucous membranes. All ages may be affected, and the incidence is equal in both sexes. This is a severe disease with a 5%–15% mortality rate. Ocular involvement, which occurs in as many as half of patients, varies from a mild mucopurulent conjunctivitis to severe perforating corneal ulcers. Blindness occasionally occurs in patients with severe late-phase corneal complications, such as ulceration, vascularization, and perforation.

Stevens-Johnson syndrome has been associated with various bacterial, viral, mycotic, and protozoal infections. Vaccines, collagen diseases, and many drugs have also been implicated. The pathogenesis consists of angiitis leading to erythematous lesions that become edematous or bullous and darken, leaving concentric rings in a target shape. When bullae are present, they are subepidermal and without acantholysis.

Clinical manifestations range from mild to severe. A prodrome of chills is followed by pharyngitis, headache, tachypnea, and tachycardia. In several days, bullous mucosal lesions develop, especially in the oropharynx. These lesions rupture and ulcerate and become covered by gray-white membranes and a hemorrhagic crust.

Ocular involvement in Stevens-Johnson syndrome begins with edema, erythema, and encrustation of the eyelids. The palpebral conjunctiva becomes hyperemic, and distinct vesicles or bullae may occur. In many instances, a concomitant conjunctivitis appears that is characterized by watery discharge with mucoid strands (Fig 17-13). Secondary infection, most commonly with *Staphylococcus* species, may develop. In severe cases, a membranous or pseudomembranous conjunctivitis may result from coalescence of fibrin and necrotic cellular debris. Symblepharon formation may occur with severe pseudomembranous conjunctivitis. Primary corneal involvement and iritis are rare ocular manifestations of Stevens-Johnson syndrome.

Late ocular complications occur in about 20% of patients and include structural anomalies of eyelid position (ectropion and entropion), trichiasis, and symblepharon. Dry eye syndrome may also result from deficiencies in the tear film—either in the aqueous layer, from scarring of lacrimal duct orifices, or, more commonly, in the mucin layer, from destruction of the conjunctival goblet cells.

Treatment

Early intervention is important in preventing the late ocular complications of Stevens-Johnson syndrome. Systemic therapy with corticosteroids is controversial. Antiviral treatment for cases associated with herpes simplex infection may be required. A discussion of systemic treatment is beyond the scope of this book. A dermatologist and pediatric infectious disease expert should be consulted.

Local measures should be instituted early in the course of the disease. Ocular lubrication with artificial tears and ointments (preferably preservative-free) should be applied regularly. Under topical anesthesia, the superior and inferior fornices should be inspected and debrided daily. A glass rod can be used for symblepharon lysis, but this may be

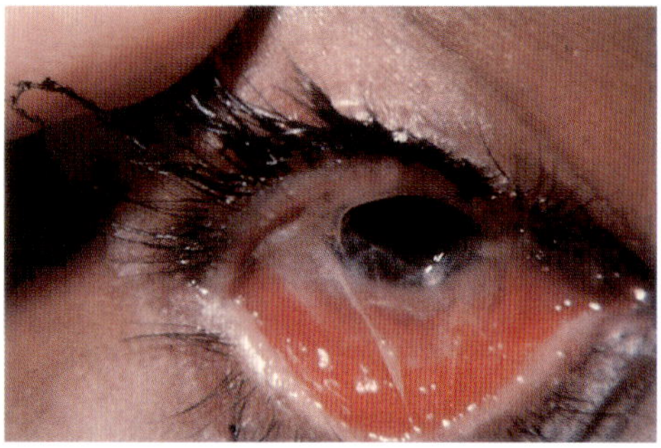

Figure 17-13 Stevens-Johnson syndrome. Early involvement of conjunctiva, right eye.

ineffective. A symblepharon ring can be useful in severe cases in cooperative patients. Surveillance cultures for microbial infection should be taken as needed. See also BCSC Section 8, *External Disease and Cornea.*

Wilkins J, Morrison L, White CR Jr. Oculocutaneous manifestations of the erythema multiforme/Stevens-Johnson syndrome/toxic epidermal necrolysis spectrum. *Dermatol Clin.* 1992;10:571–582.

Kawasaki Disease

Kawasaki disease, also known as *mucocutaneous lymph node syndrome,* is a febrile illness primarily affecting children younger than 5 years. The cause is unknown. The diagnostic criteria are an unexplainable fever lasting 5 or more days and at least 4 of the following:

- bilateral conjunctival injection
- mucous membrane changes of injected or fissured lips, injected pharynx, or "strawberry tongue"
- extremity changes involving erythema of the palms or soles, edema of the hands or feet, or generalized or periungual desquamation
- rash
- cervical lymphadenopathy

The most significant complication of Kawasaki disease is coronary artery aneurysm. Coronary artery evaluation by 2-dimensional echocardiography is therefore indicated.

Anterior uveitis during the acute phase of the illness is common but generally self-limited. Conjunctival scarring can occur, and bilateral retinal ischemia has been observed histopathologically.

Treatment is mainly supportive, and aspirin is considered the drug of choice. Corticosteroid therapy is contraindicated because of its association with an increased rate of coronary artery aneurysm formation.

Blatt AN, Vogler L, Tychsen L. Incomplete presentations in a series of 37 children with Kawasaki disease: the role of the pediatric ophthalmologist. *J Pediatr Ophthalmol Strabismus.* 1996;33:114–119.

CHAPTER 18

The Lacrimal Drainage System

Tear fluid enters the lacrimal drainage system through the *puncta*, small (approximately 0.3 mm) round openings located in the upper and lower eyelids near the inner canthus, just nasal to the most medial of the meibomian gland orifices. The lower punctum is slightly more temporally located than the upper, and both are normally positioned so as to contact the surface of the eye. Each punctum continues as a *canaliculus* that runs vertically for about 1 mm and then turns nasally, parallel to the eyelid margin. The canaliculi are lined with stratified squamous epithelium and surrounded by a layer of elastic tissue that permits considerable dilation. The tarsal plate does not extend into the portion of the eyelid containing the canaliculus, which consequently is easily torn. The upper and lower canaliculi join to form a very short *common canaliculus* before entering the *lacrimal sac* at the *valve of Rosenmüller.*

The lacrimal sac occupies the lacrimal fossa, which is formed by the lacrimal bone and the frontal process of the maxilla. The medial canthal ligament, which attaches at the anterior lacrimal crest, lies in front of the upper portion of the sac. The epithelial lining of the sac is composed of a superficial columnar layer and a deeper layer of flattened cells, as well as numerous mucus-secreting goblet cells. Similar epithelium lines the *nasolacrimal duct (NLD)*, which is the continuation of the sac, extending downward in a slightly lateral and posterior direction through the short, bony nasolacrimal canal to enter the lateral portion of the nose beneath the inferior turbinate at the *valve of Hasner.*

The lacrimal drainage components arise embryologically from a solid epithelial cord formed by invagination of surface ectoderm and canalize toward the end of gestation. Persistence of a thin tissue membrane across the lower end of the duct at birth is very common and is responsible for most obstructions.

Developmental Anomalies

Atresia of the Lacrimal Puncta or Canaliculi

Atresia of the lacrimal puncta results from failure of the upper end of the developing lacrimal structures to canalize. Symptoms are typically limited to accumulation and overflow of clear tears; mucopurulence is not seen to the degree typical of an obstruction of the lacrimal duct. A similar obstruction in the canaliculi causes symptoms similar to those of punctal atresia.

Often, only a thin epithelial punctal membrane obstructs a well-developed canalicular system. The site is easily identified in such cases, and perforating the membrane with a needle or fine probe, followed by dilation, usually is curative. If this is not successful, more elaborate surgery is required, ranging from an incisional punctoplasty combined with silicone intubation to conjunctivodacryocystorhinostomy in extreme cases.

Supernumerary Puncta

Supernumerary puncta occasionally occur nasal to the normal opening; they do not disturb tear drainage and require no treatment.

Congenital Lacrimal Fistula

A congenital lacrimal fistula is an epithelial-lined tract extending from the common canaliculus or lacrimal sac to the skin surface of the lower eyelid, usually just inferonasal to the medial canthus. Discharge from the fistula often is associated with NLD obstruction and may cease after the lower drainage system becomes patent. Persistence of bothersome symptoms despite adequate drainage necessitates surgical excision of the entire fistulous tract.

Toda C, Imai K, Tsujiguchi K, et al. Three different types of congenital lacrimal fistula. *Ann Plast Surg.* 2000;45:651–653.

Dacryocele

Congenital *dacryocele* (sometimes called *mucocele, dacryocystocele*, or *amniotocele*) of the lacrimal sac is an unusual condition that occurs when a distal blockage, usually membranous, causes a distention of the sac that also kinks and closes off the entrance to it of the common canaliculus, thereby preventing decompression by retrograde discharge of accumulated secretions. Involvement occasionally is bilateral.

Clinical Features

Dacryocele presents as a bluish swelling just below and nasal to the medial canthus (Fig 18-1). The appearance is distinctive, but there is the possibility of confusion with hemangioma, dermoid cyst, or encephalocele. Hemangiomas often increase in size when the infant is held in a head-down position and are generally less firm to the

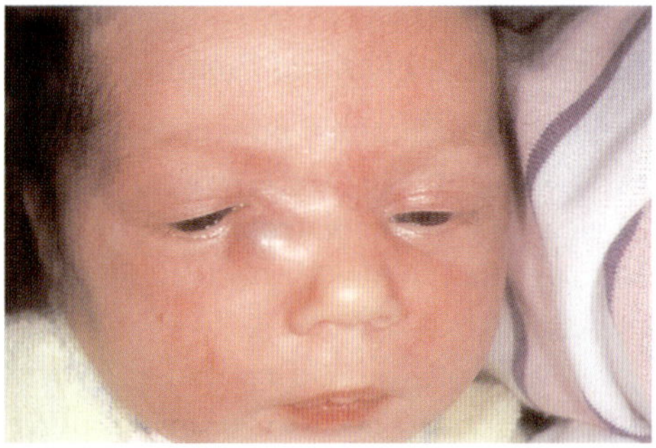

Figure 18-1 Congenital dacryocystocele, right eye, in a newborn infant. Note typical location and bluish discoloration of the overlying skin.

touch. Dermoid cysts and encephaloceles present most often above the medial canthal ligament, in contrast to dacryoceles.

Associated nasal mucocele (bulging of mucosa at the lower end of the NLD into the nasal cavity) can significantly compromise the airway. This finding also can be seen with NLD obstruction that does not result in a dacryocele. If the condition does not resolve spontaneously, infection with obvious local inflammatory changes usually develops within the first few weeks of life.

Management

A dacryocele sometimes can be decompressed by careful digital massage. Most pediatricians would employ full-dose systemic antibiotics as well, because of concern for systemic infection in these very young infants. If dacryocystitis shows no improvement 24–48 hours after initiation of intravenous antibiotics, decompression of the sac usually is necessary. This can be accomplished initially by gently passing a probe or lacrimal cannula through a canaliculus into the distended sac, to interrupt the valvelike action of the sac on the common canalicular entrance and allow the contents to reflux externally. The presence of an intranasal mucocele should be ruled out by inspection of the nasal passage.

Permanent and complete relief requires elimination of associated NLD obstruction, for which probing should be performed when the inflammation has substantially decreased. If present, an associated nasal mucocele can be marsupialized to facilitate drainage into the nose. Nasal endoscopy facilitates this treatment. Incision and drainage of an infected dacryocele through the skin should be avoided because of the danger of creating a persistent fistulous tract.

Lueder GT. Endoscopic treatment of intranasal abnormalities associated with nasolacrimal duct obstruction. *J AAPOS.* 2004;8:128–132.

Paysse EA, Coats DK, Bernstein JM, et al. Management and complications of congenital dacryocele with concurrent intranasal mucocele. *J AAPOS.* 2000;4:46–53.

Schnall BM, Christian CJ. Conservative treatment of congenital dacryocele. *J Pediatr Ophthalmol Strabismus.* 1996;33:219–222.

Nasolacrimal Duct Obstruction

The more typical nonemergency obstruction of drainage below the lacrimal sac occurs in about 5% of full-term newborns. Usually, a thin mucosal membrane at the lower end of the NLD is the cause. Symptoms become manifest by age 1 month in 80%–90% of such cases.

Clinical Features

The most severe cases of NLD obstruction resemble congenital dacryocele in showing a distended lacrimal sac that can be seen and palpated beneath the skin, just inferior to the medial canthal ligament. Unlike with congenital dacryocele, however, digital pressure usually results in retrograde discharge of mucopurulent material. Milder cases with low-grade chronic inflammation typically present with epiphora and a sticky mucoid or mucopurulent discharge that accumulates on the eyelid margins and lashes (Fig 18-2). The severity of these manifestations may vary considerably from day to day. Applying fluorescein solution to the tear film and noting significant retention after 5–10 min and failure of dye to appear in the nose or pharynx after 10–15 min is another way to confirm the blockage. Culture of the discharge typically indicates the presence of multiple strains of bacteria, but this information is not necessary for clinical management. Bilateral involvement is common.

The differential diagnosis of lower NLD obstruction includes the following disorders:

- conjunctivitis, in which the lacrimal sac is not enlarged to palpation and there is no reflux of fluid or fluorescein retention
- blepharitis, characterized by dry crusting on the eyelid margins
- congenital glaucoma, in which epiphora caused by hypersecretion of tears is associated with nasal wetness, photophobia, and corneal enlargement or clouding, features that are absent from the clinical picture of lacrimal obstruction

Nonsurgical Management

The most important initial measure in NLD obstruction is digital massage of the lacrimal sac. Instillation of topical antibiotics several times per day over a period of 1–2 weeks may clear the secondary infection but should be considered adjunctive treatment that does not address the underlying problem. The antimicrobial agent should cover a broad spectrum of bacteria.

Massage serves 2 purposes: it empties the sac, reducing the opportunity for bacterial growth; and it applies hydrostatic pressure to the obstruction, which occasionally opens the duct and permanently relieves the condition. To create sufficient pressure to accomplish the latter goal, it is preferable to compress the sac while initially occluding the canaliculi. The parent is instructed to place a finger above the medial canthus and then firmly press and slide downward.

Surgical Management

Congenital NLD obstruction resolves spontaneously with conservative management in a large majority of cases. Published series have shown clearing without the necessity of

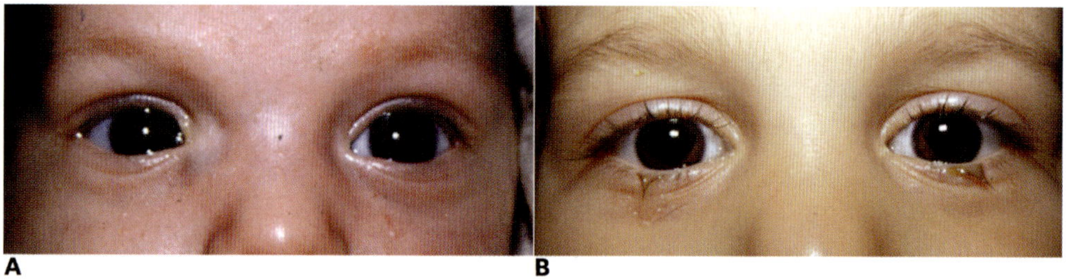

A B

Figure 18-2 Nasolacrimal duct obstruction. **A,** Lacrimal sac enlargement, right eye, similar to congenital dacryocele. **B,** Milder bilateral obstruction. Wetness and mucus accumulation without evidence of inflammation. *(Photographs courtesy of Edward L. Raab, MD.)*

probing in 50%–90% of patients during the first 6 months of life, and in about 70% by age 1 year. Accordingly, the timing of surgery for congenital NLD obstruction is controversial.

Early probing (before age 1 year) reduces the duration of bothersome symptoms, the burden of conservative management, and the potential for chronic infection. However, delaying probing beyond age 1 year may avoid surgery altogether, despite the classic view that the rate of spontaneous resolution is significantly reduced and the likelihood of permanent damage to the lacrimal drainage system from chronic infection increases with this decision. More recent studies have shown that although extensive delay is not the treatment of choice, cases with membranous (ie, uncomplicated) obstruction persisting after the first year of life have success rates with simple probing comparable to those of younger infants.

A small proportion of newborns with congenital NLD obstruction have anatomical variants that are unlikely to resolve spontaneously or be relieved by simple probing. Children with Down syndrome have a higher rate of canalicular stenosis and narrow ducts than of distal membranous obstruction. (See also Chapter 14 of BCSC Section 7, *Orbit, Eyelids, and Lacrimal System*).

Coats DK, McCreery KM, Plager DA, et al. Nasolacrimal outflow drainage anomalies in Down's syndrome. *Ophthalmology.* 2003;110:1437–1441.

Kushner BJ. The management of nasolacrimal duct obstruction in children between 18 months and 4 years old. *J AAPOS.* 1998;2:57–60.

Probing

Probing can be done in the office under topical anesthesia in the youngest patients, with the infant securely immobilized, avoiding the risk of general anesthesia and the trouble and expense of even brief hospitalization. Probing under general anesthesia in the operating room setting allows for increased control and provides the additional advantages of allowing evaluation and treatment of an obstructing inferior turbinate or an intranasal mucocele and of employing balloon dilation or intubation if indicated.

The clinician initiates probing by dilating either the upper or the lower punctum and canaliculus and attempting to irrigate a small amount of saline under moderate pressure from a syringe attached to a blunt-tipped cannula introduced into the lacrimal sac. Reflux is prevented by compression of the canaliculi. This maneuver occasionally relieves the obstruction.

If it does not, a Bowman probe (usually nos. 0–2) is advanced along the canaliculus toward the sac (Fig 18-3). When the probe tip encounters the nasal wall of the sac and underlying bone, the probe is pivoted to direct it downward toward the floor of the nose. If there is distal membranous obstruction, as the probe slides through the NLD, a sudden decrease in resistance is felt when the obstruction is overcome. Many surgeons confirm the presence of the probe tip in the nose by introducing a second probe underneath the inferior turbinate and observing movement of the first probe as the second probe rubs directly against it (Fig 18-4). Alternatively, direct inspection with a nasal speculum and headlamp or with a nasal endoscope can determine the precise position of the probe.

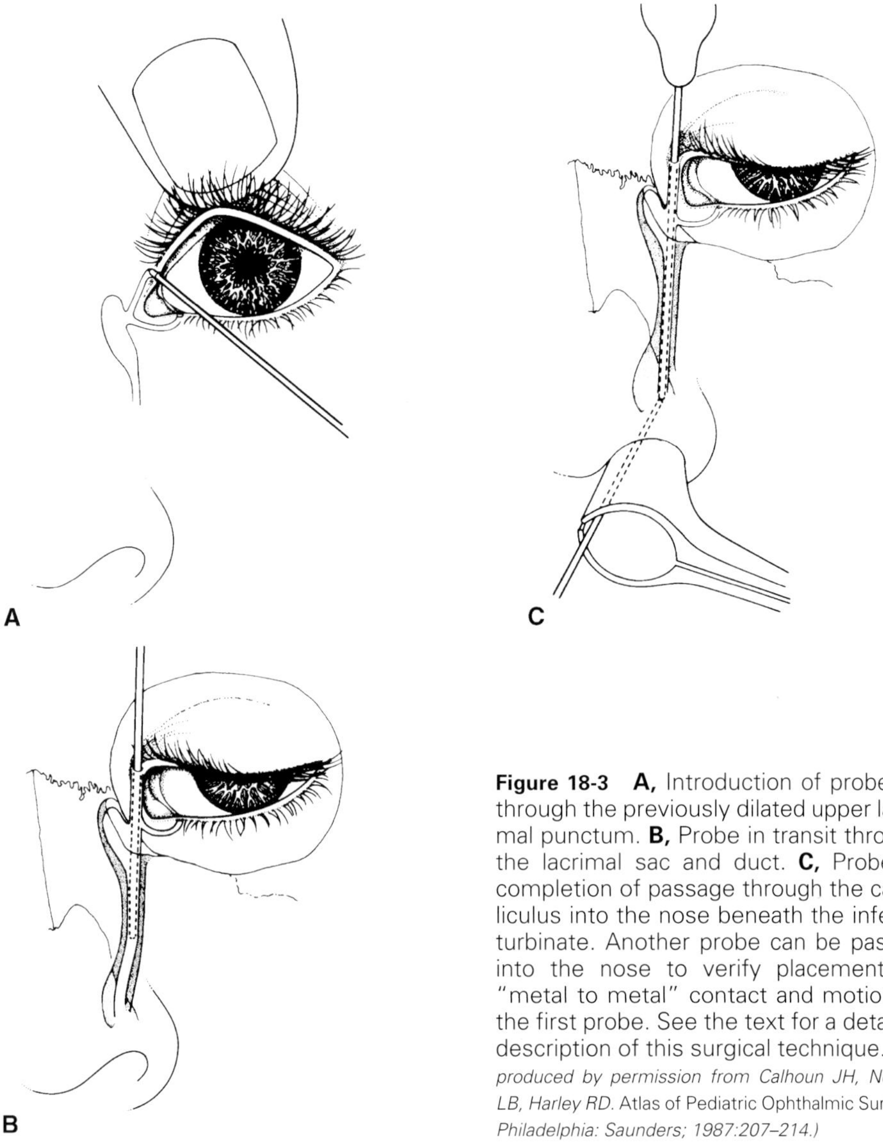

Figure 18-3 **A,** Introduction of probe tip through the previously dilated upper lacrimal punctum. **B,** Probe in transit through the lacrimal sac and duct. **C,** Probe at completion of passage through the canaliculus into the nose beneath the inferior turbinate. Another probe can be passed into the nose to verify placement by "metal to metal" contact and motion of the first probe. See the text for a detailed description of this surgical technique. *(Reproduced by permission from Calhoun JH, Nelson LB, Harley RD.* Atlas of Pediatric Ophthalmic Surgery. *Philadelphia: Saunders; 1987:207–214.)*

Gardiner JA, Forte V, Pashby RC, et al. The role of nasal endoscopy in repeat pediatric nasolacrimal duct probings. *J AAPOS.* 2001;5:148–152.

Minor bleeding from the nose or into the tears sometimes occurs but requires no treatment. Optional postoperative medications include antibiotic drops, corticosteroid drops, or both 2 to 4 times per day for up to 2 weeks. Phenylephrine 1/8% nose drops can be used concurrently for 3–5 days to promote tear drainage by minimizing edema of the nasal mucosa. Because transient bacteremia can occur after probing, systemic antibiotic

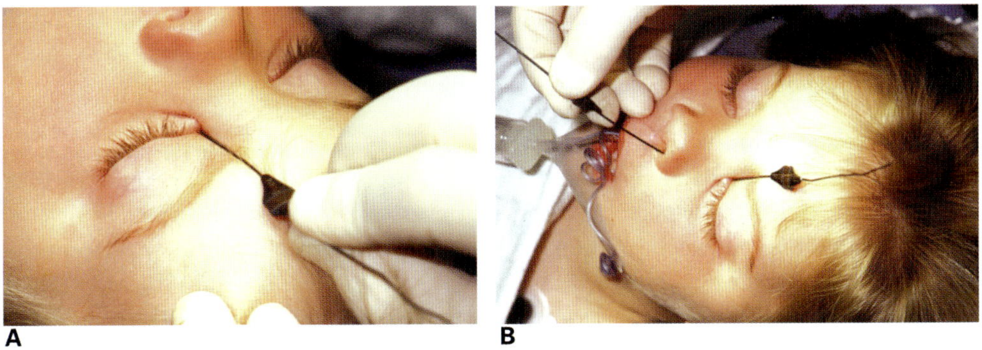

Figure 18-4 Probing for lacrimal obstruction. **A,** Probe advancing through the lacrimal sac and nasolacrimal duct, in this instance via the lower canaliculus. **B,** Instrument introduced into the nose beneath the inferior turbinate confirms the presence of the probe tip in the nose by direct contact. *(Photographs courtesy of Edward L. Raab, MD.)*

prophylaxis should be considered for the patient with congenital heart disease. Some surgeons recommend that massage over the lacrimal sac be continued for 1–2 weeks.

Resolution of symptoms is usually rapid after probing, but the full effect of the procedure may not be immediately evident. Evaluation of the results is more accurate 1 week or more after discontinuing postoperative treatment. Recurrence after unsuccessful probing usually is evident within 1 month. If the initial attempt to relieve congenital NLD obstruction with probing is unsuccessful, it is appropriate to repeat the procedure. The success rate of properly performed initial probing for congenital NLD obstruction exceeds 90% in infants up to 15 months old. Surgery first performed after age 24 months fails to relieve symptoms with simple probing in as many as one third of cases in some series.

The most common undesired outcome of probing is creation of a false passage into the nose, either from faulty manipulation of the probe or because of anatomical variations. The usual consequence of false passage is simply postoperative persistence of symptoms, but damage to the tissue lining the canaliculus or NLD can cause scarring that increases the difficulty of subsequent efforts to relieve obstruction. Significant complications of probing are otherwise rare.

In some cases, mild epiphora still occurs occasionally, particularly outdoors in cold weather or in conjunction with an upper respiratory infection. This probably is attributable to a patent but narrow lacrimal drainage channel that becomes occluded when the nasal mucosa swells. Usually no treatment is required. Spontaneous improvement over time is likely.

Infracture of the inferior turbinate

Some surgeons routinely perform infracture of the inferior turbinate at the initial probing, irrespective of the nature of the obstruction. Most reserve this procedure for use when firm resistance is felt as the advancing probe approaches the lowest portion of the bony nasolacrimal canal, for cases with crowding of the inferior meatus, or for subsequent procedures after initial probing fails.

Infracture is accomplished by placing a small periosteal elevator beneath the turbinate or by grasping it with a hemostat, then rotating the instrument inward. The value of this maneuver with mere membranous obstructions is debatable.

Balloon catheter dilation

In recent years, an inflatable balloon carried on a probe has become a popular method for dilating a lacrimal drainage system that appears to be blocked by scarring or constriction rather than merely by a distal membrane. Some surgeons routinely perform this procedure in all previously untreated cases, even when the case is within the age window considered to be timely. Many observers think that this method increases the success rate of delayed treatment at any age.

The technique also can be employed as an adjunct to intubation (see the following section). It probably would not be valuable in cases with a prominent bony abnormality. Although the original proponents of this procedure have advocated prolonged pre- and posttreatment use of systemic antibiotics and corticosteroids, most ophthalmologists do not employ these measures.

Gunton KB, Chung CW, Schnall BM, et al. Comparison of balloon dacryocystoplasty to probing as the primary treatment of congenital nasolacrimal duct obstruction. *J AAPOS.* 2001;5:139–142.

Lueder GT. Balloon catheter dilation for treatment of older children with nasolacrimal duct obstruction. *Arch Ophthalmol.* 2002;120:1685–1688.

Intubation

Silicone intubation of the lacrimal system is usually recommended when 1 or more simple probings or balloon dilations have failed. No method of intubation offers the ideal combination of ease of placement and removal along with high resistance to accidental displacement.

In the most commonly employed technique, once the probe, with its attached silicone tubing, is passed into the nose, the probe tip is engaged with a specially configured hook and withdrawn from the nares, bringing the tubing with it. A variation of the procedure employs a probe of a different design (Ritleng), which is said to facilitate recovery of the threaded stenting material from the nose. Both the upper and lower branches are intubated, leaving a small loop of silicone tubing between the puncta. A variety of measures is employed to secure the ends of the tubing in the nose, such as placing knots in the tubing, passing the tubing through a bolster, or suturing the tubes to the lateral nasal wall to prevent retrograde entry into the nasolacrimal duct.

An alternative method involves intubation via one canaliculus only. The supposed advantages of this method are ease of insertion and removal of the tube and easily achieved fixation in the intended location once passed. Acceptance of this technique may be influenced by the prominent rate of corneal complications.

Crawford JS. Intubation of the lacrimal system. *Ophthal Plast Reconstr Surg.* 1989;5:261–265.

Goldstein SM, Goldstein JB, Katowitz JA. Comparison of monocanalicular stenting and balloon dacryoplasty in secondary treatment of congenital nasolacrimal duct obstruction after failed primary probing. *Ophthal Plast Reconstr Surg.* 2004;20:352–357.

Pe MR, Langford JD, Linberg JV, et al. Ritleng intubation system for treatment of congenital nasolacrimal duct obstruction. *Arch Ophthalmol.* 1998;116:387–391.

Parents should be cautioned about the possibility of punctal lacerations. When they occur, early removal is necessary. Occasionally, the tubing becomes dislodged and protrudes excessively out of the nose or the puncta. In such situations, attempts should be made to reposition the tubing. A tube laterally displaced at the puncta sometimes can be repositioned by rethreading, although usually it must be removed.

Ideally, the silicone tubing should be left in place for 3–6 months, but shorter periods of intubation can be successful. The technique chosen for tube removal depends on the age of the patient, how the tubing was secured, and its position (in place or partially dislodged).

Dacryocystorhinostomy

Dacryocystorhinostomy may be necessary when the procedures described in the preceding sections cannot be accomplished or when symptoms persist or recur despite the measures described. BCSC Section 7, *Orbit, Eyelids, and Lacrimal System*, discusses intubation and the other procedures covered in this chapter.

CHAPTER 19

Diseases of the Cornea and Anterior Segment

This chapter focuses on corneal and anterior segment problems that begin in infancy and childhood. To understand how developmental anomalies affect the cornea and anterior segment, it is helpful to review the embryology of these regions of the eye.

Embryology of the Cornea and Anterior Segment

The lens vesicle separates from the surface ectoderm by the sixth week of gestation. The optic cup, which arises from neural ectoderm, has reached the periphery of the lens by this time, and a triangular mass of undifferentiated neural crest cells overrides the rim of the cup and surrounds the anterior periphery of the lens. Three waves of tissue move forward between the surface ectoderm and the lens. The first of these layers differentiates into the primordial corneal endothelium by the eighth week and subsequently produces Descemet's membrane. The second wave of tissue produces the stroma of the cornea, and the third wave gives rise to the pupillary membrane and the iris stroma. The pigment epithelial layer of the iris develops in later months from neural ectoderm.

By the beginning of the fifth fetal month, a complete endothelial lining overlies the primitive anterior chamber, creating a closed cavity. In addition, the iris insertion is now well anterior to the neural crest tissue destined to become the trabecular meshwork. The endothelial lining undergoes fenestration in the final weeks of gestation and the first weeks after birth. The iris insertion also repositions posteriorly to gradually uncover the developing trabecular meshwork. This repositioning, or posterior sliding, probably occurs secondary to differential growth rates and is not merely the result of a cleavage or an atrophy of tissue. At birth, the iris insertion has normally reached the level of the scleral spur. Posterior migration of the iris normally continues for about the first year of life.

A spectrum of anterior segment dysgenesis syndromes can result from abnormalities of neural crest cell migration, proliferation, or differentiation. A developmental arrest late in gestation can result in retention of primordial endothelium and incomplete posterior iris migration. BCSC Section 2, *Fundamentals and Principles of Ophthalmology*, discusses these issues in greater detail with illustrations in Part II, Embryology.

Congenital Corneal Anomalies

Abnormalities of Corneal Size and Shape

The normal horizontal corneal diameter in the newborn is 9.5–10.5 mm. The average 12-mm adult corneal diameter is reached by age 2 years. Abnormalities of corneal size and shape in childhood include simple megalocornea, keratoglobus, keratoconus, and microcornea. (See also the discussion of congenital anomalies in BCSC Section 8, *External Disease and Cornea.*)

Megalocornea

If the horizontal diameter is greater than 13 mm (or 12 mm in the newborn), megalocornea is present. The most common type of megalocornea is *anterior megalophthalmos,* which is X-linked recessive and bilateral. In this condition, the normal-sized lens is too small for the enlarged ciliary ring, which may result in subluxation. The iris is hypoplastic, with defects visible by transillumination, and the pupil is often ectopic. There is a greatly increased risk of glaucoma. Simple megalocornea is a rare condition in which both corneas exceed 13 mm in horizontal diameter, but associated abnormalities are absent. This condition must be differentiated from congenital glaucoma.

Keratoglobus

In keratoglobus, the cornea is thinner than normal and arcs high over the iris, creating a deeper than normal anterior chamber. Spontaneous breaks in Descemet's membrane may produce acute corneal edema, and the cornea is easily ruptured by minor blunt trauma. Patients with keratoglobus should be advised to wear protective lenses indefinitely. This rare autosomal recessive disorder can be part of the Ehlers-Danlos type VI syndrome, which is characterized by generalized thinning and anterior bulging of the cornea, accompanied by hyperextensible joints, blue sclera, and gradually progressive neurosensory hearing loss.

Keratoconus

In keratoconus, the central or paracentral cornea undergoes progressive thinning and bulging, so that the cornea takes on the shape of a cone. The disease can present and progress during the adolescent years. Keratoconus is associated with Down syndrome, other conditions with mental retardation, and atopic disease. There is a hereditary component in some families.

Microcornea

Microcornea is usually defined as a corneal diameter less than 9 mm in the newborn and less than 10 mm after 2 years of age (Fig 19-1). Even if both corneal diameters are within the normal range for age, if 1 cornea is significantly smaller than the other, it is usually abnormal. A study using the Orbscan II to accurately measure white-to-white diameters in the eyes of people age 8 years and older found the average corneal diameter to be 11.71 ± 0.42 mm. There were no significant differences between males and females. No infants or young children were included in the study.

Microcornea may follow a pattern of autosomal dominant inheritance, particularly as part of the oculodentodigital dysplasia syndrome, or it may appear sporadically. Microcornea may be accompanied by many other abnormalities of the eye, including cataracts, colobomas, high myopia, or persistent hyperplastic primary vitreous (PHPV). Microcornea can be seen in nanophthalmos, in which the entire eye is smaller than normal without other major structural abnormalities.

Rufer F, Schroder A, Erb C. White-to-white corneal diameter: normal values in healthy humans obtained with the Orbscan II topography system. *Cornea.* 2005;25(3):259–261.

Anterior Segment Dysgenesis: Peripheral Developmental Abnormalities

The spectrum of developmental anomalies known as anterior segment dysgenesis is sometimes called *mesenchymal dysgenesis* and was previously known as *anterior chamber cleavage syndrome* or *mesectodermal dysgenesis.*

Alward WL. Axenfeld-Rieger syndrome in the age of molecular genetics. *Am J Ophthalmol.* 2000;130:107–115.

Posterior embryotoxon

Posterior embryotoxon is seen as a central thickening and displacement of Schwalbe's line. Posterior embryotoxon is visible with the slit lamp as an irregular white line just concentric with and anterior to the limbus (Fig 19-2). Gonioscopically, the condition

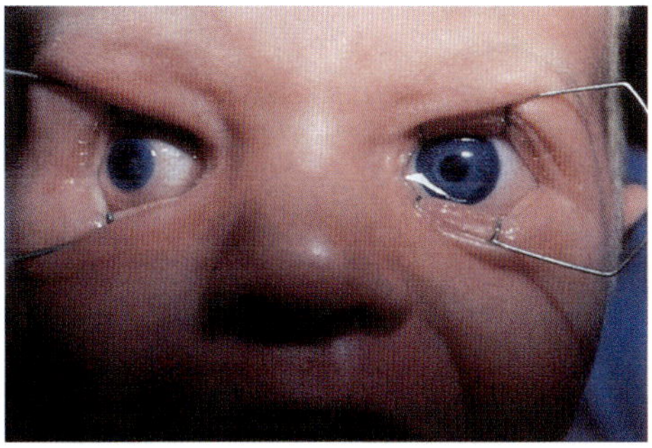

Figure 19-1 Microcornea, right eye.

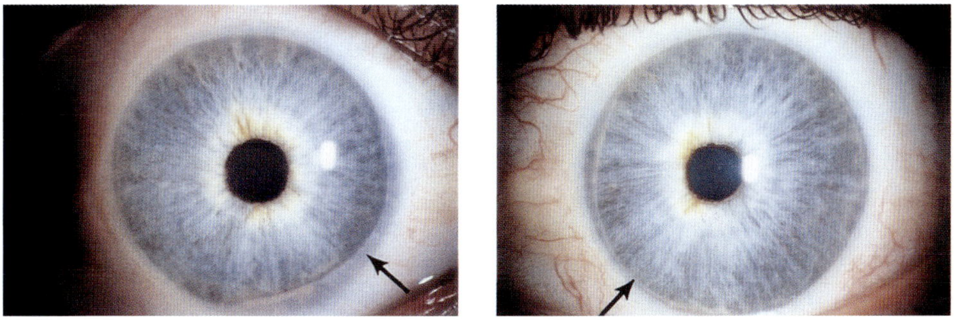

Figure 19-2 Posterior embryotoxon *(arrows)*, bilateral, in Axenfeld-Rieger syndrome.

appears as a continuous or broken ridge protruding into the anterior chamber. Posterior embryotoxon often has pigmented spots on the internal surface of this ridge. This anomaly is also called a *prominent Schwalbe's ring*. It is most often associated with Axenfeld-Rieger syndrome but is also found in arteriohepatic dysplasia (Alagille syndrome) and velocardiofacial syndrome (22q deletion) and may be an isolated finding in 15% of normal patients.

Axenfeld-Rieger syndrome

Axenfeld-Rieger syndrome represents a spectrum of developmental disorders characterized by an anteriorly displaced Schwalbe's line (posterior embryotoxon), with attached iris strands, iris hypoplasia, and anterior chamber dysgenesis leading to glaucoma in childhood or adulthood in 50% of cases (Figs 19-3, 19-4, 19-5). The conditions, previously called *Axenfeld anomaly, Rieger anomaly, Rieger syndrome, iridogoniodysgenesis anomaly and syndrome, iris hypoplasia*, and *familial glaucoma iridogoniodysplasia*, all have genotypic and phenotypic overlap and are now considered a single entity known as *Axenfeld-Rieger syndrome*. With the identification of several causative genes and loci for these disorders, it is now known that there are cases in which the same ocular appearance

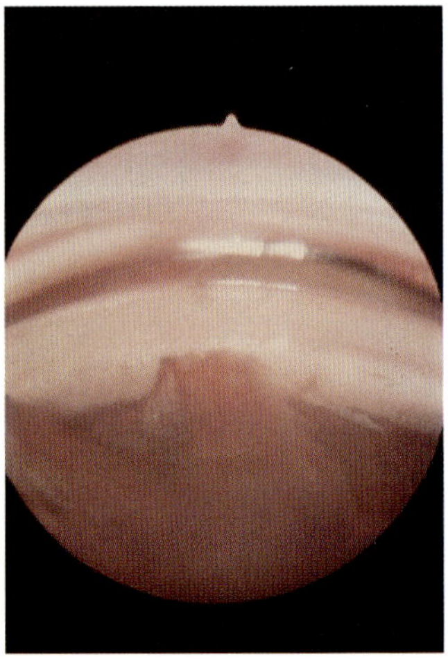

Figure 19-3 Gonioscopic view in Axenfeld-Rieger syndrome.

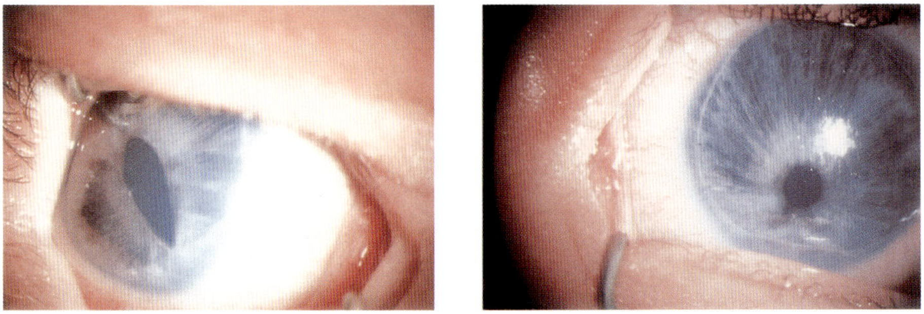

Figure 19-4 Axenfeld-Rieger syndrome, bilateral.

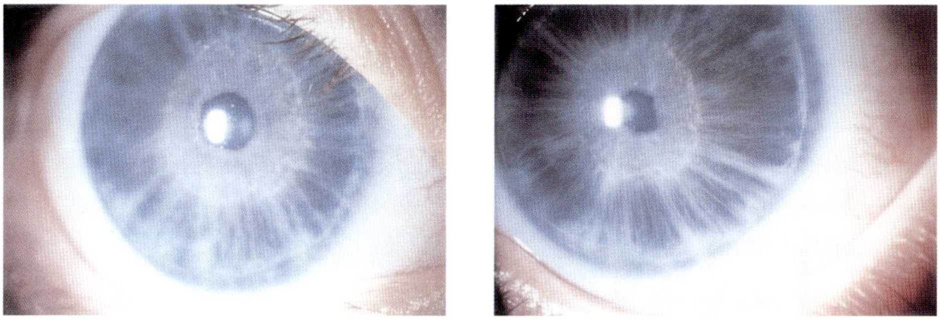

Figure 19-5 Iridogoniodysgenesis, bilateral. *(Photographs courtesy of Jane D. Kivlin, MD.)*

is caused by different genes, and others in which very different ocular presentations, which previously would have been confidently classified as Peters anomaly versus Rieger anomaly versus primary glaucoma, for example, are caused by the same mutated gene.

Axenfeld-Rieger syndrome may include a smooth, cryptless iris surface and a high iris insertion, sometimes accompanied by iris transillumination. Iris hypoplasia can range from mild stromal thinning to marked atrophy with hole formation, corectopia, and ectropion uveae. Posterior embryotoxon, megalocornea, or microcornea can occur. Most important, glaucoma develops in 50% of cases. Teeth may be small in size or reduced in number. Redundant periumbilical skin, hypospadias, and anomalies in the region of the pituitary gland have also been reported. Autosomal dominant inheritance is most common. Mutations in the *RIEG1/PITX2* gene on chromosome 4q25 have been identified. This is a paired homeobox gene that regulates expansion of other genes during embryonic development. Patients with mutations of *PITX2* have been reported with phenotypes of aniridia, Peters anomaly, Rieger anomaly, and Axenfeld anomaly. The nonocular findings are actually more consistent and should be sought with any of these ocular phenotypes. Mutations in the forkhead transcription factor gene *FOXC1* (formerly called *FKHL7*) also cause Axenfeld-Rieger syndrome, with features such as autosomal dominant iris hypoplasia, juvenile glaucoma, Rieger anomaly and syndrome, posterior embryotoxon, Peters anomaly, and primary congenital glaucoma. *FOXC1* is also expressed in the heart, and some patients have cardiac valve abnormalities. Two other loci for Axenfeld-Rieger have been identified, at 13q14 and 16q24, but the causative genes are not yet known. Mutations, deletions, and duplications of loci have been noted to cause Axenfeld-Rieger syndrome.

Alward WL. Axenfeld-Rieger syndrome in the age of molecular genetics. *Am J Ophthalmol.* 2000;130:107–115.

Lines MA, Kozlowski K, Walter MA. Molecular genetics of Axenfeld-Rieger malformations. *Hum Mol Genet.* 2002;11:1177–1184.

Perveen R, Lloyd IC, Clayton-Smith J, et al. Phenotypic variability and asymmetry of Rieger syndrome associated with PITX2 mutations. *Invest Ophthalmol Vis Sci.* 2000;41:2456–2460.

Central Corneal Developmental Abnormalities

With central corneal developmental abnormalities, the basic finding is a localized loss or attenuation of the corneal endothelium or Descemet's membrane, which is usually associated with an overlying stromal and epithelial opacity. The mnemonic "STUMPED" has been used to help generate a differential diagnosis for congenital corneal opacities. Credited to George Waring, MD, it stands for *s*clerocornea, *t*ears in Descemet's membrane (usually forceps or congential glaucoma), *u*lcers, *m*etabolic (eg, mucopolysaccharidosis), *P*eters anomaly, *e*dema [congenital hereditary endothelial dystrophy (CHED), posterior polymorphous dystrophy (PPMD), glaucoma], *d*ermoid.

Posterior corneal depression

Posterior corneal depression (central posterior keratoconus), a discrete posterior corneal indentation, is best detected with a retinoscope or direct ophthalmoscope that reveals an abnormal red reflex. This condition can also be diagnosed with the slit lamp by moving the beam across the defect to discern increased convexity of the posterior corneal surface. Sometimes, pigment deposits appear on the border of the posterior defect. The anterior curvature of the cornea is normal. This defect usually causes irregular astigmatism and can result in amblyopia if the refractive error is not corrected.

Peters anomaly

Peters anomaly consists of a posterior corneal defect with stromal opacity and often adherent iris strands. In many cases, the stromal opacity decreases with time. In some cases, lysis of adherent iris strands may improve corneal clarity. The size and density of the opacity can range from a faint stromal opacity to a dense opaque central leukoma. In extreme cases, the central leukoma may be vascularized and protrude above the level of the cornea. The strands from the iris to the borders of this defect vary in number and density. A more severe variety of this condition involves adherence of the lens to the cornea at the site of the central defect (Fig 19-6). Peters anomaly is the end result of many defects, including—but not limited to—the genetic Axenfeld-Rieger syndrome (see previous section) and nongenetic conditions such as congenital rubella.

Bilateral Peters anomaly is often associated with a syndrome. When associated with microphthalmia and reddish linear skin lesions, Peters anomaly may be part of a syndrome called *microphthalmia with linear skin defects* (*MLS*) that includes life-threatening

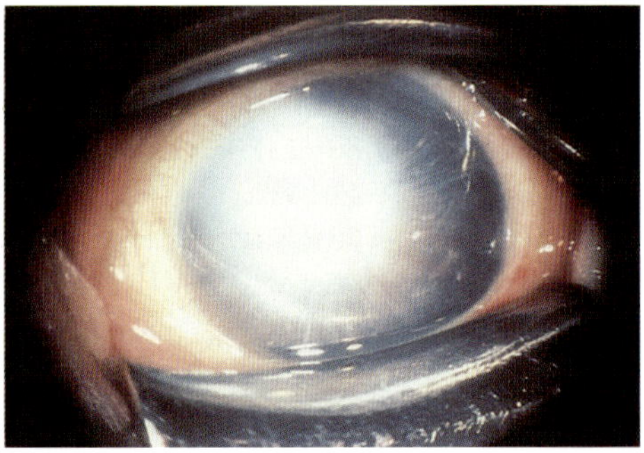

Figure 19-6 Peters anomaly, left eye.

cardiac arrhythmias. Bilateral cases warrant complete genetic and systemic workup. Unilateral cases are usually isolated.

Doward W, Perveen R, Lloyd IC, et al. A mutation in the RIEG1 gene associated with Peters' anomaly. *J Med Genet.* 1999;36:152–155.

Hanson IM, Fletcher JM, Jordan T, et al. Mutations at the PAX6 locus are found in heterogeneous anterior segment malformations including Peters' anomaly. *Nat Genet.* 1994;6:168–173.

Infantile Corneal Opacities

Peters anomaly has already been discussed. Table 19-1 lists the other possible infantile corneal opacities to be considered in a differential diagnosis.

Sclerocornea

In *sclerocornea*, a congenital condition, the cornea is opaque and resembles the sclera, making the limbus indistinct. The central cornea is clearer than the periphery in nearly all cases, in contradistinction to Peters anomaly, in which the periphery is generally clearer. Severe cases show no increased corneal curvature and no apparent scleral sulcus. Sclerocornea is often associated with other ocular or systemic abnormalities.

Tears, breaks, or ruptures of Descemet's membrane

Injuries to Descemet's membrane may be caused by forceps trauma to the eye during delivery. Rupture of Descemet's membrane leads to stromal and sometimes epithelial edema. Other signs of trauma are frequently apparent on the child. In most cases, the stromal and epithelial edema regresses, but the edges of the broken Descemet's membrane persist indefinitely and can be seen as ridges protruding slightly from the posterior corneal surface. Severe amblyopia may result from the corneal opacity. The high astigmatism induced by the trauma can cause severe amblyopia even if the cornea clears quickly. Aggressive optical correction and patching should be attempted.

Lambert SR, Drack AV, Hutchinson AK. Longitudinal changes in the refractive errors of children with tears in Descemet's membrane following forceps injuries. *J AAPOS.* 2004;8:368–370.

Mucopolysaccharidosis and mucolipidosis

The varied systemic findings and ultrastructural abnormalities of the lysosomal disorders mucopolysaccharidosis and mucolipidosis are beyond the scope of this discussion (see Table 29-1 in this volume; BCSC Section 8, *External Diseease and Cornea*; and BCSC Section 12, *Retina and Vitreous*). However, corneal clouding and haziness may be present in early life in at least 3 of these conditions: in *mucopolysaccharidosis I H,* or *Hurler I S,* or *Scheie syndrome*, corneal clouding occurs by age 6 months (see Fig 19-7). In *mucopolysaccharidosis I S,* or *Scheie syndrome*, corneal clouding occurs by age 12–24 months. In *mucolipidosis IV*, corneal clouding has been reported as early as age 6 weeks. Enzymatic and DNA analyses usually can identify the metabolic defect. Conjunctival biopsies show abnormal cytoplasmic inclusions on electron microscopy.

Table 19-1 Differential Diagnosis of Infantile Corneal Opacities

Entity	Location and Description of Opacity	Other Signs	Method of Diagnosis
Sclerocornea	Peripheral opacity, clearest centrally; unilateral or bilateral	Flat cornea	Inspection
Forceps injury	Central opacity; unilateral	Breaks in Descemet's membrane	History
Mucopolysaccharidosis, mucolipidosis	Diffuse opacity; bilateral	Smooth epithelium	Conjunctival biopsy; biochemical testing
Posterior corneal defects	Central opacity; unilateral or bilateral	Iris adherence to cornea; posterior keratoconus	Inspection
Congenital hereditary endothelial dystrophy (CHED)	Diffuse opacity; bilateral	Thickened cornea	Inspection
Dermoid	Temporal opacity; unilateral; raised; hair on surface; keratinized	Associated with Goldenhar syndrome	Inspection
Infantile glaucoma	Diffuse opacity; unilateral or bilateral	Enlarged cornea; breaks in Descemet's membrane	Elevated intraocular pressure
Congenital hereditary stromal dystrophy (CHSD)	Diffuse opacity; bilateral	Stromal opacities, normal thickness, normal epithelium	Autosomal dominant; examine family members

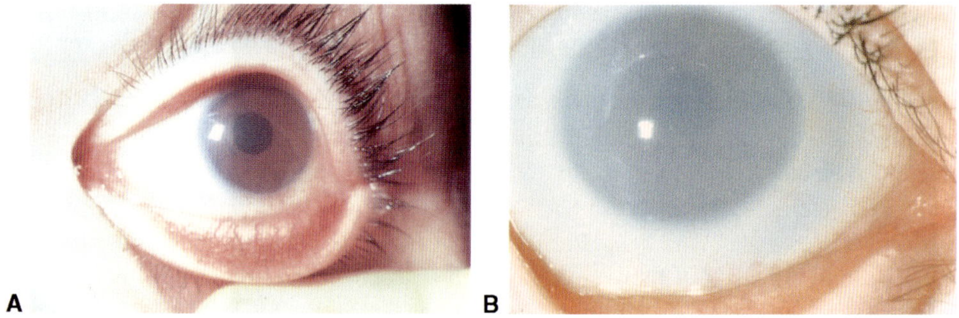

Figure 19-7 Hurler syndrome. **A,** Early corneal clouding. **B,** Late corneal clouding. *(Photographs courtesy of Jane D. Kivlin, MD.)*

Congenital hereditary endothelial dystrophy

Congenital hereditary endothelial dystrophy (CHED) is an uncommon corneal dystrophy with onset at birth or shortly thereafter. The cornea is diffusely and uniformly edematous because of a defect of the corneal endothelium and Descemet's membrane. The edema involves both the stroma and epithelium. The hallmark of CHED is increased corneal thickness. The appearance of the cornea is similar to that in congenital glaucoma but without increased corneal diameter and elevated intraocular pressure. CHED can be inherited in an autosomal dominant or autosomal recessive manner. The dominant and recessive forms are caused by different genes. The dominant form maps to the same genetic locus as posterior polymorphous dystrophy on pericentromeric chromosome 20. The autosomal recessive form maps to another locus on chromosome 20.

Hand CK, Harmon DL, Kennedy SM, et al. Localization of the gene for autosomal recessive congenital hereditary endothelial dystrophy (CHED2) to chromosome 20 by homozygosity mapping. *Genomics.* 1999;61:1–4.

Dermoids

A corneal *dermoid* is a choristoma composed of fibrofatty tissue covered by keratinized epithelium. Dermoids sometimes contain hair follicles, sebaceous glands, and sweat glands. Dermoids can range up to 8–10 mm in diameter and usually straddle the limbus. They may extend into the corneal stroma and adjacent sclera but seldom occupy the full thickness of either cornea or sclera. Most dermoids are on the inferior temporal limbus. Many produce a lipoid infiltration of the corneal stroma at their leading edge.

Limbal dermoids are often seen with Goldenhar syndrome (see Chapter 28). They are sometimes continuous with subconjunctival lipodermoids that involve the upper outer quadrant of the eye and extend into the orbit under the lateral aspect of the upper eyelid. Large dermoids can cover the visual axis; small dermoids can produce astigmatism with secondary amblyopia. Surgical excision may result in scarring and astigmatism, which can also lead to amblyopia. In some cases, however, excision may be helpful, especially for very elevated lesions (Fig 19-8).

Congenital or infantile glaucoma

Glaucoma in an infant can make the cornea edematous, cloudy, and enlarged. Chapter 21 discusses pediatric glaucoma in more detail.

Congenital hereditary stromal dystrophy

Congenital hereditary stromal dystrophy is a very rare congenital stationary opacification of the cornea transmitted in an autosomal dominant manner. Flaky or feathery clouding of the stroma, which is of normal thickness, is covered by a smooth, normal epithelium. These features are in contrast with those of CHED, which has a thickened stroma and epithelial edema.

Treatment of Corneal Opacities

The treatment of congenital corneal opacities is difficult and often visually unrewarding. If bilateral dense opacities are present, keratoplasty should be considered for 1 eye as

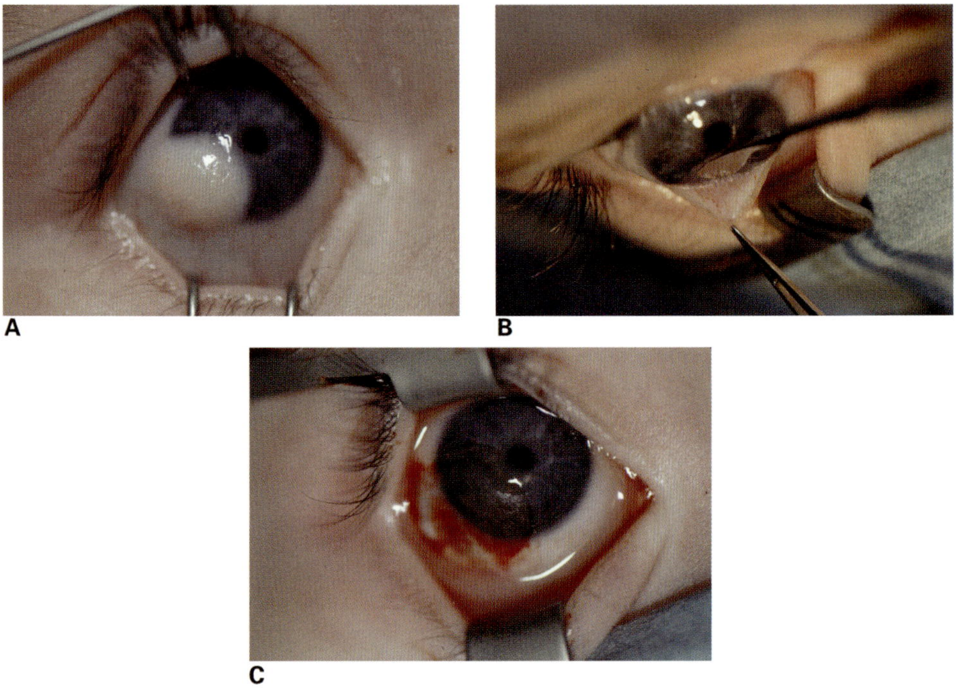

Figure 19-8 Limbal dermoid before **(A)**, during **(B)**, and after **(C)** surgical excision. Although the cornea will likely heal with a scar, it will be less irritating and noticeable than the original dermoid. *(Photographs courtesy of David Plager, MD.)*

soon as possible. If the opacity is unilateral, the decision is more difficult. Keratoplasty should be undertaken only if the family and the physicians involved in the care of the child are prepared for the tremendous commitment of time and effort needed to combat the corneal graft rejection that often occurs in children, as well as with amblyopia. The team should include ophthalmologists skilled in the management of pediatric corneal surgery, pediatric glaucoma, amblyopia, and strabismus. Contact lens expertise is important for fitting infants with small eyes and large refractive errors. Repeated examinations under anesthesia are often required, and infectious keratitis may occur.

Although there is ample evidence that deprivation amblyopia must be reversed before the age of 3 months to achieve excellent vision, it may be appropriate, in some cases of Peters anomaly, to delay corneal transplantation until the child is older. One study found better final vision in patients treated at about the age of 1 year as opposed to age 3 months because older children showed less rejection and ultimately had a clearer cornea. Very few patients in either group achieved good vision, however.

Other modalities, such as lamellar keratoplasty or laser procedures, may be indicated in some cases, but there are few data for children.

Cosar CB, Laibson PR, Cohen EJ, et al. Topical cyclosporine in pediatric keratoplasty. *Eye Contact Lens.* 2003;29:103–107.

Yang LL, Lambert SR, Lynn MJ, et al. Long-term results of corneal graft survival in infants and children with Peters anomaly. *Ophthalmology.* 1999;106:833–848.

Systemic Diseases With Corneal Manifestations in Childhood

The mucopolysaccharidoses are discussed in a previous section. Several of the mucopolysaccharidoses may involve deposits in the cornea, leading to some degree of clinical corneal clouding.

Cystinosis

Cystinosis, a metabolic disease characterized by elevated levels of cystine within the cell, is rare. French Canada has the highest incidence in the world. Cystine crystals are deposited in various places throughout the body. In the infantile form of the disease, the major presenting symptoms are failure to thrive; rickets; and progressive renal failure, collectively called *Fanconi syndrome*. The ocular findings are pathognomonic. Iridescent elongated corneal crystals appear at approximately age 1 year, first in the peripheral part of the cornea and the anterior part of the stroma. These crystals are also present in the uvea and can be seen with the slit lamp on the surface of the iris (Fig 19-9). Severe photophobia can make a slit-lamp examination almost impossible without anesthesia. Cystine can be found in conjunctival biopsy specimens, although diagnosis is typically made with a blood test. Oral cysteamine has been shown to help the systemic problems but not the corneal crystal deposition. Topical cysteamine drops must be applied every 1–2 hours, have an unpleasant odor, and are difficult to obtain; however, they can markedly reduce crystal deposition in the cornea.

Kaiser-Kupfer MI, Fujikawa L, Kuwabara T, et al. Removal of corneal crystals by topical cysteamine in nephropathic cystinosis. *N Engl J Med.* 1987;316:775–779.

Khan AO, Latimer B. Successful use of topical cysteamine formulated from the oral preparation in a child with keratopathy secondary to cystinosis. *Am J Ophthalmol.* 2004;138:674–675.

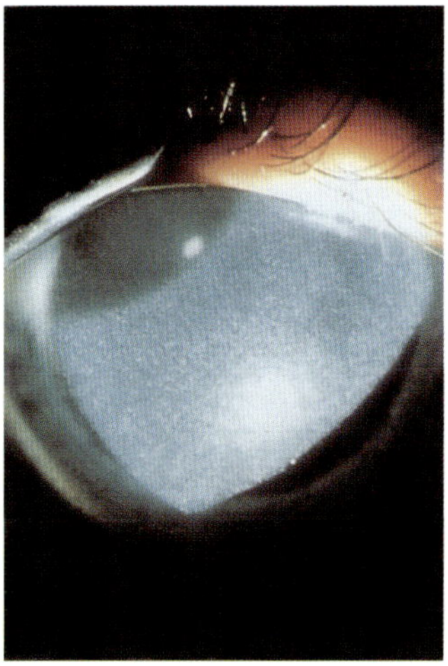

Figure 19-9 Cystinosis with corneal involvement.

Hepatolenticular degeneration

Hepatolenticular degeneration (Wilson disease), an autosomal recessive inborn error of metabolism, results in excess copper deposition in the liver, kidneys, and basal ganglia of the brain, leading to cirrhosis, renal tubular damage, and a Parkinson-like defect of motor function. The characteristic copper-colored Kayser-Fleischer ring is limited to Descemet's membrane and is thus separated from the limbus. The ring may be several millimeters in width. The initial deposits are in the corneal periphery at 12 and 6 o'clock. This arc of deposits spreads, eventually encircling the entire cornea. The ring resolves with treatment. Because it can develop fairly late, laboratory tests for serum copper and ceruloplasmin are better than an eye examination for early diagnosis.

Congenital syphilis

Interstitial keratitis may occur in the first decade of life secondary to congenital syphilis. The keratitis presents as rapidly progressive corneal edema followed by abnormal vascularization in the deep stroma adjacent to Descemet's membrane. Intense vascularization may give the cornea a salmon-pink color—hence the term *salmon patch.* Blood flow through these vessels gradually ceases over several weeks to several months, leaving empty "ghost" vessels in the corneal stroma (Fig 19-10). Immune-mediated uveitis, arthritis, and hearing loss may also develop and recur, even after syphilis treatment. Immunosuppression may be needed to decrease sequelae.

Familial dysautonomia

Familial dysautonomia (Riley-Day syndrome), a complex autosomal recessive condition, occurs largely in children of Eastern European Jewish (Ashkenazi) descent. It is characterized by autonomic dysfunction, relative insensitivity to pain, temperature instability, and absence of the fungiform papillae of the tongue. Exposure keratitis and corneal ulcers with secondary opacification are frequent problems because of the abnormal lacrimation and decreased corneal sensitivity. Preventive measures include supplemental artificial tears and tarsorrhaphies. The gene has been mapped to chromosome 9q.

Blumenfeld A, Slaugenhaupt SA, Liebert CB, et al. Precise genetic mapping and haplotype analysis of the familial dysautonomia gene on human chromosome 9q31. *Am J Hum Genet.* 1999;64:1110–1118.

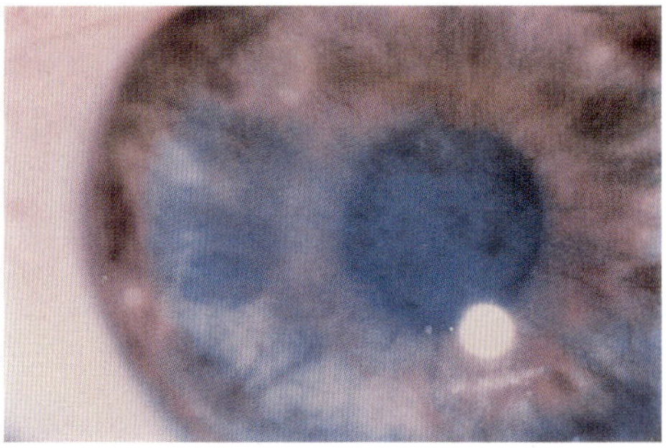

Figure 19-10 Interstitial keratitis secondary to congenital syphilis.

CHAPTER 20

Iris Abnormalities

Dyscoria

The term *dyscoria* refers to an abnormality of the shape of the pupil and is usually reserved for congenital malformations. Acquired inflammatory conditions can lead to posterior synechiae, which can also produce a misshapen pupil. Colobomatous iris defects that produce a dyscoric pupil are discussed later in the chapter. Iris hypoplasia, especially if sectorial, can produce dyscoria as well as corectopia (discussed later in the chapter). Slitlike pupils have been described in the Axenfeld-Rieger syndrome (see Fig 19-4), in ectopia lentis et pupillae (see the discussion of corectopia later in the chapter), and, rarely, as an isolated condition with normal visual acuity. Some patients with congenital cataracts have an associated microcoria. Microcoria or irregular pupil can also develop with progressive fibrosis of the plaque in persistent fetal vasculature (PFV).

Aniridia

Aniridia is a panocular, bilateral disorder. The term *aniridia* is a misnomer, because at least a rudimentary iris is always present. Variations range from almost total absence to only mild hypoplasia of the iris. In addition to iris involvement, foveal hypoplasia is usually present, with nystagmus and visual acuity less than 20/100. Glaucoma, optic nerve hypoplasia, and cataracts are common. Corneal opacification often develops later in childhood and may lead to progressive deterioration of visual acuity. The cornea appears to develop a pannus, which gradually encroaches on central vision. The condition is due to a stem cell deficiency and therefore must be treated with keratolimbal allograft stem cell transplantation rather than corneal transplantation.

The typical presentation of aniridia is an infant with nystagmus who appears to have absent irides or dilated, unresponsive pupils. Photophobia may also be present. Examination findings commonly include small anterior polar cataracts, at times with attached persistent pupillary membrane strands (Fig 20-1).

A defect in the *PAX6* gene on chromosome 11p13 is the cause of aniridia, which can be sporadic or familial. The familial form is autosomal dominant with complete penetrance but variable expressivity. There are reports of autosomal dominant pedigrees in which patients have severe glaucoma but normal maculae and good central vision. Two thirds of all aniridic children have affected parents. The *PAX6* gene is the master control gene for eye morphogenesis. This gene is probably involved in the complex inductive

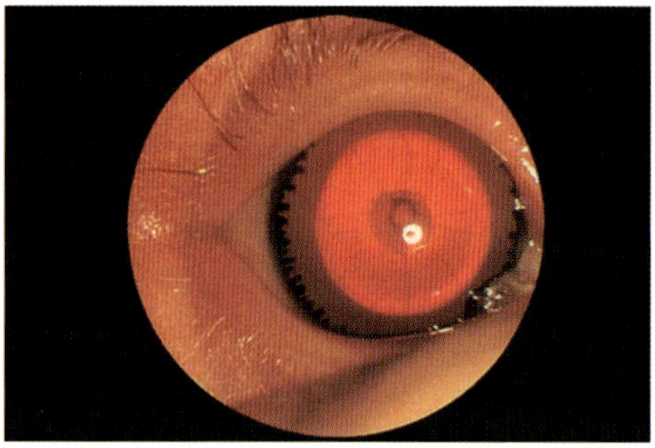

Figure 20-1 Aniridia in an infant. Both the ciliary processes and the edge of the lens are visible. Also present are persistent pupillary membrane fibers and a small central anterior polar cataract.

interactions between the optic cup, surface ectoderm, and neural crest during formation of the iris and other ocular structures. Many different mutations of the *PAX6* gene have been reported. It is likely that they cause aniridia due to a reduction in the amount of functional PAX6 protein. Parts II (Embryology) and III (Genetics) of BCSC Section 2, *Fundamentals and Principles of Ophthalmology*, discuss aniridia.

Sporadic aniridia is associated with Wilms tumor (nephroblastoma) in as many as one third of cases. When associated with aniridia, Wilms tumor is diagnosed before patients reach age 5 in 80% of cases. The combination of aniridia and Wilms tumor represents a contiguous gene syndrome in which the adjacent *PAX6* and Wilms tumor *(WT1)* genes are both deleted. Some deletions create the WAGR complex of *W*ilms tumor, *a*niridia, *g*enitourinary malformations, and mental *r*etardation. All children with sporadic aniridia should undergo chromosomal analysis for the Wilms tumor gene defect. Positive results necessitate consultation with an oncologist along with repeated abdominal ultrasonographic and clinical examinations. Patients with familial aniridia are rarely at risk for Wilms tumor.

Holland EJ, Djalilian AR, Schwartz GS. Management of aniridic keratopathy with keratolimbal allograft: a limbal stem cell transplantation technique. *Ophthalmology.* 2003;110:125–130.

Wolf MT, Lorenz B, Winterpacht A, et al. Ten novel mutations found in aniridia. *Hum Mutat.* 1998;12:304–313.

Coloboma of the Iris

Iris colobomas are classified as "typical" if they occur in the inferonasal quadrant and can thus be explained by failure of the embryonic fissure to close in the fifth week of gestation. With a typical iris coloboma, the pupil is shaped like a lightbulb, keyhole, or inverted teardrop (Fig 20-2). Typical colobomas may involve any or all of the following: the ciliary body, choroid, retina, optic nerve. These colobomas are part of a continuum that extends to microphthalmos and anophthalmos. Nystagmus may be present if both optic nerves or both maculae are involved. Isolated colobomatous microphthalmia may be inherited as an autosomal dominant trait in about 20% of cases. Parents of an affected child may have small, previously undetected chorioretinal or iris defects in an inferonasal location, so careful examination of family members is indicated.

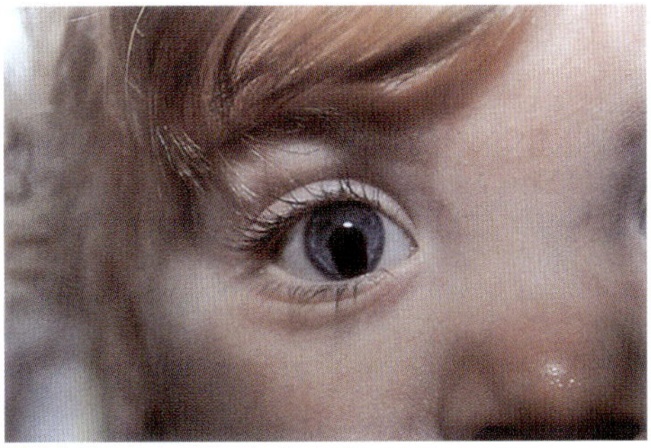

Figure 20-2 Typical iris coloboma, right eye.

Atypical iris colobomas occur in areas other than the inferonasal quadrant and are not usually associated with more posterior uveal colobomas. These colobomas probably result from fibrovascular remnants of the anterior hyaloid system and pupillary membrane.

Any child with a coloboma and at least one other organ system abnormality should undergo karyotypic analysis with extended banding. Although iris colobomas can be associated with almost any chromosomal abnormality, the most common associations are

- triploidy, especially trisomy 13 (cat's-eye syndrome) or 18
- 4p- (Wolf-Hirschhorn syndrome)
- 11q-
- 18r (ring)
- 13r
- Klinefelter syndrome
- Turner syndrome (rarely)

In addition, many well-characterized syndromes are associated with uveal colobomas. These syndromes include

- CHARGE association (ocular *c*oloboma, *h*eart defects, choanal *a*tresia, mental *r*etardation, and *g*enitourinary and *e*ar anomalies), which accounts for about 15% of cases
- Lenz microphthalmos syndrome
- Goltz focal dermal hypoplasia
- basal cell nevus syndrome
- Meckel syndrome
- Warburg syndrome
- Aicardi syndrome
- Rubinstein-Taybi syndrome
- linear sebaceous nevus syndrome
- Goldenhar syndrome

Mets MB, Erzurum SA. Uveal tract in infants. In: Isenberg SJ, ed. *The Eye in Infancy.* 2nd ed. St Louis: Mosby; 1994:308–317.

Onwochei BC, Simon JW, Bateman JB, et al. Ocular colobomata. *Surv Ophthalmol.* 2000;45:175–194.

Wright KW, ed. *Pediatric Ophthalmology and Strabismus.* 2nd ed. St Louis: Mosby; 2003.

Iris Nodules

Lisch Nodules

Lisch nodules are neural crest hamartomas commonly associated with neurofibromatosis type 1 (NF1). These nodules are raised and usually tan in color but can vary significantly in appearance (Fig 20-3). (See also Chapter 27.) The incidence of Lisch nodules in NF1 increases with age, being approximately 10 times the patient's age (up to 9 years). For example, by age 8 years, Lisch nodules are present in approximately 80% of patients. Lisch nodules tend to be distributed more in the lower iris than in other areas, leading some authors to propose that exposure to sunlight may play a role.

Beauchamp G. Neurofibromatosis type 1 in children. *Trans Am Ophthalmol Soc.* 1995;93: 445–472.

Nichols JC, Amato JE, Chung SM. Characteristics of Lisch nodules in patients with neurofibromatosis type 1. *J Ped Ophthalmol Strabismus.* 2003;40:293–296.

Juvenile Xanthogranuloma

Juvenile xanthogranuloma is primarily a cutaneous disorder with a predilection for the head and face. Vascular iris lesions may occur as discrete yellowish or reddish nodules or as diffuse infiltration causing heterochromia. Spontaneous hyphema can occur. (See also Chapter 26.)

Iris Mamillations

Iris mamillations, also called *iris folliculi* or *diffuse iris nodular nevi,* may be unilateral or bilateral. They appear as numerous, diffuse, tiny pigmented nodules on the surface of the iris (Fig 20-4). They are more common in darkly pigmented eyes and are usually of the same color as the iris. They may be bilateral, autosomal dominant, and isolated, or associated with oculodermal melanocytosis or phakomatosis pigmentovascularis type IIb (nevus flammeus with persistent aberrant Mongolian spots). They have also been re-

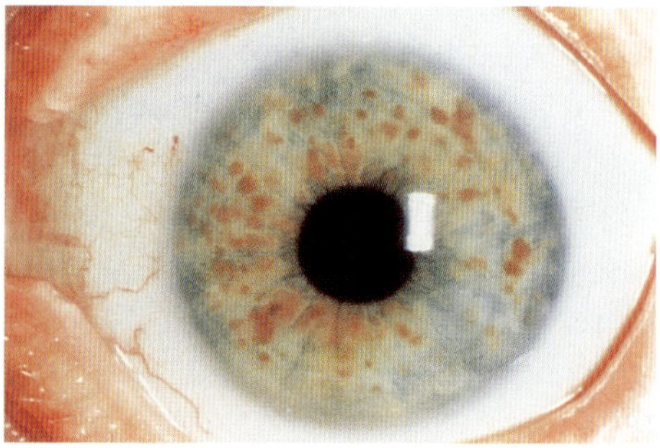

Figure 20-3 Lisch nodules in neurofibromatosis type 1.

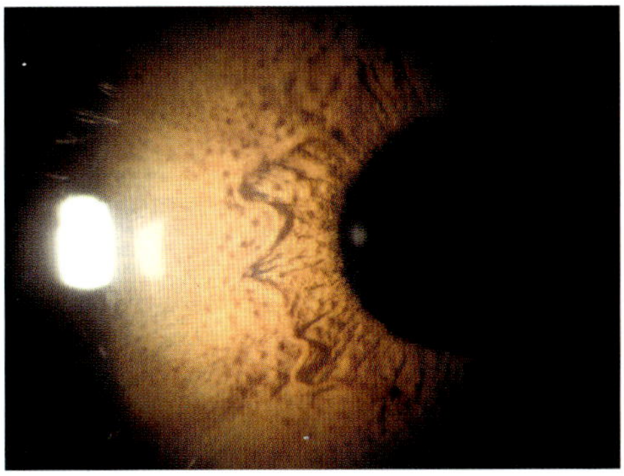

Figure 20-4 Iris mamillations or folliculi. Nodules are diffuse and are the same color as the iris, as opposed to Lisch nodules, which are lighter or darker than the surrounding iris. *(Photograph courtesy of Arlene Drack, MD.)*

ported in cases of ciliary body tumor and choroidal melanoma. Iris mamillations must be differentiated from Lisch nodules; the mamillations are usually dark brown, smooth, uniformly distributed, and equal in size or slightly larger near the pupil. The incidence of iris mamillations in NF1 is increased, but they are not diagnostic, as are Lisch nodules.

Gunduz K, Shields CL, Shields JA, et al. Iris mammillations as the only sign of ocular melanocytosis in a child with choroidal melanoma. *Arch Ophthalmol.* 2000;118:716–717.

Ticho BH, Rosner M, Mets MB, et al. Bilateral diffuse iris nodular nevi. Clinical and histopathologic characterization. *Ophthalmology.* 1995;102:419–425.

Primary Iris Cysts

Cysts of Iris Pigment Epithelium

Spontaneous cysts of the iris pigment epithelium result from a separation of the 2 layers of epithelium anywhere between the pupil and ciliary body (Fig 20-5). Clinically, these cysts tend to be stable and rarely cause ocular complications. They are usually not diagnosed until the teenage years.

Central (Pupillary) Cysts

Pigment epithelial cysts at the pupillary border are sometimes hereditary. They are usually diagnosed in infancy. They may enlarge slowly but generally remain asymptomatic and rarely require treatment. Rupture of these cysts can result in iris flocculi. Potent cholinesterase-inhibiting eyedrops such as phospholine iodide may produce similar pupillary cysts, especially in young phakic people. Discontinuation of the drug or concomitant administration of phenylephrine generally results in improvement.

Cysts of Iris Stroma

Primary iris stromal cysts are often diagnosed in infancy. They are most likely caused by sequestration of epithelium during embryologic development. The epithelium-lined stromal cysts usually contain goblet cells, and they may enlarge, causing obstruction of the visual axis, glaucoma, corneal decompensation, or iritis from cyst leakage. Numerous

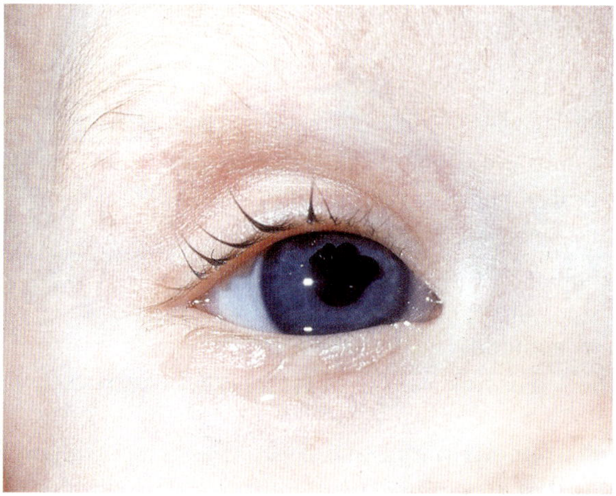

Figure 20-5 Cysts of the pigmented epithelium of the iris.

treatment modalities have been described, including cyst aspiration and photocoagulation or photodisruption, but the sudden release of cystic contents may result in transient iritis and glaucoma. Because of inherent complications or frequent cyst recurrences with other methods, surgical excision may be the preferred treatment method. Iris stromal cysts account for about 16% of childhood iris cysts.

Secondary Iris Cysts

Secondary iris cysts have been reported in childhood after trauma and associated with tumor or iris nevus.

Shields JA, Shields CL, Lois N, et al. Iris cysts in children: classification, incidence, and management. The 1998 Torrence A Makley Jr Lecture. *Br J Ophthalmol.* 1999;83:334–338.
Sidoti PA, Valencia M, Chen N, et al. Echographic evaluation of primary cysts of the iris pigment epithelium. *Am J Ophthalmol.* 1995;120:161–167.

Brushfield Spots

Focal areas of iris stromal hyperplasia surrounded by relative hypoplasia occur in up to 90% of patients with Down syndrome, in whom these areas are known as *Brushfield spots.* These are hypopigmented spots. Essentially identical areas, known as *Wofflin nodules,* occur in 24% of patients who do not have Down syndrome. Neither condition is pathologic.

Heterochromia Iridis

The differential diagnosis of pediatric *heterochromia iridis* is extensive. Causes can be classified on the basis of whether the condition is congenital or acquired and whether the affected eye is hypopigmented or hyperpigmented (Fig 20-6; Table 20-1). Trauma, chronic iridocyclitis, intraocular surgery, and topical prostaglandin analogs are important causes of acquired hyperpigmented heterochromia in children. Whether congenital or acquired, hypopigmented heterochromia, if associated with a more miotic pupil on the ipsilateral side, should prompt a workup for Horner syndrome. This may be related to a benign entity, such as shoulder dystocia at birth or previous neck-thoracic surgery, or a life-threatening one, such as neuroblastoma along the sympathetic chain.

Persistent Pupillary Membranes

Persistent pupillary membranes are the most common developmental abnormality of the iris. They are present in about 95% of newborns, and trace remnants are common in older children and adults. Persistent pupillary membranes are rarely of any visual significance.

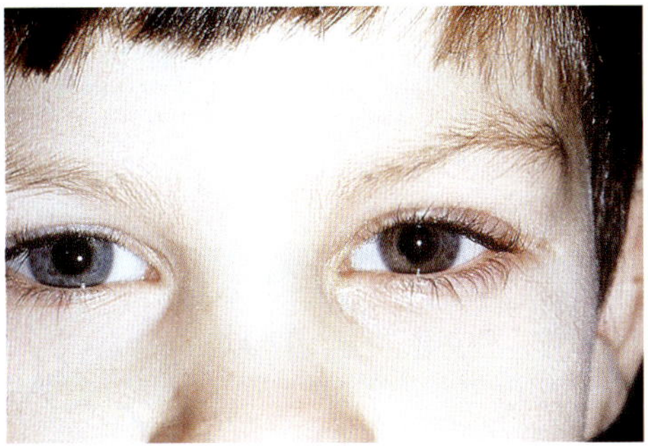

Figure 20-6 Heterochromia iridis. The left iris has become darker after developing a traumatic cataract. *(Photograph courtesy of John W. Simon, MD.)*

Table 20-1 Pediatric Heterochromia Iridis

Hypochromic heterochromia
Horner syndrome (congenital or early in life)
Incontinentia pigmenti (rare)
Fuchs heterochromia
Waardenburg-Klein syndrome
Nonpigmented tumors
Hypomelanosis of Ito
Hyperchromic heterochromia
Oculodermal melanocytosis (associated with glaucoma in nonwhite adults)
Pigmented tumors
Siderosis
Iris ectropion syndrome
Extensive rubeosis

Modified from Roy FH. *Ocular Differential Diagnosis.* 3rd ed. Philadelphia: Lea & Febiger; 1984.

However, if especially prominent, they can adhere to the anterior lens capsule, causing a small anterior polar cataract. They may also be associated with various other anterior segment abnormalities (Fig 20-7). See the discussion of posterior synechiae at the end of this chapter.

Abnormalities in the Size, Shape, or Location of the Pupil

Congenital Miosis

Congenital miosis, or *microcoria*, may represent an absence or malformation of the dilator pupillae muscle. Congenital miosis can also occur secondary to contracture of fibrous material on the pupil margin from remnants of the tunica vasculosa lentis or neural crest cell anomalies. The condition may be unilateral or bilateral and sporadic or hereditary. Severe cases require surgical pupilloplasty.

The pupil diameter rarely exceeds 2 mm, is often eccentric, and reacts poorly to mydriatic drops. Some patients with eccentric microcoria also have lens subluxation and are therefore part of the spectrum of ectopia lentis et pupillae. Congenital miosis may be associated with microcornea, cataract, megalocornea, iris atrophy, iris transillumination, myopia, and glaucoma. Congenital miosis can also be seen with congenital rubella syndrome and hereditary ataxia and in 20% of patients with Lowe oculocerebrorenal syndrome.

Toulemont PJ, Urvoy M, Coscas G, et al. Association of congenital microcoria with myopia and glaucoma. A study of 23 patients with congenital microcoria. *Ophthalmology.* 1995;102: 193–198.

Congenital Mydriasis

Congenitally dilated and fixed pupils with normal-appearing irides have been reported under the names *familial iridoplegia* and *congenital bilateral mydriasis.* Iris sphincter trauma, pharmacologic mydriasis, and acquired neurologic disease affecting the parasympathetic innervation to the pupil must also be considered. Many cases of congenital mydriasis may fall within the aniridia spectrum, especially if the central iris structures from the collarette to the pupillary sphincter are absent. Congenital heart defects may be associated.

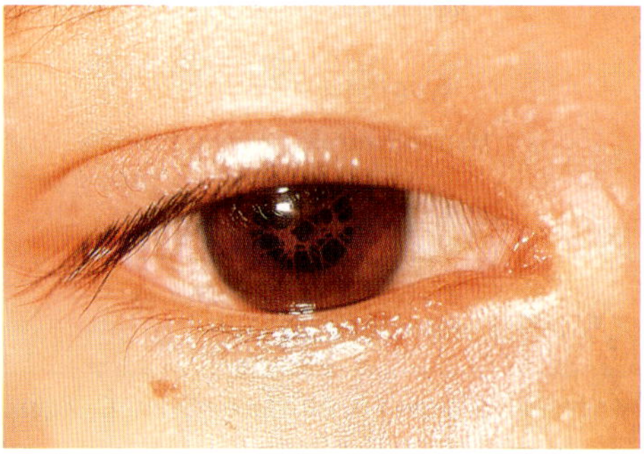

Figure 20-7 Persistent pupillary membrane. Uncorrected visual acuity is 20/40.

Bergstrom CS, Saunders RA, Hutchinson AK, et al. Iris hypoplasia and aorticopulmonary septal defect: a neurocristopathy. *J AAPOS.* 2005;9:264–267.

Sjaastad O, Lindboe CF, Schaanning J, et al. Familial mydriasis, cardiac arrythmia, respiratory failure, muscular weakness and hypohidrosis. *Acta Neurol Scand Suppl.* 2000;174:3–31.

Corectopia

Corectopia refers to displacement of the pupil. Normally, the pupil is situated about 0.5 mm inferonasally from the center of the iris. Minor deviations up to 1 mm are usually cosmetically insignificant and should probably not be considered abnormal. Sector iris hypoplasia or other colobomatous lesions can lead to corectopia, and isolated noncolobomatous autosomal dominant corectopia has also been reported. More commonly, however, corectopia is associated with lens subluxation, and this combination is called *ectopia lentis et pupillae.* The condition is almost always bilateral, with the pupils and lenses displaced in opposite directions.

The pupils may be oval or slit-shaped, and they often dilate poorly. Iris transillumination may occur, and microspherophakia has been reported.

Progressive corectopia can be associated with the Axenfeld-Rieger spectrum as well as iridocorneal endothelial (ICE) syndrome. Visual acuity may be good, even with eccentric pupils.

Polycoria and Pseudopolycoria

True *polycoria,* which must by definition include a sphincter mechanism in each pupil, is very rare. The vast majority of accessory iris openings can be classified as *pseudopolycoria.* These iris holes may be congenital or may develop in response to progressive corectopia and iris hypoplasia in Axenfeld-Rieger syndrome or ICE syndrome (Fig 20-8). Pseudopolycoria can also result from trauma, surgery, or persistent pupillary membranes.

Congenital Iris Ectropion

Ectropion of the posterior pigment epithelium onto the anterior surface of the iris is called *ectropion uveae* in much of the literature. This term is a misnomer, however, because the iris posterior epithelium is derived from neural ectoderm and is not considered part of the uvea. This iris ectropion can occur as an acquired tractional abnormality,

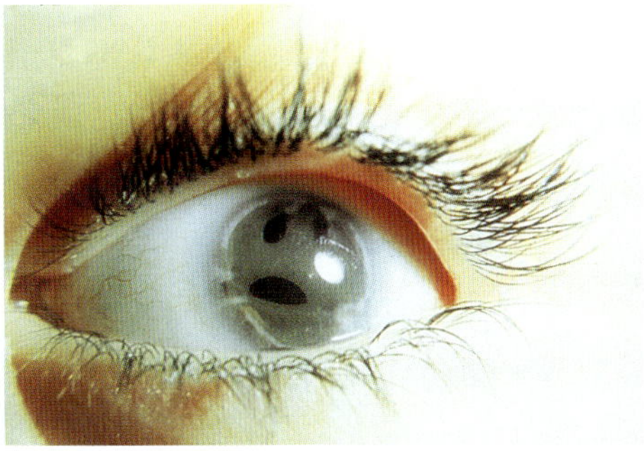

Figure 20-8 Pseudopolycoria that is secondary to Axenfeld-Rieger syndrome. *(Photograph courtesy of John W. Simon, MD.)*

often associated with rubeosis iridis, or as a congenital nonprogressive abnormality. The combination of unilateral congenital iris ectropion; a glassy smooth, cryptless iris surface; a high iris insertion; dysgenesis of the drainage angle; and glaucoma has been called *congenital iris ectropion syndrome* (Fig 20-9). In some cases, congenital iris ectropion has been associated with neurofibromatosis and has been reported more rarely with facial hemihypertrophy and Prader-Willi syndrome.

Iris Transillumination

In albinism, *iris transillumination* results from the absence of pigmentation in the posterior epithelial layers. Iris hypoplasia can also lead to iris transillumination, especially as part of Axenfeld-Rieger or ICE syndrome. Iris transillumination has also been reported in Marfan syndrome, ectopia lentis et pupillae, and microcoria. Patchy areas of transillumination can also be seen after trauma, surgery, or uveitis. Scattered iris transillumination defects may also be a normal variant in people with very lightly pigmented irides. Diffuse iris transillumination is characteristic of albinism.

Posterior Synechiae

Congenital adhesions between the iris margin and lens capsule may occur in association with cataracts, aniridia, intrauterine inflammation, or other developmental abnormalities. These adhesions can also be isolated, benign remnants of the tunica vasculosa lentis. Acquired posterior synechiae secondary to iridocyclitis occur more frequently. In pediatric sarcoidosis, inflammatory iris nodules (Koeppe or Busacca) may be associated with posterior synechiae.

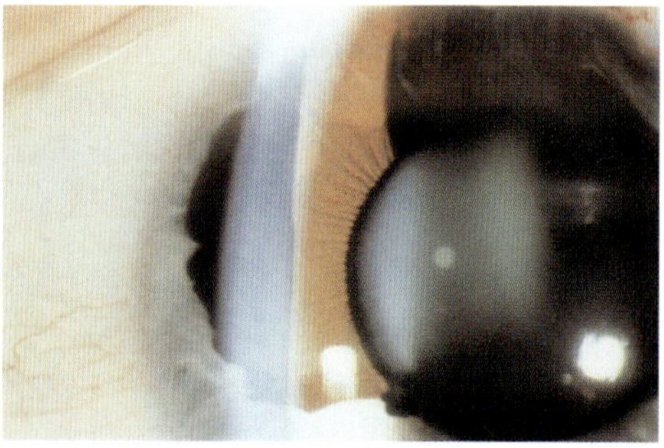

Figure 20-9 Congenital iris ectropion syndrome. A glassy-smooth, cryptless iris surface is present along with marked ectropion of the posterior pigmented epithelium onto the anterior iris surface.

CHAPTER 21

Pediatric Glaucomas

Pediatric glaucomas constitute a heterogeneous group of diseases that may result from an intrinsic disease or structural abnormality of the aqueous outflow pathways (primary glaucoma) or from abnormalities affecting other regions of the eye (secondary glaucoma). A variety of systemic abnormalities are also associated with pediatric glaucoma.

Genetics

Primary congenital glaucoma usually occurs sporadically or is inherited as an autosomal recessive trait. One gene, *CYP1B1*, at the GLC3A locus on chromosome 2p21, has been shown to cause primary congenital glaucoma. Populations in which consanguinity is common have a higher incidence of congenital glaucoma, especially those in which the carrier rate of the *CYP1B1* gene is high. A second location, GLC3B on 1p36, has also been identified.

Juvenile-onset glaucoma is inherited as an autosomal dominant trait and has been linked to the *GLC1A TIGR/Myocilin (MYOC)* gene, a gene also known to be responsible for some adult open-angle glaucomas. Affected individuals can have genetic testing performed to identify the *MYOC* mutation.

The neurocrestopathy/anterior segment dysgenesis syndromes (eg, Axenfeld-Rieger) are also inherited in an autosomal dominant fashion. Mutations causing these disorders have been linked to *PITX2* on chromosome 4q25 and *FOXC1* on chromosome 6p25.

Finally, defects in the *PAX6* gene can cause aniridia. See further discussion later in the chapter.

When no family history of congenital glaucoma exists, the chance of an affected parent having an affected child is approximately 5%. If the first child is affected, the risk of a second child being affected is still approximately 5%, rising to approximately 25% per subsequent offspring if 2 siblings are affected. Primary congenital glaucoma does not appear to be associated with adult primary open-angle glaucoma; the incidence of steroid-induced intraocular pressure (IOP) elevation is no higher in parents of affected children than in controls.

Sarfarazi M, Stoilov I. Molecular genetics of primary congenital glaucoma. *Eye.* 2000;14: 422–428.

Traboulsi EI, ed. *A Compendium of Inherited Disorders and the Eye.* New York: Oxford University Press; 2005.

Primary Congenital Glaucoma

Primary congenital open-angle glaucoma is also commonly called *congenital*, or *infantile, glaucoma*. Primary congenital glaucoma occurs in about 1 out of 10,000 births and results in blindness in 2%–15% of cases. Visual acuity is worse than 20/50 in at least 50% of cases. This condition is bilateral in about two thirds of patients and occurs more frequently in males (65%) than in females (35%).

Although diagnosis is made in only 25% of affected infants at birth, disease onset occurs within the first year of life in more than 80% of cases. If this disease presents later in childhood (after about age 3–4 years), it is considered *primary juvenile open-angle glaucoma*, a disease that appears to have a different genetic origin (see the preceding section) and often responds to therapy classically used for adult open-angle glaucoma (see BCSC Section 10, *Glaucoma*).

Buckley EG. Primary congenital open angle glaucoma. In: Epstein DL, Allingham RR, Schuman JS, eds. *Chandler and Grant's Glaucoma.* 4th ed. Baltimore: Williams & Wilkins; 1997:598–608.

deLuise VP, Anderson DR. Primary infantile glaucoma (congenital glaucoma). *Surv Ophthalmol.* 1983;28:1–19.

Pathophysiology

The basic pathologic defect in primary congenital glaucoma remains obscure. Although Barkan originally proposed a thin, imperforate membrane that covered the anterior chamber angle and blocked aqueous outflow, the site of obstruction is now thought to be the trabecular meshwork itself. This disease may represent a developmental arrest of anterior chamber tissue derived from neural crest cells during the late embryologic period.

Anderson DR. The development of the trabecular meshwork and its abnormality in primary infantile glaucoma. *Trans Am Ophthalmol Soc.* 1981;79:458–485.

Beck AD, Lynch MG. Pediatric glaucoma. *Focal Points: Clinical Modules for Ophthalmologists.* San Francisco: American Academy of Ophthalmology; 1997, module 5.

Walton DS. Primary congenital open angle glaucoma: a study of the anterior segment abnormalities. *Trans Am Ophthalmol Soc.* 1979;77:746–768.

Clinical Manifestations and Diagnosis

Primary congenital glaucoma usually presents in the neonatal or infantile period with a combination of signs and symptoms. Epiphora, photophobia, and blepharospasm constitute the classic "clinical triad" of primary congenital glaucoma. Other signs include clouding and enlargement of the cornea (Fig 21-1).

Corneal edema results from elevated intraocular pressure (IOP) and may be gradual or sudden in onset. Corneal edema is often the presenting sign in infants younger than 3 months. Microcystic edema initially involves the corneal epithelium but later extends also to the stroma, often accompanied by one or more curvilinear breaks in Descemet's membrane *(Haab striae)*. Although edema may resolve with IOP reduction, a scar will

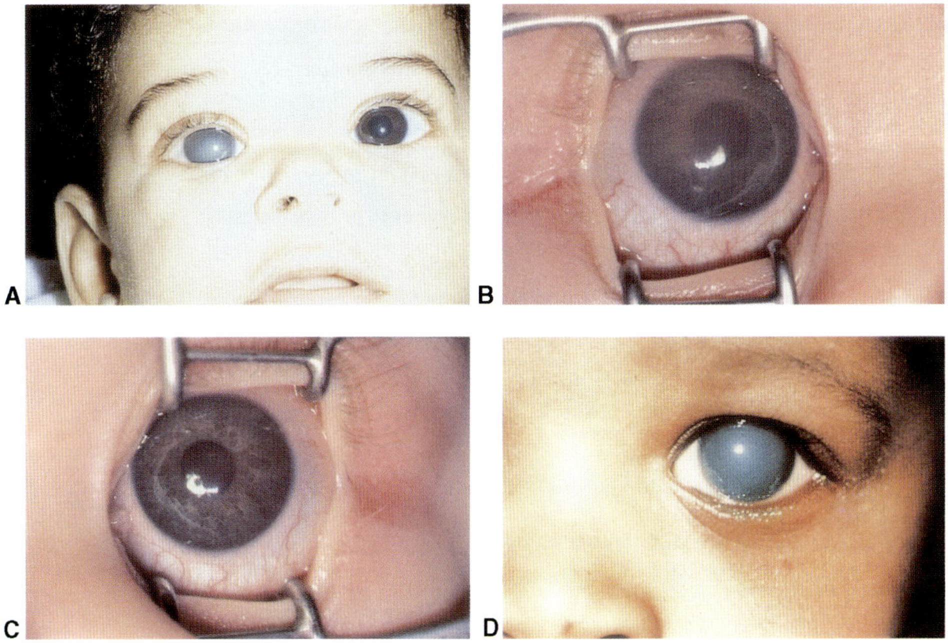

Figure 21-1 **A,** Congenital glaucoma, right eye. **B,** Right cornea larger and hazy. **C,** Left cornea clear. **D,** Late congenital glaucoma, left eye.

remain permanently at the site of Haab striae. Photophobia, epiphora, and blepharospasm result from the glare and epithelial abnormalities associated with corneal edema and opacification.

Corneal enlargement occurs with gradual stretching of the cornea as a result of elevated IOP and often appears in slightly older infants up to about age 2–3 years. The normal newborn has a horizontal corneal diameter of 9.5–10.5 mm; a diameter of greater than 11.5 mm is suggestive of glaucoma. By age 1 year, normal corneal diameter is 10.0–11.5 mm; a diameter greater than 12.5 mm suggests abnormality. Glaucoma should be suspected in any child with a corneal diameter greater than 13.0 mm.

The signs and symptoms described for primary congenital glaucoma can also occur in infants with other primary developmental and secondary glaucomas as a nonspecific result of expansion of the infant eye when faced with high IOP. Nonglaucomatous conditions may also cause some of the signs and symptoms seen in primary congenital glaucoma (Table 21-1) (see also BCSC Section 10, *Glaucoma*).

Diagnostic examination

A full ophthalmic examination of every child suspected of glaucoma is imperative. Vision is often poorer in the affected eye in unilateral cases and may be poor in both eyes when glaucoma is bilateral. The child's ability to fix and follow and the presence of nystagmus should also be noted. Refraction, when possible, often reveals myopia or astigmatism (or both) from eye enlargement and corneal irregularity.

Table 21-1 Differential Diagnosis of Signs in Primary Congenital Glaucoma

Conditions sharing signs of epiphora and red eye
Conjunctivitis
Congenital nasolacrimal duct obstruction
Corneal epithelial defect/abrasion
Ocular inflammation (uveitis, trauma)
Conditions sharing signs of corneal edema or opacification
Corneal dystrophy
Congenital hereditary endothelial dystrophy
Posterior polymorphous dystrophy
Obstetric birth trauma with Descemet's tears
Storage disease
Mucopolysaccharidoses
Cystinosis
Congenital anomalies
Sclerocornea
Peters anomaly
Keratitis
Maternal rubella keratitis
Herpetic
Phlyctenular
Idiopathic (diagnosis of exclusion only)
Conditions sharing sign of corneal enlargement
Axial myopia
Megalocornea
Conditions sharing sign of optic nerve cupping (real or apparent)
Physiologic optic nerve cupping
Optic nerve coloboma
Optic atrophy
Optic nerve hypoplasia
Optic nerve malformation

Reproduced with modification from Buckley EG. Primary congenital open angle glaucoma. In: Epstein DL, Allingham RR, Schuman JS, eds. *Chandler and Grant's Glaucoma*. 4th ed. Baltimore: Williams & Wilkins; 1997:598–608.

Corneal inspection The cornea should be examined for size, clarity, and Haab striae. A penlight, slit lamp, millimeter ruler or calipers, direct ophthalmoscope, and retinoscope are useful. Inspection can often reveal even a half-millimeter difference in corneal diameter between the eyes. Haab striae are often seen well against the red reflex after pupil dilation (Fig 21-2).

Tonometry and intraocular pressure IOP is best measured using topical anesthesia in a cooperative child; in a struggling child, IOP may be falsely elevated and unpredictably altered (usually lowered) when systemic sedatives and anesthetics are administered. A useful technique is to bring the child in slightly hungry and then bottle-feed at the time of pressure measurement. The Perkins applanation tonometer and the Tono-Pen are useful for infants and young children, and Goldmann applanation readings can frequently be taken in older children.

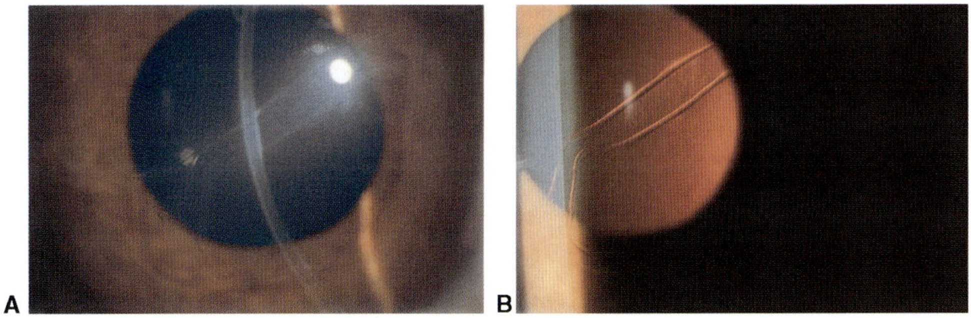

Figure 21-2 **A,** Breaks in Descemet's membrane (Haab striae), right eye. **B,** Retroillumination, same eye.

In primary congenital glaucoma, IOP commonly ranges between 30 and 40 mm Hg, and it is usually greater than 20 mm Hg even under anesthesia.

The normal IOP in infants and young children is lower than the normal IOP of adults; mean IOP is between 10 and 12 mm Hg in newborn infants and reaches approximately 14 mm Hg by age 7–8 years. Asymmetric IOP readings in a quiet or anesthetized child should also raise suspicion of glaucoma in the eye with the higher IOP. Conscious sedation with chloral hydrate (50 mg/kg PO, up to 1000 mg maximum dose) allows IOP readings that are minimally altered from those in an awake state. When conscious sedation is performed, the child's vital signs should be closely monitored, as should oxygenation by pulse oximetry.

Anterior segment examination After tonometry has been attempted, the portable slit lamp allows detailed inspection of the anterior segments. An abnormally deep anterior chamber and relative peripheral iris stromal hypoplasia are characteristic of primary congenital glaucoma.

Gonioscopy provides important information regarding the mechanism of glaucoma. It is best performed using a Koeppe contact lens and portable slit lamp or loupes. Often, a preliminary examination can be performed on a quiet infant in the office, with more detailed assessment possible in the operating room under anesthesia. The anterior chamber angle of a normal infant differs from that of an adult in the following ways:

- The trabecular meshwork is more lightly pigmented.
- Schwalbe's line is often less distinct.
- The uveal meshwork is translucent so that the junction between the scleral spur and ciliary body band is often not well seen.

In congenital glaucoma, the iris often shows an insertion more anterior than that of the normal angle, and the translucency of the uveal meshwork is altered, making ciliary body band, trabecular meshwork, and scleral spur indistinct. (The membrane described by Barkan may indeed be these translucent uveal meshwork cells.) The scalloped border of the iris-pigmented epithelium is often unusually prominent, especially when peripheral iris stromal hypoplasia is present (Fig 21-3). In contrast, the open angle usually appears normal in juvenile open-angle glaucoma.

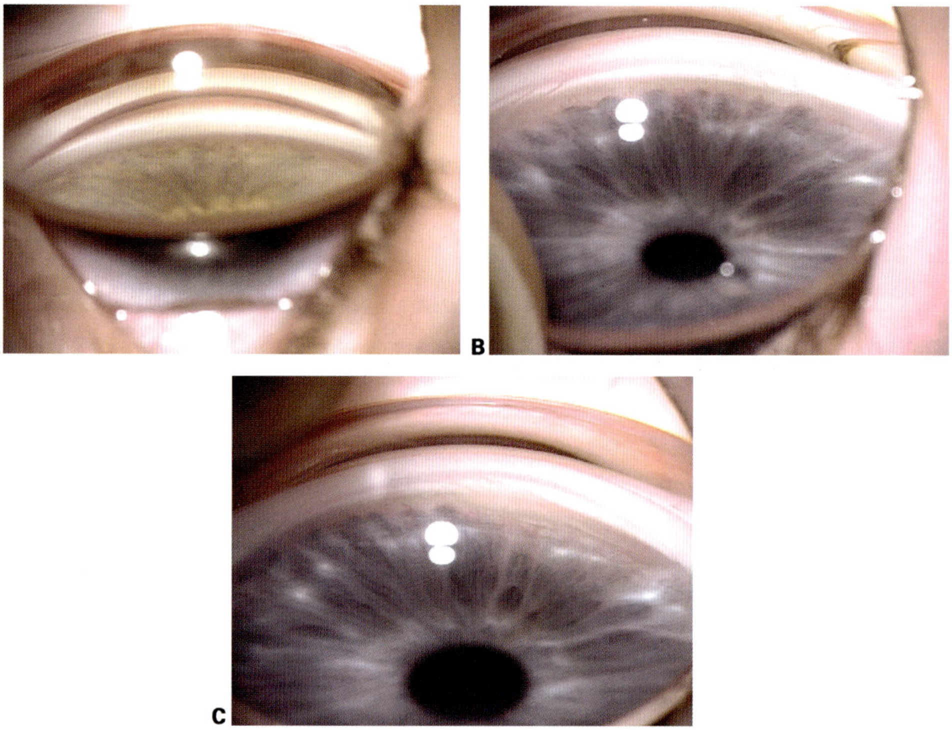

A B C

Figure 21-3 **A,** Normal gonioscopic angle in young infant. **B,** Typical appearance of infant angle with congenital glaucoma. **C,** Same angle as in **B** after trabeculotomy. Note deepening of angle appearance after procedure. *(Photographs courtesy of David A. Plager, MD.)*

Optic nerve examination The optic nerve, when visible, usually shows an increased cup–disc ratio, which can improve with successful treatment and lowering of IOP. The pattern of generalized enlargement of the optic cup seen in very young patients with glaucoma has been attributed to stretching of the optic canal and backward bowing of the lamina cribrosa, which can be reversible (Fig 21-4). In most cases of primary congenital glaucoma, the cup–disc ratio exceeds 0.3; in contrast, most normal newborn eyes show a cup–disc ratio of less than 0.3. Cup–disc asymmetry between the 2 eyes of an infant is also suspicious for glaucoma on the more cupped side.

Axial length If A-scan ultrasonography is available, serial measurement of axial length is another useful parameter to follow in evaluating the progression of disease in infant eyes. Excessive growth in an eye, especially when compared to the fellow eye, can be an indicator that the IOP control in the eye is not adequate.

Buckley EG. Primary congenital open angle glaucoma. In: Epstein DL, Allingham RR, Schuman JS, eds. *Chandler and Grant's Glaucoma.* 4th ed. Baltimore: Williams & Wilkins; 1997:598–608.

Stamper RL, Lieberman MF, Drake MV. *Becker-Shaffer's Diagnosis and Therapy of the Glaucomas.* 7th ed. St Louis: Mosby; 1999.

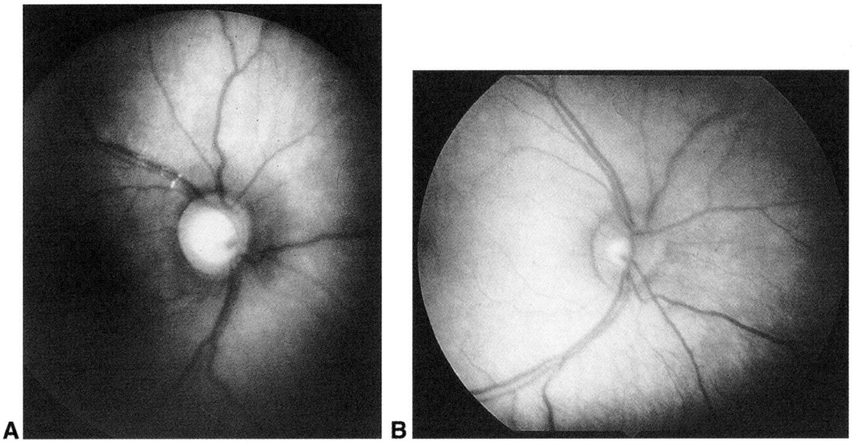

Figure 21-4 Optic nerve changes after treatment for congenital glaucoma. **A,** Preoperative enlarged optic disc cup. **B,** Resolution of disc cupping after pressure is reduced by goniotomy. *(Photographs courtesy of Sharon Freedman, MD.)*

Natural History

In almost all cases of untreated primary congenital glaucoma, the disease progresses and leads to blindness. The cornea becomes irreversibly opacified and may vascularize. It may continue to enlarge through the first 2–3 years of life, reaching a diameter of up to 16–17 mm. As the entire eye enlarges, pseudoproptosis and an "ox eye" appearance, called *buphthalmos,* may result. Scleral thinning and myopic fundus changes may occur, and spontaneous lens dislocation can result. Optic nerve cupping also increases and may finally lead to complete blindness.

Secondary Pediatric Glaucomas

All other types of glaucomas can be considered secondary glaucomas—mainly secondary to other ocular structural anomalies or secondarily associated with a systemic condition. Other secondary glaucomas include those associated with mechanical factors and aphakia. Some of the more common secondary glaucomas are discussed in the following sections.

Secondary to Ocular Anomalies

Aniridia

Aniridia is a bilateral, congenital condition that can be sporadic or inherited. The signal ocular abnormality—complete or nearly complete absence of the iris—is usually readily apparent. Other associated abnormalities include glaucoma, cataract, corneal pannus, foveal hypoplasia, and nystagmus. The inherited form involves a mutation of the *PAX6* gene located on the 11p13 region. The association between the sporadic form of aniridia and a potentially fatal renal tumor, Wilms tumor, is well known and must be considered in these patients. Up to one third of patients with sporadic aniridia develop a Wilms tumor, so these children need to be referred for serial abdominal ultrasound surveillance starting in infancy.

Anterior segment dysgenesis

Anterior segment dysgenesis (eg, Axenfeld-Rieger) includes entities known as *Axenfeld anomaly/syndrome, Rieger anomaly/syndrome*, and *Peters anomaly*. This spectrum of disorders involves abnormalities in anterior segment development. The disorders are sometimes categorized as distinct clinical entities, but they are not. Among the more common presentations are

- *Axenfeld anomaly/syndrome.* Characterized by a prominent, anteriorly displaced Schwalbe's line (posterior embryotoxon) with iridocorneal adhesions and glaucoma. It is usually inherited as an autosomal dominant trait. When only the posterior embryotoxon is present, it is referred to as *Axenfeld anomaly.*
- *Rieger anomaly/syndrome.* Includes iris stromal hypoplasia and atrophy, corectopia, and ectropion uvea, and may include the Axenfeld anomaly. Systemically, the Rieger syndrome includes dental and facial anomalies.
- *Peters anomaly.* Manifested by a central corneal opacification with iridocorneal adhesions to the edges of the leukoma.

Other glaucomas

The following are less common secondary ocular glaucomas seen in childhood:

- congenital iris ectropion
- sclerocornea
- posterior polymorphous dystrophy
- congenital hereditary endothelial dystrophy

Secondary to Systemic Disease

Sturge-Weber syndrome

Sturge-Weber syndrome (SWS), also known as *nevus flammeus* or *port-wine stain*, is a phakomatosis that includes a port-wine stain of the face, intracranial calcifications, and glaucoma, although the presence of a port-wine stain alone has been associated with the development of glaucoma. The glaucoma is invariably on the side of the port-wine stain and is thought to be more likely if the port-wine stain involves the upper eyelid.

Neurofibromatosis

Glaucoma associated with neurofibromatosis type 1 (NF1) can be bilateral or unilateral. See Chapter 27 for more detail about NF1.

Lowe syndrome

Lowe syndrome (oculocerebralrenal syndrome) is suggested by the presence of coexistent glaucoma and cataract at initial presentation. The cataractous lens is distinctly flattened and disc-like, and the pupils tend to be miotic. Children with this disorder have progressive renal tubular dysfunction and mental retardation. The syndrome is transmitted as an X-linked recessive disorder.

Secondary Mechanical Glaucomas

Glaucoma can also be caused by mechanical factors obscuring or obstructing aqueous outflow. These include

- *lens-associated disorders:* homocystinuria, Weill-Marchesani, microspherophakia, Marfan syndrome
- *posterior segment abnormalities:* persistent fetal vasculature (PFV; formerly known as *persistent hyperplastic primary vitreous, PHPV*); retinopathy of prematurity (ROP); familial exudative vitreoretinopathy (FEVR); tumors (eg, retinoblastoma in advanced stages can cause a forward shift of the lens–iris diaphragm and secondary glaucoma)
- *topirimate (Topamax):* This medication, which is used to control seizures, can cause an acute, usually bilateral, secondary angle-closure glaucoma due to ciliary effusion. Peripheral iridectomy is not effective for treatment of this angle closure, but cessation of the medication is.

Other Secondary Glaucomas

Other causes of secondary glaucoma include the following:

- uveitis
- steroids
- trauma

Walton DS. Unusual pediatric glaucomas. In: Epstein DL, Allingham RR, Schuman JS, eds. *Chandler and Grant's Glaucoma.* 4th ed. Baltimore: Williams & Wilkins; 1997:623–638.

Aphakic Glaucoma

Aphakic glaucoma deserves special comment, as it is perhaps the most common cause of secondary glaucoma in childhood. The incidence of open-angle aphakic glaucoma after removal of congenital cataracts varies from 15% to 50% or higher. Mean age to onset of aphakic glaucoma is 5 years after cataract surgery, although it can occur only weeks to months after surgery and remains a lifelong risk.

The mechanism for aphakic glaucoma is uncertain. The angle is usually open on gonioscopy; the outflow channels are compromised by some combination of abnormal development of the anterior chamber angle, early surgery, and perhaps susceptibility of the infant eye to surgically induced inflammation, loss of lens support, or vitreous factors. It is clear that children at substantial risk of developing aphakic glaucoma are those with congenital cataracts (nuclear, PFV, total) associated with any degree of microcornea (Fig 21-5). The majority of children with these cataracts has surgery in early infancy, although whether the age at surgery is an independent risk factor is uncertain. Because aphakic children are at lifelong risk for glaucoma, they need regular, careful examination (including IOP evaluation).

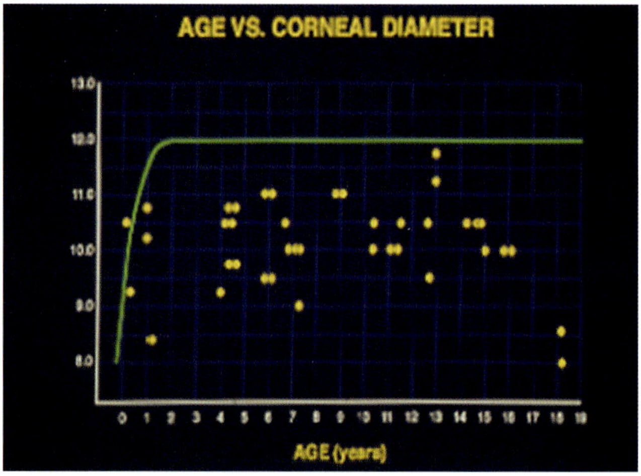

Figure 21-5 Graph showing corneal diameters of patients with aphakic glaucoma plotted against a line showing normal corneal diameter for age. *(Reproduced with permission from Wallace DK, Plager DA. Corneal diameter in childhood aphakic glaucoma.* J Pediatr Ophthalmol Strabismus. *1996;33:230–234.*

Pseudophakic glaucoma in children has been rarely reported, but this is probably due to selection bias in that children selected for IOL placement have largely been those at lower risk for glaucoma. As more infants with small eyes have IOLs implanted, the number of cases of pseudophakic glaucoma can be expected to increase.

Acute or subacute angle closure with iris bombé is a rare form of aphakic glaucoma. Although it usually occurs soon after surgery, onset can be delayed by a year or more. The diagnosis should be apparent with a slit lamp, but this can be challenging to accomplish in the young age group at risk for this complication. Treatment consists of anterior vitrectomy to relieve the pupillary block, often with surgical iridectomy and goniosynechialysis.

Chen TC, Walton DS, Bhatia LS. Aphakic glaucoma after congenital cataract surgery. *Arch Ophthalmol.* 2004;122:1819–1825.

Wallace DK, Plager DA. Corneal diameter in childhood aphakic glaucoma. *J Pediatric Ophthalmol Strabismus.* 1996;33:230–234.

Treatment

In terms of treatment, there are essentially 2 types of glaucomas in childhood: (1) primary congenital (infantile) glaucoma and (2) everything else. Primary congenital glaucoma is usually effectively treated with angle surgery (goniotomy or trabeculotomy). Although angle surgery is sometimes used in some secondary glaucomas—most notably Axenfeld syndrome, Sturge-Weber, and aniridia—the utility of such surgery in these entitities is more controversial and less successful. Most secondary glaucomas in childhood are treated more like open-angle or secondary glaucomas in adults. Frequently, medical control is attempted before surgery to improve outflow by creating new outflow channels or to decrease aqueous production with some form of cyclodestruction.

Surgical Therapy

Surgical intervention is the treatment of choice for primary congenital glaucoma presenting in infancy and early childhood. BCSC Section 10, *Glaucoma*, also covers the procedures discussed in this chapter.

Angle surgery is the preferred initial surgical intervention in these cases. *Goniotomy* is performed by making an incision across the trabecular meshwork under direct gonioscopic visualization. *Trabeculotomy* uses an external approach to identify, cannulate, and then connect Schlemm's canal with the anterior chamber by incising the trabecular meshwork from the outside. A modification of this technique uses a 6-0 Prolene suture to cannulate and open Schlemm's canal for its entire 360° circumference in 1 surgery. If the cornea is clear, either a goniotomy or trabeculotomy can be performed at the surgeon's discretion. If the view through the cornea is compromised, trabeculotomy is the preferred intial procedure.

In approximately 80% of infants with primary congenital glaucoma presenting from 3 months to 1 year of age, IOP is controlled with 1 or 2 angle surgeries. If the first angle surgery is not sufficient, at least 1 additional angle surgery is performed prior to proceeding with another surgical strategy.

For children in whom angle surgery is not successful or is not indicated (many secondary glaucomas), and medical therapy (see the next section) is inadequate to control IOP and glaucoma, additional options are available, including trabeculectomy with or without antifibrinolytic therapy (eg, mitomycin C), glaucoma implant procedures, or cycloablative procedures.

Trabeculectomy with the use of mitomycin C is successful in approximately 50%–95% of children. The reported success rates vary considerably with the characteristics of the patient and the eye, as well as the follow-up length. Patients younger than 1 year and those who are aphakic often do not fare as well. Although the success rate of trabeculectomy can be increased with antifibrinolytic agents such as mitomycin C, the long-term risk of bleb leaks, breakdown, and endophthalmitis also increase. These devastating complications have made some surgeons more reticent to use mitomycin C augmentation for children.

The reported success rate of glaucoma implant surgery with the Molteno, Baerveldt, and Ahmed implants has varied between 54% and approximately 80%–85%. Although most of these children must remain on adjunctive topical medical therapy to control IOP after surgery, their blebs are thicker and may be less prone to leaking and infection than those of mitomycin-augmented trabeculectomy. However, long-term risks of shunt failure, tube erosion and migration, restrictive strabismus, and endophthalmitis are persistent concerns in children with tube shunts.

Cycloablation using the Nd:YAG laser, the diode laser, or cyclocryotherapy is generally reserved for extremely resistant cases or those not amenable to the intraocular surgeries noted earlier. These techniques decrease ciliary body production of aqueous humor. *Cyclocryotherapy* (freeze treatment to the ciliary body through the sclera) has a reported success rate of about 33%, and the complication rate is high. Repeat applications are the rule, and the risk of phthisis and blindness is significant (approximately 10%). *Transscleral laser cycloablation* with the Nd:YAG or the diode laser has also been used in refractory cases. Short-term success is about 50%, with a retreatment rate of about 70% reported with either laser.

More recently, *endoscopic cyclophotocoagulation (ECP)* has been used in both adults and children with difficult glaucomas. This method of diode laser treatment uses a microendoscope to apply the laser energy directly to ciliary processes under direct observation (Fig 21-6). Up to 50% success rates have been reported; the rate is higher with repeat applications. Although this is an intraocular procedure, the complication rates have been lower than those observed with some of the less-controlled external cyclodestructive procedures. Use of the microendoscope is especially advantageous in eyes with abnormal anterior segment anatomy, including those with previous unsuccessful laser or cryoablative procedures. Some studies have shown especially encouraging results for aphakic glaucoma.

Carter BC, Plager DA, Neely DE, et al. Endoscopic diode laser cyclophotocoagulation in the management of aphakic and pseudophakic glaucoma in children. *J AAPOS.* 2007;11:34–40.

Medical Therapy

The menu of glaucoma medications continues to expand. See also BCSC Section 10, *Glaucoma.*

Topical medications

Topical beta-blocker therapy, which has been used in children since the 1970s, often lowers IOP 20%–30%. Six beta-blockers are currently available for use in the United States: timolol maleate (Timoptic, Timoptic XE), betaxolol hydrochloride (Betoptic S), levobunolol (Betagan), timolol hemihydrate (Betimol), metipranolol (OptiPranolol), and carteolol (Ocupress). The major risks of this therapy are respiratory distress caused by apnea or bronchospasm and bradycardia, which occurs mostly in very tiny infants and in children with a history of bronchospasm. Betaxolol is a cardioselective B1 antagonist

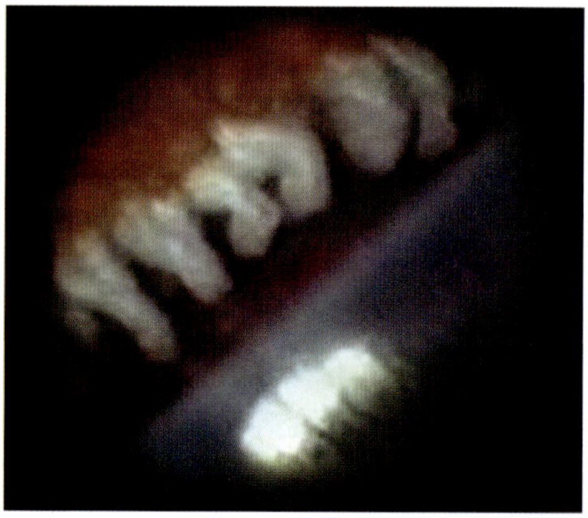

Figure 21-6 Endoscopic view of ciliary processes during ECP procedure. The white structure at bottom right of the photo is the lens. *(Photograph courtesy of Endo Optiks, Little Silver, NJ.)*

and should have less pulmonary and systemic side effects, although its pressure-lowering effect may be less than with the nonselective agents. Timolol (or its equivalent) or betaxolol (Betoptic S) should be used at 0.25% strength twice a day for initial therapy. The parent should be instructed how to perform nasolacrimal occlusion with these drugs. The gel-forming preparations of timolol (Timoptic XE) seem effective in some children but should be avoided in eyes with aphakic contact lenses.

The *topical carbonic anhydrase inhibitors (CAIs)* dorzolamide 2% (Trusopt) and brinzolamide 1% (Azopt) are available as solutions. Studies using topical CAIs 3 times a day indicate that the drugs can be effective in children, although they produce a smaller reduction in IOP (<15%). There is no increased utility in using a topical CAI in a child already on an oral CAI.

A *combined beta antagonist-CAI* (Cosopt) combines timolol and dorzolamide in a single drop. It has been used effectively at a b.i.d. dose in children requiring dual therapy for IOP control.

Prostaglandin analogues latanaprost 0.005% (Xalatan) and travoprost 0.004% (Travatan) and a prostamide bimatoprost 0.03% (Lumigan) have shown effectiveness in some pediatric patients. Use of this class of medications is generally discouraged in association with inflammatory conditions.

Miotic therapy is rarely effective in cases of primary congenital glaucoma, perhaps because of the high iris insertion in these cases. Long-acting or slow-release miotics such as pilocarpine (Pilopine gel and Ocusert) and echothiophate (Phospholine iodide, for aphakic patients) can be helpful, particularly in cases of juvenile open-angle glaucoma and some secondary childhood glaucomas.

Adrenergic agents such as epinephrine or dipivefrin (Propine) are not usually effective in children, particularly when a nonselective beta-blocker is already in use. The α_2-adrenergic agonist apraclonidine (Iopidine) has been useful when short-term IOP reduction is essential, but this drug shows a high incidence of tachyphylaxis and allergy in young children. The α_2-adrenergic agonist brimonidine (Alphagan) effectively reduces IOP in some cases of pediatric glaucoma, but this agent can produce severe systemic side effects in infants and small children (among them lethargy, hypotonia, hypothermia, and serious CNS depression) and therefore is contraindicated in children under age 2 years.

Oral medications

Carbonic anhydrase inhibitors have been used for many years as aqueous suppressants in children, and they may be quite effective. Acetazolamide (Diamox), the most commonly used agent, is effective at oral doses of 10–20 mg/kg/day divided into 3 or 4 doses. Care must be taken to watch for weight loss, lethargy, or metabolic acidosis, although many children tolerate this medication well. Methazolamide (Neptazane) is also an effective oral CAI.

See BCSC Section 10, *Glaucoma*, for a more detailed discussion of medical glaucoma therapy agents.

Freedman SF, Buckley EG. Goniotomy and trabeculectomy. In: Buckley EG, Freedman SF, Shields MB, et al, eds. *Atlas of Ophthalmic Surgery.* Vol 3, *Strabismus and Glaucoma.* St Louis: Mosby; 1995.

Prognosis and Follow-Up

If primary congenital glaucoma presents at birth, the prognosis for IOP control and visual preservation is poor, with at least half of these eyes becoming legally blind. With a corneal diameter greater than 14 mm at diagnosis, the visual prognosis is similarly poor. Up to 80%–90% of cases in the "favorable prognostic group" (onset 3–12 months) can be controlled with angle surgery. The remaining 10%–20% of these cases, and many of the remaining cases of primary and secondary glaucomas, often present a lifelong challenge.

Visual loss in childhood glaucoma is multifactorial. It may result not only from corneal scarring and opacification or optic nerve damage but also from significant myopic astigmatism and associated anisometropic and strabismic amblyopia, especially in unilateral cases. Myopia results from axial enlargement of the eye in the setting of high IOP; astigmatism often results from unequal expansion of the anterior segment, corneal scarring and opacification, or dislocation of the lens. Careful assessment of vision, refraction, and amblyopia therapy are needed to optimize visual function in these children.

All cases of childhood glaucoma require diligent follow-up, which should also be performed when glaucoma is suspected but cannot yet be confirmed. After any given surgical intervention or change in medical therapy, control of IOP should be assessed within 1–2 weeks. The status of the cornea in terms of its size and clarity, the appearance of the optic nerve, and the refractive error can all often provide clues regarding improved IOP control. If IOP cannot be determined in the office, examination may require sedation with chloral hydrate or general anesthesia. The IOP should be considered not as an isolated finding but rather in conjunction with other features of the examination. If the IOP is less than 20 mm Hg under anesthesia but clinical evidence shows persistent corneal edema or enlargement, progressive optic nerve cupping, or myopic progression, further intervention should be pursued despite the IOP reading. In contrast, IOP of about 20 mm Hg in a young child who shows evidence of clinical improvement may be followed carefully in the short term without any other intervention.

Careful repeated follow-up of all parameters associated with glaucoma in children is the only way to ensure disease control and optimal preservation of visual function. Even those children apparently "cured" after angle surgery can experience relapse years later with elevated IOP and subsequent visual loss. Although helpful in following disease progression in older children, visual fields are rarely useful in children younger than 6–8 years. Optic nerve photographs should be taken whenever possible; these can be helpful for comparison during later examinations. As discussed earlier, refractive error and corneal size and clarity are also helpful to follow as evidence of ocular stability over time. If available, serial axial length measurement with A-scan ultrasonography can be a very helpful parameter to follow for relative growth of the eyes, particularly in cases of unilateral glaucoma.

CHAPTER 22

Childhood Cataracts and Other Pediatric Lens Disorders

Disorders of the pediatric lens include, in addition to cataract, abnormalities in shape, size, location, and development. Such abnormalities constitute a significant source of visual impairment in children (Table 22-1). The incidence is approximately 6:10,000 infants. Abnormalities of the pediatric lens may be associated with diseases of the central nervous system, urinary tract, skeletal system, and skin. Pediatric lens abnormalities must be treated promptly to avoid lifelong visual loss. BCSC Section 11, *Lens and Cataract*, also covers conditions and procedures discussed in this chapter.

Pediatric Cataracts

Congenital cataracts are responsible for nearly 10% of all visual loss in children worldwide, and it is estimated that 1 in 250 newborns has some form of cataract. Cataracts in children can be

- isolated or part of a systemic condition
- congenital or acquired

Table 22-1 Congenital Lens Abnormalities

Opacification	**Shape**
Lamellar	Spherophakia
Speckled	Coloboma
Membranous	
Pulverulent	
Polar	**Location**
Zonular	Subluxed
Subcapsular	Luxed
Nuclear	
Total	
Lenticonus/lentiglobus	**Development**
	Persistent fetal vasculature (PFV, or PHPV)
Size	
Microspherophakia	
Disciform	

- inherited or sporadic
- unilateral or bilateral
- partial or complete
- stable or progressive

Systemic Implications

Cataracts in children can be isolated or can be associated with myriad systemic conditions, including chromosomal abnormalities; craniofacial, mandibulofacial, and skeletal syndromes; metabolic disorders; congenital infection; dermatologic, CNS, musculoskeletal, or renal disease; or external factors such as trauma or radiation. In almost all cases of cataract associated with systemic disease, the cataracts are bilateral (although not all bilateral cataracts are associated with systemic disease). See Table 22-2.

Cataracts can also be associated with other ocular anomalies, including persistent fetal vasculature, coloboma, anterior segment dysgenesis, and aniridia.

Table 22-2 Etiology of Pediatric Cataracts

Bilateral cataracts
- Idiopathic
- Familial (hereditary), usually autosomal dominant
- Chromosomal abnormality
  - Trisomy-21 (Down), -18 (Edward), -13 (Patau)
  - Other translocations, deletions, and duplications
- Craniofacial syndromes
  - Hallerman-Streiff, Rubenstein-Taybi, Smith-Lemli-Opitz, others
- Musculoskeletal
  - Conradi, Albright, myotonic dystrophy
- Renal
  - Lowe, Alport
- Metabolic
  - Galactosemia, Fabry, Wilson, mannisidosis, diabetes
- Maternal infection (TORCH diseases)
  - Rubella
  - Cytomegalovirus
  - Varicella
  - Syphilis
  - Toxoplasmosis
- Ocular anomalies
  - Aniridia
  - Anterior segment dysgenesis syndrome
- Toxic
  - Corticosteroids
  - Radiation (may also be unilateral)

Unilateral cataracts
- Idiopathic
- Ocular anomalies
  - Persistent fetal vasculature (PFV)—formerly, persistent hyperplastic primary vitreous (PHPV)
  - Anterior segment dysgenesis
  - Posterior segment tumors
- Traumatic (rule out child abuse)

Onset

Pediatric cataracts can be congenital or acquired. Lens opacities that are visually significant prior to the development of the fixation reflex—that is, before 2–3 months of age—have much more impact on the child's visual development than those acquired later. In general, the earlier the onset during the amblyopia-susceptible age range, the more amblyogenic the cataract will be.

A visually significant unilateral congenital cataract should be detected and treated very early (<2 months of age) in order to promote optimal visual development.

Similarly, for bilateral cataracts, once sensory-deprivation nystagmus has developed (2–3 months of age), the visual potential decreases markedly.

Inheritance

When inherited, familial cataracts are usually autosomal dominant and always bilateral. X-linked and autosomal recessive inheritance has been reported but is rare (Table 22-3).

Laterality

Pediatric cataracts can be unilateral or bilateral, although significant asymmetry can be present in bilateral cases.

Morphology

Cataracts can involve the entire lens (total or complete cataract) or can involve only part of the lens structure. The location in the lens and morphology of the cataract provide a great deal of information about its onset, etiology, laterality, and prognosis (Table 22-4).

Table 22-3 Hereditary Factors in Pediatric Cataracts

Type	OMIM Number	Gene/Gene Map
Aculeiform	115700	2q33-q35
Anterior polar 1 (CTAA1)	115650	14q24-qter
Anterior polar 2 (CTAA2)	601202	17p13
Cerulean type I (CCA1)	115660	17q24
Cerulean type II (CCA2)	601547	*CRYBB2*/22q
Congenital total	302200	Xp
Autosomal dominant		*CRYAA*/21q22.3
Coppock-like (CCL)		*CRYGA*/2q33-q35
Marner type (CAM)	116800	16q22.1
Posterior polar (CPP)	116600	1pter-p36.1
Volkmann type	115665	1p36
Dominant, zonular pulverulent (CZP3)	601885	*GJA3*/13q11-q12
Lamellar, zonular pulverulent (CZP1), Coppock (CAE)	116200	*GJA8*/1q21.1
Zonular with sutural opacities (CCZS)	600881	17q11-q12

Reproduced with permission from Traboulsi EI, ed. *A Compendium of Inherited Disorders and the Eye.* New York: Oxford University Press; 2005.

The clinically most common and important morphologies of partial cataracts are discussed in the following sections.

Anterior polar cataract

Anterior polar cataracts (APCs) are common, appearing as small white dots in the center of the anterior lens capsule. They are typically 1 mm in diameter but can be smaller or, rarely, larger. They are thought to be a remnant of persistent tunica vasculosa lentis. These opacities are usually not visually significant and are not expected to enlarge or progress, therefore rarely require surgery. They are congenital and usually sporadic and can be bilateral or unilateral. Anisometropia is common, so careful refraction is indicated. See Figure 22-1.

Table 22-4 Pediatric Cataracts: Selected Typical Cataract Appearances

Cataract Morphology	Diagnosis	Other Possible Findings
Spokelike	Fabry syndrome	Corneal whorls
	Mannosidosis	Hepatosplenomegaly
Vacuoles	Diabetes	Blood glucose level increased
Multicolor	Hypoparathyroidism	Decreased serum calcium
flecks	Myotonic dystrophy	Characteristic facial features, tonic "grip"
Green "sunflower"	Wilson disease	Kayser-Fleischer corneal ring
Thin disciform	Lowe syndrome	Hypotonia, glaucoma

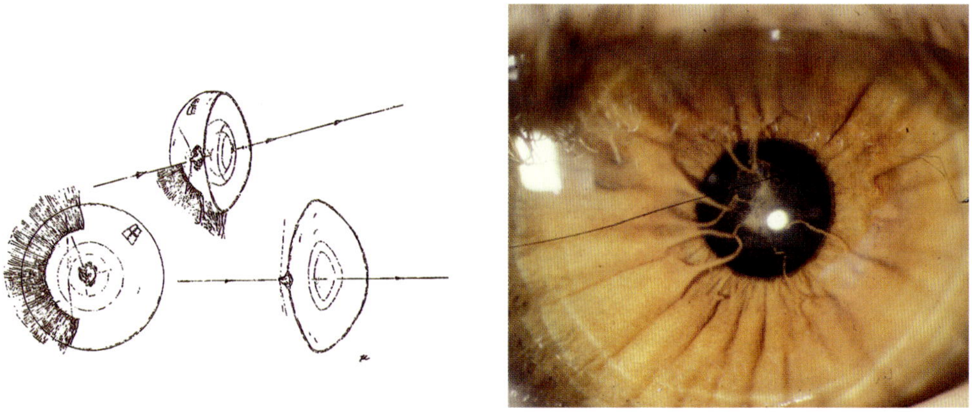

Figure 22-1 Anterior polar cataract. *(Illustration courtesy of Alan Y. Chow, MD; photograph courtesy of David A. Plager, MD.)*

Nuclear cataract

Nuclear cataracts are opacities that involve the center, or nucleus, of the lens. They are typically approximately 3 mm in diameter, but the irregularity of lens fibers can extend out farther peripherally. Density is variable. These opacities tend to be stable but can progress in density and can become slightly larger in size. They can be unilateral or bilateral, inherited or sporadic. They are congenital but may not be significantly dense at birth (Fig 22-2).

Importantly, eyes harboring nuclear cataracts usually have some degree of microcornea (corneal diameter less than normal for age). This is most readily apparent in unilateral cases. These eyes are at increased risk for developing aphakic glaucoma after cataract surgery, and the children need to be monitored carefully throughout life.

Lamellar cataract

Lamellar cataracts, which can be identified by their discrete, round (lenticular) shape, affect 1 or more of the "rings" in the developing lens cortex. The opacities are larger in diameter than nuclear cataracts, being typically 5 mm or more. They are always bilateral but can be asymmetric in density; hence, there is the possibility of amblyopia. Lamellar opacities are usually acquired but can be inherited. These eyes are normal size and normal in corneal diameter (Fig 22-3).

Because onset is usually after the child's fixation reflex has been established, the visual prognosis may be excellent following surgery.

Posterior lenticonus/lentiglobus

Posterior lenticonus/lentiglobus is caused by a relative thinning of the central or paracentral posterior capsule. This thinning initially causes an "oil droplet" appearance on red reflex. With time, as the outpouching of the lens progresses, the cortical fibers stretch and gradually opacify. This process can take many years and progress almost imperceptibly,

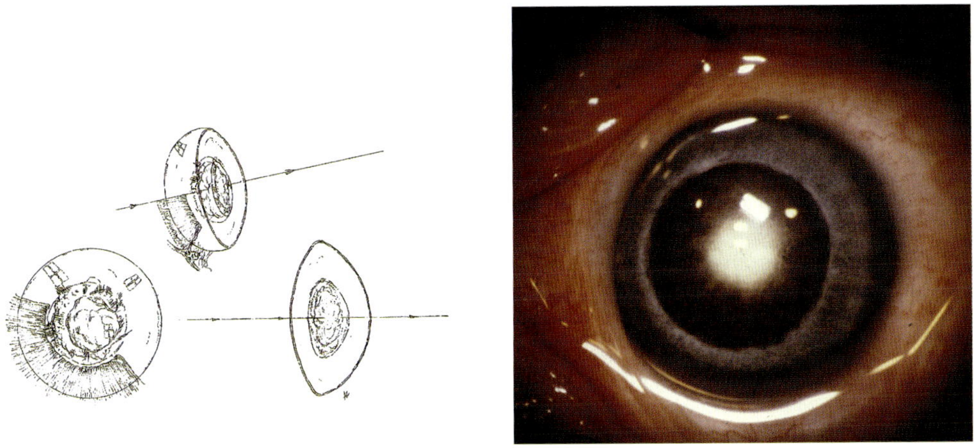

Figure 22-2 Nuclear cataract. *(Illustration courtesy of Alan Y. Chow, MD; photograph courtesy of Marshal M. Parks, MD.)*

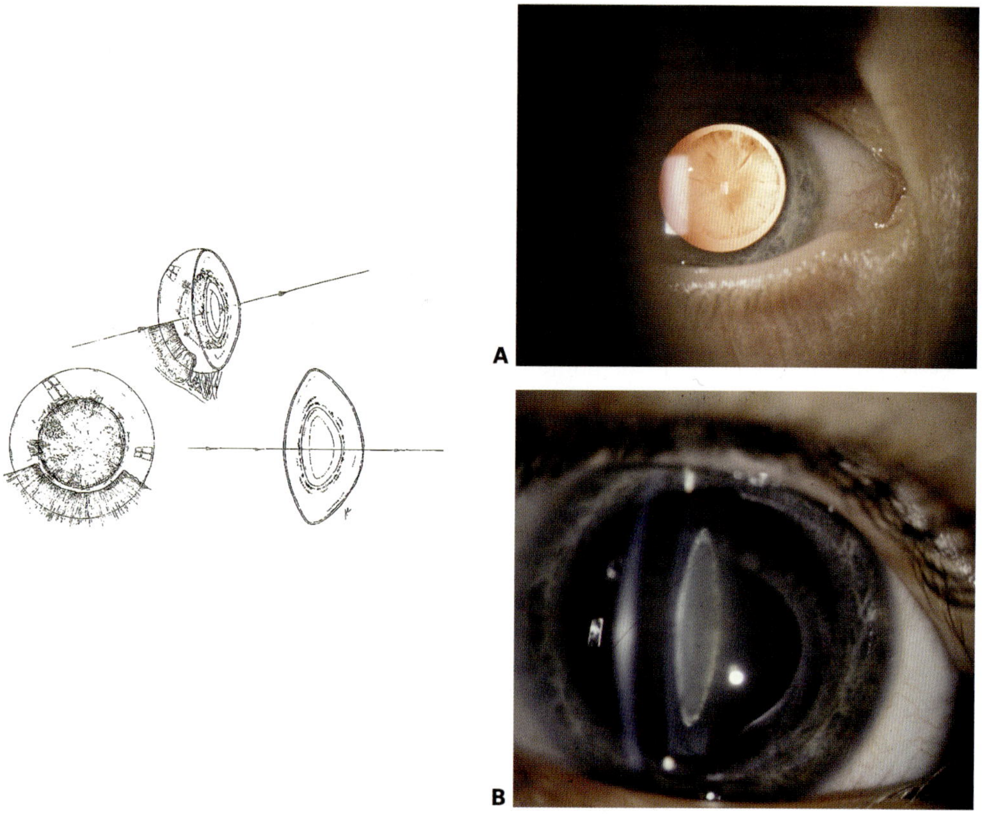

Figure 22-3 Lamellar cataract. **A,** Retroillumination shows size of the lamellar opacity. **B,** Slit-lamp view shows lamellar opacity surrounding clear nucleus. *(Illustration courtesy of Alan Y. Chow, MD; photographs courtesy of David A. Plager, MD.)*

but if the capsule tears, it can cause total opacification of the lens literally overnight (Fig 22-4).

Posterior lenticonus opacities are almost always unilateral, and the affected eye is equal in size to the unaffected eye. These opacities are not typically inherited, and although the weakness in the posterior capsule may be congenital, the cataract usually does not form until later and therefore behaves like an acquired cataract. Visual prognosis after surgery (when indicated) can be favorable.

Persistent fetal vasculature

Persistent fetal vasculature (PFV) is caused by failure of the fetal hyaloid vascular complex to regress. Historically, this entity has been referred to as *persistent hyperplastic primary vitreous (PHPV)*, but in recent years the more anatomically accurate term *persistent fetal vasculature* has been preferred. Clinically, there is a retrolental membrane of varying size and density attached to the posterior lens surface. The membrane can be small and centrally located or may extend out to attach to the ciliary processes for 360° (Fig 22-5).

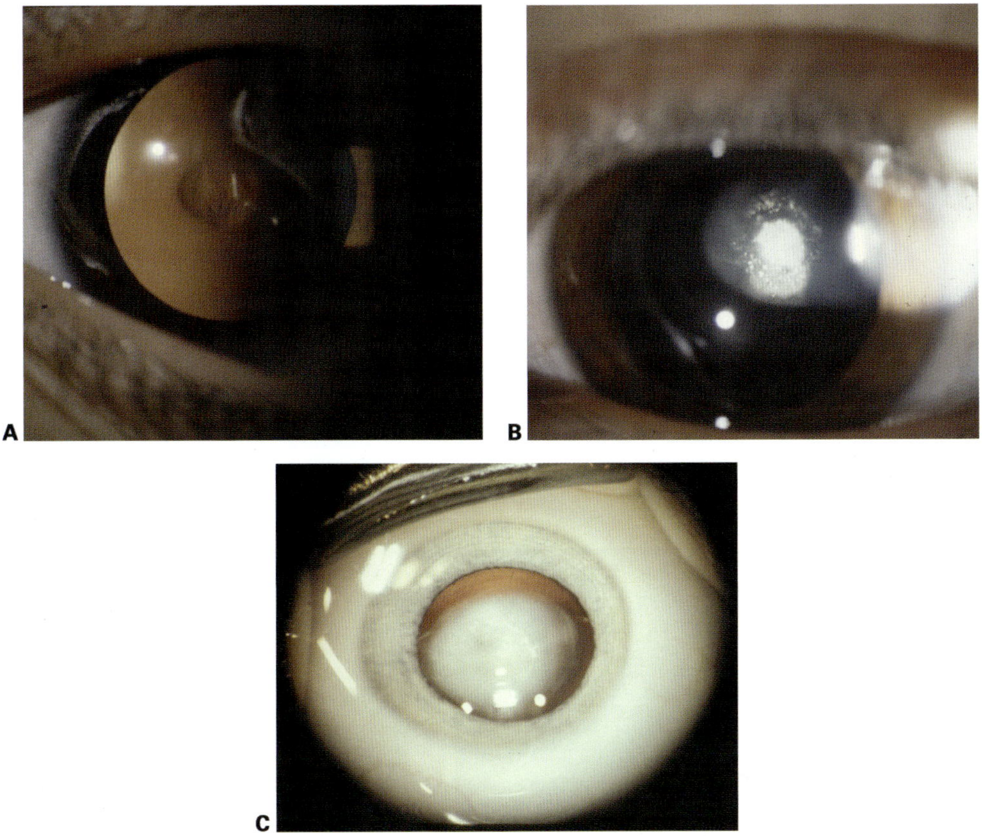

Figure 22-4 Posterior lenticonus/lentiglobus. **A,** Early central clear defect in posterior capsule and **(B)** early opacification of central defect. **C,** Advanced opacity. *(Photographs courtesy of David A. Plager, MD.)*

Like nuclear cataracts, PFV is congenital; these eyes are nearly always microphthalmic (microcornea) to some degree (if a PFV eye is not smaller than the fellow, normal eye, be suspicious of elevated IOP and secondary enlargement of the eye). Like posterior lenticonus, PFV is almost always unilateral. The persistent hyaloid vessel may connect the retrolental membrane to the optic nerve, but often the vessel regresses, leaving only the membrane. In severe cases, the lens may be pushed forward, flattening the anterior chamber and causing secondary glaucoma.

Posterior subcapsular cataract

Posterior subcapsular cataracts (PSCs) are not common in children. When present, they are acquired, bilateral, and tend to be progressive. Secondary causes for the cataracts, such as exogenous or endogenous steroids, uveitis, or retinal degeneration, should be sought. PSCs can also be seen with delayed onset following radiation of ocular, orbital, or craniofacial tumors. A type of PSC cataract can be seen with neurofibromatosis type 2, which may be the first observable manifestation of this systemic disorder.

See Table 22-5 for a summary of characteristics of select cataract morphologies.

Miscellaneous

Some other, less common cataract morphologies that may be encountered are shown in Figure 22-6.

Evaluation

All newborns deserve screening eye examinations, which should include an evaluation of the red reflexes. Examination of the red reflex can reveal even minute opacities. Detailed evaluation of the normally symmetric red reflexes is easily accomplished in a darkened room by shining a bright direct ophthalmoscope into both eyes simultaneously. This test, which is called the *illumination test, red reflex test,* or *Brückner test,* can be used for routine ocular screening by nurses, pediatricians, and family practitioners. Retinoscopy through the child's undilated pupil is helpful for estimating visual significance of

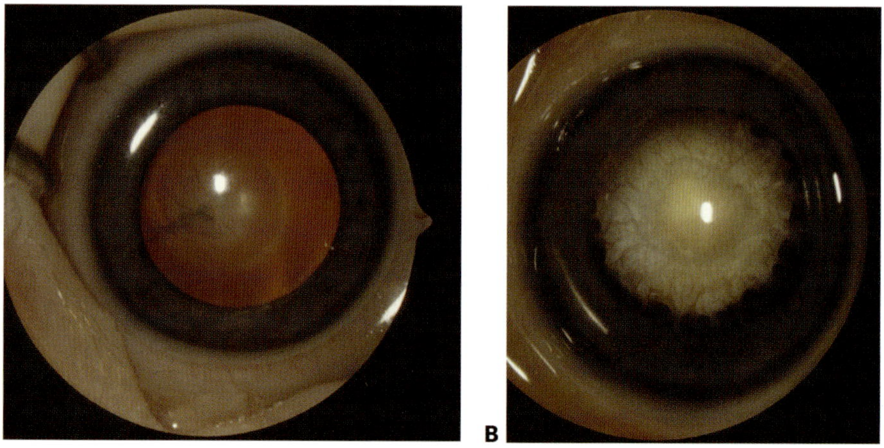

A B

Figure 22-5 Persistent fetal vasculature (formerly, *persistent hyperplastic primary vitreous*). **A,** Mild variant with central retrolental membrane. **B,** Severe PFV variant with traction on ciliary processes. *(Photographs courtesy of David A. Plager, MD.)*

Table 22-5 Characteristics of Specific Pediatric Cataract Morphologies

	Congenital or Acquired	Inherited or Sporadic	Unilateral or Bilateral	Stable or Progressive	Microphthalmic
Anterior polar	Congenital	Sporadic	Either	Stable	No
Nuclear	Congenital	Either	Either	Stable	Yes
Lamellar	Acquired	Either	Bilateral	Either	No
Posterior lenticonus	Acquired	Sporadic	Unilateral	Progressive	No
PFV	Congenital	Sporadic	Unilateral	Stable	Yes
PSC	Acquired	Sporadic	Bilateral	Progressive	No

PFV = persistent fetal vasculature; *PSC* = posterior subcapsular

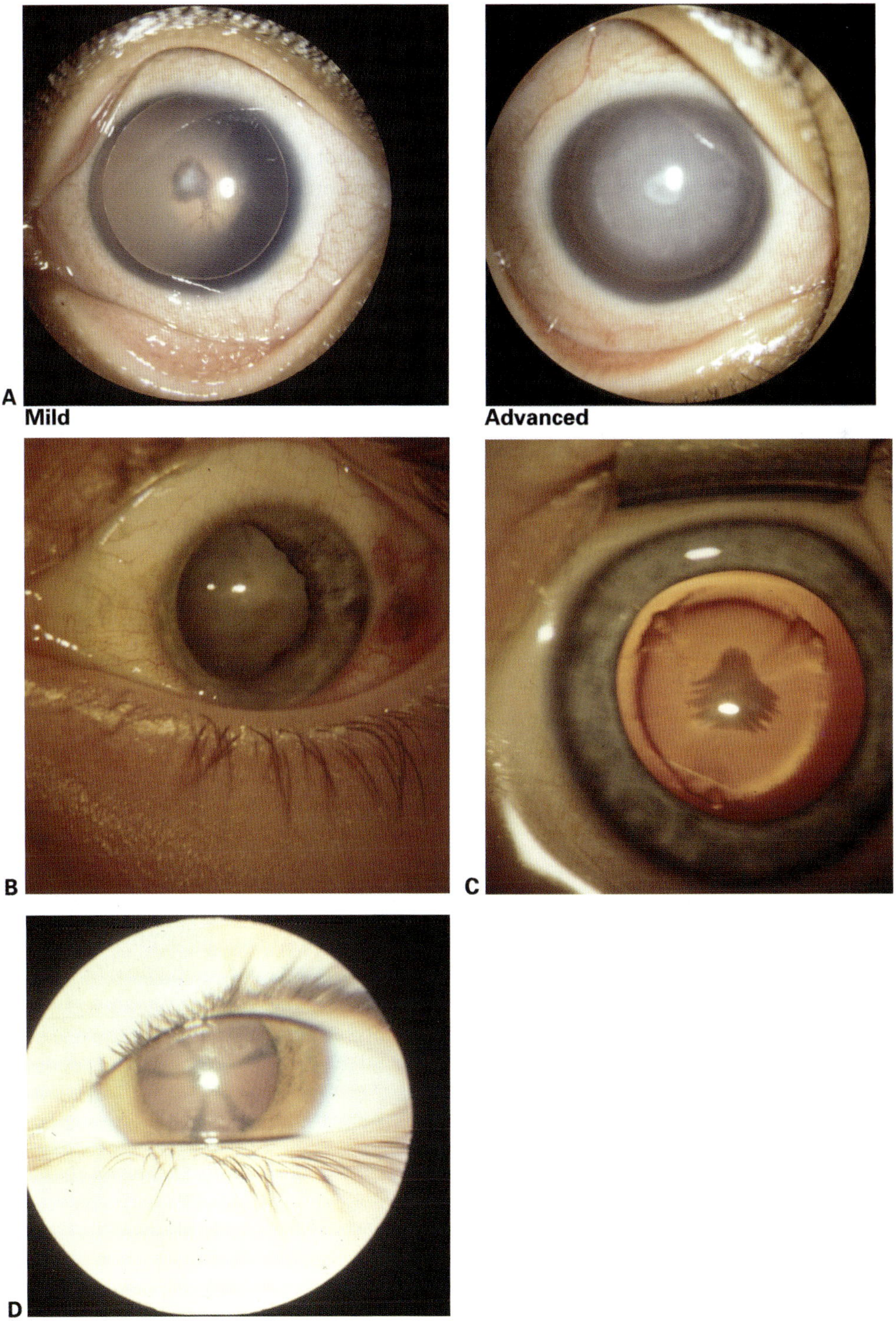

Figure 22-6 Miscellaneous cataracts in childhood. **A,** Aniridia. **B,** Traumatic (from air bag). **C,** Christmas tree. **D,** Starfish cataract. *(Photographs courtesy of David A. Plager, MD.)*

an axial lens opacity in a preverbal child. Any central opacity or surrounding cortical distortion greater than 3 mm can be assumed to be visually significant.

History

A detailed history of the child's growth, developmental milestones, feeding and digestive behavior, other developmental anomalies, skin lesions, and family history should be elicited. A slit-lamp examination of immediate family members can reveal small, previously undiagnosed lens opacities that are visually insignificant but may reveal an inherited cause for the child's cataracts.

Visual Function

The presence of a cataract in a child should stimulate a detailed evaluation to determine the etiology and establish any associated systemic implications for the child. However, the mere presence of a cataract does not imply that surgery to remove it is indicated. That determination requires assessment of the visual significance of the lens opacity.

In infants less than 2 months of age, a normal fixation reflex is not developed, and therefore its absence in an infant with a cataract is not necessarily abnormal. In general, anterior capsular opacities are not visually significant unless they occlude the entire pupil, blocking out the red reflex. Central or posterior lens opacities of sufficient density that are greater than 3 mm in diameter are usually visually significant. Opacities that have a significant area of red reflex around them and opacities that have clear areas within them frequently allow for good visual development in infancy and can be observed. Strabismus in unilateral cataract and nystagmus in bilateral cataracts are both late signs that the opacities are visually significant and that the optimal time for treatment is past, although surgery can still result in significant improvement.

In preverbal children older than 3 months of age, standard clinical assessment of fixation behavior, fixation preference, and objection to occlusion provide additional evidence of the visual significance of the cataract(s). For bilateral cataracts, an assessment of the child's visual behavior, with input from observations at home from the family, helps determine the level of visual function. Special tests such as preferential looking cards and visual evoked potential can provide additional quantitative information, but these are generally not necessary to determine the visual significance of a cataract.

In school-age and older children, surgery for bilateral cataracts should be suggested when the child's level of visual function interferes with his or her visual needs. For instance, a child in kindergarten may function well with vision in the 20/70–100 range. This level of vision may not be adequate for a grade school child, but 20/50 may be. Many young children perform well in school with these levels of vision, but later, during the teen years, they may opt for cataract surgery to help them meet the visual requirements for obtaining a driver's license.

For unilateral cataracts, cataract surgery is suggested for vision that cannot be improved past the 20/50–70 range with optical and amblyopia treatment alone.

Ocular Examination

A slit-lamp examination can help to classify the morphology of the cataract and to examine any associated abnormalities of the cornea, iris, lens, and anterior chamber. Infants can be held in place at a conventional slit lamp, but a portable handheld slit lamp is very helpful for examining infants and young children.

If the cataract allows some view of the posterior segment, careful observation of the optic nerve head, retina, and fovea should be obtained. If no view is present, B-scan ultrasonography can help rule out posterior segment pathology.

Workup

Unilateral cataracts are not usually associated with occult systemic or metabolic disease, and expensive laboratory tests are not warranted.

Bilateral cataracts, however, can be associated with many systemic and metabolic diseases (Fig 22-7). If a positive family history of infantile or childhood cataracts can be elicited or examination of the parents' lenses shows congenital lens opacities, a systemic and laboratory evaluation can be obviated. A basic laboratory evaluation for bilateral cataracts of unknown etiology in apparently healthy children will include

- urine for reducing substances
- TORCH titer and VDRL (if not done already in a newborn screen)
- blood for calcium and phosphorus and perhaps red cell galactokinase level
- serum ferritin

See Table 22-6.

Any further workup should be directed by other abnormalities in growth and development, and input should be sought from a pediatric geneticist, metabolism expert, or developmental pediatrician.

Surgery

Lensectomy Without Intraocular Lens

In children for whom contact lenses or spectacles are the chosen means of aphakic optical correction (ie, they will have no intraocular lens), lensectomy is performed through a small limbal or pars plana incision with a vitreous-cutting instrument or a manual aspirating device. Irrigation can be provided by an integrated infusion sleeve or by a separate cannula for bimanual surgery (Fig 22-8A). Lens cortex and nucleus are generally soft in children of all ages; ultrasonic phacoemulsification is not required (Fig 22-8B). Tough, fibrotic plaques, such as those encountered in some severe PVF cases, may occasionally require manually excising the plaques with intraocular scissors and forceps. A large, round anterior capsulectomy is performed either before or after complete cortical removal.

Because posterior capsule opacification occurs rapidly in young children, a controlled moderate posterior capsulectomy and anterior vitrectomy should be performed at the

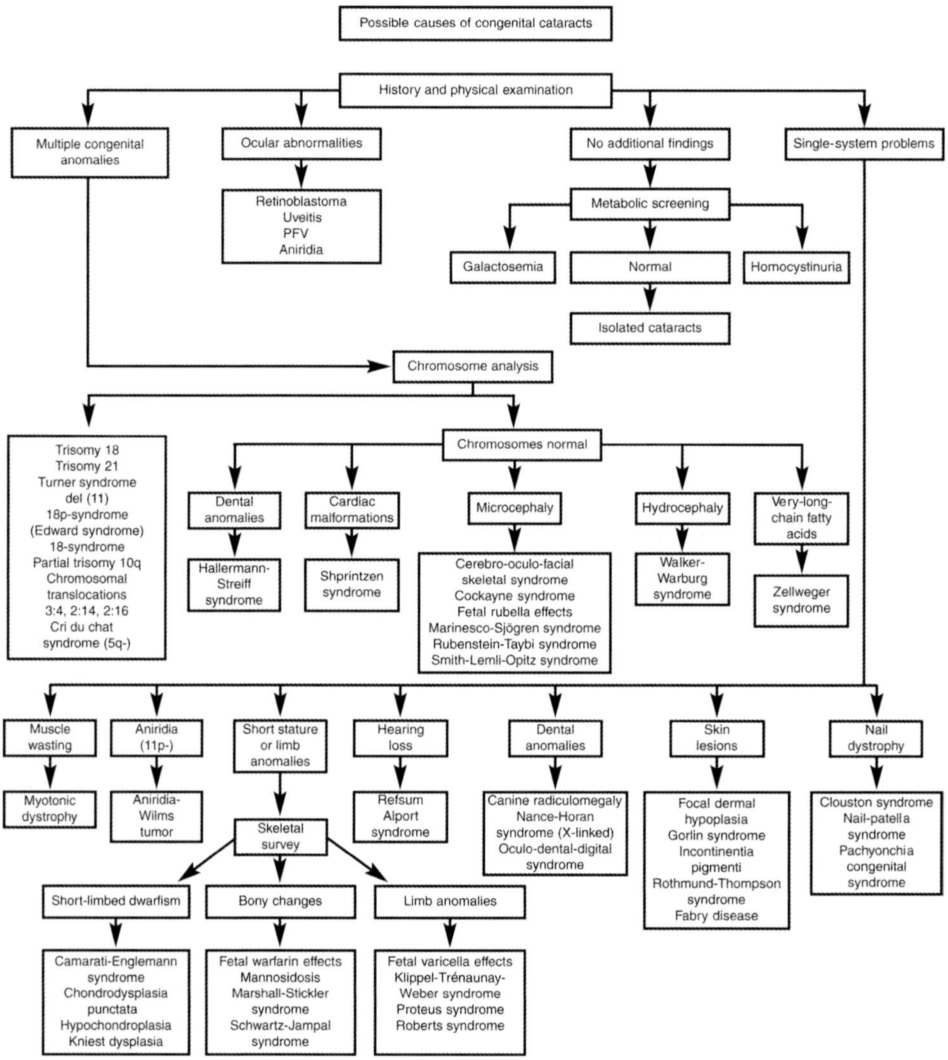

Figure 22-7 Causes of congenital cataracts. *PFV* = persistent fetal vasculature. *(Adapted from Buckley EG. Pediatric cataracts. In: Parrish R, ed.* Bascom Palmer Eye Institute's Atlas of Ophthalmology. *Philadelphia: Current Medicine; 2000.)*

time of surgery, particularly in infants (Fig 22-8C). This technique allows for rapid, permanent establishment of a clear visual axis for retinoscopy and prompt fitting and monitoring of aphakic optical correction, which is important in the age group subject to amblyopia. Sufficient peripheral posterior capsular remnants should be left, if possible, to facilitate secondary posterior chamber IOL implantation at a later date.

Table 22-6 Evaluation of Pediatric Cataracts

Family history (autosomal dominant or X-linked)
Pediatric physical examination
Ocular examination including
Corneal diameter
Iris configuration
Anterior chamber depth
Lens position
Cataract morphology
Posterior segment
Rule out posterior mass.
Rule out retinal detachment.
Rule out optic nerve stalk to lens.
Intraocular pressure
Laboratory studies
Bilateral cataracts
Urine for reducing substance
TORCH titer and VDRL
Optional: Urine for amino acids, blood for calcium and phosphorus, red-cell galactokinase level

Lensectomy With Intraocular Lens

If an IOL is going to be placed primarily at the time of cataract extraction, 2 basic techniques can be used, depending on whether the posterior capsule will be left intact. Many pediatric cataract surgeons leave the posterior capsule intact if the child is approaching the age when a YAG capsulotomy could be performed without anesthesia. Studies have shown that pediatric capsules in the post-infant years will opacify in 18–24 months postsurgery on average, although considerable variation from this average can occur.

Technique with posterior capsule intact (older children)

The technique leaving the posterior capsule intact is similar to that described earlier for a lensectomy. An anterior capsulotomy is made either manually with a continuous curvilinear capsulorrhexis or with an automated vitrector. The surgeon should be aware that the tearing characteristics of the more elastic pediatric capsule are significantly different from those of adult capsules. This requires that the pulling force be directed closer to 90° from the direction of intended tear (Fig 22-9). The capsule should be regrasped frequently to maintain optimal control over the direction of tear. The toughness and elasticity of the capsule is greatest in younger patients, especially infants. Visibility of the anterior capsule can be enhanced in difficult cases with the application of capsule stain. Trypan blue ophthalmic solution 0.06% (Vision Blue, Dutch Ophthalmic, USA, Kingston, NH) has been used for this application worldwide and has recently become available in the United States.

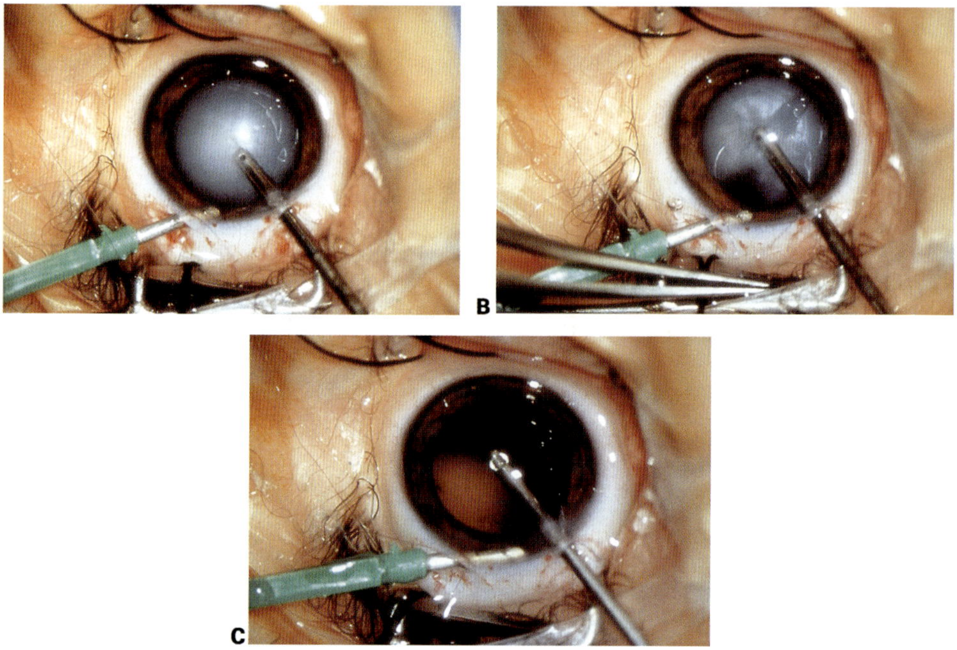

A B C

Figure 22-8 **A,** Unlike cataractous adult lenses, the pediatric lens is soft and can easily be aspirated through a small port. This avoids the large corneal or limbal opening required for extracapsular extraction or phacoemulsification. A 2-port closed system technique with an infusion source and a separate aspiration instrument or vitrector is ideal and allows the instrument to be switched from 1 side to the other, thereby facilitating cortical removal. An anterior capsule opening can be created with a vitrector. **B,** Both nucleus and surrounding cortex are aspirated. Complete cortical removal is important because remaining pediatric lens fibers will quickly proliferate, causing opacification and adhesions. **C,** After lens removal a large posterior capsulectomy and limited anterior vitrectomy are necessary to minimize the development of recurrent pupillary membranes, iris capsular adhesions, and posterior membranes. A small rim of capsule should be left to support possible secondary intraocular lens implants in the future. *(Photographs courtesy of Edward G. Buckley, MD.)*

The cortex is then aspirated with either the vitrector or a manual irrigation/aspiration handpiece. Ultrasonic phacoemulsification is not necessary in pediatric cataract surgery. It is important to remove all cortical material because of the propensity of pediatric lens epithelial cells to reproliferate. The clear corneal or scleral tunnel incision is enlarged to allow placement of the IOL. Single-piece acrylic foldable lenses, which can be placed through a 3-mm incision, have become very popular among pediatric cataract surgeons, although some prefer to use larger single-piece polymethylmethacrylate (PMMA) lenses. Placement of the IOL in the capsular bag is thought to be far superior to sulcus fixation for long-term stability and safety. All viscoelastic material should be removed to prevent postoperative IOP spikes, especially because it can be difficult to measure IOP in the early postoperative period in young children. Closure of 3-mm clear cornea incisions with 10-0 absorbable suture has been shown to be safe and astigmatically neutral in children.

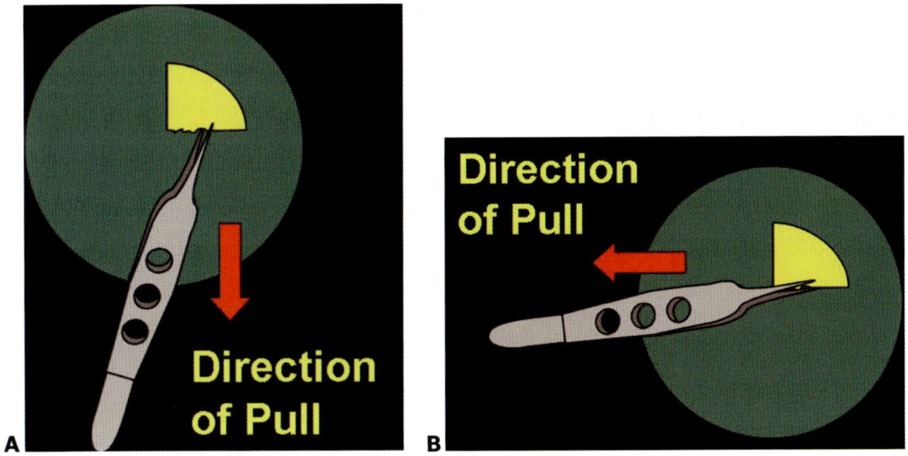

Figure 22-9 Schematics showing the different force vectors used in tearing a capsulorrhexis in **(A)** a teenage eye and **(B)** an infant eye. *(Schematics courtesy of David A. Plager, MD.)*

Bradfield YS, Plager DA, Neely DE, et al. Astigmatism after small incision cataract surgery and intraocular lens implantation in children. *J Cataract Refract Surg.* 2004;30:1948–1952.

Technique for IOL and primary posterior capsulectomy (younger children)

In children under 3–4 years of age or older children who are predicted to maintain a limited level of cooperation, a primary posterior capsulectomy with vitrectomy should generally be performed at the time of cataract/IOL surgery. The posterior capsulectomy/vitrectomy can be performed either before or after IOL placement.

Posterior capsulectomy/vitrectomy before IOL placement After lensectomy, the vitrector settings should be changed to the low-suction, high-cutting rate appropriate for vitreous surgery, and the posterior capsulectomy with anterior vitrectomy is performed. The anterior incision is enlarged to an appropriate size for the IOL, and the lens is implanted into the capsular bag. Care must be exercised to ensure that the capsulotomy does not extend, the IOL does not go through the posterior opening, and vitreous does not become incorporated with the IOL or anterior chamber.

Posterior capsulectomy/vitrectomy after IOL placement Many pediatric cataract surgeons prefer the security of placing the IOL in the intact capsular bag, closing the anterior incision, and approaching the posterior capsule through the pars plana. Irrigation can be maintained through the same anterior infusion cannula used during lensectomy. A small conjunctival opening is made over the pars plana, and a sclerotomy is made with an MVR blade 1.5–2.5 mm posterior to the limbus. This provides good access to the posterior capsule, and a wide anterior vitrectomy can be performed. The sclerotomy is closed with a single suture and the conjunctiva with absorbable 8-0 suture (Fig 22-10).

A third technique is also possible. The IOL is placed into the intact capsular bag and the posterior capsulectomy/vitrectomy is performed through the anterior incision by

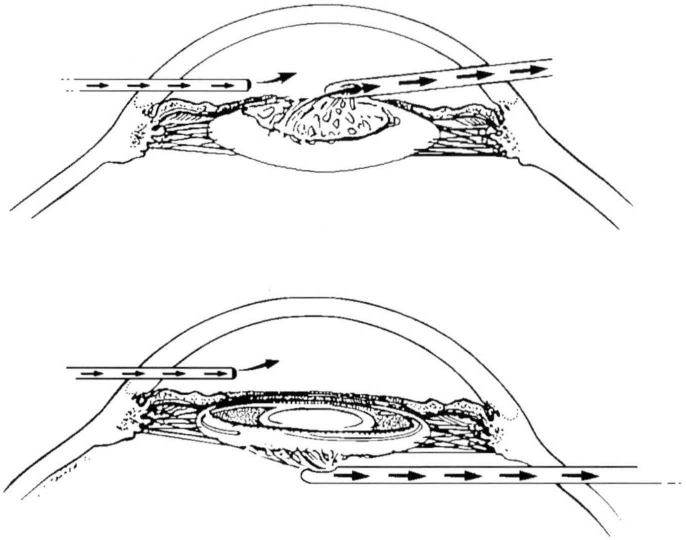

Figure 22-10 The posterior capsule can be removed primarily either (1) before the lens implantation from an anterior approach or (2) after lens implantation in 1 of 2 ways: anteriorly from the limbus or posteriorly via the pars plana. The pars plana approach has the advantage that the IOL is implanted with an intact posterior capsule. The technique involves maintaining an anterior chamber infusion source, which helps bow the posterior capsule backward. A pars plana incision made approximately 2 mm from the limbus is performed. The vitrector is set at a low-cut, high-suction rate and the capsule is opened in the center and enlarged to approximately 4 mm. *(Illustrations courtesy of Edward G. Buckley, MD.)*

carefully inserting the vitrector over the iris and edge of the anterior capsulotomy, around, then behind, the IOL and into the posterior capsule and vitreous. Because this technique allows only limited access to the vitreous cavity; is technically difficult; and risks dislodging the IOL, tearing the capsulorrhexis, or bringing vitreous into the anterior chamber, it is a less popular alternative.

Wilson ME, Trivedi RH, Pandey SK. *Pediatric Cataract Surgery: Techniques, Complications, and Management.* Philadelphia: Lippincott Williams & Wilkens; 2005.

Postoperative Optical Rehabilitation

The choice of optical device for correction of aphakia depends on various factors. Aphakic spectacles are the safest method available and can be easily changed to accommodate the refractive shifts that occur with growth. These spectacles are not ideal in monocular aphakia but can be used when other options are not suitable. Until the child can use a bifocal lens, the power selected should make the child slightly myopic when wearing the glasses. Contact lenses are the most popular method and are excellent for monocular cases. The power change for lenses is relatively easy, and some lenses can be worn 24 hours a day. Unfortunately, contact lenses are easily displaced by eye rubbing and can be expensive to replace. In addition, spectacle correction (bifocal) is necessary if a clear image is desired for both distance and near functions. Contact lenses also pose a risk of recurring infections and corneal ulcers.

Intraocular Lens Implant

Intraocular lens implantation has gained widespread acceptance, and numerous studies have documented the safety and efficacy of this procedure in selected children down to the toddler age group. Many questions still remain, however, including what IOL power should be implanted in the growing child's eye and what the lowest age group is for which the advantages of IOLs outweigh their potential risks or disadvantages when compared to conventional contact lens or spectacle correction.

IOL power selection

Because the child's eye continues to elongate throughout the first decade and beyond, the selection of an appropriate IOL power is complicated. Studies have shown that the refractive error of aphakic children undergoes a variable myopic shift of approximately 7–8 D from age 1 to age 10. This would suggest that if a child is made emmetropic at age 1 with an IOL, refraction at age 10 would be expected to be up to –8 D or greater (refractive change below age 1 year is even more unpredictable). This approach assumes that presence of an IOL does not alter this normal aphakic growth curve, an assumption that is probably not valid based on both animal and early human studies. Clearly, however, lens implantation in children requires a compromise that accounts for the age of the child and the target refraction at the time of surgery. Most surgeons implant IOLs with powers that are expected to be required in adulthood, allowing the child to grow into the power selection of the lens. Thus, the child is undercorrected and requires hyperopic spectacles of decreasing powers until the teenage years. Other surgeons strive for emmetropia at the time of lens implantation, especially in unilateral situations, to avoid anisometropia and facilitate development of binocular function. However, these children can be expected to become progressively more myopic with time and eventually require a secondary procedure in order to eliminate the increasing anisometropia.

Crouch ER, Crouch ER Jr, Pressman SH. Prospective analysis of pediatric pseudophakia: myopic shift and postoperative outcomes. *J AAPOS.* 2002;6:277–282.

Plager DA, Kipfer H, Sprunger DT, et al. Refractive change in pediatric pseudophakia: 6-year follow-up. *J Cataract Refract Surg.* 2002;28:810–815.

Superstein R, Archer SM, Del Monte MA. Minimal myopic shift in pseudophakic versus aphakic pediatric cataract patients. *J AAPOS.* 2002;6:271–276.

IOL lens material

Both single-piece PMMA and foldable acrylic lenses have been widely used in pediatric cataract surgery in recent years. Many studies have shown them to be well tolerated. Silicone lenses have not been well studied in children.

IOL use in infants

The role of IOLs in infants is controversial. Small studies have shown IOLs can be implanted in infants, but the complication rate, particularly reopacification of the visual axis, is much higher in infants than in older children. Other complicating factors peculiar to infants include the following:

- The eyes are small and soft, making surgery technically challenging.
- Most of the growth in axial length and corneal curvature is yet to occur, making optimal IOL power difficult to determine.

A multicenter, randomized clinical trial of IOL implantation versus conventional contact lens correction of aphakia in unilateral congenital cataract (Infant Aphakia Treatment Study) was begun in 2005. The results of this study are anticipated to provide much needed scientific data regarding the optimal role of IOL use in infants.

Lambert SR, Lynn M, Drews-Botsch C, et al. Optotype acuity and re-operation rate after unilateral cataract surgery during the first 6 months of life with or without IOL implantation. *Br J Ophthalmol.* 2004;88:1387–1390.

Postoperative Care

Medical therapy

If all cortical material is adequately removed, postoperative inflammation in children without a lens implant is usually very mild. Postoperative topical antibiotics and steroid drops are commonly used for a couple of weeks. In aphakic children, mydriasis should be continued for several weeks with atropine or other dilating agent.

Topical steroids need to be used much more aggressively in children if an IOL is placed. Some surgeons opt for oral steroids, especially in very young children and children with heavily pigmented irides.

Amblyopia management

Amblyopia therapy, if necessary, should begin as soon as possible after surgery. For patients who become aphakic, corrective lenses—contact lenses for unilateral or bilateral aphakia, spectacles for bilateral aphakia—can be dispensed as early as 1 week after surgery. Patching of the better eye is frequently indicated in cases of unilateral cataracts or asymmetric bilateral cataracts. The amount of patching should be titrated to the degree of amblyopia and the age of the child. Part-time occlusion in the neonatal period may allow stimulation of binocular vision and may help to prevent associated strabismus. One popular regimen is to patch 1 hour per month of age per day, up to 8 months of age—for example, 2 hours per day for a 2-month-old, 5 hours per day for a 5-month-old, and so on up to a maximum of 8 hours per day.

Complications

Complications after lens extraction are different in children than in adults. Retinal detachments, macular edema, and corneal abnormalities are rare in children. The incidence of postoperative infections and bleeding is similar in adults and in children. Glaucoma associated with pediatric aphakia may develop many years after lens extraction. The use of IOLs in older children has been associated with a very low rate of glaucoma. This rate can be expected to increase as the number of infants with congenital cataracts receiving lens implants increases. See Chapter 21 for a discussion of aphakic and pseudophakic glaucoma.

Visual Outcome After Cataract Extraction

Good visual outcome after cataract surgery depends on many factors, including age of onset and type of cataract, the timing of surgery, optical correction, and treatment of amblyopia. For dense congenital cataracts, visual acuity is best in patients who undergo surgery before age 2 months and who comply with amblyopia treatment. Early surgery by itself does not ensure good outcome. Optimal visual acuity requires careful postoperative management to treat amblyopia. Conversely, even when congenital cataracts are detected late (after age 4 months), cataract removal combined with a strong postoperative visual rehabilitation program can achieve good vision in some eyes (Fig 22-11).

In general, young children with bilateral aphakia do much better visually in the affected eye(s) than children with monocular aphakia, and both experience worse visual outcomes than adults. This poor outcome is undoubtedly due to the effect of aphakia on the developing visual system. Patients with monocular aphakia have the added difficulty of interocular competition, which invariably results in better vision in the phakic eye. The early data in infants comparing contact lenses with IOLs indicate slightly better results with IOLs; however, selection biases may explain this finding.

Birch EE, Stager DR. The critical period for surgical treatment of dense congenital unilateral cataract. *Invest Ophthalmol Vis Sci.* 1996;37:1532–1538.

Seaber JH, Buckley EG. Functional outcome of monocular and binocular congenital cataract. Part I: visual acuity. *Am Orthoptic J.* 1997;47:29–38.

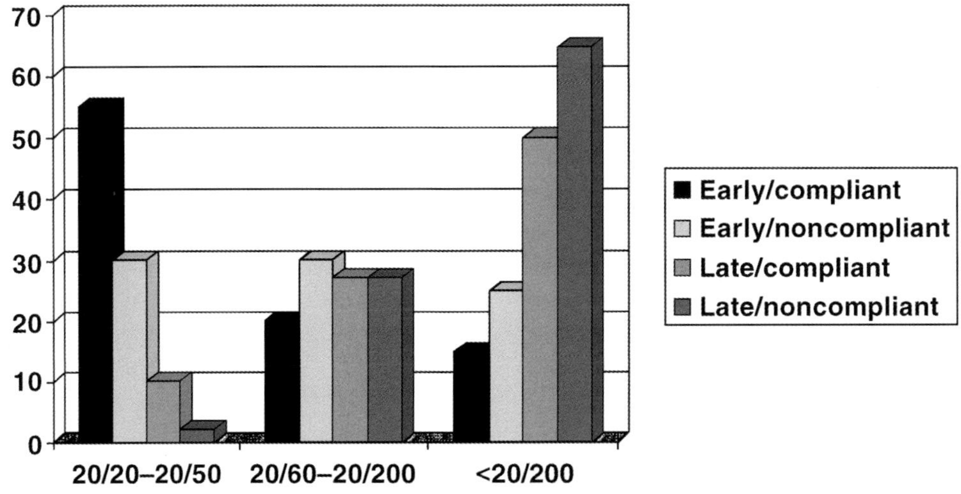

Figure 22-11 Visual outcomes in monocular dense congenital cataracts. *(Adapted from Seaber JH, Buckley EG. Functional outcome of monocular and binocular congenital cataract. Part 1: visual acuity.* Am Orthopt J. *1997;47:29–38.)*

Structural or Positional Lens Abnormalities

Congenital Aphakia

Congenital aphakia, the absence of the lens at birth, is rare. This condition is usually associated with a markedly abnormal eye.

Spherophakia

A lens that is spherical and smaller than a normal lens is called *spherophakic.* This condition is usually bilateral. The lens may dislocate, causing secondary glaucoma (Fig 22-12).

Coloboma

A lens coloboma (a misnomer) involves flattening or notching of the lens periphery (Fig 22-13). A coloboma can be associated with a defect in the iris, optic nerve, or retina and is due to the abnormal closure of the embryonic fissure. The coloboma is usually located inferonasally, and zonular fibers are typically absent in the colobomatous area, resulting in a flattening of the lens at that location without any dislocation. In significant colobomatous defects, lens dislocations occur superiorly and temporally. Most colobomatous lenses do not worsen progressively.

Dislocated Lenses in Children

When the lens is not in its normal anatomical position, it is said to be *dislocated, subluxed, subluxated, luxed, luxated*, or *ectopic.* Luxed or luxated lenses are completely detached from the ciliary body and are either loose in the posterior chamber or vitreous or can prolapse to the anterior chamber. The amount of dislocation can vary from only slight displacement with minimal *iridodonesis* (tremulousness of the iris) to severe displacement, with the edge of the lens totally out of the pupillary margin. Lens dislocation can

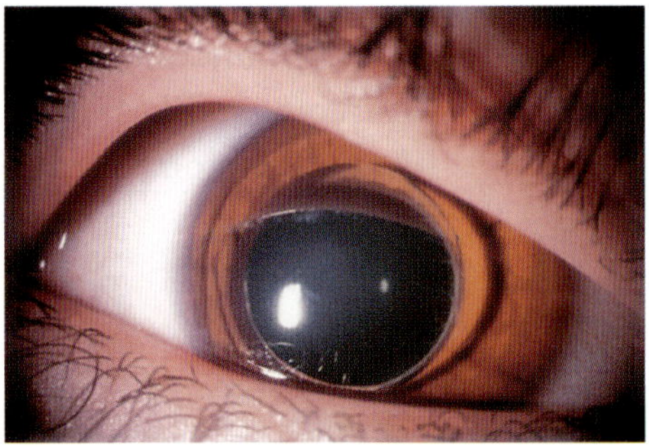

Figure 22-12 Spherophakia with lens dislocation into anterior chamber, left eye.

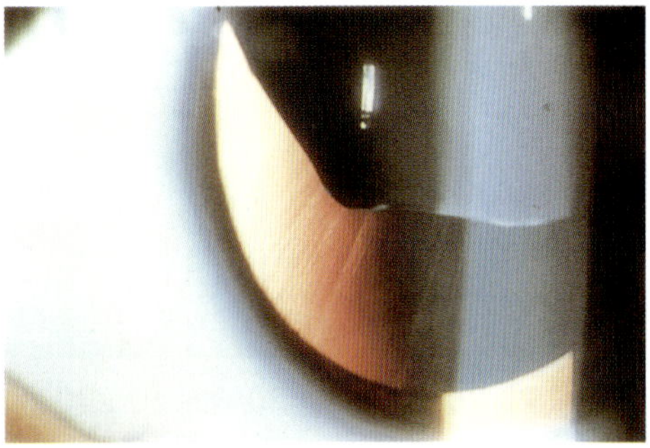

Figure 22-13 Lens equator flattening (with dislocation), which may be referred to as *lens coloboma.*

be familial or sporadic or be associated with multisystem disease or an inborn error of metabolism (Table 22-7). Lens dislocation can occur with trauma, although this is not common and usually involves a significant injury to the eye. Spontaneous lens dislocation has been reported in aniridia and, rarely, with exfoliation syndrome and buphthalmos (secondary to congenital glaucoma).

Simple Ectopia Lentis

Simple ectopia lentis is usually bilateral and symmetric, with upward and temporal lens displacement. Autosomal dominant inheritance is most common. The onset may be congenital or the condition may develop later. Glaucoma is common in the late-onset type.

Ectopia Lentis Et Pupillae

Ectopia lentis et pupillae is a rare autosomal recessive condition. It is manifested by bilateral displacement of the pupil, usually inferotemporally, with lens dislocation in the opposite direction (Fig 22-14). Patients have microspherophakia, miosis, and poor pupillary dilation with mydriatics. This condition is thought to be due to a defect in neuroectodermal

Table 22-7 Subluxed Lenses

Systemic Conditions
Marfan syndrome
Homocystinuria
Weill-Marchesani syndrome
Hyperlysinemia
Sulfite oxidase deficiency
Syphilis
Ehlers-Danlos syndrome
Ocular Conditions
Aniridia
Iris coloboma
Trauma
Hereditary ectopia lentis
Congenital glaucoma

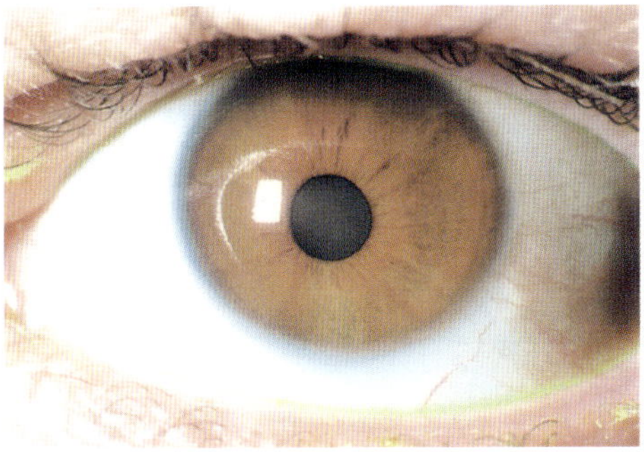

Figure 22-14 Ectopia lentis et pupillae, left eye.

tissue development because the pigmented layers of the iris, zonules, and iris dilator are all involved. Some family members may have only subluxation without the pupillary displacement. The condition is nonprogressive.

Marfan Syndrome

Marfan syndrome is the systemic disease most commonly associated with dislocated lenses. The syndrome consists of abnormalities of the cardiovascular, musculoskeletal, and ocular systems. It is inherited as an autosomal dominant trait, but family history is negative in 15% of cases. Marfan syndrome is caused by mutations in the fibrillin gene on chromosome 15. These patients are characteristically tall, with long limbs and fingers *(arachnodactyly)*; loose, flexible joints; scoliosis; and chest deformities. Cardiovascular abnormalities are a source of significant mortality and manifest as enlargement of the aortic root, dilation of a descending aorta, dissecting aneurysm, and floppy mitral valve. The life expectancy of patients with Marfan syndrome is about half that of the normal population. Ocular abnormalities occur in over 80% of patients, with lens dislocation being the most common. In approximately 75% of cases, the lens is upwardly dislocated (Fig 22-15). Typically, the zonules that are visible are intact and unbroken, in contradistinction to the broken zonules seen in homocystinuria. Examination of the iris usually shows iridodenesis and may reveal transillumination defects that are more marked near the iris base. The pupil is small and dilates poorly. The axial length is increased, and the

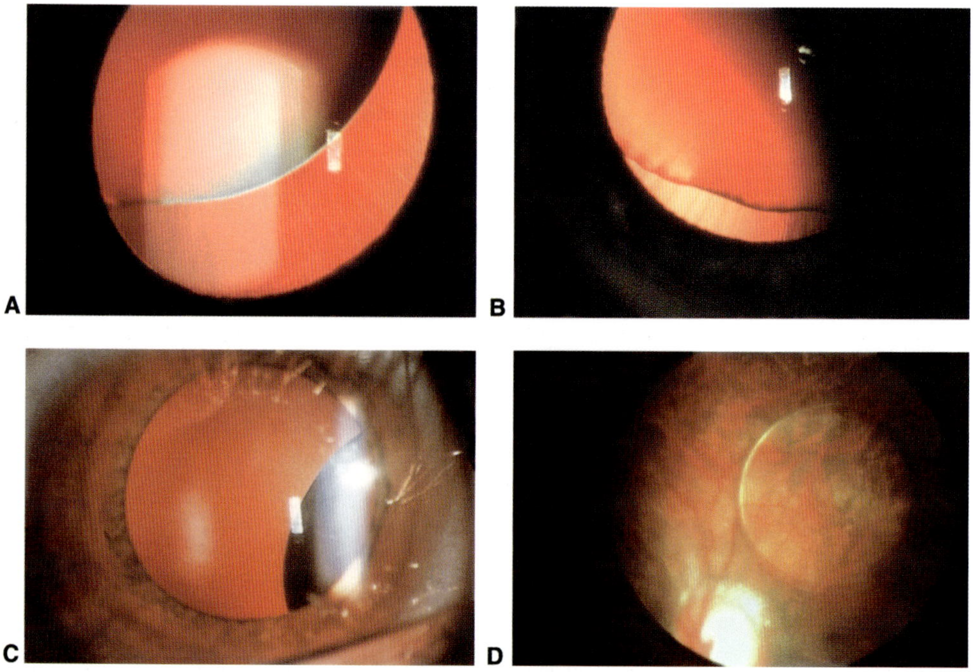

Figure 22-15 Marfan syndrome. **A** and **B,** Superotemporal displacement of lenses, bilateral. **C,** Inferonasal displacement, right eye. **D,** Lens dislocation into vitreous, left eye.

patients are usually myopic. Retinal detachment can occur spontaneously, commonly in the second and third decades of life.

Homocystinuria

Homocystinuria is a rare autosomal recessive condition. The classic form is caused by an abnormality in the enzyme cystathionine β-synthase, although it can be caused by other enzyme defects. This abnormality causes homocystine to accumulate in the plasma and be excreted in the urine. Homocystinuria occurs in approximately 1 in 100,000 births.

The clinical manifestations of homocystinuria vary markedly, affecting the eye, skeletal system, central nervous system, and vascular system. Most of the abnormalities develop after birth and become progressively worse with age. Ocular findings consist mainly of dislocated lenses (frequently downward, although the direction of subluxation is not invariable or diagnostic), a condition that typically occurs between the ages of 3 and 10 years. The lenses may dislocate into the anterior chamber, a finding suggestive of homocystinuria (Fig 22-16).

Systemically, vascular complications are common and secondary to thrombotic disease, which affects large or medium-sized arteries and veins anywhere in the body. Partial or complete vascular obstruction is present in various organs, and hypertension, cardiac murmurs, and cardiomegaly are common. Anesthesia carries a higher risk for patients with homocystinuria because of thromboembolic phenomena, and therefore this diagnosis must be ruled out before patients undergo general anesthesia. These patients are usually tall, with osteoporosis, scoliosis, and chest deformities. Central nervous system abnormalities occur in approximately 50% of patients, with mental retardation and seizures being the most common.

Diagnosis is confirmed by detecting disulfides, including homocystine, in the urine. The medical management of homocystinuria is directed toward normalizing the biochemical abnormality. Dietary management (low methionine and high cystine) has been attempted, and coenzyme supplements (pyridoxine or vitamin B6) are effective in about 50% of cases.

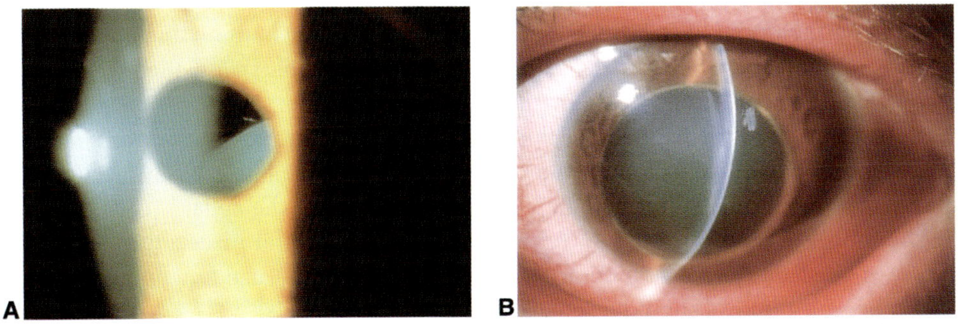

Figure 22-16 Homocystinuria. **A,** Inferonasal lens dislocation, right eye. Note broken and absent zonules, a typical finding in homocystinuria. **B,** Lens may dislocate into anterior chamber with acute pupillary block glaucoma (same patient).

Weill-Marchesani Syndrome

Patients with Weill-Marchesani syndrome characteristically are short, with short fingers and limbs; they can be thought of as clinical opposites of patients with Marfan syndrome. Inheritance can be autosomal dominant or recessive. The lenses are also small and nearly round *(microspherophakia)*. With time, the lens dislocates anteriorly and pupillary block glaucoma may occur. Because of this, prophylactic laser peripheral iridectomy has been recommended, although lensectomy may be required.

Hyperlysinemia

Hyperlysinemia is the result of a deficiency of lysine α-ketoglutarate reductase; it has been found in mentally retarded patients, some of whom have had dislocated lenses. However, the same biochemical abnormality and enzyme deficiency have been found in normal persons identified through newborn screening. The association between hyperlysinemia and dislocated lenses is not clearly documented.

Sulfite Oxidase Deficiency

Sulfite oxidase deficiency is a very rare hereditary disorder of sulfur metabolism manifested by severe neurologic disorders and ectopia lentis. The enzyme deficiency interferes with conversion of sulfite to sulphate, resulting in increased urine secretion of sulfite. The diagnosis can be confirmed by the absence of sulfite oxidase activity in skin fibroblasts. Neurologic abnormalities include infantile hemiplegia, choreoathetosis, and seizures. Irreversible brain damage and death usually occur by age 5.

Maumenee IH. The eye in the Marfan syndrome. *Trans Am Ophthalmol Soc.* 1981;79: 684–733.

Neely DE, Plager DA. The management of ectopia lentis in children. *Ophthalmol Clin North Am.* 2001;14:493–499.

Treatment

Optical correction

Optical correction of the refractive error caused by lens dislocation is often difficult. Depending on the extent of the dislocation, the patient may see better with a myopic astigmatic correction or an aphakic correction. With very mild subluxation, the patient may be only myopic and corrected visual function may be good. More severe amounts of dislocation cause optical distortion because the patient is looking through the far peripheral part of the lens. Because the resultant myopic astigmatism is difficult to measure accurately by retinoscopy or automated refractometry, visual acuity using the aphakic correction may be superior. Pre- and postdilation refractions are often helpful in deciding on the best choice. If satisfactory visual function cannot be obtained or if visual function is worsening over time, lens removal should be considered.

Surgery

Subluxed lenses can be removed either from the anterior segment through a limbal incision or through the pars plana. In most circumstances, complete lensectomy is indicated. Postoperative visual rehabilitation can be achieved using contact lenses or glasses, and postoperative visual results are quite good. The use of sutured intraocular lenses, lens capsular bag expanders, or other types of lens-supporting maneuvers has undergone limited testing in children. Caution should be exercised in patients with Marfan syndrome because there is an increased risk of retinal detachment, which may occur years after surgery.

Plager DA, Parks MM, Helveston EM, et al. Surgical treatment of subluxed lenses in children. *Ophthalmology.* 1992;99:1018–1023.

CHAPTER 23

Uveitis in the Pediatric Age Group

Uveitis in the pediatric age group is relatively uncommon, occurring at an annual rate of 6:100,000 and accounting for only 5%–10% of the total cases of uveitis seen in tertiary care centers. Nevertheless, uveitis in children can present unique challenges to the physician. Children may not verbalize symptoms until disease is advanced. Therapeutic options may be limited by the potential side effects of medications, the need for general anesthesia, or poor compliance with self-administered medications. In addition, the rate of complications may be increased in children. Finally, the risk of amblyopia is unique to children. This chapter focuses on the features of uveitis specific to children. See BCSC Section 9, *Intraocular Inflammation and Uveitis*, for a description of the clinical features of uveitis and mechanisms of inflammation and for more details about many of the conditions mentioned here.

Classification

As in adults, uveitis in children can be classified by a number of methods, including anatomical location (anterior, posterior, intermediate, or panuveitis); pathology (granulomatous, nongranulomatous); course (acute, chronic, recurrent); or cause (traumatic, immunologic, infectious, masquerade syndromes, idiopathic). Anatomical location can be helpful in determining etiology (Table 23-1). Traditionally, posterior uveitis has been thought to account for 40%–50% of uveitis cases in children; anterior uveitis, 30%–40%; intermediate uveitis, about 20%; and panuveitis, less than 10%. These percentages are based on studies published by tertiary care centers. In contrast, recent population-based studies suggest that the majority of children with uveitis have disease that is restricted to the anterior segment. Nevertheless, posterior uveitis probably accounts for a greater proportion of uveitis cases in children than in adults.

In many cases, uveitis in children is idiopathic, but *juvenile idiopathic arthritis (JIA)* is the most common identifiable underlying systemic disease. Infections including toxoplasmosis, toxocariasis, and herpesviruses are relatively common in children with uveitis. Malignancies that can mimic uveitis in children include retinoblastoma and leukemia.

Table 23-1 Differential Diagnosis of Uveitis

Anterior uveitis
Juvenile idiopathic arthritis
Trauma
Sarcoidosis
Herpes and other viruses
Syphilis
Lyme disease
Fuchs heterochromic iridocyclitis
Kawasaki syndrome
Tubulointerstitial nephritis and uveitis syndrome
Behçet syndrome
Unknown cause
Intermediate uveitis
Pars planitis (idiopathic)
Sarcoidosis
Tuberculosis
Toxocariasis
Juvenile xanthogranuloma
Lyme disease
Unknown cause
Posterior uveitis and panuveitis
Toxoplasmosis
Toxocariasis
Herpetic disease, rubella, rubeola, measles
Histoplasmosis
Syphilis
Sympathetic ophthalmia
Sarcoidosis
Bartonella
Candida
Lyme disease
Familial juvenile systemic granulomatosis (Blau syndrome)
Diffuse unilateral subacute neuroretinitis (DUSN)
Tuberculosis
Vogt-Koyanagi-Harada syndrome
Behçet syndrome
Unknown cause

Anterior Uveitis

Juvenile Idiopathic Arthritis

Nomenclature

Ophthalmologists may be confused by the different terminology used for chronic childhood arthritis. The criteria of the European League of Associations of Rheumatology (EULAR) are used in Europe, where the disease is referred to as *juvenile chronic arthritis*; the criteria of the American College of Rheumatology (ACR) are used in the United States, where it is called *juvenile rheumatoid arthritis.* The main differences between the EULAR and ACR criteria are the duration of joint symptoms necessary for the diagnosis of arthritis and inclusion versus exclusion of certain disease conditions, such as juvenile ankylosing spondylitis and juvenile psoriatic arthritis.

Recently, a new set of criteria was published by the International League of Associations of Rheumatology (ILAR), which includes all idiopathic childhood arthritides under the name *juvenile idiopathic arthritis (JIA)*. We have chosen to use the term *JIA* in this chapter. The 3 sets of criteria for childhood chronic arthritis are shown in Table 23-2, and the subtypes of JIA are listed in Table 23-3.

Occurrence of uveitis in JIA

The categories of JIA (see Table 23-3) that are particularly important with regard to uveitis are oligoarthritis, rheumatoid factor (RF)-negative polyarthritis, psoriatic arthritis, and enthesitis-related arthritis. Uveitis almost never occurs in children with systemic arthritis and is very rare in those with RF-positive polyarthritis.

Oligoarthritis is the most frequent type of chronic arthritis in children in North America and Europe. Oligoarthritis occurs predominantly in young girls and is defined as a persistent arthritis lasting more than 6 weeks and affecting 4 or fewer joints during the first 6 months of the disease. Chronic insidious anterior uveitis is most likely to occur with this type of uveitis; it has been reported in 10%–30% of children with the disease

Table 23-2 Comparison of the European League of Associations of Rheumatology (EULAR), American College of Rheumatology (ACR), and International League of Associations of Rheumatology (ILAR) Criteria

	EULAR	ACR	ILAR
Age of patients (years)	0–15	0–15	0–15
Disease duration	3 months	6 weeks	6 weeks
JAS, JpsA, IBD	Included	Excluded	Included

JAS = juvenile ankylosing spondylitis; *JpsA* = juvenile psoriatic arthritis; *IBD* = arthropathy associated with inflammatory bowel disease.

Used with permission from Kotaniemi K, Savolainen A, Karma A, et al. Recent advances in uveitis of juvenile idiopathic arthritis. *Surv Ophthalmol.* 2003;48:489–502.

Table 23-3 Subtypes of Juvenile Idiopathic Arthritis

	Disease Type
I	Systemic arthritis
II	Oligoarthritis
	a. persistent
	b. extended
III	Polyarthritis, rheumatoid factor (RF)-negative
IV	Polyarthritis, rheumatoid factor (RF)-positive
V	Psoriatic arthritis
VI	Enthesitis-related arthritis
VII	Other forms of arthritis

Used with permission from Kotaniemi K, Savolainen A, Karma A, et al. Recent advances in uveitis of juvenile idiopathic arthritis. *Surv Ophthalmol.* 2003;48:489–502.

and is usually diagnosed in the first 4 years of the disease. Laboratory markers include a high frequency of nonspecific low-titer antinuclear antibodies (ANA). RF is almost always absent. Human leukocyte antigen (HLA) associations include –A2, –DR5, –DR8, –DR11, and –DP2.1.

RF-negative polyarthritis probably represents a heterogeneous group of disorders. Children with this disorder have more than 4 inflamed joints during the first 6 months of the disease. It is more common in girls, but mean age at onset is higher than in children with oligoarthritis. Uveitis occurs in about 10% of affected children. ANA may be present, but RF is absent. Strong HLA associations have not been consistently documented.

Psoriatic arthritis may resemble oligoarthritis or RF-negative polyarthritis and, for this reason, is probably underdiagnosed. The diagnosis is suggested by the presence of arthritis and 2 of the following: nail pitting or onycholysis, dactylitis, or a history of psoriasis in a first-degree relative. Insidious and chronic anterior uveitis is seen in 10% of affected children.

Enthesitis-related arthritis is a chronic arthritis that is associated with inflammation of entheses, which are the sites of attachment to bone of ligaments, tendons, fascia, and capsule. This type of arthritis typically affects older boys. In these children, uveitis is sudden and symptomatic; it may be unilateral; and it is more common in older children and adults. Most patients are HLA-B27 positive, and many will eventually develop lumbosacral spine disease and sacroiliitis.

The cause of juvenile arthritis and the mechanism of anterior uveitis remain unknown, although immunologic processes most likely play a role. Correlation between the course of arthritis and uveitis is uncertain. Although 90% of patients with JIA who develop uveitis do so within 7 years of the onset of arthritis, the interval may be longer. Occasionally, uveitis is diagnosed before the onset of joint symptoms; these patients often have a poorer prognosis. Other features associated with more aggressive uveitis include short time interval between the onset of arthritis and uveitis, and severe uveitis at the first examination.

The uveitis associated with most types of JIA is usually asymptomatic and chronic. Such uveitis is characterized by anterior chamber cells and flare. Prolonged inflammation may lead to posterior synechiae, band keratopathy, cataract, ciliary membrane formation, hypotony, and glaucoma (Fig 23-1). Vitritis and macular edema occur infrequently.

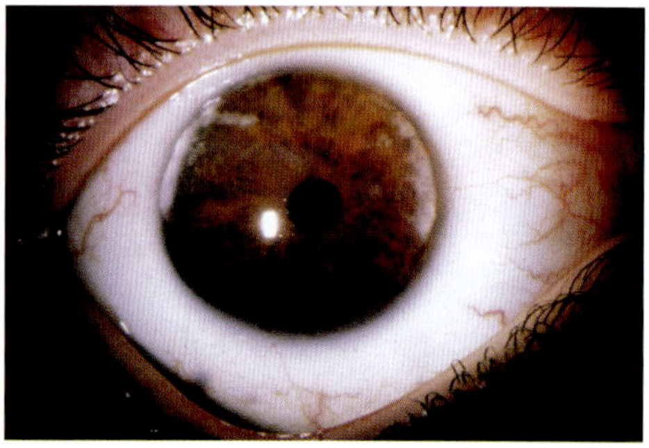

Figure 23-1 Slit-lamp photograph showing the left eye of a patient with JIA-associated uveitis. As is characteristic, the conjunctiva is "white." Band keratopathy is present. *(Photograph courtesy of Amy Hutchinson, MD.)*

Because many patients are asymptomatic, the disease may be advanced at diagnosis. Visual loss in JIA may be associated with multiple factors, including amblyopia in susceptible patients.

Recognition of the importance of screening for uveitis in children with JIA has probably resulted in improved prognosis over the years. Nevertheless, visual impairment is seen in as many as 40% of children with JIA-associated uveitis, and blindness has been reported in as many as 10% of affected eyes. Screening guidelines continue to undergo revision but are generally based on 3 factors believed to predispose children with arthritis to uveitis:

1. type of arthritis
2. age at onset of arthritis
3. presence of ANA

Table 23-4 outlines an eye examination schedule for children with juvenile rheumatoid arthritis developed by the American Academy of Pediatrics.

Kotaniemi K, Savolainen A, Karma A, et al. Recent advances in uveitis of juvenile idiopathic arthritis. *Surv Ophthalmol.* 2003;48:489–502.

Smith JR, Rosenbaum JT. Immune-mediated systemic diseases associated with uveitis. *Focal Points: Clinical Modules for Ophthalmologists.* San Francisco: American Academy of Ophthalmology; 2003, module 11.

Sarcoidosis

Sarcoidosis is an uncommon but well-known cause of uveitis in children. It is important to note that its presentation in young children tends to be different from that found in adults and older children. Young children with sarcoidosis are less likely to have pulmonary involvement and are more likely to have skin involvement and arthritis. Chest roentgenograms are thus less likely to be of value in evaluating children for possible sarcoidosis. Serum angiotensin-converting enzyme (ACE) levels are normally higher in children and can be misleading. If sarcoidosis is suspected, children should undergo careful rheumatologic evaluation for systemic disease, including of the skin and joints; roentgenograms of the hands may be helpful.

Anterior uveitis is the most common manifestation of ocular sarcoidosis in children; it is more common in younger children than in older children and adults. It can sometimes be difficult to distinguish sarcoidosis in children from JIA-associated uveitis, but unlike JIA-associated uveitis, juvenile sarcoidosis can involve all segments of the eye.

Shetty AK, Gedalia A. Sarcoidosis: a pediatric perspective. *Clin Pediatr.* 1998;37:707–717.

Tubulointerstitial Nephritis and Uveitis Syndrome

Tubulointerstitial nephritis and uveitis syndrome (TINU) is a distinct clinical entity that may be underrecognized and may account for some cases of unexplained chronic or recurrent uveitis in children. Renal disease is characterized by acute interstitial nephritis, and ocular disease is most often a bilateral uveitis that may occur before, simultaneously with, or after renal disease. The median age of onset is 15 years, and there is a 3:1 female-to-male

Table 23-4 Examination Schedule for Children With JRA Without Known Iridocyclitis

JRA Subtype	Age at Onset <7 years	Age at Onset ≥7 years
Pauciarticular		
Positive ANA		
Less than 4 years' duration	Every 3–4 months	Every 6 months
4–7 years' duration	Every 6 months	Annually
More than 7 years' duration	Annually	Annually
Negative ANA		
Less than 4 years' duration	Every 6 months	Every 6 months
4–7 years' duration	Every 6 months	Annually
More than 7 years' duration	Annually	Annually
Polyarticular		
Positive ANA		
Less than 4 years' duration	Every 3–4 months	Every 6 months
4–7 years' duration	Every 6 months	Annually
More than 7 years' duration	Annually	Annually
Negative ANA		
Less than 4 years' duration	Every 6 months	Every 6 months
4–7 years' duration	Every 6 months	Annually
More than 7 years' duration	Annually	Annually
Systemic	Annually, regardless of duration	Annually, regardless of duration

Adapted from American Academy of Pediatrics, Sections on Rheumatology and Ophthalmology. Guidelines for Ophthalmic Examinations in Children With Juvenile Rheumatoid Arthritis. *Pediatrics.* 1993;92:295–296.

ratio. Prognosis is generally good, although long-term follow-up is required because the disease often recurs.

Mandeville JT, Levinson RD, Holland GN. The tubulointerstitial nephritis and uveitis syndrome. *Surv Ophthalmol.* 2001;46:195–208.

Other Causes of Anterior Uveitis

Anterior uveitis may also be associated with a variety of infectious and noninfectious diseases, including herpesviruses, syphilis, trauma, Kawasaki syndrome, Fuchs heterochromic iridocyclitis, Lyme disease, and Behçet syndrome. These conditions are discussed in more detail in Chapter 17 and in BCSC Section 9, *Intraocular Inflammation and Uveitis.*

Intermediate Uveitis

The term *intermediate uveitis*, which is a diagnosis based on the anatomical location of inflammation, is preferred by the International Committee on Uveitis Nomenclature. Intermediate uveitis accounts for 5%–15% of all cases of uveitis and about 25% of uveitis in the pediatric age group. Intermediate uveitis is associated with a variety of conditions in children, including sarcoidosis, Lyme disease, toxocariasis, juvenile xanthogranuloma, and tuberculosis. Idiopathic disease, known as *pars planitis* (Fig 23-2), accounts for 85%–90% of cases. The distinction between pars planitis and intermediate uveitis is not always clear in common usage, and the 2 terms are often used interchangeably. The clinical features, diagnosis, and treatment of intermediate uveitis are discussed in Chapter 8 of BCSC Section 9, *Intraocular Inflammation and Uveitis.*

Posterior Uveitis

Toxoplasmosis

Toxoplasmosis is the most common cause of posterior uveitis in children. The diagnosis, clinical manifestations, and treatment of toxoplasmosis are discussd in Chapter 17 of this volume.

Toxocariasis

The nematode larvae of a common intestinal parasite of dogs *(Toxocara canis)* and cats *(Toxocara cati)* cause ocular toxocariasis, which is a common cause of posterior uveitis in children. *Toxocara canis* has been identified in up to 80% of puppies 2–6 months old and in 10%–30% of soil samples from public parks and playgrounds. Children contract the disease by ingesting the ova from dirt contaminated by dog or cat feces. Infection can also result from eating improperly cleaned foods. Systemic infection is referred to as *visceral larval migrans (VLM)*; it is most common in children age 6 months to 3 years and can be asymptomatic or associated with fever, cough, malaise, and anorexia.

Ocular involvement can occur simultaneously with VLM or may appear years later. Eye involvement is almost always unilateral and can present as a posterior pole granuloma, a peripheral granuloma with macular traction (Fig 23-3), or as endophthalmitis. Ocular toxocariasis can be confused with retinoblastoma in children; detection of eosinophilia and ELISA testing of serum or intraocular fluid for antibodies to the *Toxocara* organism are helpful in making the distinction.

Treatment includes observation of peripheral lesions, periocular or systemic steroids for posterior lesions and endophthalmitis, or surgical intervention to address retinal traction, cataract, glaucoma, or cyclitic membranes. Laser photocoagulation or systemic antihelminthics to destroy a motile nematode can cause a severe inflammatory reaction

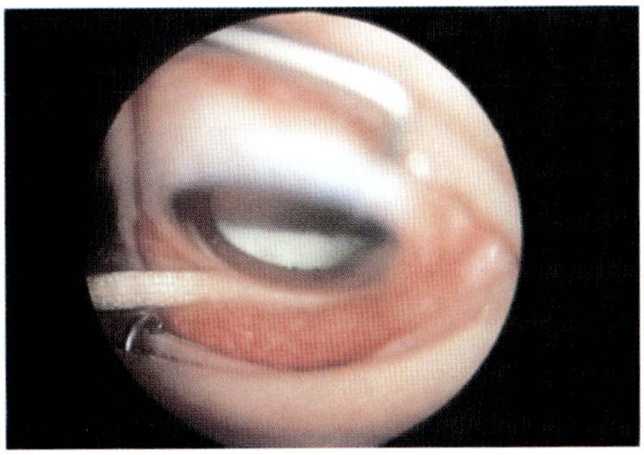

Figure 23-2 Intermediate uveitis with inferior snowbank formation, right eye.

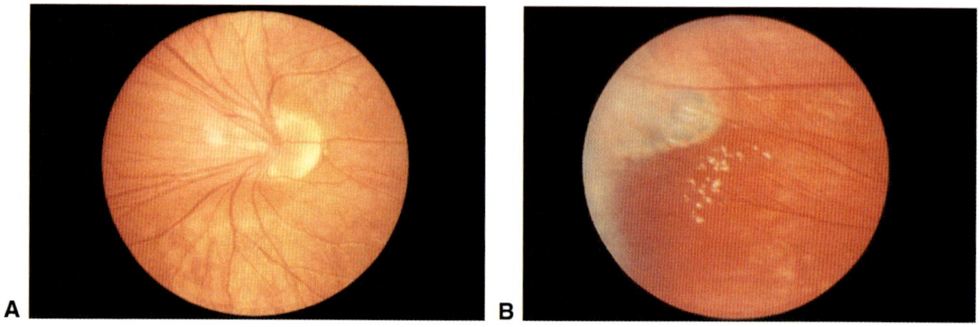

Figure 23-3 Toxocariasis, right eye. **A,** Distortion of posterior pole vessels. **B,** Peripheral granuloma.

and, if used, should be combined with steroids. See also BCSC Section 9, *Intraocular Inflammation and Uveitis*, Chapter 9.

Shields JA. Ocular toxocariasis. A review. *Surv Ophthalmol.* 1984;28:361–381.

Diffuse Unilateral Subacute Neuroretinitis

Diffuse unilateral subacute neuroretinitis (DUSN) is caused by an immunologic reaction to a motile nematode and may be an underrecognized cause of posterior uveitis in children, especially those living in tropical climates. See BCSC Section 9, *Intraocular Inflammation and Uveitis*, for a description of this condition.

Familial Juvenile Systemic Granulomatosis

Familial juvenile systemic granulomatosis (Blau syndrome) is an autosomal dominantly inherited disease that includes granulomatous arthritis, uveitis associated with multifocal choroiditis, and vasculitic rash. The disease usually presents during childhood. It resembles sarcoidosis, but pulmonary involvement and adenopathy are absent. Chronic panuveitis associated with multifocal choroiditis is the most common ocular presentation, but uveitis can be limited to the anterior segment in some cases, and the disease is often misdiagnosed as JIA or sarcoidosis. A positive family history is helpful in making the diagnosis. The gene has been linked to chromosome 16. Ocular complications such as cataract, glaucoma, band keratopathy, and visual loss are common.

Latkany PA, Jabs DA, Smith JR, et al. Multifocal choroiditis in patients with familial juvenile systemic granulomatosis. *Am J Ophthalmol.* 2002;134;897–904.

Vogt-Koyanagi-Harada Syndrome

Vogt-Koyanagi-Harada syndrome is a chronic progressive bilateral panuveitis that is associated with exudative retinal detachments and may be accompanied by signs of meningeal irritation, auditory disturbances, and skin changes. It is rare in children but is associated with a higher frequency of ocular complications such as cataract and glaucoma and with a poorer visual prognosis than in adults.

Tabbara KF, Chavis PS, Freeman WR. Vogt-Koyanagi-Harada syndrome in children compared to adults. *Acta Ophthalmol Scand.* 1998;76:723–726.

Other Causes of Posterior Uveitis

Other infectious and noninfectious causes of posterior uveitis include herpes, rubella, rubeola and measles viruses, syphilis, Bartonella, tuberculosis, Lyme disease, histoplasmosis, *Candida albicans*, sympathetic ophthalmia, sarcoidosis, and Behçet syndrome (see BCSC Section 9, *Intraocular Inflammation and Uveitis*). When posterior uveitis is associated with significant anterior chamber inflammation, it is designated panuveitis.

Masquerade Syndromes

Other conditions can simulate uveitis in the pediatric age group. These masquerade syndromes are listed together with their diagnostic features in Table 23-5.

Diagnosis of Pediatric Uveitis

Establishing the correct diagnosis is the essential first step in managing a pediatric patient with uveitis, although some ophthalmologists prefer to postpone workup of isolated anterior uveitis unless it is recurrent or unresponsive to initial therapy. Making an accurate diagnosis relies on obtaining a history and performing a complete ophthalmic examination and selected laboratory tests. The child's parent or guardian may have to provide the history, and an examination under anesthesia may be needed to identify subtle clinical findings. Laboratory investigations are selected on the basis of history and examination to support or refute a proposed diagnosis (see Table 23-5; Table 23-6).

Treatment of Pediatric Uveitis

The goal of uveitis treatment in children is to decrease the number of anterior chamber cells in order to prevent the sequelae of ongoing inflammation; chronic flare is less responsive to therapy and does not require treatment in the absence of cells.

Infectious disease and malignancies should be identified and treated appropriately. Currently accepted medical and surgical treatment of noninfectious uveitis is discussed in the following sections.

Medical Management

Anterior segment inflammation is treated with topical corticosteroid and mydriatic/cycloplegic agents. Because topical corticosteroids do not penetrate well into the vitreous or posterior segment, sub-Tenon injections of a corticosteroid may be useful in treating older children with intermediate or posterior uveitis. Injections may also be useful for patients who are noncompliant with topical therapy or for whom topical therapy is ineffective. Short courses of oral corticosteroids may be used, but long-term use should be avoided because of significant side effects in young children.

Table 23-5 Masquerade Syndromes

Disease	Age (Years)	Signs of Inflammation	Diagnostic Studies
Anterior segment			
Retinoblastoma	<15	Flare, cells, pseudohypopyon	Ultrasound; CT
Leukemia	<15	Flare, cells, heterochromia	Bone marrow, peripheral blood smear
Intraocular foreign body	Any age	Flare, cells	X-ray, ultrasound
Malignant melanoma	Any age	Flare, cells	Fluorescein angiography, ultrasound
Juvenile xanthogranuloma	<15	Flare, cells, hyphema	Examination of skin, iris biopsy
Peripheral retinal detachment	Any age	Flare, cells	Ophthalmoscopy
Posterior segment			
Retinitis pigmentosa	Any age	Cells in vitreous	ERG, EOG, visual fields
Reticulum cell sarcoma	15+	Vitreous exudate, retinal hemorrhage or exudates, retinal pigment epithelium infiltrates	Cytology study of aqueous and vitreous
Lymphoma	15+	Retinal hemorrhage or exudates, vitreous cells	Node biopsy, bone marrow, physical examination
Retinoblastoma	<15	Vitreous cells, retinal exudates	Ultrasound, CT
Malignant melanoma	15+	Vitreous cell	Fluorescein angiography, ultrasound
Multiple sclerosis	15+	Periphlebitis	Neurologic examination

CT, computed tomography; ERG, electroretinogram; EOG, electro-oculogram.

Glaucoma and cataract formation are 2 of the most serious ocular side effects of corticosteroid therapy. In general, the most potent corticosteroids are those most likely to produce an increase in intraocular pressure. Periocular injections of corticosteroids can produce elevations in intraocular pressure weeks to months after injection. Children appear to develop posterior subcortical cataracts following oral corticosteroid therapy sooner and at lower doses than adults, but these cataracts may be reversible after cessation of treatment.

Other risks of long-term systemic corticosteroid use in children include retardation of skeletal maturation and growth, osteoporosis and bone fractures, cushingoid appearance, diabetes, peptic ulcers, myopathy, hypertension, altered mental status, pseudotumor cerebri, and increased mortality from infection. Patients may also require increased doses of corticosteroids during times of stress to avoid an Addisonian crisis.

Naproxen and tolmetin are 2 nonsteroidal anti-inflammatory drugs (NSAIDs) that are commonly used to treat arthritis in children and may have some efficacy in treating uveitis. Potential complications of NSAIDs include gastrointestinal irritation, renal toxicity, skin rashes, and CNS reactions.

Table 23-6 Laboratory Tests for Various Types of Uveitis

Anterior
- Complete blood count (to rule out leukemia)
- Antinuclear antibody (to subtype JRA)
- Serum lysozyme (to rule out sarcoidosis)
- Serum protein electrophoresis (to look for $alpha_2$ globulin fraction in sarcoidosis)
- FTA-ABS (to rule out syphilis)
- HLA-B27 (to rule out ankylosing spondylitis and Reiter syndrome)
- PCR, ELISA, IFA, for Lyme disease
- Tuberculin skin test, chest x-ray (to rule out sarcoidosis and tuberculosis)
- GI series (if ulcerative colitis or regional enteritis [Crohn disease] is suspected)
- Angiotensin-converting enzyme (ACE)

Intermediate
- Serum lysozyme (to rule out sarcoidosis)
- FTA-ABS (to rule out syphilis)
- Chest x-ray (to rule out sarcoidosis or tuberculosis)
- Tuberculin skin test
- PCR, ELISA for toxocariasis
- Angiotensin-converting enzyme

Posterior
- PCR, ELISA for toxoplasmosis
- PCR, ELISA for toxocariasis
- Serum lysozyme (to rule out sarcoidosis)
- FTA-ABS (to rule out syphilis)
- PCR, blood cultures, viral cultures, or antibody levels if cytomegalovirus, herpes simplex (especially in a newborn), or rubella is suspected
- PCR, ELISA, IFA, for Lyme disease
- Angiotensin-converting enzyme

Systemic immunosuppressive therapy may be beneficial in treating both uveitis and arthritis. It can sometimes reduce or eliminate the need for steroids. The therapy should be undertaken in cooperation with a pediatric specialist familiar with the use of immunosuppressive and immunomodulatory medications and their side effects.

Methotrexate is an antimetabolite that is commonly used in low doses to treat arthritis and uveitis in children. Less commonly used antimetabolites include azathioprine, mycophenolate mofetil, and leflunomide. These agents inhibit nucleic acid synthesis by a variety of mechanisms. Gastrointestinal disturbance is the most common side effect of methotrexate; this can be alleviated by concurrent oral folic acid administration or by switching to subcutaneous injections. Hepatic toxicity and interstitial pneumonitis are rare but serious complications.

Cyclosporine is a fungal metabolite with substantial immunosuppressive effect. It has limited efficacy as monotherapy for uveitis, but it can be used in combination with steroids and methotrexate. Renal toxicity, hypertension, gingival hyperplasia, gastrointestinal disturbance, and neurologic symptoms are potential side effects.

Alkylating agents, including chlorambucil and cyclophosphamide, cause cross-linking of DNA and prevent cell replication. Because of their serious adverse effects, including bone marrow suppression, infection, infertility, and secondary malignancies, they are usually not used in children. However, they may occasionally be used in the most severe cases threatening blindness.

A number of newer therapies are under investigation for the treatment of uveitis. Tumor necrosis factor α is a proinflammatory cytokine. Its inhibitors etanercept and infliximab are used to treat inflammatory diseases including uveitis. Other medications under investigation include daclizumab, a humanized murine anti–interleukin-2 receptor, and oral chicken collagen type II.

Children receiving immunosuppressive drugs should receive a yearly influenza vaccine and, if susceptible, varicella-zoster virus immunoglobulin upon close exposure to chickenpox. If the $CD4^{+}$ T-lymphocyte count is less than 200 cells per microliter, then *Pneumocystis carinii* prophylaxis should be considered. An infectious diseases (ID) specialist should be consulted regarding the use of live attenuated viral vaccines in children receiving high-dose corticosteroids or immunosuppressive drugs.

Agle L, Vazquez-Cobian LB, Lehman TJ. Clinical trials in pediatric uveitis. *Curr Rheumatol Rep.* 2003;5:477–481.

Jabs DA, Rosenbaum JT, Foster CS, et al. Guidelines for the use of immunosuppressive drugs in patients with ocular inflammatory disorders: recommendations of an expert panel. *Am J Ophthalmol.* 2000;130:492–513.

Smith JR. Management of uveitis in pediatric populations: special considerations. *Paediatr Drugs.* 2002;4:183–189.

Surgical Treatment

Band keratopathy can often be alleviated by removal of corneal epithelium followed by chelation with ethylenediaminetetraacetic acid (EDTA). Several treatments may be needed.

Cataract surgery in patients with uveitis can be complicated by hypotony, glaucoma, synechiae formation, cystoid macular edema, and retinal detachment. In patients with JIA, a combined lensectomy/vitrectomy appears to give better results than cataract extraction alone. Uveitis must be aggressively treated so that it is under control both before and after surgery. IOL implantation in children with uveitis is controversial.

Glaucoma surgery may become necessary in children with uveitis. Many different techniques have been used, and long-term success rates vary. Standard trabeculotomy is associated with a high rate of failure due to scarring. Intraoperative application of mitomycin C may improve outcomes, but the risk of postoperative infection and bleb leaks over the lifespan of a child is of concern. Goniotomy or trabeculotomy may be of use in some children. The use of drainage devices is currently the most popular technique for surgical management of pediatric uveitic glaucoma.

Holland GN, Stiehm ER. Special considerations in the evaluation and management of uveitis in children. *Am J Ophthalmol.* 2003;135:867–878.

CHAPTER 24

Vitreous and Retinal Diseases and Disorders

Vitreous and retinal disorders in children are often associated with an underlying systemic disorder. A careful family history, a history of growth and development, and any details about other sensory or health problems should be part of the evaluation of these children.

Drack AV. Patterns of retinal disease in children. In: Wright KW, Spiegel PH, eds. *Pediatric Ophthalmology and Strabismus*. 2nd ed. New York: Springer; 2003.

Leukocoria

The term *leukocoria* means "white pupil." Depending on the lesion, the pupil may appear normal in room light but have no red reflex on ophthalmoscopy or flash photography. The differential diagnosis of leukocoria includes

- retinoblastoma
- persistent fetal vasculature, also known as persistent hyperplastic primary vitreous
- retinopathy of prematurity—stage 5, with total retinal detachment and fibrous membrane
- cataract
- chorioretinal colobomas
- uveitis
- toxocariasis
- congenital retinal folds
- Coats disease
- vitreous hemorrhage
- retinal dysplasia
- other tumors (eg, hamartomas, choroidal hemangiomas, diktyomas)

The major retinal causes are discussed in this chapter with the exception of retinoblastoma, which is covered in Chapter 26. See also BCSC Section 12, *Retina and Vitreous*, for more information about these conditions.

Persistent Fetal Vasculature

Persistent fetal vasculature (PFV) is the more accurate term for the condition referred to for many years as *persistent hyperplastic primary vitreous (PHPV)*. This is a congenital, usually unilateral, isolated, sporadic malformation of the eye. Bilateral cases may be associated with systemic or neurologic abnormalities and syndromes. Bilateral retinal folds or familial exudative vitreoretinopathy (FEVR) may be phenocopies. The spectrum of severity is broad. Mild cases feature eyes with prominent hyaloid vessel remnants, large Mittendorf dots, and Bergmeister papillae. At the other end of the spectrum are microphthalmic eyes with progressive shallowing of the anterior chamber and angle-closure glaucoma from fibrovascular invasion of the lens through a defect in the posterior lens capsule. Some authors believe that most unilateral congenital cataracts are associated with PFV.

Peripheral and posterior central retinal detachments may also occur in more severely involved eyes. The hyaloid artery may be replaced by a thick fibrous stalk. The ciliary processes may be elongated and visible through the dilated pupil, and prominent radial vessels are often noted on the iris surface (Fig 24-1). The retrolental plaque is usually densest centrally, and it may contain cartilage as well as fibrovascular tissue. Eccentric plaques may also occur.

The natural history of more severely affected untreated eyes is usually one of relentless, progressive cataract formation with concomitant shallowing of the anterior chamber, eventually resulting in angle-closure glaucoma. Retinal detachment, intraocular hemorrhage, ciliary body detachment, and angle-closure glaucoma are the severest complications in PFV. The hemorrhages presumably originate in the fibrovascular membrane in the retrolental space. Affected eyes are usually smaller than the normal fellow eye, although this finding may be apparent only by ultrasonography or careful caliper measurement of the corneal diameters. It is important to document microphthalmos because retinoblastoma is rarely found in microphthalmic eyes, and retinoblastoma may be part of the initial differential diagnosis. The presence of a cataract is also evidence against the diagnosis of retinoblastoma, although lens opacities may develop in advanced cases.

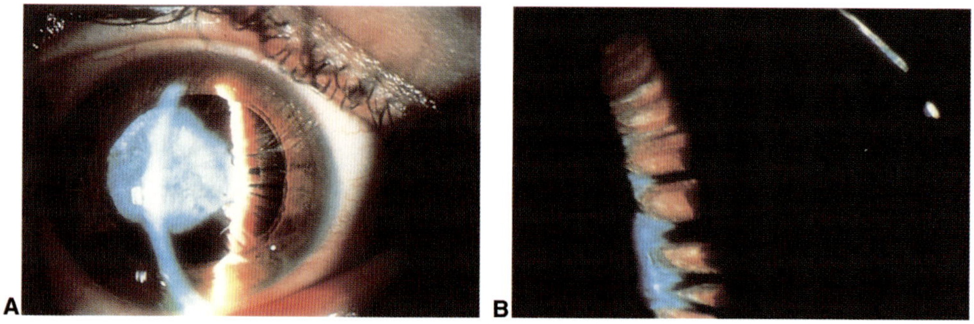

Figure 24-1 Persistent fetal vasculature (formerly called *persistent hyperplastic primary vitreous*). **A,** Elongated ciliary processes are adherent to lens. Note the dense fibrous plaque on the lens. **B,** Close-up of ciliary processes dragged into the pupillary axis.

Many eyes with PFV can be saved by early cataract surgery combined with membrane excision. In cases without significant posterior involvement, it is possible to obtain some degree of central vision if early surgical intervention is followed by consistent contact lens wear, combined with carefully monitored patching of the uninvolved eye. The visual prognosis often depends on the degree of retinal involvement and whether glaucoma develops.

Various surgical approaches to the management of PFV have been described. In most cases, the retrolenticular tissues can be removed by vitreous-cutting instruments and/or intraocular scissors, with intraocular cautery as necessary. Both limbal and pars plicata/pars plana approaches have been successfully employed. An anterior approach may decrease the chance of retinal detachment, as the pars plicata may be abnormally anterior. If the macula and optic nerve appear normal postoperatively, a vigorous effort should be made to correct aphakia optically and to patch, as would be done with a unilateral cataract.

Goldberg MF. Persistent fetal vasculature (PFV): an integrated interpretation of signs and symptoms associated with persistent hyperplastic primary vitreous (PHPV). LIV Edward Jackson Memorial Lecture. *Am J Ophthalmol.* 1997;124:587–626.

Karr DJ, Scott WE. Visual acuity results following treatment of persistent hyperplastic primary vitreous. *Arch Ophthalmol.* 1986;104:662–667.

Mullner-Eidenbock A, Amon M, Hauff W, et al. Surgery in unilateral congenital cataract caused by persistent fetal vasculature or minimal fetal remnants: age-related findings and management challenges. *J Cataract Refract Surg.* 2004;30:611–619.

Paysse EA, McCreery KM, Coats DK. Surgical management of the lens and retrolenticular fibrotic membranes associated with persistent fetal vasculature. *J Cataract Refract Surg.* 2002;8:816–820.

Retinopathy of Prematurity

Retinopathy of prematurity (ROP) is the current designation for what was previously called *retrolental fibroplasia.* ROP includes the acute disease seen in the nursery and the cicatricial disease seen later.

Normally, retinal vascular development begins during week 16 of gestation. Mesenchymal tissue containing spindle cells is the source of retinal vessels. The mesenchyme grows centrifugally from the optic disc, reaching the nasal ora serrata in the eighth month of gestation and the temporal ora serrata up to 1–2 months later. Premature birth may trigger the onset of ROP, in which normal retinal vascular development is altered and abnormal neovascularization occurs. The pathologic process may stop or reverse itself at any point, or the disease may eventually progress to fibroglial proliferation and lead to vitreoretinal traction and retinal detachment.

ROP is rare in infants with a birth weight greater than 2000 g. Premature infants weighing less than 1500 g at birth are at risk for serious visual sequelae from ROP, and the risk increases as gestational age and birth weight decrease. In the multicenter trial of cryotherapy for ROP (CRYO-ROP Study), 37% of infants weighing less than 750 g developed severe (stage 3; see the following discussion) ROP, whereas only 21.9% of those weighing 750–999 g and 8.5% of those weighing 1000–1250 g did so.

In the 1960s, as smaller and smaller premature babies were surviving, it was noted that delivering high doses of supplemental oxygen to these babies caused ROP. This has been demonstrated in animal models as well. Curtailment of oxygen was attempted and did decrease rates of ROP; however, rates of death and cerebral palsy increased. As pulse oximetry became widespread, allowing better regulation of oxygen administration, low birth weight and gestational age became better predictors of ROP than oxygen exposure, signifying the complex interaction of factors that cause disease development. Recent studies, using improved oxygenation monitors and avoidance of fluctuation in fraction of inspired oxygen, have shown more promising results, with reduction in rate of severe ROP without increased morbidity or mortality. Regulation of vascular endothelial growth factor (VEGF) at the retinal level appears to play a role.

Factors other than oxygen have also been examined. Several studies have used vitamin E (α-tocopherol) as a preventive treatment, with conflicting results. Intraventricular hemorrhage, necrotizing enterocolitis, and death have been associated with high-dose IV vitamin E use. The possibility of premature exposure to light as a factor was also raised but was not substantiated in a multicenter trial.

The ultimate prevention of ROP would be prevention of premature birth itself. Good early prenatal care can greatly affect the incidence of premature birth.

Gestational age and birth weight are inversely correlated with the development of ROP. The amount of time in oxygen therapy is a strong correlate, but the level of oxygenation is a weaker correlate. Other characteristics that correlate with the development of ROP are multiple births and transfer after birth to a hospital with a neonatal intensive care unit. Severe ROP is also more prevalent in white newborns, especially males.

Among infants who develop ROP, certain diseases are common, particularly various forms of respiratory distress syndrome, including hyaline membrane disease, pulmonary interstitial emphysema, pneumothorax, and bronchopulmonary dysplasia. Other disease entities observed include patent ductus arteriosus, apnea and bradycardia, intracranial hemorrhage, suspected sepsis, anemia, and jaundice.

Classification

The 1984 international classification of ROP describes the disease by stage, zone, and extent. The classification functioned very well in the CRYO-ROP Study and will probably be the standard classification for many years (Table 24-1; Figs 24-2 through 24-6). BCSC Section 12, *Retina and Vitreous*, discusses this classification in detail. Plus disease is defined by a standard photo and refers to arteriolar tortuosity and venous engorgement of the posterior pole (see Fig 24-6).

Management

Fundus examination of the premature infant must be performed with extreme care; these infants are fragile, and the examination is stressful. The recommended solution to be used in the examination is Cyclomydril (0.2% cyclopentolate and 1.0% phenylephrine). Phenylephrine 10% (Neo-Synephrine) should never be used because of its potential to cause hypertension. For examinations in the NICU, a nurse should be present, because many infants experience bradycardia during the examination. If an examination must be

Table 24-1 International Classification of Acute Stages of Retinopathy of Prematurity

Location—Zones II and III are based on convention rather than strict anatomy (Fig 24-7)

Zone I (posterior pole)—Circle with radius of 30°, twice disc-macula distance

Zone II—From edge of zone I to point tangential to nasal ora serrata and around to area near the temporal equator

Zone III—Residual crescent anterior to zone II

Extent—Specified as hours of the clock as observer looks at each eye

Staging the disease

Stage 1—Demarcation line (see Fig 24-2)

Stage 2—Ridge, ± small tufts of fibrovascular proliferation (popcorns) (see Fig 24-3)

Stage 3—Ridge with extraretinal fibrovascular proliferation (see Fig 24-4)

- Mild fibrovascular proliferation
- Moderate fibrovascular proliferation
- Severe fibrovascular proliferation

Stage 4—Subtotal retinal detachment (see Fig 24-5)

A. Extrafoveal
B. Retinal detachment including fovea

Stage 5—Total retinal detachment

Funnel:	Anterior	Posterior
	Open	Open
	Narrow	Narrow

Plus disease—Plus (+) is added when vascular shunting is so marked that the veins are enlarged and the arteries tortuous in the posterior pole (see Fig 24-6).

Modified from the Committee for Classification of Retinopathy of Prematurity: An international classification of retinopathy of prematurity. *Arch Ophthalmol.* 1984;102:1130–1134.

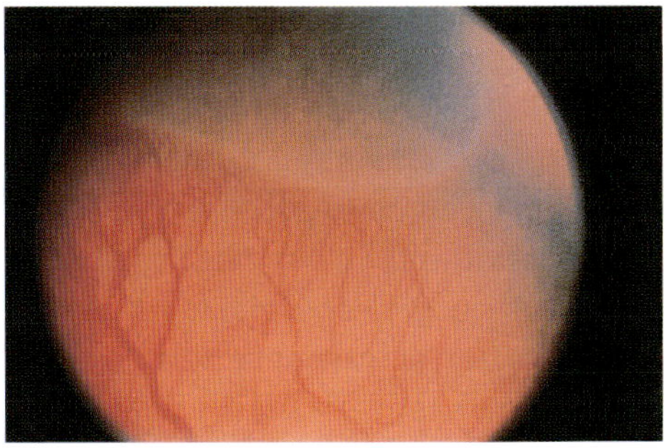

Figure 24-2 Late stage 1 ROP. Demarcation line has no height. *(Reproduced courtesy of Oregon Health Sciences University Ophthalmic Photography Department.)*

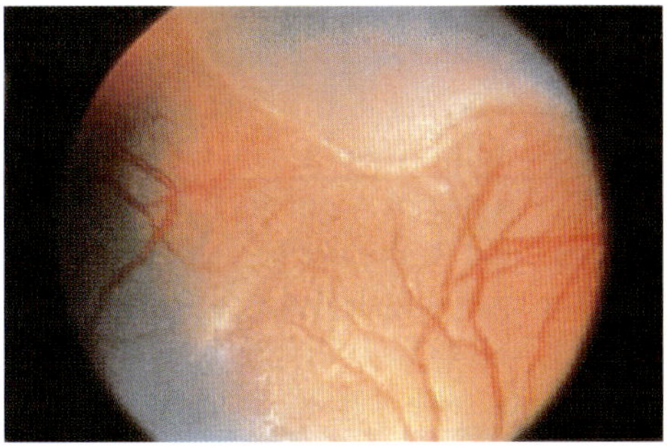

Figure 24-3 Early stage 2 ROP. Demarcation height and width, creating a ridge. *(Reproduced courtesy of Oregon Health Sciences University Ophthalmic Photography Department and CRYO-ROP Cooperative Group.)*

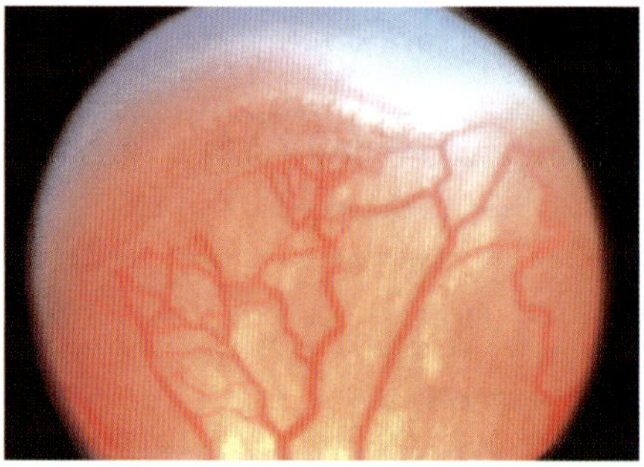

Figure 24-4 Stage 3 ROP. Ridge with extraretinal fibrovascular proliferation (top right shows stage 2). *(Reproduced by permission from* Arch Ophthalmol. *1984;102:1132. ©1988 American Medical Association.)*

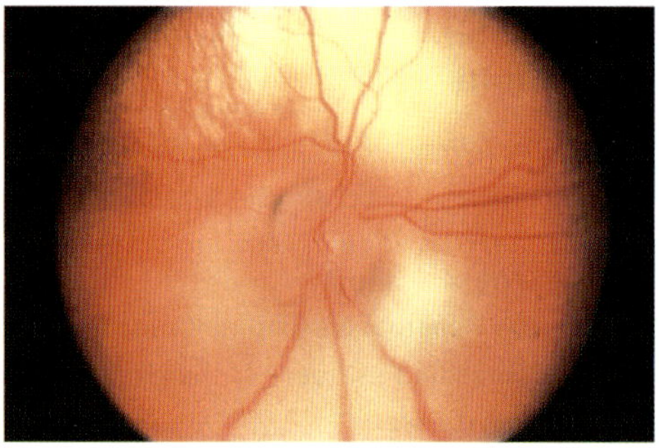

Figure 24-5 Stage 4 ROP. Subtotal retinal detachment. *(Reproduced by permission from* Arch Ophthalmol. *1984;102:1134. ©1988 American Medical Association.)*

postponed, the postponement and medical reason should be documented in the patient's chart.

It has been recommended that a fundus examination be performed on infants born at or below 30 weeks'* gestation or weighing less than 1500 g at birth. The joint statement on ROP by the American Academy of Pediatrics, American Association for Pediatric Ophthalmology and Strabismus, and the American Academy of Ophthalmology (given at the end of this chapter) recommends screening all babies born at less than 30 weeks' gestation and/or less than 1500 g at birth. These recommendations may change based on new data; the most current version should be consulted on the web sites of the American Academy of Pediatrics, the American Association for Pediatric Ophthalmology and Strabismus, and the American Academy of Ophthalmology. In the past, babies who required more than 48 hours of supplemental oxygen were recommended for screening, but now, determining whether to screen unstable infants whose age and weight are older and larger than the parameters is left to the discretion of the neonatology team. The first examination should be done at 4 weeks after birth or when the corrected gestational age is 31 weeks, whichever is later. If the retina is fully vascularized, which is true on the first examination in only a minority of infants, the baby should be seen again in 3 months to evaluate for other sequelae of prematurity. Great care should be taken to ensure that retinal vessels truly extend to the ora serrata—very immature retinas with no line or ridge can be difficult to distinguish from complete vascularization. It is safest to see infants whose eyes are believed to be fully vascularized on the first examination at least once more within 1 to 2 weeks to be certain. If there is any ROP or incomplete vascularization, examinations should be repeated at 1- to 2-week intervals, or sometimes more frequently, until either the retina is fully vascularized or the eye reaches threshold or type 1 (see the following discussion for definitions).

The screening clinician is initially looking for ROP and retinal vessel development. Regardless of the presence or absence of ROP, if the normal retinal vessels do not extend past zone I on early examinations, the chance that treatment will be needed becomes

*Corrected per *Pediatrics*. 2006;118:1324. Erratum.

much higher. For infants weighing less than 1000 g at birth who are not vascularized beyond zone I, weekly examinations are advisable even if no ROP is present. Such infants are predisposed to *Rush disease,* in which plus disease and retinal detachment develop rapidly, without intervening stages. On follow-up examinations, the patient is observed for development of ROP, spontaneous resolution of ROP, or progression to threshold disease. *Threshold disease* is defined by the CRYO-ROP Study as stage 3+ ROP in zone I or II, involving at least 5 contiguous clock-hour sectors or at least 8 interrupted clock-hour sectors. The Early Treatment for Retinopathy of Prematurity (ETROP) Study recently reported that more eyes can be saved by treating at earlier than threshold. These eyes are classified as type 1, including zone I and any ROP with plus; zone I, any stage 3 with or without plus; and zone II, any stage 2 or 3 with plus (Table 24-2, Fig 24-7). The iris vessels can become visibly congested just prior to the development of threshold disease (Fig 24-8).

The CRYO-ROP Study has shown that 6% of infants with a birth weight less than 1251 g will develop threshold disease and that 45% of these will have vision of 20/200 or worse at age 3½ years if not treated. If cryotherapy is applied to the avascular areas of

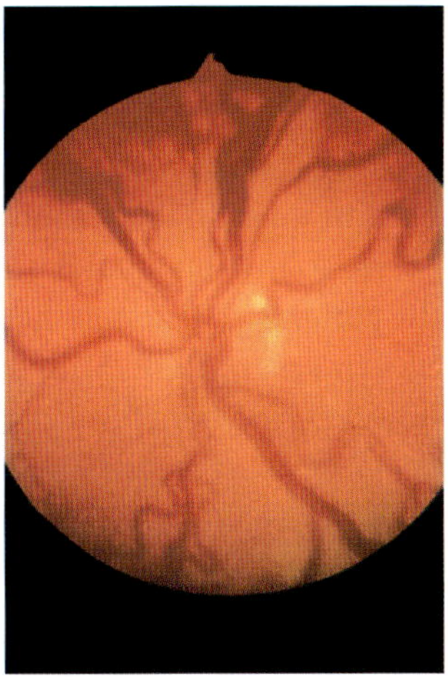

Figure 24-6 Classic plus disease.

Table 24-2 Examination and Treatment Schedule for Premature Infants (Birth Weight <1500 g)

Prethreshold disease/Type 2

- 1-week or less follow-up: stage 1 or 2 ROP, zone I; stage 3 ROP, zone II
- 1- to 2-week follow-up: immature vascularization, zone I (no ROP); stage 2 ROP, zone II; regressing ROP, zone I
- 2-week follow-up: stage 1 ROP, zone II; regressing ROP, zone II
- 2- to 3-week follow-up: immature vascularization, zone II (no ROP); stage 1 or 2 ROP, zone III; regressing ROP, zone III

Type 1 ROP

- Zone I, any ROP with plus
- Zone I, any stage 3
- Zone II, any stage 2 or 3 with at least 2 quadrants of plus
- If type 1 or threshold (5 continuous or 8 discontinuous clock-hours of stage 3+), do laser photocoagulation or cryotherapy within 72 hours.

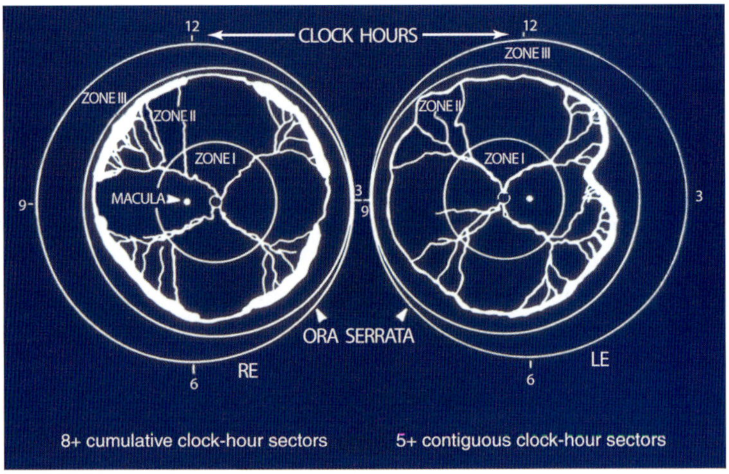

Figure 24-7 Diagram of ROP zones. *(Reproduced by permission from* Arch Ophthalmol. *1988;106:472. ©1988 American Medical Association.)*

retina in these eyes (Fig 24-9), only 26% of these patients will have vision of 20/200 or worse at age 3½ years. Therefore, cryotherapy reduces severe vision loss by about half. The study showed that at age 5½ years, treated eyes were still much less likely to have very poor vision. However, more of the untreated eyes with quantifiable vision had vision of 20/40 or better than did the treated eyes. Longer-term follow-up studies are necessary to see whether this trend persists, particularly after the patients go through the teenage years, a common time for secondary retinal detachments in severe ROP. Mild constriction of visual field has been measured in treated eyes; however, the benefit of preserved acuity outweighs this disadvantage.

The median age at which eyes reached threshold disease in the CRYO-ROP Study was 36.9 weeks postconception; 90% of cases reached threshold between 33.6 and 42 weeks postconception. This age can coincide with the age at which the patient is transferred to another facility or discharged to home. If a child has worsening ROP at this age, the discharge plans should include consideration of follow-up and treatment possibilities.

Laser photocoagulation has largely replaced cryotherapy as the treatment of choice for ROP in the United States. Laser has been shown in studies to be equally or more effective, less inflammatory, easier to apply to posterior disease, and perhaps less likely to cause severe myopia. Potential complications from laser treatment include an intense inflammatory response, hyphema, cataract, and glaucoma. For this reason, follow-up and a postoperative regimen of topical steroids and cycloplegia are imperative for the first week. Cataracts are often accompanied by hypotony, and the eye may be lost.

Sequelae of advanced ROP, either treated or spontaneously resolved, can include both peripheral and posterior retinal changes. Therefore, a child who has had ROP requires periodic ophthalmic examinations beyond the newborn period to reach maximum visual function. Vitreoretinal traction may cause retinal detachment in the first or second decade of life. Retinal folds and dragging of the macula can also occur, causing visual impairment (Fig 24-10). Amblyopia may be present as a result of high myopia, macular dragging, or strabismus. Pseudostrabismus caused by dragging of the macula can occur, often giving the appearance of an exotropia as a result of a large positive angle kappa (Fig 24-11). These children need particular attention paid to their development and education because they are often multiply handicapped beyond their visual problems.

When laser or cryotherapy has not prevented the progression of ROP to stage 4 or retinal detachment, scleral buckling and vitrectomy may be indicated. Anatomical success is as high as 83% in some studies, but visual results may be disappointing, particularly with stage 5 eyes. Even with treatment, several hundred babies are blinded by this disease in the United States yearly.

Other late changes associated with stage 5 ROP include microphthalmos, cataract, glaucoma, and phthisis bulbi. Glaucoma is caused by peripheral anterior synechiae and

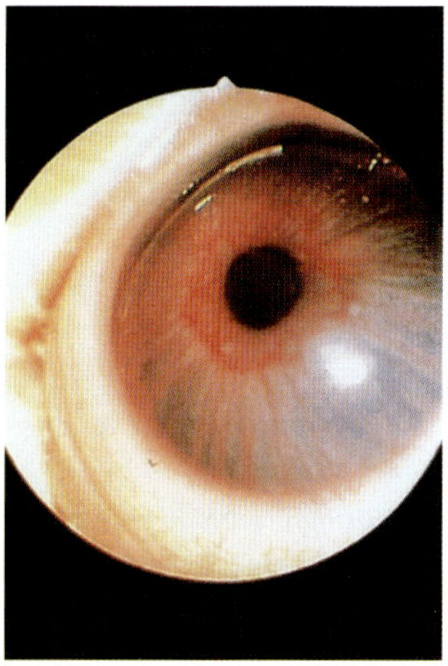

Figure 24-8 Congested iris vessels associated with stage 3+ ROP.

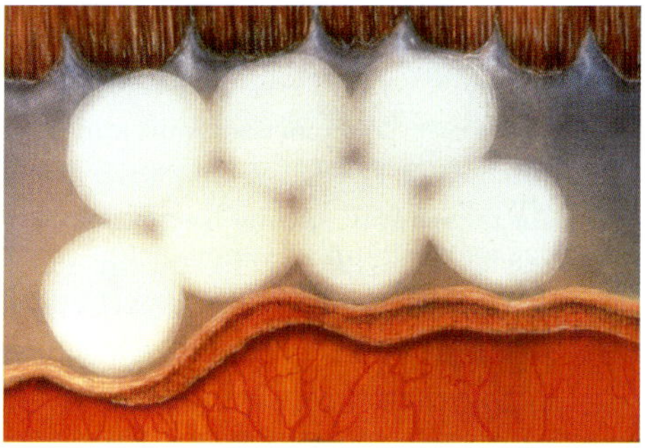

Figure 24-9 Cryotherapy as a row at ora serrata extending posteriorly to anterior edge of ridge. *(Reproduced by permission from* Arch Ophthalmol. *1988;106:474. ©1988 American Medical Association.)*

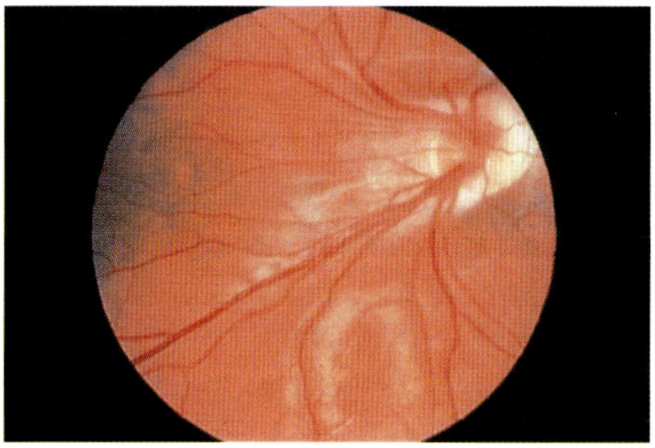

Figure 24-10 Posterior pole traction/dragging, a sequela of ROP, right eye. Central acuity is usually diminished in such eyes.

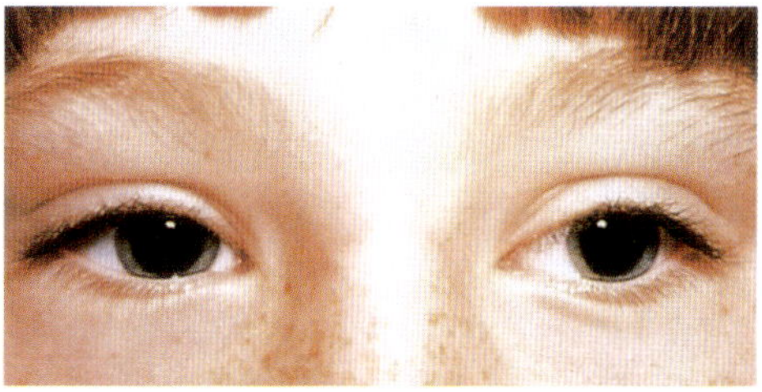

Figure 24-11 Pseudoexotropia in a fixating left eye in ROP. Patient has a positive angle kappa as a result of macular dragging.

angle closure resulting from forward movement of the lens–iris diaphragm. Such eyes are often blind but may be preserved by cycloplegic agents, steroids, lensectomy, and iridectomy. In seeing eyes, progressive myopia may indicate progression of lens movement and rounding and may be a harbinger of angle closure. In blind eyes, enucleation is sometimes necessary for pain relief.

See the end of this chapter for the joint statement on ROP screening approved by the American Academy of Pediatrics, the American Association for Pediatric Ophthalmology and Strabismus, and the American Academy of Ophthalmology.

Chow LC, Wright KW, Sola A, et al. Can changes in clinical practice decrease the incidence of severe retinopathy of prematurity in very low birth weight infants? *Pediatrics.* 2003;111:339–345.

ET-ROP Cooperative Group. Revised indications for the treatment of retinopathy of prematurity: results of the early treatment for ROP randomized trial. *Arch Ophthalmol.* 2003;121:1684–1694.

Multicenter trial of cryotherapy for retinopathy of prematurity: Snellen visual acuity and structural outcome at 5½ years after randomization. Cryotherapy for Retinopathy of Prematurity Cooperative Group. *Arch Ophthalmol.* 1996;114:417–424.

Prenner JL, Capone A Jr, Trese MT. Visual outcomes after lens-sparing vitrectomy for stage 4A retinopathy of prematurity. *Ophthalmology.* 2004;111:2271–2273.

Quinn GE, Young TL. Retinopathy of prematurity. *Focal Points: Clinical Modules for Ophthalmologists.* San Francisco: American Academy of Ophthalmology; 2001, module 11.

Reynolds JD, Dobson V, Quinn GE, et al. Evidence-based screening criteria for retinopathy of prematurity: natural history data from the CRYO-ROP and LIGHT-ROP studies. *Arch Ophthalmol.* 2002;120:1470–1476.

Reynolds JD, Hardy RJ, Kennedy KA, et al. Lack of efficacy of light reduction in preventing retinopathy of prematurity. Light Reduction in Retinopathy of Prematurity (LIGHT-ROP) Cooperative Group. *N Engl J Med.* 1998;338:1572–1576.

Coats Disease

Coats disease is an important mimicker of retinoblastoma. The definition of this condition has been narrowed, and Coats disease is now understood to mean the presence of abnormal retinal vessels with a fundus picture showing yellow subretinal exudates. The term *telangiectasia* is frequently used to indicate these anomalous grapelike clusters of vessels. The macular area is a favored site for exudation. Once the fovea is detached and the subretinal exudate becomes organized, the prognosis for restoration of central vision is poor. See also BCSC Section 12, *Retina and Vitreous.*

Males are affected more frequently than females, and the condition is usually, but not always, unilateral. When *idiopathic retinal telangiectasia with exudation* was considered as a spectrum, with the most severe group corresponding to typical Coats disease, the average age at diagnosis was 6–8 years in a study by Cahill et al (2001), but the disease has also been observed in infants (Fig 24-12; see also BCSC Section 12, *Retina and Vitreous*). The most widely held theory for this is that the subretinal exudation originates from the leaking anomalous vessels. Hence, the diagnosis of Coats disease requires the presence of the abnormal retinal vessels, which occasionally are small and difficult to

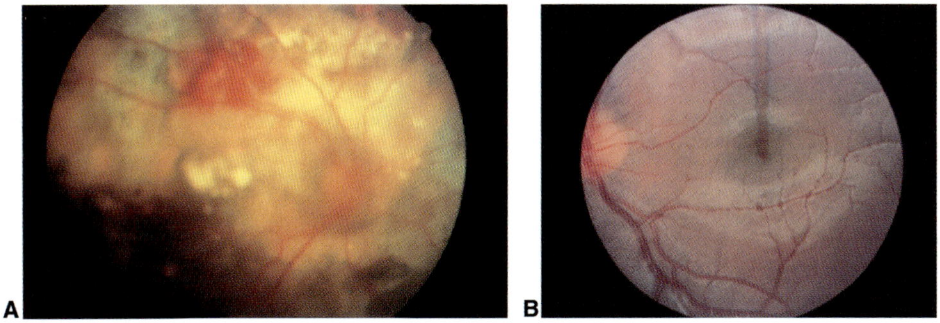

Figure 24-12 Coats disease. **A,** Affected right eye. Note extensive subretinal exudate and exudative retinal detachment. **B,** Normal left eye.

find. Fluorescein angioscopy and angiography may be helpful in demonstrating leakage from the telangiectatic vessels and in assessing the effectiveness of therapy.

The differential diagnosis includes angiomatosis retinae, retinoblastoma, PFV, ROP, toxocariasis, metastatic retinitis, familial exudative vitreoretinopathy, massive retinal fibrosis, Eales disease, sickle cell retinopathy, leukemia, anemia, and cavernous retinal hemangioma.

Treatment is directed at obliterating the abnormal vessels and includes cryotherapy or laser photocoagulation. The disease is stopped when the leaking vessels are destroyed. Eyes with progressive disease develop exudative retinal detachments and subretinal fibrosis. Scleral buckling may be used on eyes with retinal detachments. Some eyes develop intractable glaucoma.

In one study, 22 untreated patients were followed for an average of 5 years. The ocular disease progressed in about half of patients, remaining stable in the other half. Ridley and coworkers (1982) reported on 43 eyes, of which 29 were treated. Of the treated group, 8 (27.5%) deteriorated, 15 (52%) stabilized, and 6 (20.5%) improved. Aggressive treatment of the abnormal vessels and prolonged follow-up were recommended.

Cahill M, O'Keefe M, Acheson R, et al. Classification of the spectrum of Coats disease as subtypes of idiopathic retinal telangiectasias with exudation. *Acta Ophthalmol Scand.* 2001;79:596–602.

Ridley ME, Shields JA, Brown GC, et al. Coats' disease. Evaluation of management. *Ophthalmology.* 1982;89:1381–1387.

Hereditary Retinal Disease

Nystagmus is the most definitive presenting sign of a hereditary retinal disorder in the preverbal child. The onset of nystagmus typically occurs between 8 and 12 weeks of age. Poor visual function can also be the presenting abnormality in a young child, and school-age children with retinal disease often fail a vision screening. Workup requires a complete ophthalmic examination. Older children can be examined further with an electroretinogram (ERG), electro-oculogram (EOG), color vision testing, visual fields, and dark adaptation testing.

Table 24-3 outlines common causes of nystagmus in the first 3 months of life. Congenital motor nystagmus, infectious diseases, and optic nerve disorders are discussed in Chapters 12, 17, and 25. Hereditary retinal diseases with onset late in childhood are much like adult hereditary retinal diseases and are thoroughly covered in BCSC Section 12, *Retina and Vitreous.*

Leber Congenital Amaurosis

Leber congenital amaurosis (LCA) is an autosomal recessive disorder that affects both rods and cones. It presents with decreased vision during the first year of life, usually manifesting as nystagmus beginning in the second or third month. Vision ranges from 20/200 to bare light perception in most patients. Hyperopic refraction and sluggish pupillary responses are characteristic findings, although some patients are myopic. Ophthalmoscopic appearance varies highly, ranging from a normal appearance, particularly in infancy, to one resembling classic retinitis pigmentosa, with bone spicules, attenuation of arterioles, and disc pallor. Other reported fundus findings include irregularity of the retinal pigment epithelium, extensive chorioretinal atrophy, macular coloboma, white dots (similar to retinitis punctata albescens), marbleized retinal appearance, and disc edema (Fig 24-13). Additional ocular abnormalities include oculodigital reflex (eye poking), cataracts, keratoconus, and keratoglobus. The incidence of neurologic and renal

Table 24-3 Causes of Nystagmus in First 3 Months of Life

Primary sensory retinal abnormality
- Leber congenital amaurosis
- Achromatopsia
- Blue-cone monochromatism
- Congenital stationary night blindness (X-linked and autosomal recessive)

Vitreoretinal abnormality
- Norrie disease
- Familial exudative vitreoretinopathy

Foveal hypoplasia
- Associated with albinism
- Associated with aniridia
- Isolated

Optic nerve disorder
- Optic nerve hypoplasia
- Optic nerve coloboma
- Optic atrophy

Infectious disease
- Congenital toxoplasmosis
- Cytomegalovirus
- Rubella
- Syphilis

Congenital motor nystagmus

Generalized central nervous system disorder
- Aicardi syndrome
- Others

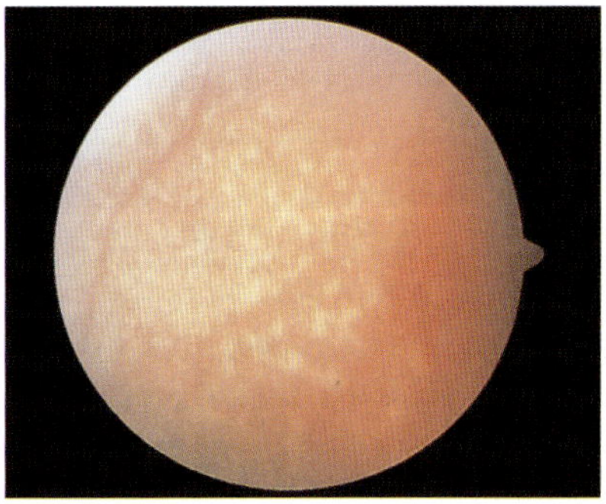

Figure 24-13 Leber congenital amaurosis, marbleized fundus type.

disorders is significant in these patients. See Familial Oculorenal Syndromes, later in this chapter.

Given such variability, the diagnosis of Leber congenital amaurosis cannot be based on fundus appearance alone and requires an ERG. However, electroretinography can be technically difficult to perform in infants, and there is a maturation of the ERG response. Thus, an ERG can appear highly abnormal in an infant who will later develop a more normal response. It is often advisable either to delay the ERG until age 6 months or to repeat the ERG after this time. General anesthesia may be required for ERG.

The characteristic clinical picture in this disorder is of an infant in the first 6 months of life presenting with nystagmus and an ERG that is nearly or essentially flat. Histologic examination shows diffuse absence of photoreceptors. Leber congenital amaurosis is genetically heterogeneous. Mutations of the photoreceptor-specific guanylate cyclase gene *(RETGC1)*, the *RPE65* gene, and the *CRX* gene account for about 27% of cases. Other genes are being sought. Patients with *RETGC1* mutations may experience a more stable course than those with *RPE65* mutations. A dog model of *RPE65* LCA has had vision restored by gene therapy with an adenovirus vector; human trials are planned for the near future.

Both Refsum disease (infantile phytanic acid storage disease) and Bassen-Kornzweig syndrome (abetalipoproteinemia) have been reported to present as Leber congenital amaurosis. Because these are potentially treatable metabolic disorders (by reduction of phytanic acid intake and vitamin A and E therapy, respectively), it is recommended that the evaluation of a new patient with findings of Leber congenital amaurosis include a complete blood lipid profile, inspection of peripheral smear for acanthocytes (Bassen-Kornzweig syndrome), and measurement of serum phytanic acid levels.

Lambert SR, Taylor D, Kriss A. The infant with nystagmus, normal appearing fundi, but an abnormal ERG. *Surv Ophthalmol.* 1989;34:173–186.

Perrault I, Rozet JM, Gerber S, et al. Leber congenital amaurosis. *Mol Genet Metab.* 1999;68: 200–208.

Achromatopsia

Achromatopsia can be difficult to distinguish initially from Leber congenital amaurosis, but infants with achromatopsia develop better visual functioning. Complete achromatopsia, or rod monochromatism, is a stationary autosomal recessive disorder in which patients have no color vision, poor central vision, nystagmus, and photophobia. The photophobia is actually a desire to avoid bright light rather than true pain or discomfort, and photophobia may be manifested by squinting or rapid fluttering of the eyelids in normal indoor illumination. It may not appear until several months of age.

Retinal examination is usually normal, with the possible exception of a decreased or absent foveal reflex. Color vision testing results are markedly abnormal, as is the ERG, which shows extinguished photopic responses. Dark glasses or red glasses that exclude short wavelengths may help. Autosomal recessive achromatopsia is associated with mutations of the *CNGA3* gene on chromosome 2. This encodes the α-subunit of the cone cyclic nucleotide-gated cation channel, which generates the light-evoked electrical responses of the cones. In the Pingelapese islanders of Micronesia, mutations have been found in the *CNBG3* gene on chromosome 8. This gene encodes the β-subunit of the cone cyclic nucleotide-gated cation channel. Incomplete autosomal recessive forms of achromatopsia occur less often.

Pokorny J, Smith VC, Pinckers AJ, et al. Classification of complete and incomplete autosomal recessive achromatopsia. *Graefes Arch Clin Exp Ophthalmol.* 1982;219:121–130.

Sundin OH, Yang JM, Li Y, et al. Genetic basis of total colour blindness among the Pingelapese islanders. *Nat Genet.* 2000;25:289–293.

Blue-Cone Monochromatism

Blue-cone monochromatism is an X-linked cone disorder that may present with nystagmus in the first few months of life. These patients are less severely affected clinically than those with complete achromatopsia. Vision may decline slowly over time. Patients have a characteristic color vision abnormality and visual acuity ranging from 20/60 to 20/200. Fundus examination appears essentially normal. Although the short-wavelength (blue) cones are functioning, the photopic ERG is essentially extinguished. Mutations in the red and green pigment gene array at Xq28 are responsible.

Ladekjaer-Mikkelsen AS, Rosenberg T, Jorgensen AL. A new mechanism in blue cone monochromatism. *Hum Genet.* 1996;98:403–408.

Congenital Stationary Night Blindness

The following classification scheme for *congenital stationary night blindness (CSNB)* was proposed by Carr (1974). Forms with normal fundi are

- autosomal dominant
- autosomal recessive
- X-linked

Forms with abnormal fundi are

- *Oguchi disease:* yellow sheen after light exposure that disappears following dark adaptation
- *fundus albipunctatus:* yellow-white dots, normal vessels

Both autosomal recessive and X-linked forms of CSNB can present in early infancy with nystagmus and normal fundi. These forms are often also associated with myopia and decreased acuity in the range of 20/200. The retina appears normal, although the optic nerve may show some temporal pallor. The ERG shows 2 characteristic patterns; in both, the scotopic b-wave amplitude is greatly reduced. Dark adaptation is abnormal in all patients. Infants with CSNB may have a flat ERG until approximately 6 months of age, when it converts to the classic negative configuration. Other forms of CSNB are discussed in BCSC Section 12, *Retina and Vitreous.*

Carr RE. Congenital stationary night blindness. *Trans Am Ophthalmol Soc.* 1974;72:448–487.

Foveal Hypoplasia

Foveal hypoplasia, or incomplete development of the fovea, is another cause of nystagmus in early infancy. This condition is most often associated with albinism or aniridia but may also be an isolated finding. The ophthalmoscopic appearance is of a decreased or absent foveal reflex with varying degrees of hypoplasia of the macula itself (patients with complete achromatopsia also show decreased foveal reflex). The ERG appears normal in these cases. Foveal hypoplasia can be familial and may be related to a defect in the *PAX6* gene.

Aicardi Syndrome

Aicardi syndrome is a disorder characterized by round or oval, widespread, depigmented chorioretinal lesions (Fig 24-14). Colobomas and microphthalmos may also occur. CT reveals agenesis of the corpus callosum. Affected patients have infantile spasms and severe mental retardation. Aicardi syndrome is an X-linked dominant disorder, lethal in males.

Aicardi J. Aicardi syndrome. *Brain Dev.* 2005;27:164–171.

Rosser T. Aicardi syndrome. *Arch Neurol.* 2003;60:1471–1473.

Van den Veyver IB. Microphthalmia with linear skin defects, Aicardi, and Goltz syndromes: are they related X-linked dominant male-lethal disorders? *Cytogenet Genome Res.* 2002;99: 289–296.

Hereditary Macular Dystrophies

The macula can be involved in a hereditary disorder in 3 possible ways:

1. The macula may appear abnormal secondary to a hereditary systemic disease (eg, the cherry-red spot seen in generalized gangliosidosis).
2. The macula may be involved in a generalized primary retinal disorder, as in some cases of Leber congenital amaurosis. Tests of overall retinal function such as the ERG reveal abnormal results in this situation.
3. The macula alone may be affected by a hereditary disorder such as Stargardt disease, Best vitelliform dystrophy, and familial drusen. The ERG may be normal.

Stargardt Disease

Stargardt disease (juvenile macular degeneration) is the most common hereditary macular dystrophy. It is usually autosomal recessive but may be autosomal dominant. It is a bilateral, symmetric, progressive condition in which acuity levels off at approximately 20/200. Vision typically begins to deteriorate between ages 8 and 15 years. The fundus appears normal early in the course of the disease, even when some vision has been lost. The first ophthalmoscopic changes observed are loss of foveal reflex, followed by development of a characteristic bull's-eye lesion. Yellow flecks in the posterior pole are characteristic, but they are not required for the diagnosis (Fig 24-15). Eventually, the macula may acquire an atrophic appearance, with a peculiar light-reflecting quality that has been described as beaten bronze. The lesion then enlarges and deepens and may finally show choroidal atrophy with prominent choroidal vessels at its base. The dark choroid sign on fluorescein angiography is distinctive but not always present. Progressive cone–rod dystrophy may present like Stargardt disease in children but has a much worse prognosis, often resulting in very little vision. Repeat ERG and acuity measurements over the first year are recommended before a definitive diagnosis is made. Stargardt disease is caused by mutations in the retina-specific ATP binding transporter gene *(ABCR)*. Interestingly, this gene is expressed in rods, not cones, although clinically Stargardt disease manifests primarily in the cones.

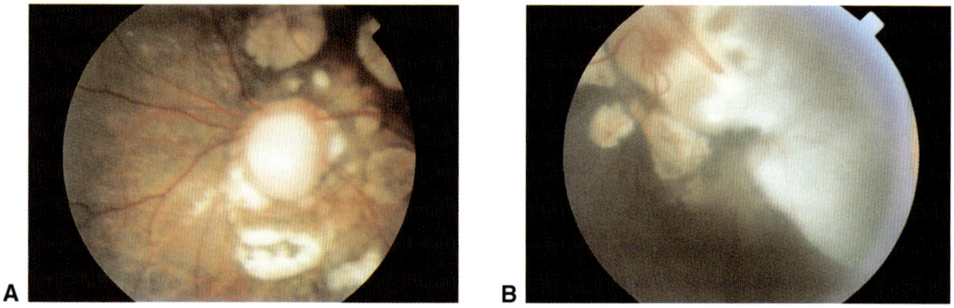

Figure 24-14 Aicardi syndrome. **A,** Fundus photograph showing disc and adjacent chorioretinal lacunae. **B,** Peripheral view of same patient showing large chorioretinal lacuna.

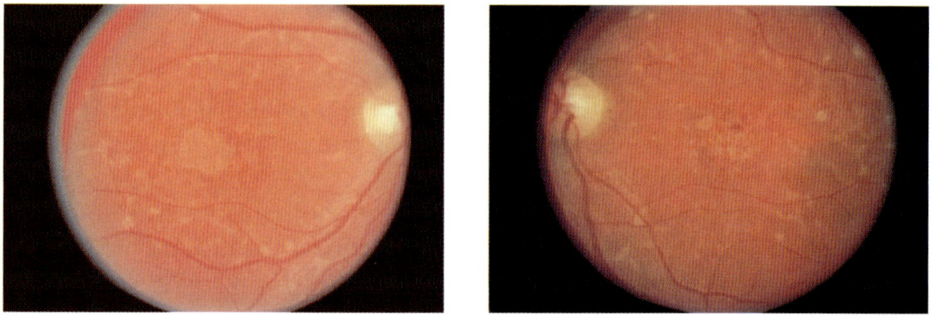

Figure 24-15 Stargardt disease, bilateral. Note atrophic, beaten-metal appearance of macula. Early in the disease, usually at presentation, the macula appears normal.

Fundus flavimaculatus

When more retinal flecks develop in the periphery and evidence suggests generalized retinal involvement, the condition has been called *fundus flavimaculatus* (Fig 24-16). ERG abnormalities are usually very mild in Stargardt disease and more significant in fundus flavimaculatus. Many clinicians now group the 2 entities together as Stargardt disease/fundus flavimaculatus because of reports of families in which both forms exist in different members with the same genetic mutations. Both disorders also map to the same genetic locus.

Rozet JM, Gerber S, Ghazi I, et al. Mutations of the retinal specific ATP binding transporter gene (ABCR) in a single family segregating both autosomal recessive retinitis pigmentosa RP19 and Stargardt disease: evidence of clinical heterogeneity at this locus. *J Med Genet.* 1999;36:447–451.

Best Vitelliform Dystrophy

The retina may at first appear normal in *Best vitelliform dystrophy* even though the EOG appears abnormal (Fig 24-17). The vitelliform stage begins between 4 and 10 years of age and is seen as a yellow-orange cystlike structure, usually in the macula, although the lesion may occur elsewhere and can occasionally be multiple. It is usually 1.5–5.0 disc

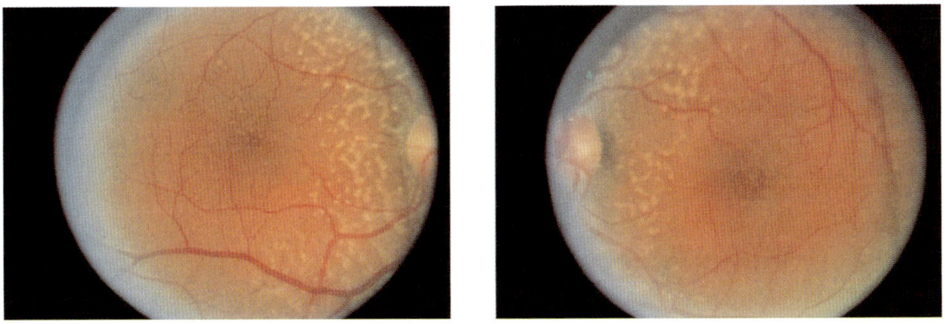

Figure 24-16 Fundus flavimaculatus. Note pisciform yellowish flecks.

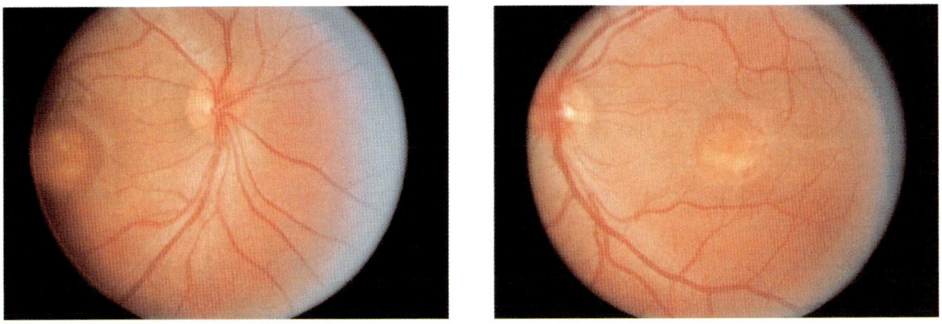

Figure 24-17 Best vitelliform dystrophy, bilateral. Even with pronounced vitelliform maculopathy as seen here, vision may be nearly normal.

diameters in size. The sunny-side-up appearance is associated with good central vision. With time, the cystic material may become granular, giving rise to the scrambled-egg stage. Central vision usually remains good.

The contents of the retinal pigment epithelial cyst may rupture and become partially resorbed, and pseudohypopyon may form with liquefaction of the cystic contents. Eventually, atrophy of the macula ensues. There may be subretinal neovascularization and serous detachment of the retinal pigment epithelium, and subretinal hemorrhage may occur. Most patients see surprisingly well for many years; eventually, however, central vision often deteriorates to 20/100 or worse.

The EOG appears abnormal in all affected patients and in carriers. This disorder is one of the few in which the EOG appears abnormal and the ERG appears normal. Carriers can be identified by the presence of an abnormal-appearing EOG in the absence of morphologic abnormalities. The condition is autosomal dominant and is caused by mutations in the *vitelliform macular dystrophy gene (VMD2)*, also called *bestrophin*, on chromosome 11. Inheritance is autosomal dominant. Commercial DNA testing is available.

Petrukhin K, Koisti MJ, Bakall B, et al. Identification of the gene responsible for Best macular dystrophy. *Nat Genet.* 1998;19:241–247.

Familial Drusen

In *familial drusen*, a dominantly transmitted disorder, drusen appear on Bruch's membrane. Decreased central acuity is rare before age 40, but macular drusen are occasionally seen in children. The drusen are small, yellow-white, and round or oval. They are similar to the lesions of fundus albipunctatus, except that familial drusen tend to form grapelike clusters. Complications in adult life include macular edema, hemorrhage, and macular degenerations of various types following subretinal neovascularization.

Hereditary Vitreoretinopathies

The vitreoretinopathies include a broad range of disease entities. The ones discussed here characteristically present in childhood.

Juvenile Retinoschisis

Foveal retinoschisis is present in almost all cases of *juvenile retinoschisis.* About 50% of patients have peripheral retinoschisis in addition to foveal involvement. The retinoschisis occurs in the nerve fiber layer. The fovea has a star-shaped or spokelike configuration that may resemble cystoid macular edema. Vitreous veils or strands are common (Fig 24-18), and vitreal syneresis is prominent. Visual acuity varies but may gradually deteriorate to the finger-counting range. Complications include vitreous hemorrhages and retinal detachments. The ERG shows a reduction of the scotopic b-wave with preservation of the a-wave; the EOG appears normal. The condition is usually transmitted as an X-linked trait. The gene is known, and gene therapy in a mouse model has shown early successes.

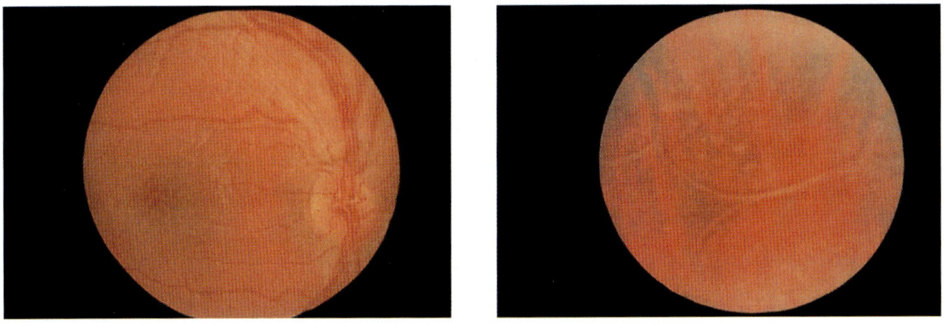

Figure 24-18 Juvenile retinoschisis. Central (macular) and peripheral schisis may be present.

Stickler Syndrome

Stickler syndrome is an autosomal dominant disease characterized by progressive arthropathy, high myopia, retinal detachment, degenerative joint changes, epiphyseal dysplasia, flat midface, progressive hearing loss, and heart defects. A single family can show great variability in expression of the syndrome, and individuals may manifest only a few of the characteristic findings. In many families, a defect in the type II procollagen gene has been found. Type II collagen is the major structural component of secondary vitreous.

A significant percentage of patients with Stickler syndrome also have the Pierre Robin sequence of cleft palate, small mandible, and backward displacement of the tongue. These patients can be detected in infancy because of their vulnerability to serious respiratory and feeding problems, but others with only ophthalmic defects may go unrecognized until later in childhood. The ophthalmic manifestations are frequent and vision-threatening. Myopia, usually of a high degree, is the most common finding, and it is often associated with a radial type of lattice retinal degeneration with pigment clumping around the retinal vessels. There is a high incidence of retinal detachment with large retinal breaks and proliferative vitreoretinopathy. Angle anomalies, ectopia lentis, cataracts, ptosis, and strabismus are less frequently associated. The incidence of vitreous loss during cataract surgery is high, as is the rate of subsequent retinal detachments. When possible, retinal folds and breaks should be treated before cataract extraction.

Early diagnosis may aid in preventing some of the severe complications of the ocular pathology and allow treatment of mild joint involvement. Although the arthropathy may not be symptomatic initially, these children often show radiographic abnormalities of long bones and joints. Progressive deafness may also develop.

Snead MP, Payne SJ, Barton DE, et al. Stickler syndrome: correlation between vitreoretinal phenotypes and linkage to COL 2A1. *Eye.* 1994;8:609–614.

Vandenberg P. Molecular basis of heritable connective tissue disease. *Biochem Med Metab Biol.* 1993;49:1–12.

Familial Exudative Vitreoretinopathy

Both vitreous traction and posterior vitreous detachment are present in *familial exudative vitreoretinopathy (FEVR).* The peripheral retina shows lack of vascularization and white areas with and without pressure. Thick peripheral exudates develop both in and under the retina. The combined effect of exudates and vitreous membranes results in retinal traction and subsequent retinal break. Early signs include decreased vision from retinal detachment and cataract. Family members can show marked variation of severity, from minimal straightening of vessels and peripheral nonperfusion to total retinal detachment. Some patients have bilateral retinal folds. The differential diagnosis includes ROP and Coats disease.

The disease is usually autosomal dominant as a result of a mutation of the *FEVR1* locus on chromosome 11. X-linked transmission has also been reported in families with a defect in the same gene that causes Norrie disease and primary retinal dysplasia. Autosomal recessive inheritance has also been reported. Cryopexy, photocoagulation, retinal detachment surgery, vitrectomy, and cataract surgery have all been used to manage this disorder.

Shastry BS, Hejtmancik JF, Trese MT. Identification of novel missense mutations in the Norrie disease gene associated with one X-linked and four sporadic cases of familial exudative vitreoretinopathy. *Hum Mutat.* 1997;9:396–401.

Norrie Disease

Norrie disease is an X-linked disorder characterized by bilateral congenital blindness associated with varying degrees of hearing impairment and mental retardation. Affected boys are typically born blind, although the external ocular appearance may initially be normal. During the first few days or weeks of life, a yellowish retinal detachment appears bilaterally, followed by a whiter mass behind the clear lens. Over time, the lenses, and later the cornea, opacify; phthisis bulbi may ensue by age 10 years or earlier. Before the end stage is reached, the retina shows dysplasia histopathologically. DNA testing is possible for genetic counseling.

Mintz-Hittner HA, Ferrell RE, Sims KB, et al. Peripheral retinopathy in offspring of carriers of Norrie disease gene mutations. Possible transplacental effect of abnormal Norrin. *Ophthalmology.* 1996;103:2128–2134.

Goldmann-Favre Vitreoretinal Dystrophy

Goldmann-Favre vitreoretinal dystrophy consists of vitreous strands and veils as well as foveal and peripheral retinoschisis. The fundus may appear similar to those seen in retinitis pigmentosa, including optic nerve pallor and attenuation of the retinal vessels. The pigmentary disturbance tends to be in a nummular, rather than a bone spicule, configuration; in some cases, little pigment is seen. Decreased central acuity and night blindness are prominent early findings in the second decade of life, and complicated cataracts subsequently develop. Inheritance is autosomal recessive.

Brown DM, Weingeist TA. Disorders of the vitreous and the vitreoretinal interface. In: Wright KW, ed. *Pediatric Ophthalmology and Strabismus.* St Louis: Mosby; 1995:467–476.

Systemic Diseases and Disorders With Retinal Manifestations

Diabetes Mellitus

Type 1, or *insulin-dependent, diabetes mellitus* was formerly called *juvenile-onset diabetes mellitus*. The prevalence of retinopathy in this condition is directly proportional to the duration of diabetes after puberty. Retinopathy rarely occurs less than 3 years after the onset of diabetes mellitus. Fundus photography or angiography reveals that about 50% of patients have nonproliferative (background) retinopathy after 7 years, although only half of these cases can be recognized by direct ophthalmoscopy. The prevalence of retinopathy increases to approximately 90% in patients who have had type 1 diabetes for 15 years or more. Proliferative diabetic retinopathy is rare in pediatric cases and is not covered in this section. For further discussion see BCSC Section 12, *Retina and Vitreous*.

A variety of nonproliferative changes may occur in the pediatric age group. These changes are thought to result from obstruction of retinal capillaries and abnormal capillary permeability. Microaneurysms are the first ophthalmoscopic sign; they may be followed by retinal hemorrhages, areas of retinal nonperfusion, cotton-wool spots, hard exudates, intraretinal microvascular abnormalities, and venous dilation. A rapid rise of blood glucose may produce myopia, and sudden reduction of blood glucose can induce hyperopia. Several weeks may be required before acuity returns to normal.

True diabetic cataracts are uncommon, occurring most often in patients with poorly controlled disease. Such cataracts resemble a snowstorm that affects the anterior and posterior cortices of young patients. Diabetic cataracts are caused by collection of sorbitol within the lens. Sorbitol concentration increases the lens osmolarity, leading to lens swelling and leakage of intralenticular contents. Diabetes mellitus, especially in young children, may be part of the DIDMOAD syndrome (*d*iabetes *i*nsipidus, *d*iabetes *m*ellitus, *o*ptic *a*trophy, and *d*eafness).

Management

Specific treatment is not indicated for nonproliferative retinopathy in children. A schedule of ophthalmic examinations proposed by the American Academy of Pediatrics includes an initial discussion between the parents and the endocrinologist regarding ocular complications and the need for surveillance; this discussion should take place within the first year after diagnosis of type 1 diabetes mellitus. An initial eye examination should be performed at age 9 if the glucose is poorly controlled or 3 years after puberty if glucose is well controlled, with annual follow-up examinations. Cataract surgery may be required if cataracts and vision do not improve after blood glucose levels are well controlled.

Leukemia

Ocular abnormalities occur in patients with leukemia. Retinopathy appears less often in children than in adults. Two series describe a poorer prognosis for children with ocular manifestations. Histopathologically, the choroid is the most frequently affected ocular tissue, but choroidal involvement is usually not apparent clinically. Indirect ophthalmoscopy sometimes reveals mildly pale fundus areas, but choroidal involvement is more accurately detected ultrasonically.

The most common eye findings are retinal hemorrhages, especially flame-shaped lesions in the nerve fiber layer. They involve the posterior fundus and can have some correlation with other aspects of the disease such as anemia, thrombocytopenia, or coagulation abnormalities. At times, these retinal hemorrhages have white centers similar to the hemorrhages described in pernicious anemia, subacute bacterial endocarditis, scurvy, and septicemia. These hemorrhages can also resemble those associated with intracranial hemorrhages and trauma in infants in that the white centers are fibrin thrombi. However, collections of leukocytes have also been found on histopathologic examination. Retinal hemorrhages have been reported as the first manifestation of leukemia. Other forms of retinal involvement include localized perivascular infiltrations, microinfarction, and discrete tumor infiltrations.

Optic nerve involvement is visible if the disc is infiltrated by leukemic cells (Fig 24-19). Translucent swelling of the disc obscures the normal landmarks; with florid involvement, only a white mass is visible in the region of the disc. A papilledema-like fundus picture may occur; such retrolaminar optic nerve involvement results in the loss of central vision. Therefore, a leukemic child with papilledema and a loss of central vision should be considered to have this complication. Early optic nerve involvement in leukemia constitutes a medical emergency because permanent loss of central vision is imminent. Generally, such patients should undergo radiation therapy as soon as possible. However, patients receiving cancer chemotherapy may be abnormally sensitive to radiation therapy; blinding optic nerve atrophy has been reported in some patients.

Leukemic infiltrates in the anterior segment may lead to heterochromia iridis; a change in the architecture of the iris; frank iris infiltrates; spontaneous hyphemas; leukemic cells in the anterior chamber; and hypopyon. Keratic precipitates may be seen, and some affected eyes develop glaucoma from tumor cells clogging the trabecular meshwork. Other possible glaucoma mechanisms include posterior synechiae formation, seclusion of the pupil, and pupillary block. Anterior chamber paracentesis for cytologic studies may be diagnostic in cases involving the anterior segment. Topical steroids and local irradiation are effective for anterior segment complications.

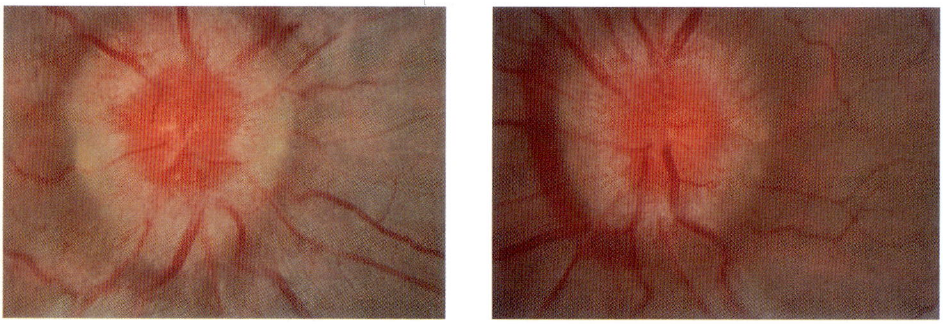

Figure 24-19 Leukemic infiltration of optic nerves, bilateral.

Leukemic involvement of the iris may be confused with juvenile xanthogranuloma. Methods for distinguishing between these 2 eye disorders of children include the following:

- biopsy of skin lesions of juvenile xanthogranuloma
- peripheral blood analysis
- bone marrow biopsy
- anterior chamber taps for cytologic studies

Leukemic infiltration of the orbit is relatively uncommon and is more characteristic of acute myelogenous leukemia. Orbital involvement may be difficult to distinguish from bacterial or fungal orbital cellulitis. Leukemic orbital infiltration may be best managed by radiation therapy. Ocular involvement is highly correlated with central nervous system involvement when the cerebrospinal fluid contains abnormal cells.

Kaikov Y. Optic nerve head infiltration in acute leukemia in children: an indication for emergency optic nerve radiation therapy. *Med Pediatr Oncol.* 1996;26:101–104.

Ohkoshi K, Tsiaras WG. Prognostic importance of ophthalmic manifestations in childhood leukaemia. *Br J Ophthalmol.* 1992;76:651–655.

Albinism

Albinism is a group of various conditions that involve the melanin system of the skin, eye, or both (Table 24-4; see also BCSC Section 12, *Retina and Vitreous*). The most common forms are oculocutaneous albinism (both tyrosinase-positive and tyrosinase-negative) and X-linked ocular albinism. The primary morbidity for most forms of albinism is ocular, so the ophthalmologist may be the physician who educates the family about heredity and skin protection from the sun.

The major ophthalmic findings in albinism are iris transillumination from decreased pigmentation, foveal aplasia or hypoplasia, and a characteristic deficit of pigment in the retina, especially peripheral to the posterior pole (Fig 24-20). Nystagmus, light sensitivity, high refractive errors, and reduced central acuity are often present, and visual acuity ranges from 20/40 to 20/200. If a child has significant foveal hypoplasia, nystagmus will begin at 2–3 months of life. The severity of the visual defect tends to be proportional to the degree of nystagmus. An abnormally large number of crossed fibers appear in the optic chiasm of patients and animals with albinism, precluding stereopsis and normal representation of space in the central nervous system. Asymmetric visually evoked cortical potentials reflect this abnormality.

All forms of albinism are heritable, and genetic counseling is important. Unlike other recessive disorders, the defective genes responsible for albinism are fairly common, so parents of the patients are usually not related. Different ethnic groups show large variations in incidence. Africans and African Americans have a much higher incidence than Caucasians but frequently have incomplete forms. Defects in the *P* gene are commonly the cause of albinism in people of African descent; mutations of the tyrosinase gene are more common in Caucasians. Albinism resulting from *P* gene mutations presents as nystagmus in a child with pigment but who is more lightly pigmented than expected for ethnicity and other family members. Because pigment is present, motor nystagmus is a

Table 24-4 Albinism

Disease	Ocular Manifestations	Systemic Manifestations	Inheritance
OCA1A (tyrosinase-negative)	Iris is thin, pale blue; characteristic orange reflex from the iris occurs because of marked transillumination defect; prominent choroidal vessels with poorly defined fovea; nystagmus; head-nodding; frequently myopic astigmatism and strabismus; vision 20/100–20/200; marked photophobia	White hair throughout life; tyrosinase absent, serum tyrosine levels normal; stage I and II melanosomes only; increased susceptibility to skin neoplasia	Autosomal recessive, chromosome 11q14–21; tyrosinase gene
OCA1B (with pigment)	At birth complete albinism with blue, translucent irides and albinotic fundal reflex; nystagmus and photophobia; increasing pigmentation with age	White hair and skin at birth; increasing pigmentation with yellow-red hair and light normal skin that tans; biochemically, intermediate reaction between tyrosinase positive and negative; stage III pheomelanosomes	Autosomal recessive; allelic with OCA1A; tyrosinase gene
OCA2 (tyrosinase-positive)	Eye color blue, yellow, or brown (age- and race-dependent); pigment cartwheel effect at pupil and limbus; transillumination minimal to absent in dark-skinned adults; moderate to severe nystagmus; photophobia; moderately severe visual defect; 20/80–20/100	Hair and skin color white at birth, darkening slightly by 2 years; melanosomes to early stage III polyphagosomes; hair bulbs develop pigmentation upon incubation in tyrosine; increased susceptibility to skin neoplasia; hyperkeratoses and freckling in exposed areas of skin	Autosomal recessive, chromosome 15q11.2–q12; *P* gene
Hermansky-Pudlak syndrome	Eye color blue-gray to brown (age- and race-dependent); iris normal to cartwheel effect; transillumination present in light-skinned individuals; mild to severe nystagmus and photophobia; slight to moderate decrease in visual acuity; high frequency in Puerto Rico	Platelet bleeding disorder, pulmonary fibrosis; hair color variable, white to dark red-brown; cream-colored skin; melanosis on exposed skin; pigmented nevi and freckles; susceptibility to skin neoplasia; serum tyrosine levels normal to decreased; platelet defect; ceroid storage, cytoplasmic bodies	Autosomal recessive, chromosome 10q2; *HPS1* gene *ADTB3A* gene
OCA3 (Brown)	Blue to brown irides; transillumination of irides; retinal hypopigmentation; nystagmus; strabismus	Skin and hair light brown; freckles present; areas of hypopigmentation	Autosomal recessive, *TRP-1* gene
Oculocerebral hypopigmentation (Cross syndrome)	Gray-blue eye color; cataracts; microphthalmos; nystagmus; blindness	White to light blond hair; white to pink skin; pigmented nevi; freckles; scanty melanosomes, stage III, some stage IV; oligophrenia; gingival fibromatosis; athetosis; urinary tract abnormalities	Autosomal recessive

Disease	Ocular Manifestations	Systemic Manifestations	Inheritance
Ocular	*X-linked form:* Marked deficiency of pigment in iris and choroid; nystagmus and myopic astigmatism; if darkly pigmented, may be limited to nystagmus, foveal hypoplasia, and tessellated fundus; mosaic pigment pattern in fundi	Normal pigmentation elsewhere; occasional hypopigmented cutaneous macules; giant melanosomes in normal skin; patients appear more lightly pigmented than their relatives	X-linked recessive, Xp22.3; *OA1* gene
	Autosomal recessive form: Ocular signs as above, females as severely affected as males, and obligate heterozygotes have normal fundi	May be the same as brown albinism	Autosomal recessive
Chédiak-Higashi syndrome	Partial albinism; diminished uveal and retinal pigmentation with photophobia and nystagmus	Early death from recurrent infections; silver tinge to hair; neutropenia with tendency toward lymphocytosis, anemia, and thrombocytopenia, hepatosplenomegaly, lymphadenopathy; leukemia, lymphoma	Autosomal recessive, chromosome 1q42–43; *LYST* gene
	On histologic examination: papilledema; lymphocytic infiltration of the optic nerve; leukocytes containing the typical metachromatic inclusion granules in the limbal area, iris, and choroid		
Temperature sensitive (OCA1TS)	Similar to findings for OCA1A	White hair on warmer parts of body including scalp, darker hair on extremities	Autosomal recessive, allelic with OCA1A form due to a temperature-sensitive tyrosinase
OCA1MP (minimal pigment)	Vision 20/50–20/200; some iris pigment develops; foveal hypoplasia and nystagmus	Minimal hair and skin pigment; low tyrosinase levels	Autosomal recessive
With deafness	Typical ocular changes	Typical albinism with nerve deafness	X-linked recessive
Dominant oculocutaneous	Fine diffuse pattern of depigmentation on irides	Hypomelanism of skin, hair	Autosomal dominant, very rare

Adapted and updated from Nelson LB, Calhoun JH, Harley RD, eds. *Pediatric Ophthalmology.* 3rd ed. Philadelphia: Saunders; 1991.

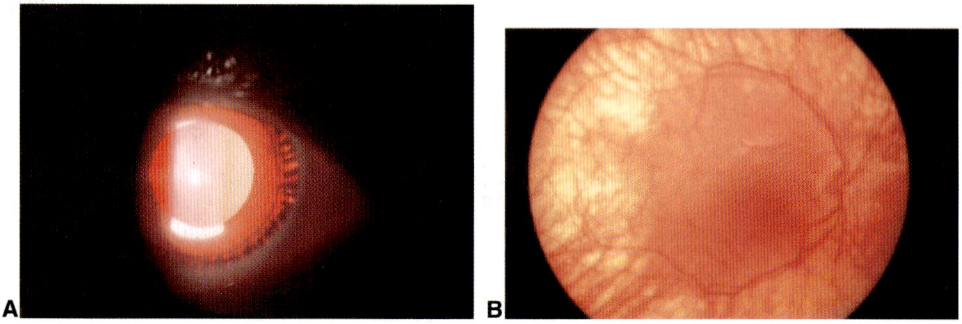

Figure 24-20 **A,** Transillumination of iris in albinism, right eye. **B,** Fundus in albinism, right eye, demonstrating complete lack of pigment and macular agenesis. In some incomplete forms of albinism, transillumination defects may be difficult to detect and retinal pigment may appear nearly normal, but the foveal reflex is absent.

common misdiagnosis. The pigment such patients possess, however, does not protect against ultraviolet damage, and skin cancer is common unless sunscreen and skin protection are used starting in childhood. All children with nystagmus should undergo a careful examination that looks for iris transillumination defects and macular hypoplasia, which are diagnostic, before motor nystagmus is diagnosed.

Most children with albinism can be mainstreamed into traditional schools with some assistance, but few see well enough to obtain a regular driver's license. Treatment is nonspecific and includes refraction, tinted glasses, and low vision aids for older patients. When either Chédiak-Higashi albinism syndrome (with susceptibility to infections) or Hermansky-Pudlak syndrome (bleeding diathesis, more common in people of Puerto Rican descent) is suspected, hematologic consultation is advised.

Dorey SE, Neveu MM, Burton LC, et al. The clinical features of albinism and their correlation with visual evoked potentials. *Br J Ophthalmol.* 2003;87:767–772.

Kerr R, Stevens G, Manga P, et al. Identification of P gene mutations in individuals with oculocutaneous albinism in sub-Saharan Africa. *Hum Mutat.* 2000;15:166–172.

Oetting WS, Summers CG, King RA. Albinism and the associated ocular defects. *Metab Pediatr Syst Ophthalmol.* 1994;17:5–9.

Familial Oculorenal Syndromes

Oculorenal syndromes include *Lowe (oculocerebral) syndrome.* This X-linked recessive disorder with renal defects presents in the first year of life, producing aminoaciduria, metabolic acidosis, proteinuria, hematuria, granular casts in the urine, and rickets. Affected children are mentally retarded, hypotonic, and areflexic. The biochemical defect is in a phosphatase important in Golgi complex vesicular transport. No specific treatment exists.

The most common eye defect is cataract. The lenses are small, thick, and opaque and may demonstrate posterior lenticonus. Congenital glaucoma may be present. Surgery is often difficult, with recurrent cyclitic membranes and recalcitrant glaucoma. Mothers of affected children may have punctate snowflake opacities within the lens cortex.

Lavin CW, McKeown CA. The oculocerebrorenal syndrome of Lowe. *Int Ophthalmol Clin.* 1993;33:179–191.

Alport syndrome is usually transmitted as an X-linked disorder but is autosomal recessive in approximately 10% of cases. It is a disorder of basement membranes that produces progressive renal failure, deafness, anterior lenticonus, cataract of the crystalline lens, and fleck retinopathy. Hematuria begins in childhood. Proteinuria and renal casts develop, with hypertension and kidney failure occurring late in the course of the disease. Mutations in collagen genes on the X chromosome or chromosome 2 are responsible for this disorder.

Colville D, Savige J, Morfis M, et al. Ocular manifestations of autosomal recessive Alport syndrome. *Ophthalmic Genet.* 1997;18:119–128.

Familial renal-retinal dystrophy is an autosomal recessive inherited condition characterized by interstitial nephritis and pigmentary retinal degeneration. Polyuria, polydipsia, and progressive azotemia are the rule. The eye signs and symptoms are characteristic of retinitis pigmentosa. Some patients who present early in life appear similar to those with Leber congenital amaurosis. Progressive anterior polar cataracts may be present.

Clarke MP, Sullivan TJ, Francis C, et al. Senior-Loken syndrome. Case reports of two siblings and association with sensorineural deafness. *Br J Ophthalmol.* 1992;76:171–172.

Warady BA, Cibis G, Alon V, et al. Senior-Loken syndrome: revisited. *Pediatrics.* 1994;94:111–112.

Ocular findings in *chronic renal disease* are often those of hypertensive retinopathy. Diffuse retinal and disc edema are common. Nonrhegmatogenous bullous retinal detachments, usually involving the inferior retina, may occur. Calcium salts may be deposited in the cornea and conjunctiva. Punctate stippling of the lens capsule occurs in many patients with chronic renal disease, and dense lens opacities develop in some patients. Steroid-induced glaucoma and cataract may follow transplantation. Cytomegalic inclusion retinitis and *Candida* retinitis may develop following renal transplantation.

Cherry-Red Spot

The appearance of a cherry-red spot in the macula is caused by loss of transparency of the perifoveal retina due to edema or deposition of abnormal materials in the retinal ganglion cells. Ophthalmologists are often consulted to determine whether a cherry-red spot is present, because such a spot may confirm the diagnosis of a number of disorders, especially some of the storage diseases. The most common causes of a cherry-red spot are

- Tay-Sachs disease (GM_2 gangliosidosis type I)
- Sandhoff disease (GM_2 gangliosidosis type II)
- Niemann-Pick disease
- sialidosis
- Farber lipogranulomatosis
- metachromatic leukodystrophy
- GM_1 gangliosidosis

- central retinal artery occlusion
- trauma (retinal edema) (See also BCSC Section 12, *Retina and Vitreous.*)

The cherry-red spot of storage diseases may disappear over time, so an absent spot should not be used to rule out a diagnosis, especially in older children. Even so, the presence of a cherry-red spot may be diagnostic. More detailed descriptions of the major storage diseases associated with a cherry-red spot follow.

Gangliosidoses

In *GM_1 type I gangliosidosis,* all 3 β-galactosidase isoenzymes (hexosaminidase A, B, and C) are absent. This severe disease often occurs with congenital edema and hepatosplenomegaly. A cherry-red spot is present in 50% of patients. Acuity is greatly diminished, and pendular nystagmus is present. Tortuous conjunctival vessels with saccular microaneurysms, optic atrophy, occasional corneal clouding, papilledema, and high myopia may be present. Other features of this disease include psychomotor retardation, hypotonia, Hurler-like facial features, kyphosis, and congestive heart failure. Affected children usually die by age 2 years.

In *GM_1 type II gangliosidosis (Derry disease),* β-galactosidase isoenzymes B and C are lacking. There is no cherry-red spot, but nystagmus, esotropia, pigmentary retinopathy, and optic atrophy have been observed. The first sign is locomotor ataxia followed by progressive psychomotor deterioration and seizures. Affected children are decerebrate and rigid by the end of their second year of life. Death occurs between the ages of 3 and 10.

GM_2 type I gangliosidosis (Tay-Sachs disease) is caused by a deficiency in isoenzyme hexosaminidase A. A foveal cherry-red spot is characteristic by age 6 months, and vision is reduced by age 12–18 months. The pathologic finding is the white ring resulting from accumulation of storage material in the ganglion cells around the normally pigmented macula. Nystagmus, optic atrophy, and narrowing of the retinal vessels develop. As the ganglion cells of the retina die, the cherry-red spot can disappear. Affected children become apathetic, hypotonic, and abnormally sensitive to sound. Seizures and progressive neurologic deterioration ensue, and patients usually die by age 24–30 months.

This disease is the most common of the gangliosidoses. It used to occur most often in persons of Eastern European Jewish (Ashkenazi) descent. An effective genetic screening and counseling program in that population has reduced the number of cases of Tay-Sachs disease by 90% in the United States. Other groups, such as French Canadians, can also be affected more often than the general population. The heterozygous condition can be identified so that carriers can be counseled, and the homozygous state can be diagnosed in utero by amniocentesis.

In *GM_2 type II gangliosidosis (Sandhoff disease),* hexosaminidase A and B are absent. Ocular findings include decreased visual acuity, strabismus, inconspicuous corneal clouding, a prominent cherry-red spot, and normal-appearing optic nerves. This disorder has an ocular and systemic course similar to that of Tay-Sachs disease. Hepatosplenomegaly is not a conspicuous feature. Most affected children die as a result of progressive psychomotor deterioration by the age of 2–12 years.

In *GM_2 type III gangliosidosis (Bernheimer-Seitelberger disease)*, hexosaminidase A is partially deficient. The eye findings include late-onset visual loss, optic atrophy, and pigmentary retinopathy. No cherry-red spot appears. The disorder begins in early childhood with progressive psychomotor retardation, locomotor ataxia, speech loss, and spasticity. This disease leads to death before the age of 15 years.

The causative genes for many of the gangliosidoses are known, and carrier detection and treatment strategies are evolving.

Many other subtypes of gangliosidoses, with differing genetic defects, occur. Most present later in life with motor problems, and few have cherry-red spots.

Chavany C, Jendoubi M. Biology and potential strategies for the treatment of GM2 gangliosidoses. *Mol Med Today.* 1998;4:158–165.

Kivlin JD, Sanborn GE, Myers GG. The cherry red spot in Tay-Sachs and other storage diseases. *Ann Neurol.* 1985;17:356–360.

SCREENING EXAMINATION OF PREMATURE INFANTS FOR RETINOPATHY OF PREMATURITY

A Joint Statement of the American Academy of Pediatrics, Section on Ophthalmology; The American Association for Pediatric Ophthalmology and Strabismus; and the American Academy of Ophthalmology

Abstract

This statement revises a previous statement on screening of premature infants for retinopathy of prematurity (ROP) published in 2001. ROP is a pathologic process that occurs only in immature retinal tissue and can progress to a tractional retinal detachment, which can result in functional or complete blindness. Recent development of peripheral retinal ablative therapy using laser photocoagulation has resulted in the possibility of markedly decreasing the incidence of this poor visual outcome, but the sequential nature of ROP creates a requirement that at-risk preterm infants be examined at proper times to detect the changes of ROP before they become permanently destructive. This statement presents the attributes on which an effective program for detecting and treating ROP could be based, including timing of initial examination and subsequent reexamination intervals.

Introduction

Retinopathy of prematurity (ROP) is a disorder of the developing retina of low birth weight preterm infants potentially leading to blindness in a small but significant percentage of those infants. In term infants, the retina is fully developed, and ROP cannot occur; however, in preterm infants, the development of the retina, which proceeds from the optic nerve head anteriorly during the course of gestation, is incomplete, the extent of the immature retina depending mainly on the degree of prematurity at birth. The Multicenter Trial of Cryotherapy for Retinopathy of Prematurity demonstrated the efficacy of peripheral retinal cryotherapy—that is, cryoablation of the immature, unvascularized peripheral retina—in reducing unfavorable outcomes. The study's 10-year follow-up report[1] confirmed these lasting benefits: unfavorable structural outcomes were reduced from 48% to 27%, and unfavorable visual outcomes (ie, best corrected visual acuity worse than 20/200) were reduced from 62% to 44%. Subsequently, laser photocoagulation has been used for peripheral retinal ablation with at least equal success.[2–5] Most recently, the Early Treatment for Retinopathy of Prematurity Randomized Trial confirmed the efficacy of treatment for severe ROP and redefined the indications for treatment.[6] Because of the sequential nature of ROP progression and the proven benefits of timely treatment in reducing the risk of visual loss, effective care now requires that at-risk infants receive carefully timed retinal examinations by an ophthalmologist experienced in the examination of preterm infants for ROP and that all pediatricians caring for these at-risk preterm infants be aware of this timing.

This statement outlines the principles on which a program to detect ROP in infants at risk might be based. The goal of an effective screening program must be to identify the relatively few preterm infants who require treatment for ROP from among the much larger number of at-risk infants while minimizing the number of stressful examinations required for these sick infants. Any screening program designed to implement an evolving standard of care has inherent defects, such as overreferral or underreferral, and cannot, by its very nature, duplicate the precision and rigor of a scientifically based clinical trial. With that in mind and on the basis of information published thus far, the sponsoring organizations of this statement suggest the following guidelines for the United States. It is important to recognize that other world locations could have very different screening parameters.[7]

Recommendations

1. Infants with birth weight of less than 1500 g or gestational age of 30 weeks* or less, as defined by the attending neonatologist, as well as selected infants with birth weight between 1500 and 2000 g or gestational age greater than 30 weeks* with an unstable clinical course, including those requiring cardiorespiratory support, who are believed by their attending pediatrician or neonatologist to be at high risk, should have retinal screening examinations performed after pupillary dilation using binocular indirect ophthalmoscopy to detect ROP. One examination is sufficient only if it unequivocally shows the retina to be fully vascularized in each eye. Effort should be made to minimize the discomfort and systemic effect of this examination by pretreatment of the eyes with a topical anesthetic agent, such as proparacaine; consideration may also be given to the use of pacifiers, oral sucrose, etc.
2. Retinal examinations in preterm infants should be performed by an ophthalmologist with sufficient knowledge and experience to enable accurate identification of the location and sequential retinal changes of ROP. The "International Classification of Retinopathy of Prematurity"[8] should be used to classify, diagram, and record these retinal findings at the time of examination.
3. The initiation of acute-phase ROP screening should be based on the infant's age. The onset of serious ROP correlates better with postmenstrual age (gestational

*Corrected per *Pediatrics*. 2006;118:1324. Erratum.

age at birth plus chronologic age) than with postnatal age.[9] That is, the youngest infants at birth take the longest time to develop serious ROP. This knowledge has been used previously in conducting a screening schedule.[10,11] Table 1 was developed from an evidence-based analysis of the Multicenter Trial of Cryotherapy for Retinopathy of Prematurity natural history data and confirmed by the Light Reduction in ROP Study conducted a decade later.[12] It represents a suggested schedule for timing of the initial eye examinations based on postmenstrual age and chronologic (postnatal) age to detect ROP before it becomes severe enough to result in retinal detachment while minimizing the number of potentially traumatic examinations.[13] Table 1 provides a schedule for detecting ROP potentially damaging to the retina with 99% confidence.

4. Follow-up examinations should be recommended by the examining ophthalmologist on the basis of retinal findings classified according to the international classification.[8] The following schedule is suggested (see Fig 1):

   1-Week or Less Follow-up
   - Stage 1 or 2 ROP – zone I
   - Stage 3 ROP – zone II

   1- to 2-Week Follow-up
   - Immature vascularization – zone I – no ROP
   - Stage 2 ROP – zone II
   - Regressing ROP – zone I

   2-Week Follow-up
   - Stage 1 ROP – zone II
   - Regressing ROP – zone II

Table 1 Timing of First Eye Examination Based on Gestational Age at Birth*

Gestational Age at Birth (wk)	Age at Initial Examination (wk) Postmenstrual	Age at Initial Examination (wk) Chronologic
22†	31	9
23†	31	8
24	31	7
25	31	6
26	31	5
27	31	4
28	32	4
29	33	4
30	34	4
31‡	35	4
32‡	36	4

*The table provides a schedule for detecting prethreshold ROP with 99% confidence, usually well before any required treatment.

†This guideline should be considered tentative rather than evidence based for infants with gestational age of 22 to 23 weeks because of the small number of survivors in these gestational age categories.

‡If necessary.

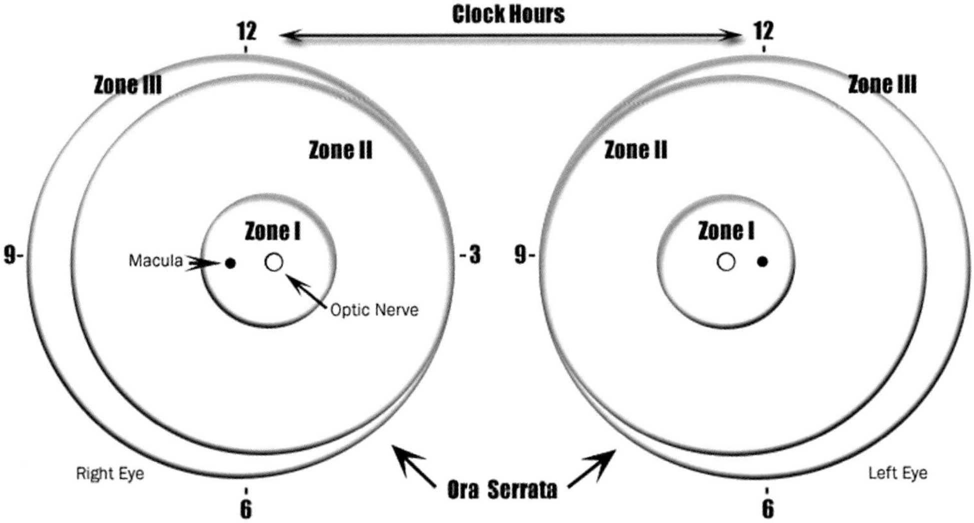

Figure 1 Scheme of retina of right eye (RE) and left eye (LE) showing zone borders and clock hours employed to describe location and extent of retinopathy of prematurity. Diagrammatic representation of the potential total area of the premature retina, with zone I, the most posterior, symmetrically surrounding the optic nerve head, the earliest to develop. A larger retinal area is present temporally (laterally) than nasally (medially), zone III. Only zones I and II are present nasally. The retinal changes discussed in recommendation 4 are usually recorded on a diagram such as this.

2- to 3-Week Follow-up

- Immature vascularization – zone II – no ROP
- Stage 1 or 2 ROP – zone III
- Regressing ROP – zone III

The presence of plus disease (defined as dilation and tortuosity of the posterior retinal blood vessels, see below) in zones I or II suggests that peripheral ablation, rather than observation, is appropriate.[13]

5. Practitioners involved in the ophthalmologic care of preterm infants should be aware that the retinal findings requiring strong consideration of ablative treatment have recently been revised according to the Early Treatment for Retinopathy of Prematurity Randomized Trial study.[6] The finding of threshold ROP, as defined in the Multicenter Trial of Cryotherapy for Retinopathy of Prematurity, may no longer be the preferred time of intervention.

   Treatment may also be initiated for the following retinal findings:

   - Zone I ROP – any stage with plus disease
   - Zone I ROP – stage 3 – no plus disease
   - Zone II – stage 2 or 3 with plus disease

   Plus disease is defined as a degree of dilation and tortuosity of the posterior retinal blood vessels as defined by a standard photograph.[8,14] Special care must be used in determining the zone of disease. The number of clock hours of disease may no longer be the determining factor in recommending ablative treatment. Treatment should generally be accomplished, when possible, within 72 hours of determination of treatable disease to minimize the risk of retinal detachment.

6. Conclusion of acute retinal screening examinations should be based on age and retinal ophthalmoscopic findings.[13] Findings that suggest that examinations can be curtailed include:
   - Zone III retinal vascularization attained without previous zone I or II ROP. If there is examiner doubt about the zone or if the postmenstrual age is less than 35 weeks, confirmatory examinations may be warranted.
   - Full retinal vascularization.
   - Postmenstrual age of 45 weeks and no prethreshold disease (defined as stage 3 ROP in zone II, any ROP in zone I) or worse ROP is present.
   - Regression of ROP.[15] Care must be taken to be sure there is no abnormal vascular tissue present capable of reactivation and progression.
7. Communication with the parents by members of the staff is very important. Parents should be aware of ROP examinations and should be informed if their child has ROP, with subsequent updates on ROP progression. The possible consequences of serious ROP should be discussed at the time a significant risk of poor visual outcome develops. Documentation of such conversations with parents in the nurse or physician notes is highly recommended.
8. Responsibility for examination and follow-up of infants at risk of ROP must be carefully defined by each neonatal intensive care unit. Unit-specific criteria with respect to birth weight and gestational age for examination for ROP should be established for each neonatal intensive care unit by consultation and agreement between neonatology and ophthalmology services. These criteria should be recorded and should automatically trigger ophthalmologic examinations. If hospital discharge or transfer to another neonatal unit or hospital is contemplated before retinal maturation into zone III has taken place, or if the infant has been treated by ablation for ROP and is not yet fully healed, the availability of appropriate follow-up ophthalmologic examination must be ensured, and specific arrangement for that examination must be made before such discharge or transfer occurs. The transferring primary physician, after communication with the examining ophthalmologist, should have the responsibility of communicating what eye examinations are needed and their required timing to the infant's new primary physician. The new primary physician should ascertain the current ocular examination status of the infant from the record and through communication with the transferring physician so that any necessary examinations by an ophthalmologist with ongoing experience and expertise in examination of preterm infants for ROP can be arranged promptly at the receiving facility or on an outpatient basis if discharge is contemplated before the need for continued examination has ceased, as outlined in recommendation 6. If responsibility for arranging follow-up ophthalmologic care after discharge is delegated to the parents, they should be

made to understand the potential for severe visual loss, including blindness; that there is a critical time window to be met if treatment is to be successful; and that timely follow-up examination is essential to successful treatment. This information should preferably be communicated both orally and in writing. If such arrangements for communication and follow-up after transfer or discharge cannot be made, the infant should not be transferred or discharged until appropriate follow-up examination can be arranged by the unit discharging the infant.

Pediatricians and other practitioners caring for infants who have had ROP, whether requiring treatment or not, should be aware that these infants may be at risk of other seemingly unrelated visual disorders, like strabismus, amblyopia, cataract, etc. Ophthalmologic follow-up for these potential problems after discharge from the neonatal intensive care unit is indicated.

THIS STATEMENT REPLACES THE PREVIOUS STATEMENT ON ROP FROM THE AMERICAN ACADEMY OF PEDIATRICS, AMERICAN ASSOCIATION FOR PEDIATRIC OPHTHALMOLOGY AND STRABISMUS, AND AMERICAN ACADEMY OF OPHTHALMOLOGY[16]; IS EVOLVING; AND MAY BE MODIFIED AS ADDITIONAL ROP RISK FACTORS, TREATMENTS, AND LONG-TERM OUTCOMES ARE KNOWN.

AAP Section on Ophthalmology, 2003–2004

Steven J. Lichtenstein, MD, Chairperson
Edward G. Buckley, MD
George S. Ellis, MD
Jane D. Kivlin, MD
Gregg T. Lueder, MD
James B. Ruben, MD
Gary T. Denslow, MD, Immediate Past Chairperson

Liaisons

Michael R. Redmond, MD
American Academy of Ophthalmology
Michael X. Repka, MD
American Association for Pediatric Ophthalmology and Strabismus
Kyle Arnoldi, CO
American Association of Certified Orthoptists

Staff

S. Niccole Alexander, MPP

Subcommittee on Retinopathy of Prematurity, 2003–2005

*Walter M. Fierson, MD, Chairperson
John Flynn, MD
William Good, MD
Dale L. Phelps, MD
James Reynolds, MD
Richard Saunders, MD

American Association for Pediatric Ophthalmology and Strabismus
American Academy of Ophthalmology

**Lead author*

References

1. Cryotherapy for Retinopathy of Prematurity Cooperative Group. Multicenter trial of cryotherapy for retinopathy of prematurity. Preliminary results. *Arch Ophthalmol.* 1988; 106:471–479.
2. Cryotherapy for Retinopathy of Prematurity Cooperative Group. Multicenter trial of cryotherapy for retinopathy of prematurity: ophthalmological outcomes at 10 years. *Arch Ophthalmol.* 2001;119:1110–1118.
3. McNamara JA, Tasman W, Brown GC, Federman JL. Laser photocoagulation for stage 3+ retinopathy of prematurity. *Ophthalmology.* 1991;98:576–580.
4. Hunter DG, Repka MX. Diode laser photocoagulation for threshold retinopathy of prematurity. A randomized study. *Ophthalmology.* 1993;100:238–244.
5. Laser ROP Study Group. Laser therapy for retinopathy of prematurity. *Arch Ophthalmol.* 1994;112:154–156.
6. Iverson DA, Trese MT, Orgel IK, Williams GA. Laser photocoagulation for threshold retinopathy of prematurity. *Arch Ophthalmol.* 1991;109:1342–1343.
7. Early Treatment for Retinopathy of Prematurity Cooperative Group. Revised indications for the treatment of retinopathy of prematurity. Results of the early treatment for retinopathy of prematurity randomized trial. *Arch Ophthalmol.* 2003;121:1684–1694.
8. Phan HM, Nguyen PN, Reynolds JD. Incidence and severity of retinopathy of prematurity in Vietnam, a developing middle-income country. *J Pediatr Ophthalmol Strabismus.* 2003;40:208–212.
9. The International Committee for the Classification of Retinopathy of Prematurity. The International Classification of Retinopathy of Prematurity revisited. *Arch Ophthalmol.* 2005;123:991–999.
10. Palmer EA, Flynn JT, Hardy RJ, et al. The Cryotherapy for Retinopathy of Prematurity Cooperative Group. Incidence and early course of retinopathy of prematurity. *Ophthalmology.* 1991;98:1628–1640.
11. LIGHT-ROP Cooperative Group. The design of the multicenter study of light reduction in retinopathy of prematurity (LIGHT-ROP). *J Pediatr Ophthalmol Strabismus.* 1999;36:257–263.
12. Hutchinson AK, Saunders RA, O'Neil JW, Lovering A, Wilson ME. Timing of initial screening examination in retinopathy of prematurity. *Arch Ophthalmol.* 1998;116:608–612.
13. Reynolds JD, Hardy RJ, Kennedy KA, Spencer R, van Heuven WA, Fielder AR. Light Reduction in Retinopathy of Prematurity (LIGHT-ROP) Cooperative Group. Lack of efficacy of light reduction in preventing retinopathy of prematurity. *N Engl J Med.* 1998; 338:1572–1576.
14. Reynolds JD, Dobson V, Quinn GE, et al. CRYO-ROP and LIGHT-ROP Cooperative Groups. Evidence-based screening criteria for retinopathy of prematurity: natural history data from the CRYO-ROP and LIGHT-ROP studies. *Arch Ophthalmol.* 2002;120:1470–1476.
15. Repka MX, Palmer EA, Tung B. Cryotherapy for Retinopathy of Prematurity Cooperative Group. Involution of retinopathy of prematurity. *Arch Ophthalmol.* 2000;118:645–659.
16. American Academy of Pediatrics, Section on Ophthalmology, American Academy of Ophthalmology, and American Association for Pediatric Ophthalmology and Strabismus. Screening examination of premature infants for retinopathy of prematurity. *Pediatrics.* 2001;108:809–811.

CHAPTER 25

Optic Disc Abnormalities

Developmental Anomalies

Morning Glory Disc Anomaly

A striking congenital abnormality of the optic disc and surrounding retina, *morning glory disc anomaly* is caused by either an abnormal closure of the embryonic fissure or abnormal development of the distal optic stalk at its junction with the primitive optic vesicle. Clinically, the anomaly appears as a funnel-shaped excavation of the posterior fundus that incorporates the optic disc. The surrounding retinal pigment epithelium is elevated, with an increased number of blood vessels looping at the edges of the disc (Fig 25-1). A central core of white glial tissue occupies the position of the normal cup. This tissue may have contractile elements, and the optic cup can actually be seen to open and close with some periodicity. Visual acuity can range anywhere from 20/20 to no light perception but in general is approximately 20/100 to 20/200. Serous retinal detachments can occur in approximately one third of affected patients, but the source of the subretinal fluid is unknown. Morning glory disc anomaly has been associated with basal encephalocele in patients with midfacial anomalies. Abnormalities of the carotid circulation can also be seen in patients with morning glory anomaly. Moyamoya disease is a well-described associated finding.

Coloboma of the Optic Nerve

Coloboma of the optic nerve may be part of a complete chorioretinal coloboma that involves the entire embryonic fissure, or the coloboma may involve only the optic disc. Mild optic disc colobomas resemble deep physiologic cupping and may be confused with

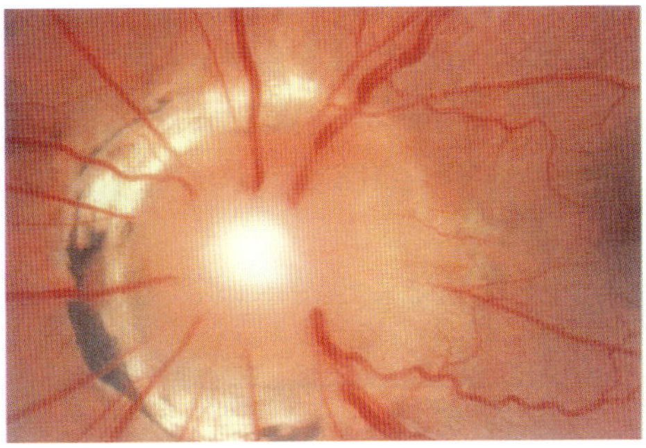

Figure 25-1 Morning glory disc anomaly, left eye.

glaucomatous damage. More extensive disorders appear as an enlargement of the peripapillary area with a deep central excavation lined by a glistening white tissue, with blood vessels crossing over the edge of this deep cavity (Fig 25-2). The defects usually extend inferonasally and are often associated with retinal coloboma in the periphery. Nonrhegmatogenous or rhegmatogenous retinal detachments may occur. This condition may be unilateral or bilateral and can be very asymmetric. Visual acuity may be mildly or severely decreased and is difficult to predict from the optic disc appearance. Ocular colobomas may also be accompanied by multiple systemic abnormalities (eg, CHARGE association: *c*oloboma, *h*eart, choanal *a*tresia, mental *r*etardation, *g*enitourinary abnormalities, and *e*ar abnormalities; see Chapter 20).

Brodsky MC. Congenital optic disk anomalies. *Surv Ophthalmol.* 1994;39:89–112.

Massaro M, Thorarensen O, Liu GT, et al. Morning glory disc anomaly and moyamoya vessels. *Arch Ophthalmol.* 1998;116:253–254.

Myelinated (Medullated) Retinal Nerve Fibers

Normal myelination starts at the lateral geniculate ganglion and stops at the lamina cribrosa. Occasionally, some of the fibers in the retina acquire a myelin sheath. Clinically, this appears as a white superficial retinal area with frayed and feathered edges that tends to follow the same orientation as the normal retinal nerve fibers (Fig 25-3). Retinal vessels that pass within the superficial layer of the nerve fibers are obscured. The myelinated fibers may occur as a single spot or as several noncontiguous isolated patches. The most common location is along the disc margin. Visual loss can occur from macular involvement or from unilateral high myopia and amblyopia. In these cases, the macula can also be hypoplastic. Treatment for amblyopia should be attempted but is often unsuccessful. Absolute scotomata correspond to the area of the myelination.

Straatsma BR, Heckenlively JR, Foos RY, et al. Myelinated retinal nerve fibers associated with ipsilateral myopia, amblyopia, and strabismus. *Am J Ophthalmol.* 1979;88:506–510.

Tilted Disc Syndrome

In *tilted disc syndrome*, or *Fuchs coloboma*, the superior pole of the optic disc may appear elevated with posterior displacement of the inferior nasal disc, or the disc can be hori-

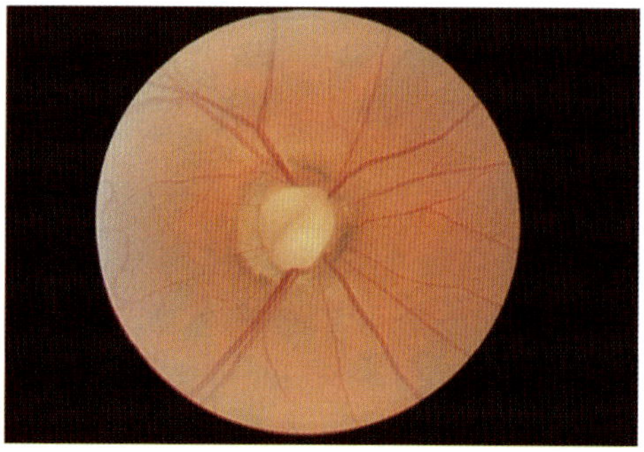

Figure 25-2 Optic nerve coloboma, right eye.

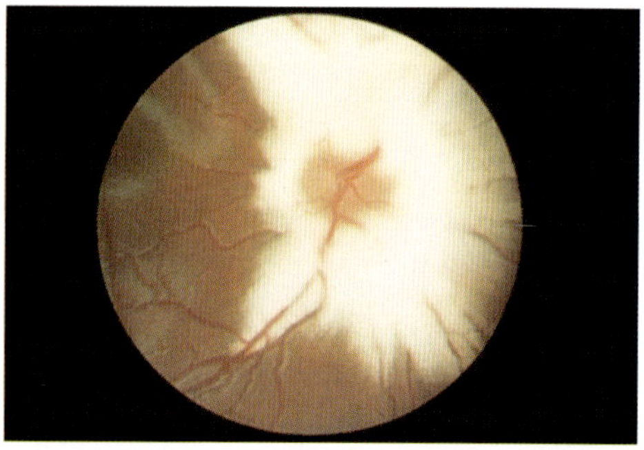

Figure 25-3 Myelinated nerve fibers of optic nerve and retina, right eye.

zontally tilted, resulting in an oval-appearing optic disc with an obliquely oriented long axis (Fig 25-4). This condition is often accompanied by a scleral crescent located inferiorly or inferonasally, situs inversus (a nasal detour of the temporal retinal vessels as they emerge from the disc before turning back temporally), and posterior ectasia of the inferior nasal fundus. Many affected eyes are myopic.

Because of the fundus abnormality, affected patients have myopic astigmatism with the plus axis oriented parallel to the ectasia. Patients may demonstrate a bitemporal hemianopia, which is typically incomplete and preferentially involves the superior quadrants. The hemianopia can usually be distinguished from a chiasmal lesion because the defect does not respect the vertical midline. Large and small isopters are fairly normal; medium-sized isopters are severely constricted. Appropriate refractive correction often results in elimination of the visual field defect. Tilted discs, myopic astigmatism, bilateral decreased vision, and visual difficulty at night should suggest the possibility of X-linked congenital stationary night blindness (see Chapter 24).

Bergmeister Papillae

To varying extents, the hyaloid artery may not be resorbed before birth. The entire artery may remain as a fine thread or cord extending from the optic disc to the lens and can be associated with *persistent fetal vasculature* (formerly called *persistent hyperplastic primary vitreous*). The hyaloid artery may be patent and contain blood where it was attached to the posterior lens capsule. In mild cases, the attachment to the posterior lens capsule is located inferonasally (Mittendorf dot) and is usually visually insignificant. When all that remains of the hyaloid artery is glial tissue on the disc in association with avascular prepapillary veils and epipapillary membranes, the term *Bergmeister papillae* is used.

Megalopapilla

Megalopapilla features an abnormally large optic disc diameter and is often associated with an increased cup–disc ratio that can be confused with normal-tension glaucoma. Visual acuity is usually normal or slightly decreased, and visual fields may demonstrate a slightly enlarged blind spot. Rarely, megalopapilla has been associated with optic nerve glioma. The condition can be unilateral or bilateral, and the cause is unknown.

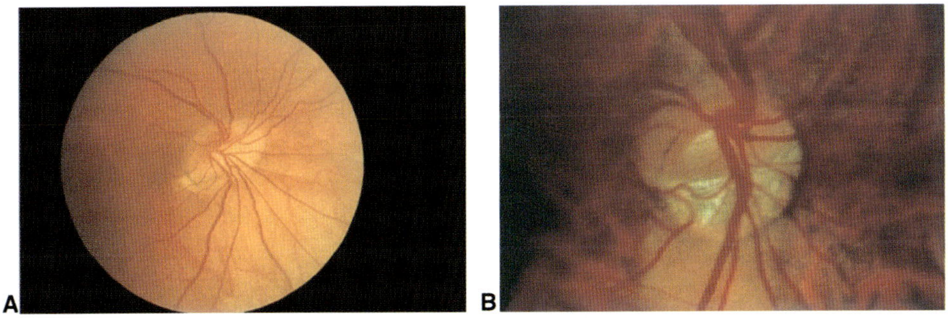

Figure 25-4 Tilted disc syndrome. **A,** Right eye. **B,** Magnified view of right eye (different patient).

Optic Nerve Hypoplasia

Histologically, optic nerve hypoplasia is characterized by a decreased number of optic nerve axons. Clinically, the disc is pale and smaller than normal. This condition can be unilateral or bilateral and is often asymmetric. It may be associated with a yellow to white ring around the disc *(double ring sign)* (Fig 25-5). Because the size of the surrounding ring often corresponds to the normal disc diameter, careful observation is necessary to avoid mistaking the entire hypoplastic disc/ring complex for a normal-sized disc. The vascular pattern is also abnormal and can be associated with too few or too many disc vessels. Retinal vascular tortuosity is common.

Visual acuity ranges from normal to light perception, and visual field defects are invariably present. Visual acuity is related to the integrity of the macular fibers and often does not correlate with the overall size of the disc. Because patients with optic nerve hypoplasia often also have strabismus, unilateral visual loss may result from amblyopia and may respond to patching therapy.

The cause of optic nerve hypoplasia is multifactorial. Usually, this condition results from an insult in the first trimester as the optic nerves are developing. Any intrauterine damage to the visual pathway can result in optic nerve hypoplasia. Segmental hypoplasia occurs in some children of mothers with insulin-dependent diabetes.

Optic nerve hypoplasia has been associated with midline central nervous system anomalies consisting of absence of the septum pellucidum and agenesis of the corpus callosum. Septo-optic dysplasia *(de Morsier syndrome)* is occasionally accompanied by manifestations of hypothalamic and pituitary dysfunction, such as growth hormone deficiency, neonatal hypoglycemia, diabetes insipidus, panhypopituitarism, hyperprolactinemia, and hypothyroidism.

MRI is preferred for evaluating central nervous system abnormalities in patients with optic nerve hypoplasia. These abnormalities include small intracranial optic nerves, absent septum pellucidum, agenesis of the corpus callosum, and cerebral hemisphere abnormalities such as schizencephaly, leukomalacia, or encephalomalacia. Absence of the septum pellucidum or agenesis of the corpus callosum is not detectable by clinical evaluation. Neurodevelopmental defects, when present, are usually the result of associated cerebral hemispheric abnormalities.

During MRI, special attention should be directed to the pituitary infundibulum, where ectopia of the posterior pituitary may be found. Posterior pituitary ectopia appears

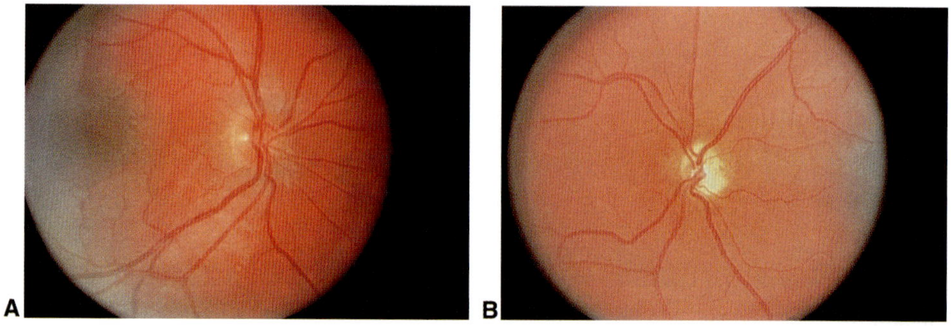

Figure 25-5 Optic nerve hypoplasia. **A,** Normal right optic nerve. **B,** Hypoplastic left optic nerve.

on MRI as an absence of the pituitary infundibulum, with an abnormal bright spot at the upper infundibulum area. This abnormality is present in approximately 15% of patients and suggests posterior pituitary hormone deficiency, requiring further endocrinologic workup.

Laboratory evaluation of patients with optic nerve hypoplasia is directed by their clinical appearance and MRI findings. A history of neonatal jaundice suggests hypothyroidism; neonatal hypoglycemia or seizures indicates possible panhypopituitarism. Patients with optic nerve hypoplasia and diabetes insipidus can have significant problems with thermal regulation and must be monitored carefully during febrile illnesses. A referral to a pediatric endocrinologist should be considered for these patients.

Children with *periventricular leukomalacia (PVL)* display an unusual form of optic nerve hypoplasia. The optic nerves demonstrate a large cup within a normal-sized optic disc. This form of optic nerve hypoplasia occurs secondary to transsynaptic degeneration of optic axons caused by bilateral lesions in the optic radiation (PVL).

Birkebaek NH, Patel L, Wright NB, et al. Endocrine status in patients with optic nerve hypoplasia: relationship to midline central nervous system abnormalities and appearance of the hypothalamic-pituitary axis on magnetic resonance imaging. *J Clin Endocrinol Metab.* 2003;88:5281–5286.

Brodsky MC, Glasier CM. Optic nerve hypoplasia. Clinical significance of associated central nervous system abnormalities on magnetic resonance imaging. *Arch Ophthalmol.* 1993;111:66–74.

Hoyt WF, Kaplan SL, Grumbach MM, et al. Septo-optic dysplasia and pituitary dwarfism. *Lancet.* 1970;1:893–894.

Optic Nerve Aplasia

Optic nerve aplasia is rare. There are no optic nerve or retinal blood vessels, making the choroidal pattern clearly visible.

Optic Pits or Holes

Optic pits (Fig 25-6) are usually unilateral and typically appear in the inferotemporal quadrant or central portion of the disc. A pit may be shallow or very deep, and it is often covered with a gray veil of tissue. Optic pits have been associated with serous retinal detachments occurring mainly during the second and third decades of life.

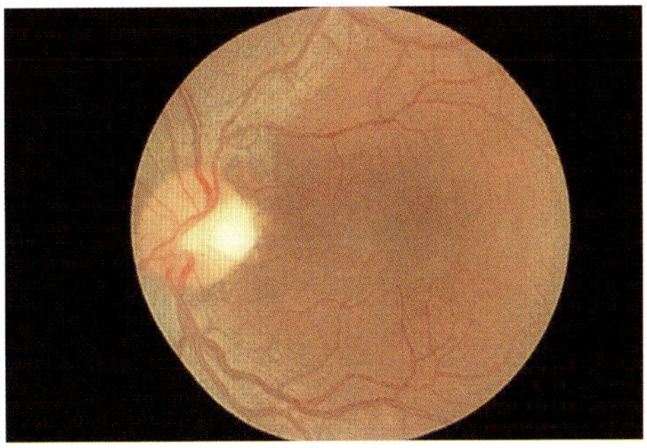

Figure 25-6 Temporal optic nerve pit with serous retinal detachment, left eye.

Peripapillary Staphyloma

Peripapillary staphyloma is a posterior bulging of the sclera in which the optic disc occupies the bottom of the bowl. The disc may be normal but is surrounded by stretched choroid, thereby exposing the white sclera encircling the disc. Visual acuity is usually poor.

Optic Atrophy

Optic atrophy in children usually results from anterior visual pathway disease (Table 25-1) such as inflammation (optic neuritis), hereditary optic atrophy, perinatal asphyxia, hydrocephalus, and optic nerve tumors. The workup should include neuroimaging in all cases of uncertain cause (negative family history, normal neurologic examination results), because a tumor or hydrocephalus is present in over 40% of these cases.

Dominant Optic Atrophy

Bilateral slow loss of central vision in childhood may be due to dominant optic atrophy. This condition usually begins before the age of 10 years with mild visual loss, ranging from 20/40 to 20/100. Visual fields show central or cecocentral scotomata with normal peripheral isopters. Color vision testing may be diagnostic, revealing a tritan dyschromatopsia. Clinically, the optic disc shows temporal pallor with an area of triangular excavation. Inheritance is usually autosomal dominant but can be recessive, and family pedigrees may be hard to elicit. Long-term prognosis is good, with visual function rarely reduced to the 20/200 level.

A rare recessive optic atrophy can occur with severe bilateral visual loss before age 5. Nystagmus is present in approximately half of these patients. Funduscopic examination reveals a pale optic disc with vascular attenuation of the type characteristically seen in retinal degeneration. ERG results are normal, however.

Behr Optic Atrophy

A hereditary disorder, Behr optic atrophy occurs mainly in males, with onset in childhood. This condition is associated with increased deep tendon reflexes, cerebellar ataxia, bladder dysfunction, mental retardation, hypotonia of the extremities, and external ophthalmoplegia.

Leber Hereditary Optic Neuropathy

A maternally inherited (mitochondrial) disease, Leber hereditary optic neuropathy (LHON) is characterized by acute or subacute bilateral loss of central vision, acquired red-green dyschromatopsia, and central or cecocentral scotomata in otherwise healthy patients (usually males) in their second to fourth decade of life. Progressive atrophy results in a flat, pale disc with a dense central scotoma. Clinically, this disorder presents as a low-grade optic neuritis with circumpapillary telangiectasia, pseudoedema of the disc, and absence of fluorescein staining. Pallor of the entire disc indistinguishable from primary atrophy generally develops within a few weeks after onset of visual disturbance.

Final visual acuity is rarely better than 20/200. Associated neurologic abnormalities may include paraplegia, dementia, deafness, migraines, vertigo, spasticity, and a cardiac preexcitation arrhythmia (Wolff-Parkinson-White) syndrome.

LHON is transmitted by female carriers and involves the mitochondrial DNA (mtDNA). The majority of cases are associated with point mutations in the mitochondrial genome responsible for complex I (NADH: ubiquinone oxidoreductase). Molecular genetic analysis of mtDNA from leukocytes is currently available, and the finding of a primary mutation is pathognomonic for the disease. No effective treatment exists, although a small percentage of patients will demonstrate spontaneous improvement.

Optic Neuritis

Optic neuritis in childhood frequently presents after systemic infections such as measles, mumps, chickenpox, and viral illnesses (Fig 25-7). It can also be associated with immunizations. Visual loss can be severe and is often bilateral. In over half of affected children, the history suggests central nervous system involvement including headache,

Table 25-1 Causes of Acquired Optic Atrophy in Childhood

Craniopharyngioma
Optic nerve/chiasmal glioma
Retinal degenerative disease
Hydrocephalus
Optic neuritis
Postpapilledema
Hereditary

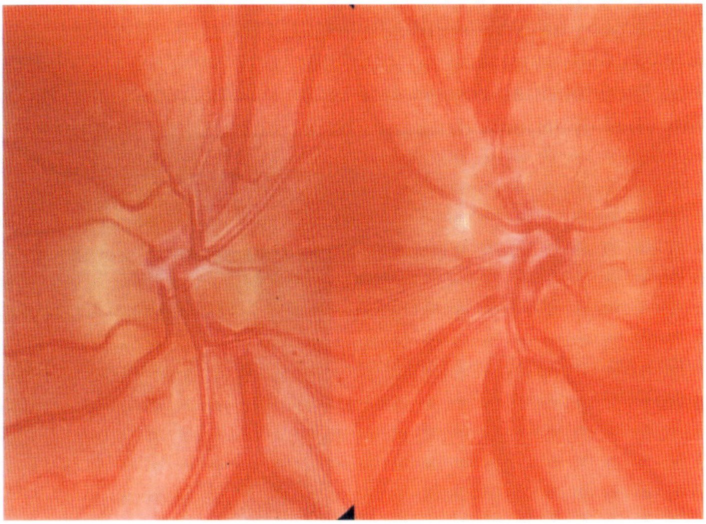

Figure 25-7 Optic neuritis, left eye. *(Photograph courtesy of Edward G. Buckley, MD.)*

nausea, vomiting, lethargy, or malaise. Disc swelling, when present, can be extensive and may result in a macular star formation (Leber idiopathic stellate neuroretinitis; Fig 25-8).

The cause of this postinfectious form of viral optic neuritis is unknown. It has been speculated that a presumed autoimmune process, triggered by previous viral infection, may result in a demyelinative injury.

The relationship between optic neuritis and the development of multiple sclerosis, which is common in adults, is less clear in children. A small subset of children with optic neuritis develops signs and symptoms consistent with multiple sclerosis within 1 year. Most of the neurologic deficits are minor, but disability can be severe.

Treatment of optic neuritis in children remains controversial. The Optic Neuritis Treatment Trial did not specifically address the issue of treatment in children. Optic neuritis in the pediatric population is a different clinical entity so it is difficult to apply the results of this study to children. BCSC Section 5, *Neuro-Ophthalmology*, discusses the treatment of optic neuritis and the relationship between optic neuritis and multiple sclerosis.

Papilledema

Increased intracranial pressure in children can be caused by hydrocephalus from a mass lesion or from pseudotumor cerebri. A full evaluation, including neuroimaging and lumbar puncture, is indicated. In infants, increased intracranial pressure results in firmness and distension of the open fontanelles. Significantly elevated pressure is usually accompanied by nausea, vomiting, and headaches. The older child may experience transient visual obscurations. Esotropia and diplopia may result from injury to the sixth nerve, which usually resolves once intracranial pressure is reduced.

Pseudotumor Cerebri

Pseudotumor cerebri, or *idiopathic intracranial hypertension*, consists of increased intracranial pressure of unknown cause and duration. The presenting symptoms are headache and visual loss. Pseudotumor cerebri can occur in children of any age and has been associated with viral infections, drug use (tetracycline, corticosteroids, vitamin A, and

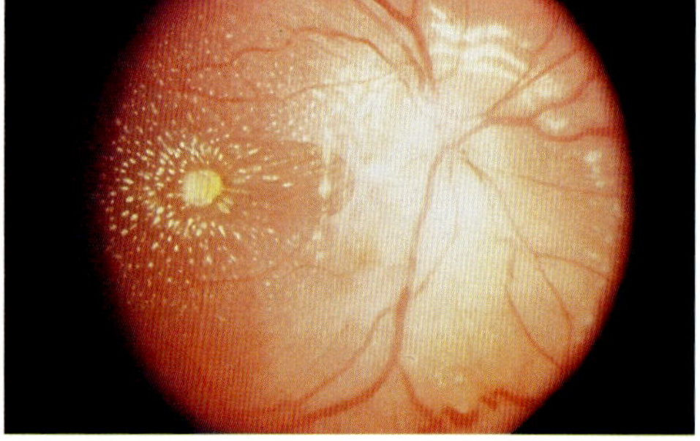

Figure 25-8 Leber idiopathic stellate neuroretinitis.

nalidixic acid), thyroid medications, growth hormone, and venous sinus thrombosis. Often the cause is not determined. Ocular examination reveals excellent visual acuity with marked swelling of both optic nerves. The patient should be monitored closely for signs of visual loss and worsening headaches. Medical treatments include acetazolamide and corticosteroids. Repeated lumbar punctures have been used to control intracranial pressure, and optic nerve sheath fenestration has been shown to reduce the incidence of visual loss. Severe cases require lumbar or ventricular shunts. The visual prognosis is excellent, although loss of vision can occur secondary to chronic papilledema; spontaneous resolution occurs in most cases within 12–18 months.

Pseudopapilledema

Pseudopapilledema refers to any elevated anomaly of the optic disc that resembles papilledema (Table 25-2). Disc anomalies that are frequently confused with papilledema in children include drusen, hyperopia, and prominent glial tissue. Pseudopapilledema can be differentiated from true papilledema by the absence of associated venous dilation and retinal hemorrhages or exudates and by the lack of any systemic findings that are usually associated with increased intracranial pressure.

Table 25-2 Conditions Associated With Pediatric Optic Disc Swelling

Papillitis
Optic neuritis (postinfectious)
Toxoplasmosis
Lyme disease
Bartonella infection
Neuroretinitis
Leber hereditary optic neuropathy
Toxocara infection of disc
Papilledema
Intracranial mass
Pseudotumor cerebri
Dural sinus thrombosis
Hypertension
Cranial synostosis
Hydrocephalus
Chiari malformation
Aqueductal stenosis
Dandy-Walker syndrome
Infection
Astrocytoma of optic disc (tuberous sclerosis)
Optic disc drusen
Hyperopia
Glial veils
Leukemia infiltrate

Drusen

Interpapillary drusen, which are the most common cause of pseudopapilledema in children, can appear within the first or second decade of life (Fig 25-9). Drusen are frequently inherited, and examination of the parents is helpful when drusen are suspected in children.

Clinically, the elevated disc does not obscure the retinal arterioles lying anteriorly and often has an irregular border suggesting the presence of drusen beneath the surface. There is no pallor, dilation of the papillary network, exudates, or hemorrhages. When drusen are not buried, they appear as shiny refractile bodies visible on the surface, with a gray-yellow translucent appearance. Visual defects are frequently associated; lower nasal field defects are most common. However, central defects, an arcuate scotoma, and concentric narrowing can also occur. These defects can be slowly progressive, and central visual acuity is rarely affected.

Although some patients with drusen can be identified by funduscopic evaluation, occasionally it is difficult to tell for certain that drusen are responsible for the swollen disc appearance. B-scan ultrasonography can be helpful in this situation. This technique permits detection of bright objects in the end of the optic nerve. CT can also detect these drusen.

Auw-Haedrich C, Staubach F, Witschel H. Optic disk drusen. *Surv Ophthalmol.* 2002;47: 515–532.

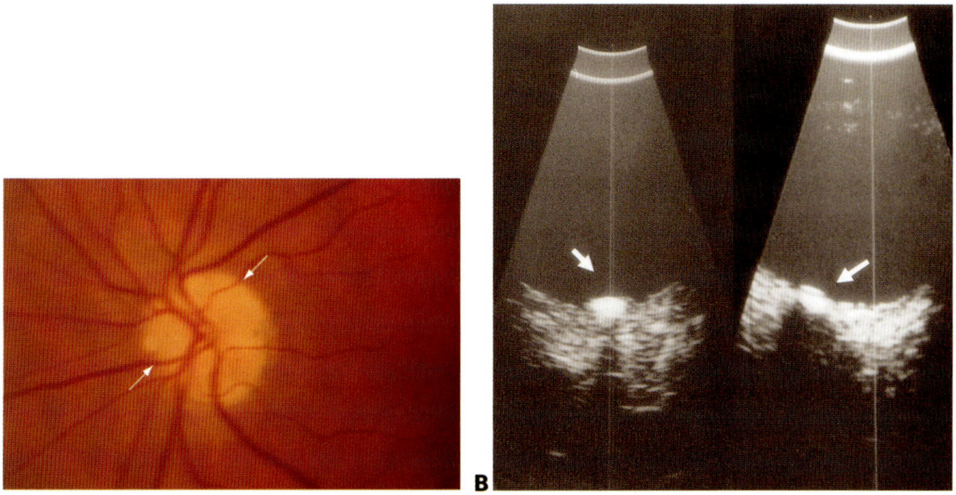

A B

Figure 25-9 **A,** Fundus photograph of optic nerve head drusen seen as refractile opacities on disc surface *(arrows).* **B,** Ultrasound image of bright spot in nerve *(arrows)* consistent with drusen. *(Part A reprinted from Volpe NJ, Liu GT, Galetta SL. Idiopathic intracranial hypertension [IIH, pseudotumor cerebri].* Focal Points: Clinical Modules for Ophthalmologists. *San Francisco: American Academy of Ophthalmology; 2004, module 3; part B photograph courtesy of Edward G. Buckley, MD.)*

CHAPTER 26

Ocular and Periocular Tumors in Childhood

Ocular and orbital tumors, both benign and malignant, occur relatively frequently in infants and children. Benign masses are much more common than malignant ones. Ocular and orbital tumors can be classified by location and type (Table 26-1). See also BCSC Section 4, *Ophthalmic Pathology and Intraocular Tumors.*

Shields JA, Shields CL. Pediatric ocular and periocular tumors. *Pediatr Ann.* 2001;30:491–501.

Orbital Tumors

A wide variety of space-occupying lesions can develop in the region of the orbit during childhood. Several of the most important pediatric malignancies show a predilection for orbital involvement. Benign (nonmalignant) adnexal masses are common and, in many cases, constitute a threat to vision. BCSC Section 7, *Orbit, Eyelids, and Lacrimal System,* and Section 4, *Ophthalmic Pathology and Intraocular Tumors,* also discuss and illustrate orbital tumors.

Differential Diagnosis

The diagnosis of space-occupying lesions in the orbit is a particular challenge because the clinical manifestations of these lesions are both nonspecific and relatively limited in variety:

- proptosis or other displacement of the globe
- swelling or discoloration of the eyelids
- palpable subcutaneous mass
- ptosis
- strabismus

The problem of differential diagnosis in childhood is compounded by the fact that in young patients, both benign and malignant tumors often enlarge very rapidly, making them difficult to distinguish from one another; from infectious and inflammatory disorders such as orbital cellulitis; and from the effects of trauma, which occurs with high frequency and often without a reliable history. Furthermore, mild to moderate proptosis can be difficult to detect in an uncooperative child with associated eyelid swelling.

Table 26-1 Ocular and Orbital Tumor Classification

- **I. Orbital lesions**
  - A. Cystic lesions
    - 1. Developmental orbital cysts
      - a. Choristoma, dermoid, epidermoid
      - b. Teratoma
      - c. Congenital cystic eye
      - d. Colobomatous cyst
    - 2. Acquired orbital cysts
      - a. Cystic vascular lesions
      - b. Epithelial appendage cysts
      - c. Epithelial implantation cysts
      - d. Lacrimal duct cysts
      - e. Optic nerve sheath meningocele
      - f. Hematic cyst
      - g. Aneurismal bone cyst
      - h. Cystic myositis
      - i. Parasitic cysts: hydatid, cysticercus cellulosae
      - j. Chocolate cyst
      - k. Cholesterol granulomatous cyst
    - 3. Adjacent structure cysts
      - a. Mucocele
      - b. Mucopyocele
      - c. Dacryocele
      - d. Cephalocele
      - e. Enterogenous cysts
      - f. Dentigerous cysts
  - B. Vascular lesions
    - 1. Capillary hemangioma
    - 2. Cavernous hemangioma
    - 3. Lymphangioma
    - 4. Orbital varix
    - 5. Arteriovenous malformation
    - 6. Hemangiopericytoma
    - 7. Malignant hemangioendothelioma
    - 8. Organizing hematoma (hematic cysts, cholesterol granuloma)
    - 9. Sturge-Weber syndrome
    - 10. Klippel-Trénaunay-Weber syndrome
  - C. Inflammatory masses
    - 1. Preseptal and orbital cellulitis
    - 2. Idiopathic orbital inflammatory syndrome
    - 3. Other orbital inflammatory syndromes
  - D. Histiocytia, hematopoietic, and lymphoproliferative masses
    - 1. Langerhans cell histiocytosis
      - a. Histiocytosis X
      - b. Hand-Schüller-Christian disease
      - c. Letterer-Siwe disease
    - 2. Juvenile xanthogranuloma (non–Langerhans cell histiocytosis)
    - 3. Sinus histiocytosis
    - 4. Leukemia and granulocytic sarcoma
    - 5. Lymphoma
  - E. Mesodermal tumors
    - 1. Fibroma
    - 2. Myofibromatosis
    - 3. Lipoma

(Continued)

Table 26-1 *(continued)*

4. Leiomyoma
5. Fibrous dysplasia
6. Juvenile ossifying fibroma
7. Giant cell (reparative) granuloma of bone
8. Aneurysmal bone cyst
9. Cartilagenous hamartoma
10. Sarcoma
    a. Osteogenic sarcoma
    b. Leiomyosarcoma
    c. Fibrosarcoma
    d. Malignant fibrous histiocytoma
    e. Alveolar soft part sarcoma
11. Rhabdomyosarcoma

F. Neurogenic tumor
1. Glioma
2. Meningioma
3. Neurofibroma
4. Schwannoma
5. Esthesioneuroblastoma
6. Paraganglioma
7. Melanotic neuroectodermal tumor of infancy

G. Lacrimal gland
1. Pleomorphic adenoma (benign mixed tumor)
2. Adenocarcinoma (malignant mixed tumor)

H. Metastatic
1. Neuroblastoma
2. Ewing sarcoma
3. Wilms tumor
4. Rhabdomyosarcoma (rarely)

II. Eyelid lesions

A. Chalazion
B. Hordeolum
C. Benign epithelial and appendage tumors: syringoma, porosyringoma, myoepithelioma, apocrine hidrocystoma (sudiferous cyst; originating from a blocked excretory duct of Moll's apocrine sweat gland), eccrine hydrocystoma (derived from lid eccrine sweat gland), sebaceous cyst (pilar cyst; retention cyst of the pilosebaceous structure), milia (cystic expansion of the pilosebaceous structure due to obstruction of the orifice), epidermal inclusion cyst, pilomatrixoma (calcifying epithelioma of Malherbe; a solid or cystic mass derived from hair matrix cells), conjunctival inclusion cyst
D. Papilloma
E. Molluscum contagiosum
F. Cutaneous horn
G. Rhabdomyosarcoma

III. Epibulbar tumors

A. Papilloma
B. Limbal dermoid
H. Choroidal osteoma
I. Choroidal melanoma
J. Teratoma
K. Rhabdomyosarcoma

Typical presentations of the common benign orbital and periorbital masses in infants and children (hemangioma, dermoid cyst) are sufficiently distinctive to permit confident clinical diagnosis in most cases. A malignant process should be suspected when proptosis and eyelid swelling suggestive of cellulitis are not accompanied by warmth of the overlying skin or when periorbital ecchymosis or hematoma develops in the absence of an unequivocal trauma history.

The current widespread availability of high-quality imaging permits orbital masses to be differentiated noninvasively in most cases. For initial diagnostic evaluation of the orbit, CT has advantages over MRI because of CT's high sensitivity to disturbances of bony architecture, avoidance of interference from the high-MRI signal intensity of orbital fat, and greater ease of use (although sedation is still generally required for young children). Dermoid cysts, teratomas, colobomatous cysts, and encephaloceles have highly distinctive appearances on CT, as do the blood-filled cavities found in acutely deteriorated lymphangiomas. The superior ability of MRI to differentiate various tissue types makes it a valuable adjunctive study in many cases, and its lack of radiation is an advantage when repeated imaging is required. In experienced hands, ultrasonography may also provide important diagnostic information about the orbit.

Definitive diagnosis still often requires biopsy. A pediatric oncologist should be consulted when appropriate, and a metastatic workup should be considered before resorting to orbital surgery, because other, more easily accessible sites can sometimes be used as tissue sources.

Pseudoproptosis can result from a mismatch between the volume of the globe and the capacity of the orbit. Examples include the elongation of the eyeball from infantile glaucoma or high myopia and the shallowness of the orbit in craniofacial syndromes with midfacial hypoplasia or plagiocephaly.

Gorospe L, Royo A, Berrocal T, et al. Imaging of orbital disorders in pediatric patients. *Eur Radiol.* 2003;13:2012–2026.

Primary Malignant Neoplasms

Malignant diseases of the orbit include primary tumors arising from orbital tissue elements, secondary growth of solid tumors originating elsewhere in the body (metastasis), and abnormally proliferating cells of the hematopoietic and lymphoreticular systems. A large majority of primary malignant tumors of the orbit in childhood are sarcomas. Tumors of epithelial origin (eg, carcinoma of the lacrimal gland) are extremely rare.

Rhabdomyosarcoma

The most common primary pediatric orbital malignancy is *rhabdomyosarcoma.* The incidence of this disease (which is found in about 5% of orbital biopsies of children and adolescents) exceeds that of all other sarcomas combined. The orbit is the origin of 10% of rhabdomyosarcomas; an additional 25% develop elsewhere in the head and neck, occasionally involving the orbit secondarily. The average age of onset is about 5–7 years, although onset can occur at any age. Rhabdomyosarcoma in infancy is more aggressive and carries a poorer prognosis.

Although ocular rhabdomyosarcoma usually originates in the orbit, it can occasionally arise in the conjunctiva, eyelid, or anterior uveal tract. Patients generally present with proptosis (80%–100%), globe displacement (80%), blepharoptosis (30%–50%), conjunctival and eyelid swelling (60%), palpable mass (25%), and pain (10%) (Fig 26-1). Onset of symptoms and signs is usually rapid. CT or MRI demonstrates an irregular but well-circumscribed mass of uniform density.

A biopsy is required for confirmation of the diagnosis whenever a rhabdomyosarcoma is suspected. Fine-needle aspiration biopsy (FNAB) should rarely, if ever, be used to make the primary diagnosis. The most common histopathologic type is embryonal, which shows few cells containing characteristic cross-striations. Second in frequency is the prognostically unfavorable alveolar pattern, showing poorly differentiated tumor cells compartmentalized by orderly connective tissue septa. Botryoid (grapelike), or well-differentiated pleomorphic tumors, are rarely found in the orbit but may originate from conjunctiva. It is now widely accepted that rhabdomyosarcoma arises independently of the muscles and probably develops from undifferentiated mesenchymal cells.

Small encapsulated or otherwise well-localized rhabdomyosarcomas should be totally excised when possible. For larger or more extensive tumors, chemotherapy and radiation are used in conjunction with surgery. Exenteration of the orbit is seldom indicated.

Much of the current information on diagnosis and treatment of rhabdomyosarcoma has been obtained through the collaborative endeavors of the Intergroup Rhabdomyosarcoma Study Group (IRSG). A staging classification of rhabdomyosarcoma is employed by the IRSG. In brief, Group I is defined as localized disease that is completely resected, Group II is microscopic disease remaining after biopsy, Group III is gross residual disease remaining after biopsy, and Group IV is distant metastasis present at onset. This classification can help in selecting treatment and in predicting prognosis. Primary orbital rhabdomyosarcoma has a relatively good prognosis, with patients with alveolar cell type having a 74% 5-year survival and patients with embryonal cell type, a 94% 5-year survival.

After completion of treatment, affected children should have a comprehensive ocular examination every 3–4 months initially, every 4–6 months for several years, and then yearly, with periodic orbital CT or MRI, depending on the clinical findings.

Shields JA, Shields CL. Rhabdomyosarcoma: review for the ophthalmologist. *Surv Ophthalmol.* 2003;48:39–57.

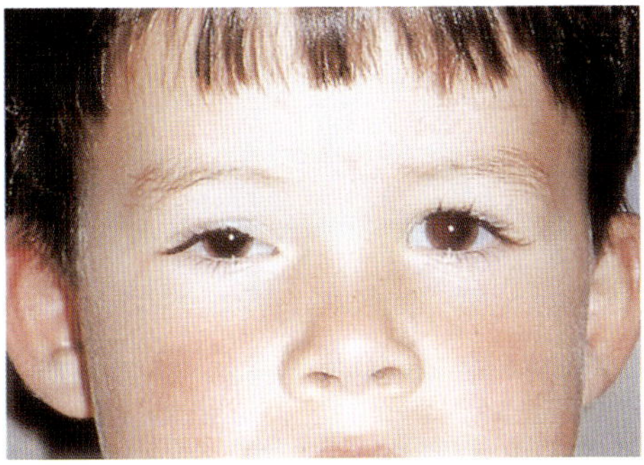

Figure 26-1 Rhabdomyosarcoma in a 4-year-old boy presenting with right upper eyelid ptosis of 3 weeks' duration and a palpable subcutaneous mass.

Other sarcomas

Osteosarcoma, chondrosarcoma, and fibrosarcoma can also develop in the orbit during childhood. The risk of sarcoma increases in children with a history of heritable retinoblastoma, particularly when external-beam radiation treatment has been given.

Metastatic Tumors

The orbit is the most common site of ocular metastasis in children, in contrast to adults, in whom the uvea is the most frequently affected.

Neuroblastoma

One of the most common childhood cancers is neuroblastoma, the most frequent source of orbital metastasis. It usually originates in either the adrenal gland or the sympathetic ganglion chain in the retroperitoneum or mediastinum. Approximately 20% of all patients with neuroblastoma show clinical evidence of orbital involvement, which is sometimes the initial manifestation of the tumor.

Unilateral or bilateral proptosis and lid ecchymosis are the classic presentations of metastatic neuroblastoma (Fig 26-2). Patients may also have eyelid swelling, ocular motility disturbances, ptosis, and Horner syndrome caused by a cervical or apical thoracic tumor (Fig 26-3). Opsoclonus, characterized by rapid, multidirectional saccadic eye movements, is a unique paraneoplastic syndrome that is not related to orbital involvement and is associated with a good prognosis for survival, although neurologic deficits may persist. Other signs and symptoms may include abdominal fullness and pain, venous obstruction and edema, hypertension caused by renal vascular compromise, and bone pain. Incisional biopsy shows small, round blue cells and confirms the diagnosis. Urinalysis for catecholamines is positive in 90%–95% of cases.

The mean age at diagnosis of patients with orbital neuroblastoma metastasis is about 2 years. Even with intensive treatment including radiation and chemotherapy, only about 10%–25% of affected patients survive. The prognosis for disseminated neuroblastoma is considerably better in infants under age 1 year than in older children.

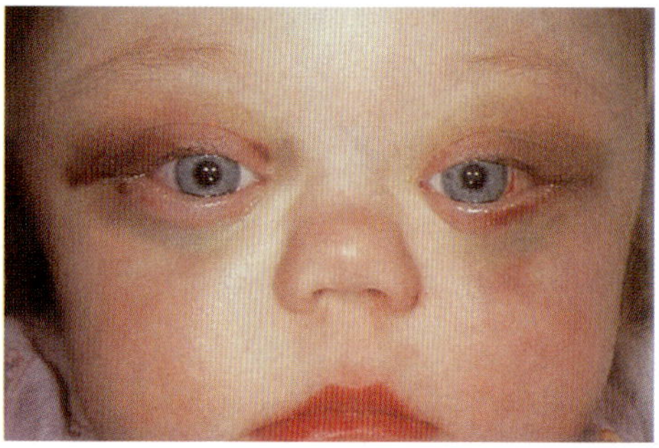

Figure 26-2 Bilateral orbital metastasis of neuroblastoma, presenting with periorbital ecchymosis in a 2-year-old girl.

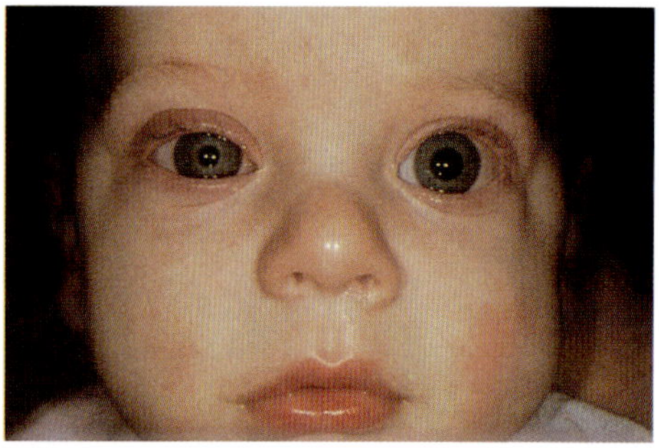

Figure 26-3 Right Horner syndrome, the presenting sign of localized intrathoracic neuroblastoma in a 6-month-old boy.

Weinstein JL, Katzenstein HM, Cohn SL. Advances in the diagnosis and treatment of neuroblastoma. *The Oncologist.* 2003;8:278–292.

Ewing sarcoma

Ewing sarcoma is a tumor composed of small, round cells that usually originates in the long bones of the extremities or the axial skeleton. Ewing sarcoma is the second most frequent solid tumor source of orbital metastasis. Contemporary treatment regimens involving surgery, radiation, and chemotherapy permit long-term survival in many cases with disseminated disease.

Leukemia

By far the most common malignancy of childhood, leukemia is acute in 95% of cases, more often lymphocytic than myelocytic. Although the most common clinical manifestation of leukemia is leukemic retinopathy, all ocular structures can be affected and orbital infiltration can cause proptosis, eyelid swelling, and ecchymosis. Infiltration of the optic nerve by leukemic cells may cause optic disc edema and loss of vision and requires prompt treatment with low-dose radiation.

Granulocytic sarcoma, or chloroma (in reference to the greenish color of involved tissue), is a localized accumulation of leukemic cells in the orbit more characteristic of myelocytic than of lymphocytic disease in childhood. This lesion may develop several months before leukemia becomes hematologically evident.

Lymphoma

In contrast with adult disease, lymphoma in children very rarely involves the orbit. Burkitt lymphoma, endemic to east Africa and uncommon in North America, is the most likely form to involve the orbit.

Histiocytosis X

Histiocytosis X (Langerhans cell histiocytosis) is the collective term for a group of disorders involving abnormal proliferation of histiocytes, often within bone. More specifically, the cells are of the dendritic type, which are considered to be immune accessory cells or antigen-processing and antigen-presenting cells, as opposed to phagocytic cells. Eosinophilic granuloma, the most localized and benign form of histiocytosis, produces bone lesions that involve the orbit, skull, ribs, and long bones in childhood or adolescence. Symptoms may include proptosis, ptosis, and periorbital swelling; localized pain and tenderness are relatively common. Radiography and CT characteristically demonstrate sharply demarcated osteolytic lesions without surrounding sclerosis (Fig 26-4). Treatment consists of observation of isolated asymptomatic lesions, excision of painful and easily accessible lesions, systemic corticosteroid administration, or low-dose radiation; all modalities have a high rate of success.

Hand-Schüller-Christian disease is a more disseminated and aggressive form of histiocytosis X that is likely to produce proptosis from involvement of the bony orbit in childhood. Diabetes insipidus is common. Chemotherapy is often required, but the prognosis is generally good. Children with this condition usually present between ages 2 and 5 years.

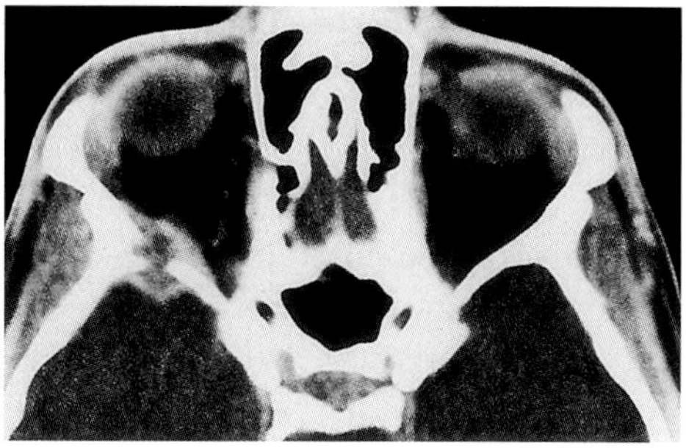

Figure 26-4 Axial CT image showing eosinophilic granuloma with partial destruction of the right posterior lateral orbital wall in a 15-year-old boy, who presented with retrobulbar pain and mild edema and erythema of the right upper eyelid.

Letterer-Siwe disease is the most severe and malignant variety of histiocytosis X, usually affecting infants younger than 2 years. It is characterized by soft tissue lesions of multiple viscera (liver, spleen) but rarely involves the eye.

Huang F, Arceci R. The histiocytoses of infancy. *Semin Perinatol.* 1999;23:319–331.

Benign Tumors

Vascular lesions: hemangiomas

Advances in the biological characterization of vascular lesions have led to a revision of their classification. The current classification of vascular lesions establishes clear clinical, histopathologic, and prognostic differences between hemangiomas and vascular malformations. The older terms *capillary* and *strawberry hemangioma* should be translated into the single term *hemangioma.* In contrast, cavernous hemangiomas, port-wine stains, and lymphangiomas all should be called "malformations." This nomenclature has been incorporated into the medical literature but has not been used consistently in the ophthalmic literature.

Hemangiomas are hamartomatous growths composed of proliferating capillary endothelial cells. They show a characteristic early phase of active growth in early infancy, with a subsequent period of regression and involution. Hemangiomas can be classified as

- superficial, arising only on the skin and immediate subjacent skin and having a bright red appearance
- deep, arising only in the deeper subcutaneous tissue and having a bluish hue (Fig 26-5)
- compound/mixed, having components of both

Hemangiomas occur in 1%–3% of term newborns and are more common in premature infants and females and after chorionic villus sampling. Most hemangiomas are clinically insignificant at birth, appearing as an erythematous macule, a telangiectasia, or no lesion at all. The natural history is rapid proliferation and growth over the first several months of life, rarely lasting beyond 1 year. During this phase, the lesion may ulcerate, hemorrhage, or cause amblyopia by inducing astigmatism or obstructing the visual axis. After the first year of life, the lesion usually begins to regress, although the rate and degree of

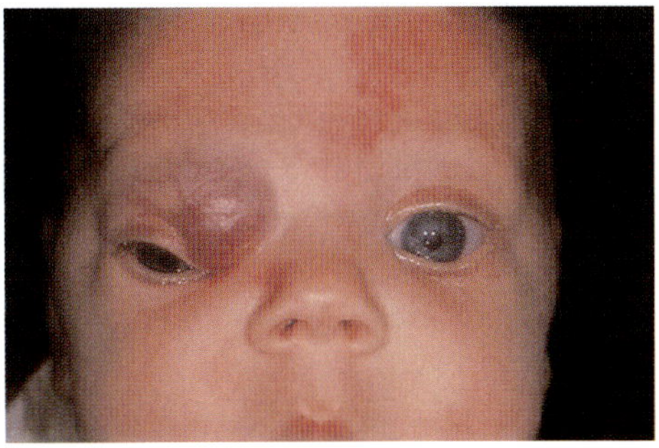

Figure 26-5 Capillary hemangioma in a 2-month-old girl involving the right upper eyelid and orbit with displacement of the globe and induction of 8 D of astigmatic refractive error.

involution vary. Children and their parents may also suffer psychologically if a marked cosmetic deformity persists.

Systemic disease associated with hemangiomas *PHACE(S)* is an acronym for *p*osterior fossa malformations, *h*emangiomas, *a*rterial anomalies, *c*o-arctation of the aorta and *c*ardiac defects, *e*ye abnormalities (including increased retinal vascularity, microphthalmia, optic nerve hypoplasia, exophthalmos, choroidal hemangiomas, strabismus, colobomas, cataracts, and glaucoma), and *s*ternal clefting and *s*upraumbilical raphe. The PHACE(S) syndrome should be considered in any infant presenting with a large, segmental, plaquelike facial hemangioma involving 1 or more dermatomes.

Kasabach-Merritt syndrome is a thrombocytopenic coagulopathy with a high mortality rate. It is caused by sequestration of platelets within a vascular lesion that is now thought not to be a true hemangioma, but 1 of 2 distinct vascular lesions, either the kaposiform hemangioendothelioma or the tufted angioma.

Diffuse neonatal hemangiomatosis is a potentially lethal condition that occurs in infants with multiple small cutaneous hemangiomas associated with visceral lesions affecting the liver, gastrointestinal tract, and brain. These hemangiomas are initially asymptomatic but can lead to cardiac failure and death within weeks. Infants with more than 3 cutaneous lesions should be evaluated for visceral lesions.

Maffucci syndrome is a rare genetic disorder affecting both males and females. It is characterized by benign enlargement of cartilage (enchondromas); bone deformities; and dark, irregularly shaped hemangiomas. About 30%–37% of enchondromas develop into a chondrosarcoma. Malignant transformation of vascular lesions is possible but exceedingly rare.

Treatment of hemangiomas If the diagnosis is unclear on clinical grounds, MRI can be useful to distinguish hemangioma from plexiform neurofibroma, lymphatic malformation, and rhabdomyosarcoma, each of which may be associated with rapid growth and proliferation or progressive proptosis. MRI may also be helpful in delineating the posterior extent of the tumor if it cannot be determined clinically.

Observation is indicated when hemangiomas are small and there is no risk of amblyopia from either obstruction of the visual axis or induced astigmatism.

Steroids are used during the proliferative phase of the tumor to arrest growth and accelerate involution of the lesion. They can be administered topically, intralesionally, or systemically. Topical clobetasol proprionate cream 0.05% may be preferred for small superficial lesions. Intralesional injections of a combination of a long-acting and a short-acting steroid are commonly used for localized periocular hemangiomas. One popular regimen is to inject a mixture of triamcinolone and betamethasone sodium phosphate directly into the tumor, using multiple injection sites to evenly distribute the medication. If the hemangioma is diffuse or extensively involves the posterior orbit, then systemic steroids may be employed, with recommended dosages of prednisone or prednisolone ranging from 2 to 5 mg/kg/day.

Steroids are associated with myriad well-known complications, the risks of which must be weighed against the potential benefits of treatment and discussed with the family. Adrenal suppression and growth retardation can occur with all routes of administration, including topical creams. Intralesional injections carry the risks of bilateral retinal embolization, subcutaneous linear fat atrophy, and eyelid depigmentation. It may also be necessary to postpone immunizations for children receiving high doses of steroids. Consultation with a child's primary care provider is recommended.

Interferon alfa-2a, although effective, has been associated with an unacceptably high side-effect profile and is usually reserved for severe, recalcitrant, or life-threatening tumors. Vincristine may be a promising alternative but is still under investigation.

A pulsed-dye laser can be used to treat superficial hemangiomas with few complications, but it has little effect on deeper components of the tumor.

Surgical excision of periocular hemangiomas is feasible for some well-localized lesions (Fig 26-6). In other cases, surgery may be used as a reconstructive tool years after medical treatment.

A 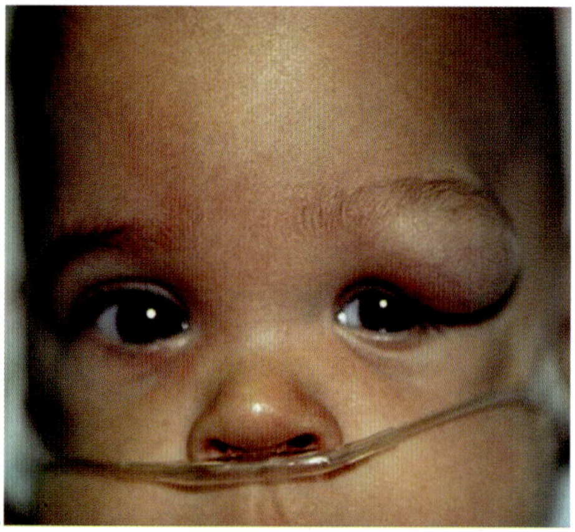

B 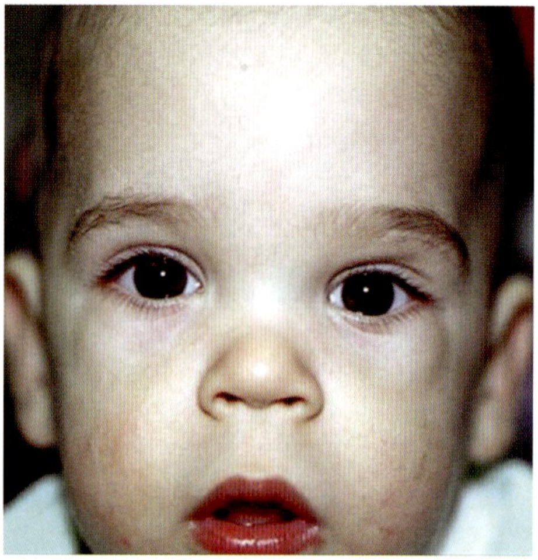

Figure 26-6 **A,** Five-month-old boy with well-circumscribed capillary hemangioma in left upper eyelid. Preoperative refraction was –6.00 + 8.00 × 40°. **B,** At 6 months postoperative, induced astigmatism has resolved and refraction was –0.25 + 0.25 ×80°. *(Photographs courtesy of David Plager, MD.)*

Vascular lesions: malformations

Vascular malformations are developmental anomalies that can be derived from capillary venous, arterial, or lymphatic vessels. In contrast to hemangiomas, vascular malformations remain relatively static, with growth of the lesion correlating to growth of the child. The age and mode of clinical presentation vary, but, in general, vascular malformations manifest later in life, although cutaneous vascular malformations such as port-wine stains are evident from birth.

Orbital lymphangioma *Orbital lymphangioma*, a lymphatic malformation, may produce proptosis at birth or, more commonly, in the second or third decade of life. Lymphangioma of the orbit is best managed conservatively. Exacerbations tend to occur during upper respiratory infections and may be managed with short-course systemic corticosteroids. Rapid expansion may also be seen in cases of intralesional hemorrhage (Fig 26-7). In these cases, partial resection and drainage may be required to manage acute orbital symptoms and compressive optic neuropathy. Because of the infiltrative character of this malformation, complete removal is considered impossible. Intralesional injection of a sclerosing agent may hold promise but requires further investigation before it can be recommended for general use.

Orbital venous malformations Orbital venous malformations, or varices, can be divided into primary and secondary types. The primary type is confined to the orbit and has no association with arteriovenous malformations (AVMs). The secondary orbital varix occurs as a result of an intracranial AVM shunt that causes the orbital veins to dilate. Orbital venous malformations usually become symptomatic after years of progressive congestion and rarely manifest before the second decade of life. Treatment is reserved for highly symptomatic lesions.

Orbital AVMs AVMs isolated to the orbit are extremely rare. Patients with congenital AVM aneurysms of the retina and midbrain, known as Wyburn-Mason syndrome (see Chapter 27, Phakomatoses), may have orbital involvement. AVMs of the bony orbit rarely manifest in childhood but are characterized by pulsatile exophthalmos, chemosis, congested conjunctival vessels, and raised intraocular pressure. AVMs may be treated by embolization, surgical resection, or both.

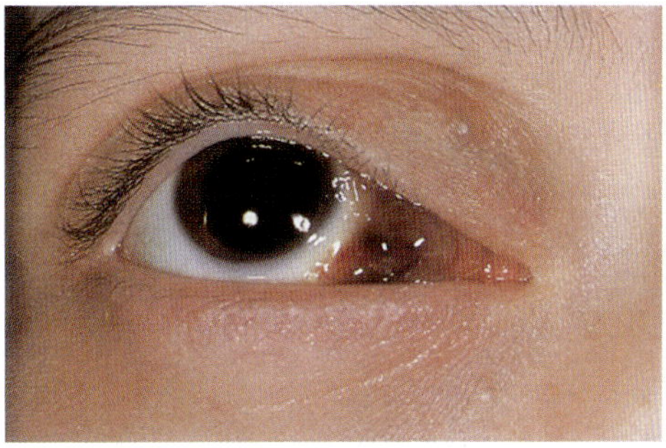

Figure 26-7 Lymphangioma with hemorrhage involving the right orbit, upper eyelid, and conjunctiva in a 15-year-old girl.

Capillary malformations Port-wine stains manifest as a flat red or pink cutaneous lesion that may lighten during the first year but then tends to become darker, thicker, and more nodular over time. Sturge-Weber syndrome, or encephalotrigeminal angiomatosis, is a capillary malformation of the leptomeninges with or without ocular or facial involvement. The classic manifestation is a port-wine stain of the face following trigeminal distribution, intraocular choroidal hemangioma, and seizures. Glaucoma can occur in affected eyes and can be difficult to treat. The development of new lasers has provided additional treatment options for patients with port-wine stains.

Ceisler EJ, Santos L, Blei F. Periocular hemangiomas: what every physician should know. *Pediatr Dermatol.* 2004;21:1–9.

Garza G, Fay A, Rubin PAD. Treatment of pediatric vascular lesions of the eyelid and orbit. *Int Ophthalmol Clin.* 2001;41:43–55.

Other vascular tumors Other orbital tumors composed of vascular elements are rare in childhood. *Hemangiopericytoma* is a benign tumor of pericytes that manifests as slow proptosis of the globe and has the potential for malignant transformation.

Tumors of bony origin

A variety of uncommon benign orbital tumors of bony origin may present during the early years of life with gradually increasing proptosis. Fibrous dysplasia and ossifying fibroma are similar disorders characterized by destruction of normal bone and replacement by fibroosseous tissue. In both conditions, orbital radiography and CT show varying degrees of lucency and sclerosis.

Fibrous dysplasia has a slow progression that ceases when skeletal maturation is complete. The most serious complication is visual loss caused by optic nerve compression, which may occur acutely. Periodic assessment of vision, pupil function, and optic disc appearance is indicated. Surgical treatment is indicated for functional deterioration or disfigurement.

Histopathologically, *ossifying fibroma* is distinguished by the presence of osteoblasts. Ossifying fibroma tends to be a more locally invasive lesion than fibrous dysplasia; some authorities recommend early excision.

Brown tumor of bone is an osteoclastic giant cell reaction resulting from hyperparathyroidism. *Aneurysmal bone cyst* is a degenerative process in which normal bone is replaced by cystic cavities containing fibrous tissue, inflammatory cells, and blood, producing a characteristic radiographic appearance.

Tumors of connective tissue origin

Benign orbital tumors originating from connective tissue are rare in childhood. *Juvenile fibromatosis* may present as a mass in the inferior anterior portion of the orbit. These tumors, sometimes called *myofibromas* or *desmoid tumors*, are composed of relatively mature fibroblasts. They tend to recur locally after excision and can be difficult to control, but they do not metastasize.

Tumors of neural origin

Optic pathway glioma is the most important orbital tumor of neural origin in childhood. Optic pathway gliomas are usually low-grade astrocytomas; however, the rate of growth with or without therapeutic intervention is unpredictable. Accordingly, the management of these tumors is controversial and depends largely on their location. About 20% of optic pathway gliomas are associated with type 1 neurofibromatosis. *Plexiform neurofibroma* nearly always occurs in the context of neurofibromatosis and not infrequently involves the eyelid and orbit. (These tumors are discussed in detail in Chapter 27.) Orbital *meningioma* and *schwannoma* (neurilemoma, neurinoma) are rare prior to adulthood and also usually appear in patients with neurofibromatosis. Meningioma typically presents with progressive visual loss, mild proptosis, and restriction of ocular motility; a large majority of patients is female. Childhood meningiomas tend to be locally aggressive and should be totally excised if possible, unless the involved eye retains good vision.

Steinbok P. Optic pathway tumors in children. *J Chin Med Assoc.* 2003;66:4–12.

Ectopic Tissue Masses

The term *choristoma* is applied to growths consisting of normal cells and tissues appearing at an abnormal location. They may result from abnormal sequestration of germ layer tissue during embryonic development or from faulty differentiation of pluripotential cells. Masses composed of such ectopic tissue growing in the orbit can also be a consequence of herniation of tissue from adjacent structures.

Cystic lesions

Dermoid cysts are benign developmental choristomas thought to be the most common space-occupying orbital lesions of childhood. These cysts are congenital, arising from primitive dermal elements that have been sequestered in fetal suture lines at the time of closure. The tissue forms a cyst lined with keratinized epithelium and dermal appendages, including hair follicles, sweat glands, and sebaceous glands. Cysts containing squamous epithelium without dermal appendages are called *epidermoid cysts.*

Orbital dermoid cysts presenting in childhood most commonly arise in the superonasal and superotemporal quadrants (Fig 26-8) but sometimes extend into the bony suture line. Clinically, the dermoid cyst in children presents as a painless mass that is unattached to overlying skin and is mobile, smooth, and nontender. Episodes of inflammation may occur with small ruptures of the cyst wall and consequent extrusion of cyst contents into the surrounding tissue. Most patients have no visual symptoms. CT confirms the diagnosis, revealing a well-circumscribed lesion with a low-density lumen and often bony remodeling. Deeper orbital lesions may show complete bony defects.

Management of dermoid cysts is surgical. Early excision may avoid the increased risk of traumatic rupture with ambulation. An infrabrow or eyelid crease incision is used and the cyst is carefully dissected. If possible, rupture of the cyst at the time of surgery is avoided to limit lipogranulomatous inflammation and scarring. If the cyst is entered, the site should be irrigated. Sutural cysts often cannot be removed intact because of their communication into or through bone. Care is taken to remove all remaining cyst lining to limit the possibility of recurrence.

Shields JA, Kaden IH, Eagle RC Jr, et al. Orbital dermoid cysts: clinicopathologic correlations, classification, and management. The 1997 Josephine E. Schueler Lecture. *Ophthal Plast Reconstr Surg.* 1997;13:265–276.

Teratomas

Choristomatous tumors that contain multiple tissues derived from all 3 germinal layers (ectoderm, mesoderm, and endoderm) are known as *teratomas.* Skin and dermal appendages, neural tissue, muscle, and bone are typically present; endodermal elements such as respiratory and intestinal tract epithelium are less consistently found. Most teratomas are partially cystic, with varying fluid content. Orbital teratomas account for a very small fraction of both orbital tumors and teratomas in general, which usually arise in the gonads or sacrococcygeal region. The clinical presentation of orbital teratomas is particularly dramatic, however, with massive proptosis evident at birth (Fig 26-9). In contrast with teratomas in other locations, which tend to show malignant growth, most orbital lesions are benign. Surgical excision, facilitated by prior aspiration of fluid, can often be accomplished without sacrificing the globe. Permanent optic nerve damage from stretching and compression usually results in poor vision in the involved eye.

Ectopic lacrimal gland

A rare choristomatous lesion, *ectopic lacrimal gland* may present with proptosis in childhood. Cystic enlargement and chronic inflammation sometimes aggravate the problem.

A

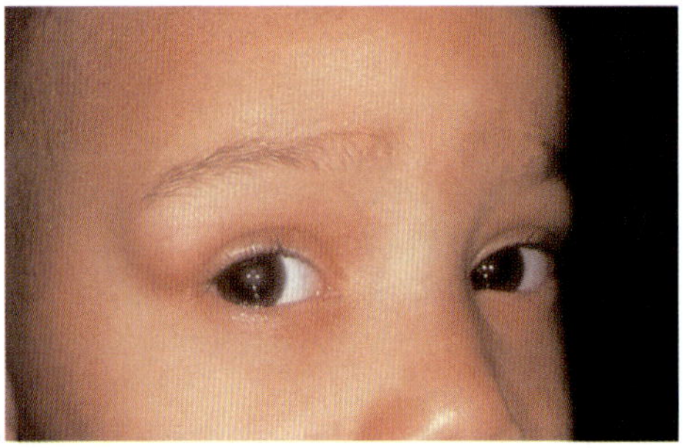

B

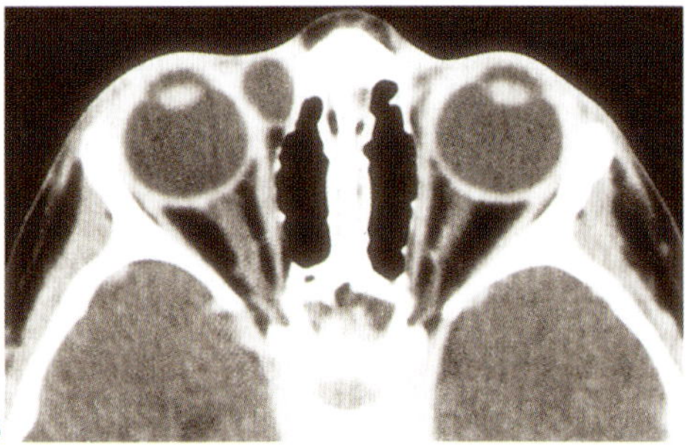

Figure 26-8 **A,** Periorbital dermoid cyst, right eye, with typical superotemporal location in a 3-year-old girl. **B,** Axial CT image showing a dermoid cyst of the superonasal anterior orbit, right eye, in a 6-year-old boy.

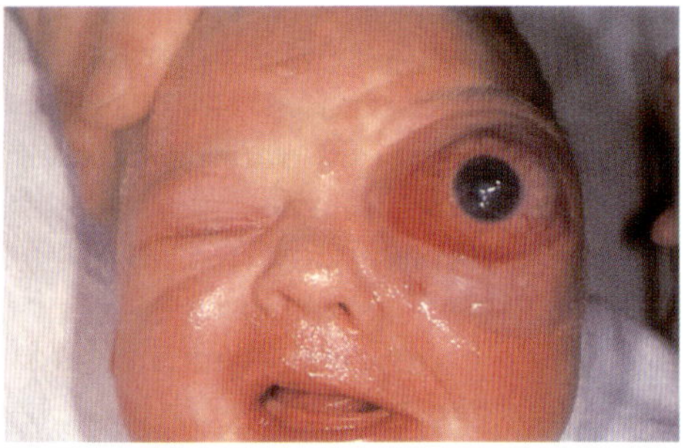

Figure 26-9 Congenital cystic teratoma originating in the left orbit of a 1-day-old girl.

Colobomatous cyst

Also known as *microphthalmos with cyst*, the *colobomatous cyst* is composed of tissues that originate from the eye wall of a malformed globe with posterior segment coloboma. Most fundus colobomas show some degree of scleral ectasia, resulting from a deficiency of tissue in the region where apposing edges of the embryonic neuroectodermal fissure have failed to fuse properly. In extreme cases, a bulging globular appendage grows to become as large as or larger than the globe itself, which is invariably microphthalmic, sometimes to a marked degree.

Like other colobomatous malformations, microphthalmos with cyst may occur either as an isolated congenital defect or in association with a variety of intracranial or systemic anomalies. Frequently, the other eye shows evidence of coloboma as well. The wall of a colobomatous cyst consists of thin sclera lined by rudimentary tissue of neuroectodermal origin, occasionally incorporating hyperplastic glial tissue accumulations; the cyst contains aqueous fluid with a few suspended cells. The usual location is inferior or posterior to the globe, with which the cyst is always in contact. The cyst interior communicates with the vitreous cavity, sometimes through a channel so small it is undetectable even with high-resolution imaging.

Posteriorly located colobomatous cysts may or may not cause proptosis, depending on the size of the globe and the cyst. Inferiorly located cysts present as a bulging of the lower eyelid or a bluish subconjunctival mass (Fig 26-10). Occasionally, the globe is pushed so far superiorly that it disappears behind the upper eyelid. If fundus examination does not make the diagnosis obvious, other possibilities can be excluded by using CT, MRI, or ultrasonography to demonstrate a cystic lesion with the uniform internal density of vitreous attached to the globe. The goal of treatment is to promote normal growth of the orbit, and a variety of methods are used, including aspiration of the cyst, surgical excision of the cyst, and orbital expanders and conformers.

McLean CJ, Rage NK, Jones RB, et al. The management of orbital cysts associated with congenital microphthalmos and anophthalmos. *Br J Ophthalmol.* 2003;87:860–863.

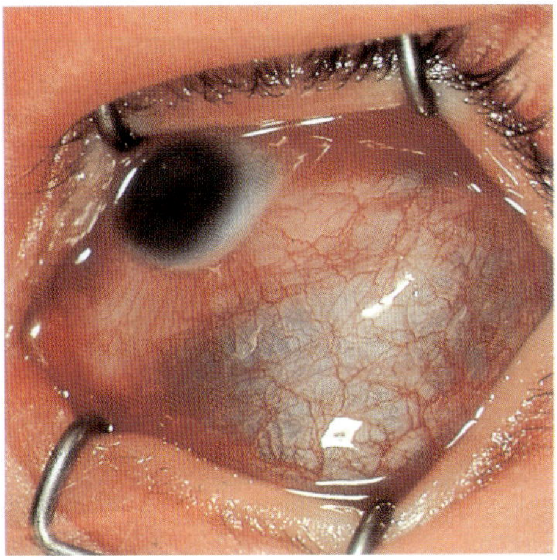

Figure 26-10 Colobomatous cyst (microphthalmos), left eye.

Mucocele

Mucoceles are cystic lesions that originate from the paranasal sinuses and may expand over time, potentially causing destruction of bone and possibly eroding into the orbit or intracranial space. These lesions most commonly arise from the frontal or anterior ethmoidal sinuses with inferior or medial displacement of the globe. The differential diagnosis includes encephalocele with skull base deformity. Treatment involves reestablishing normal sinus drainage and removing the cyst wall.

Encephalocele or meningocele

Encephaloceles or *meningoceles* in the orbital region may result from a congenital bony defect that permits herniation of intracranial tissue or may develop after trauma that disrupts the bone and dura mater of the anterior cranial fossa. Intraorbital location leads to proptosis or downward displacement of the globe. Anterior presentation takes the form of a subcutaneous mass, typically located above the medial canthal ligament. Pulsation of the globe or the mass from the transmission of intracranial pulse pressure is characteristic. Neuroimaging readily confirms the diagnosis of this rare condition.

Childhood Orbital Inflammations

Several noninfectious, nontraumatic disorders that may simulate an orbital mass lesion deserve brief mention. Graves disease, the most common cause of proptosis in adults, rarely occurs in prepubescent children but occasionally affects adolescents (Fig 26-11). (See also Chapter 11.)

Idiopathic orbital inflammatory disease

Idiopathic orbital inflammatory disease (orbital pseudotumor) is an inflammatory cause of proptosis in childhood that differs significantly from the adult form. The typical pediatric presentation is acute and painful, resembling orbital cellulitis more than tumor or Graves ophthalmopathy (Fig 26-12). Bilaterality and episodic recurrence are common, as are associated systemic manifestations such as headache, nausea and vomiting, and lethargy. Uveitis is common and occasionally constitutes the dominant manifestation. Imaging studies may show increased density of orbital fat, thickening of posterior sclera and Tenon's layer, or enlargement of extraocular muscles. Treatment with a systemic corticosteroid usually provides prompt and dramatic relief, but recurrent disease is common.

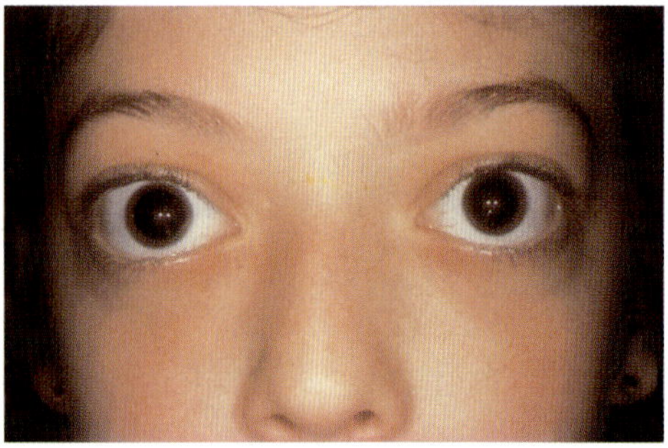

Figure 26-11 Graves disease with bilateral exophthalmos in a 15-year-old girl.

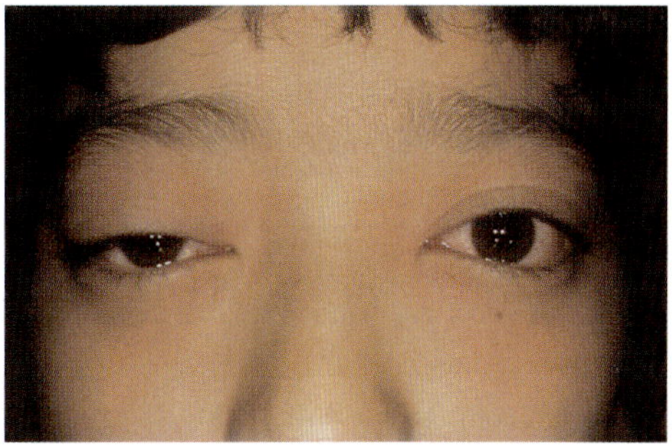

Figure 26-12 Bilateral idiopathic orbital inflammatory disease (orbital pseudotumor) in an 11-year-old boy with a 1-week history of eye pain. Ocular rotation was markedly limited in all directions. CT confirmed proptosis and showed enlargement of all extraocular muscles. Laboratory workup was negative for thyroid disease and rheumatologic disorders. Complete resolution occurred after 1 month of corticosteroid treatment.

Orbital myositis

Orbital myositis describes idiopathic orbital inflammatory disease that is confined to 1 or more extraocular muscles. The clinical presentation depends on the amount of inflammation. Diplopia, conjunctival chemosis, and orbital pain are common. Symptoms can be subacute for weeks or can progress quite rapidly. Visual function is rarely involved unless massive muscle enlargement is present. CT or MRI findings consist of diffusely enlarged muscles with the enlargement extending all the way to the insertion (unlike with thyroid myopathy, which mainly involves the muscle belly). Corticosteroid treatment usually results in resolution of symptoms, but prolonged treatment (4–6 weeks) is often necessary and recurrence is common.

Eyelid and Epibulbar Lesions

Malignant tumors arising from eyelid skin or conjunctiva (basal cell carcinoma, squamous cell carcinoma, melanoma) are relatively common in adults, but they are extremely rare in childhood. These tumors are discussed elsewhere in the BCSC (see Section 4, *Ophthalmic Pathology and Intraocular Tumors*; Section 7, *Orbit, Eyelids, and Lacrimal System*; and Section 8, *External Disease and Cornea*). Pediatric cases are likely to be associated with underlying systemic disorders that predispose to malignancy, such as basal cell nevus syndrome or xeroderma pigmentosum. In addition, rhabdomyosarcoma may present atypically as an eyelid or conjunctival mass.

Benign lesions of the ocular surface and surrounding skin are common, and these may be classified as originating from epithelium, melanocytes, or vascular tissue.

Papillomas

Papillomas are benign epithelial proliferations that usually appear as sessile masses at the limbus or as pedunculated lesions of the caruncle, fornix, or palpebral conjunctiva. Papillomas may be transparent, pale yellow, or salmon-colored, sometimes speckled with red dots. Papillomas in children usually result from viral infection and are likely to disappear spontaneously. Surgical excision is indicated if there is persistent associated conjunctivitis or keratitis or if new lesions continue to appear. Recurrence following surgical excision is possible.

Conjunctival Epithelial Inclusion Cysts

Usually resulting from surgery or trauma, conjunctival epithelial inclusion cysts are filled with clear fluid. Excision is indicated only if they are a source of bothersome symptoms.

Epibulbar Limbal Dermoid Tumors

Although both are classified as choristomas, dermoid tumors are completely distinct from dermoid cysts. Epibulbar limbal dermoid tumors are evident at birth as whitish dome-shaped masses, straddling the limbus in the inferotemporal quadrant in about three quarters of cases, with a diameter of about 2–10 mm and a thickness of 1–3 mm. They are composed of keratinizing surface epithelium with an underlying dermal layer that frequently contains a few hair follicles and a small amount of fatty tissue. Little if any postnatal growth occurs. Apart from their undesirable appearance, epibulbar limbal dermoids may cause ocular irritation and interfere with vision by inducing astigmatism or haziness of adjacent clear cornea.

There is no urgency to remove epibulbar dermoid tumors unless irritating symptoms persist. Epibulbar dermoid tumors are removed by excising the episcleral portion flush with the plane of surrounding tissue. In general, the surgeon need not remove underlying clear corneal tissue, mobilize surrounding tissue, or apply a patch graft over the resulting surface defect; however, because some lesions may extend into the anterior chamber, tissue should be available in the event that a patch graft is required. Cornea and conjunctiva heal within a few days to several weeks, generally with some scarring and imperfect corneal transparency; nevertheless, the appearance can be improved considerably.

Lipodermoid

A conjunctival lesion, the *lipodermoid (dermolipoma)* is usually located near the temporal fornix and is composed of adipose tissue and dense connective tissue. The overlying conjunctival epithelium is normal, and hair follicles are absent. Lipodermoids may be extensive, sometimes involving orbital tissue, lacrimal gland, and extraocular muscle. Both epibulbar limbal dermoid tumors and conjunctival lipodermoids are frequently associated with Goldenhar syndrome (Fig 26-13). In patients with Goldenhar syndrome, the lesions are accompanied by a variety of other anomalies, including ear deformities (preauricular appendages, aural fistulas), maxillary or mandibular hypoplasia (hemifacial microsomia), vertebral deformities, notching of the upper eyelid, and Duane syndrome.

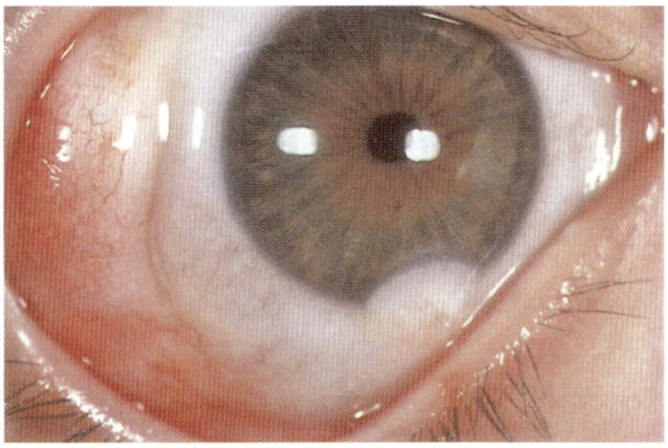

Figure 26-13 Small inferior limbal dermoid and larger lipodermoid involving the temporal conjunctival fornix, right eye, in a child with Goldenhar syndrome.

Lipodermoids rarely require excision. If surgery is undertaken, the surgeon should attempt to remove only the portion of the lesion visible within the palpebral fissure, disturbing conjunctiva and Tenon's layer as little as possible to minimize scarring. Even with a conservative operative approach, cicatrization may be a problem that requires surgical revision.

Conjunctival Nevi

Conjunctival nevi are relatively common in childhood. The lesions may be flat or elevated. Histopathologically, most of these nevi are compound (nevus cells are found in both epithelium and substantia propria); others are junctional (nevus cells confined to the interface between epithelium and substantia propria). The color is typically brown, but approximately one third are nonpigmented, having a pinkish appearance. The lesions are occasionally noted at birth but more commonly develop during later childhood or adolescence (Fig 26-14).

Malignant melanoma of the conjunctiva and primary acquired melanosis, a premalignant nevoid lesion of adulthood, are extremely rare in childhood.

Congenital Nevocellular Nevi of the Skin

Congenital nevocellular nevi can occur on the eyelids and may cause amblyopia or undergo malignant transformation (Fig 26-15). The risk of malignant transformation increases with the size of the lesion, with large lesions (>20 cm) having a 5%–20% risk of malignant transformation. Observation is often recommended for small (<1.5 cm) and medium-sized (1.5–20 cm) lesions.

Ocular Melanocytosis

A congenital pigmentary lesion, *ocular melanocytosis (melanosis oculi)* is characterized by unilateral patchy but extensive slate-gray or bluish discoloration of the sclera (not conjunctiva). Intraocular pigmentation is also increased, which contributes to a higher incidence of glaucoma and increases the risk of malignant melanoma. Some patients, particularly persons of Asian ancestry, may have associated involvement of eyelid and adjacent skin with dermal hyperpigmentation that produces brown, bluish, or black discoloration without thickening or other abnormality (oculodermal melanocytosis, nevus of Ota). Small patches of slate-gray scleral pigmentation, typically bilateral and without clinical

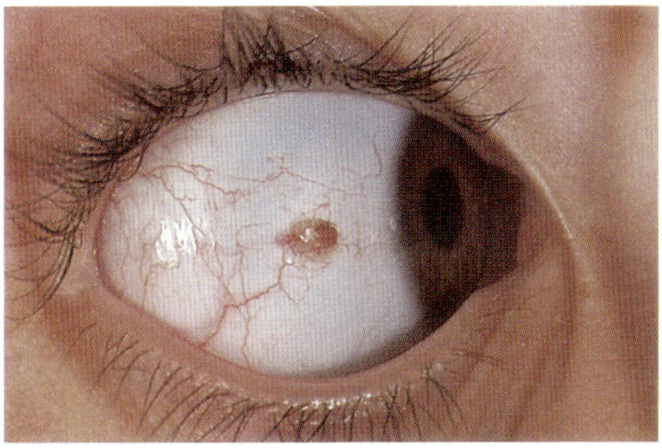

Figure 26-14 Pigmented nevus of the bulbar conjunctiva, right eye, recently developed in a 4-year-old girl.

significance, are common in black and Asian children. Melanosis of skin and sclera is occasionally associated with Sturge-Weber syndrome and Klippel-Trénaunay-Weber syndrome (Fig 26-16).

Akor C, Greenburg MF, Pollard ZF, et al. Conjunctival melanoma in a child. *J Pediatr Ophthalmol Strabismus.* 2004;41:56–58.

Inflammatory Conditions

Inflammatory masses of the eyelids and ocular surface are much more common than tumors. *Chalazia* are caused by blockage of the meibomian glands, and *hordeola* arise from blocked eccrine and apocrine glands. Treament of both includes eyelid hygiene and warm compresses, with surgical treatment reserved for large, painful, or chronic lesions. Doxycycline can be used safely in children who are at least 8 years old but should be avoided in younger children. Pyogenic granuloma is a pedunculated, fleshy pink growth of granulation tissue that develops, sometimes rapidly and exuberantly, from the conjunctiva overlying a chalazion or site of trauma.

Phlyctenular keratoconjunctivitis and *ligneous conjunctivitis* are 2 uncommon inflammatory disorders of the conjunctiva that typically occur in young patients and may result in formation of ocular surface masses. *Nodular episcleritis* occasionally is seen in childhood. Eyelid and epibulbar lesions can develop in juvenile xanthogranuloma, which is discussed later in the chapter. See also BCSC Section 8, *External Disease and Cornea.*

Intraocular Tumors

Iris and Ciliary Body Lesions

Both primary and secondary malignant tumors of the iris are very rare in children. Leukemic infiltration of iris tissue may create a mass lesion, which is one of the less common ocular manifestations of pediatric leukemia. Solid tumors almost never metastasize to the uveal tract in childhood.

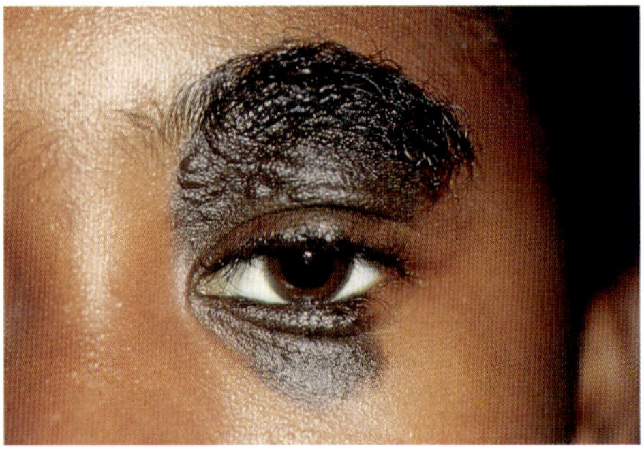

Figure 26-15 Congenital nevocellular nevus of the eyelid, present since birth. *(Photograph courtesy of Amy Hutchinson, MD.)*

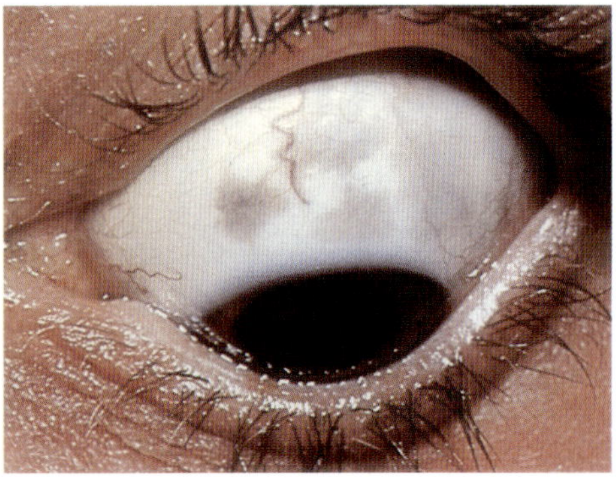

Figure 26-16 Congenital ocular melanocytosis.

A number of relatively common and entirely benign iris lesions may generate concern about the possibility of malignancy in childhood. Pigmented iris nevi and freckles large enough to be noticed by family members or primary care physicians sometimes require repeated observation to provide reassurance concerning their harmless nature. Children with type 1 neurofibromatosis occasionally develop melanocytic lesions similar to the common Lisch nodule that are large enough to be considered benign tumors. Nodules of iris-pigmented epithelium at the pupillary margin may be present as an insignificant congenital anomaly or may develop after prolonged use of miotic drops (eg, echothiophate for treatment of strabismus).

Juvenile xanthogranuloma

Juvenile xanthogranuloma is a nonneoplastic histiocytic proliferation that develops in infants younger than 2 years. It is characterized by the presence of Touton giant cells. Skin involvement is typically but not invariably present in the form of one or more small round papules, orange or tan in color. Iris lesions are relatively rare and virtually always unilateral. The fleshy yellow-brown mass may be small and localized or diffusely infiltrative of the entire iris, with resulting heterochromia. Spontaneous bleeding with hyphema is a characteristic clinical presentation. Secondary glaucoma may cause acute pain and photophobia and ultimately significant visual loss (Fig 26-17).

Juvenile xanthogranuloma is a self-limited condition that usually regresses spontaneously by age 5 years, but treatment is indicated for ocular involvement to avoid complications. Topical corticosteroids and pharmacologic agents to lower intraocular pressure, given as necessary, are generally sufficient to control the problem; surgical excision or radiation should be considered if intractable glaucoma is present.

Medulloepithelioma

A *medulloepithelioma (diktyoma)* originates from the nonpigmented epithelium of the ciliary body and most often presents as an iris mass during the first decade of life. Secondary glaucoma, hyphema, and ectopia lentis are less frequent initial manifestations. This rare lesion shows a spectrum of clinical and pathologic characteristics, ranging from benign to malignant. Although metastasis is rare, local invasiveness can lead to death. Teratoid elements are often present. Enucleation is usually required and is curative in a large majority of cases.

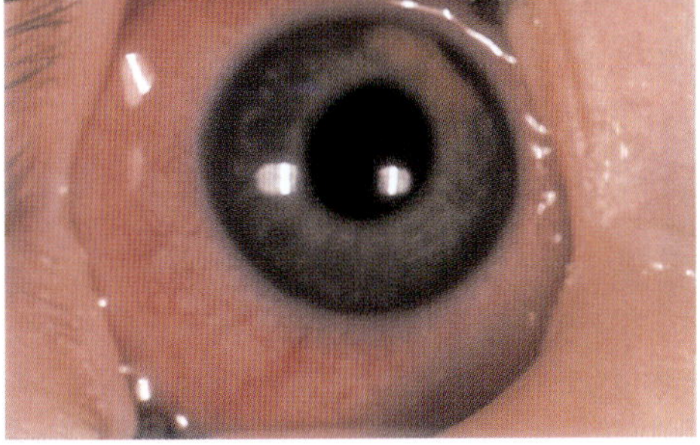

Figure 26-17 Juvenile xanthogranuloma of iris, right eye, in a 1-year-old boy with a 3-day history of redness and light sensitivity. Note small hyphema layered superonasally adjacent to the tan-colored iris lesion. Intraocular pressure was 30 mm Hg. The lesion regressed without further complications over 6 months with topical corticosteroid treatment.

Choroidal and Retinal Pigment Epithelial Lesions

A pigmented fundus lesion in a child is usually benign. Flat choroidal nevi are common as an incidental fundus finding in children and need not be viewed as a particular cause for concern. Patients with neurofibromatosis type 1 often have flat, tan-colored spots in the choroid.

Congenital hypertrophy of the retinal pigment epithelium (CHRPE) is a sharply demarcated, flat, hyperpigmented lesion that may be isolated or multifocal. Such lesions are sometimes grouped, in which case they are also known as *bear tracks.* A specific subgroup of these lesions has been associated with familial adenomatous polyposis (Gardner syndrome) (Fig 26-18). Patients with Gardner syndrome are at very high risk for adenocarcinoma of the colon by age 50 years. The CHRPE lesions associated with Gardner syndrome have a halo of surrounding depigmentation with a tail of depigmentation that is oriented radially and directed toward the optic nerve. Patients with Gardner syndrome may also have skeletal hamartomas and various other soft tissue tumors. The presence of 4 or more CHRPE lesions not restricted to 1 sector of the fundus or bilateral involvement should raise suspicion of familial polyposis syndrome.

Combined hamartoma of the retina and retinal pigment epithelium is an ill-defined, elevated, variably pigmented tumor that may be either juxtapapillary or located in the retinal periphery. In the peripheral location, dragging of the retinal vessels is a prominent feature. Tumors have a variable composition of glial tissue and retinal pigment epithelium. This condition can be associated with neurofibromatosis type 2, incontinentia pigmenti, X-linked retinoschisis, and facial hemangiomas.

Melanocytoma is a darkly pigmented tumor with little or no growth potential that usually involves the optic disc and adjacent retina (Fig 26-19). Malignant melanoma of the choroid is extremely rare in children.

Choroidal osteoma is a benign bony tumor of the uveal tract that may occur in childhood, usually presenting with decreased visual acuity.

Isolated localized choroidal hemangioma is extremely rare in childhood. Diffuse hemangioma of the choroid associated with Sturge-Weber syndrome is discussed in Chapter 27.

Leukemia

Childhood leukemias can be associated with tumor infiltration of the retina, optic disc, and uvea. Optic disc edema, retinal and choroidal thickening with hemorrhage, and retinal detachment may be observed. Intraocular leukemic infiltrates may respond to systemic chemotherapy and irradiation, but the prognosis is poor.

Retinoblastoma

Retinoblastoma is the most common malignant ocular tumor of childhood and one of the most common pediatric solid tumors, with an incidence of 1:14,000–1:20,000 live births. Retinoblastoma is typically diagnosed during the first year of life in familial and bilateral cases and between ages 1 and 3 in sporadic unilateral cases. Onset later than age 5 is rare but can occur. The most common initial sign is leukocoria (white pupil), which is usually first noticed by the family and described as a glow, glint, or cat's-eye appearance

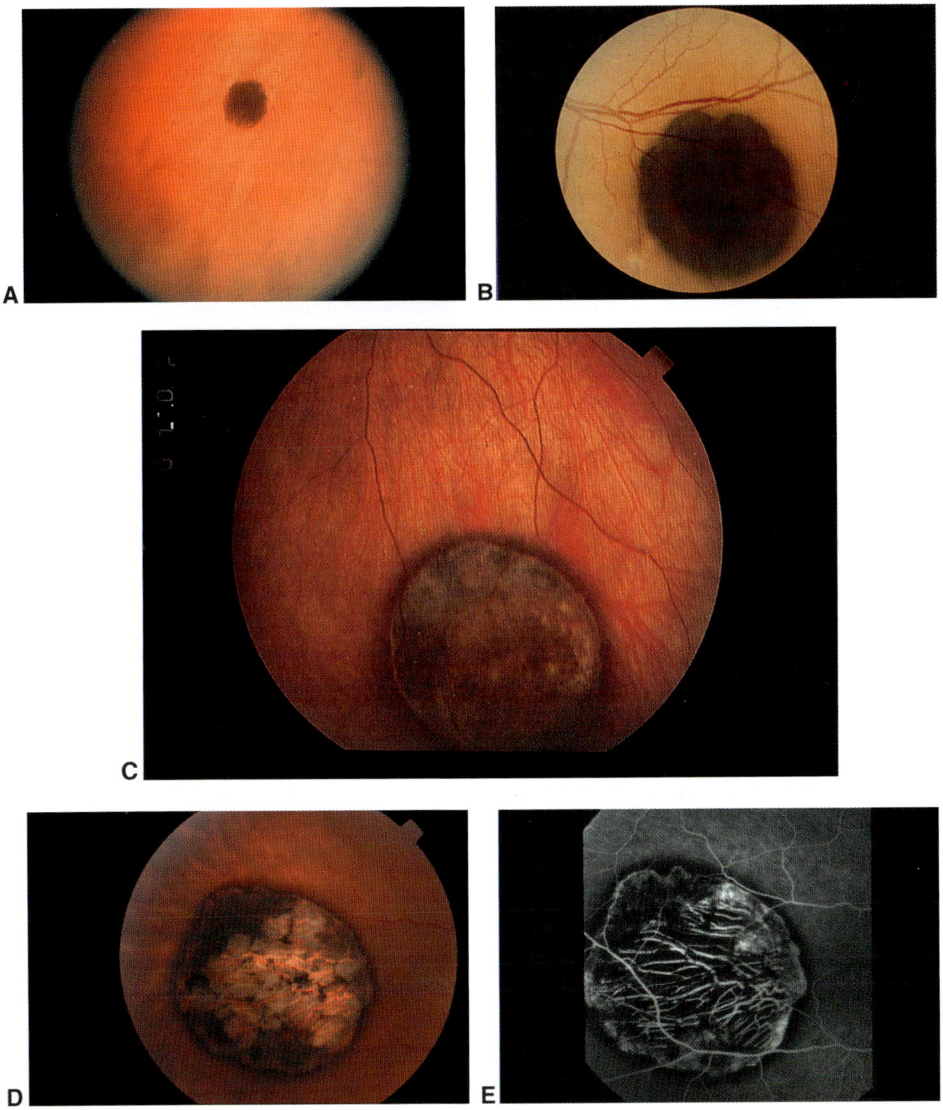

Figure 26-18 Congenital hypertrophy of the RPE (CHRPE). Examples of varying clinical appearances. **A,** Small CHRPE. **B,** Medium-sized CHRPE; note the homogeneous black color and well-defined margins of this nummular lesion. **C,** Large CHRPE. This lesion exhibits pigment loss with the formation of central depigmented lacunae. **D, E,** Color fundus photograph and corresponding fluorescein angiogram of a large CHRPE. Note the loss of RPE architecture and highlighted choroidal vasculature. *(Parts A, D, and E courtesy of Timothy G. Murray, MD.)*

(Fig 26-20A). Approximately 25% of cases present with strabismus (esotropia or exotropia). Less common presentations include vitreous hemorrhage, hyphema, ocular or periocular inflammation, glaucoma, proptosis, and hypopyon. BCSC Section 4, *Ophthalmic Pathology and Intraocular Tumors*, also discusses retinoblastoma.

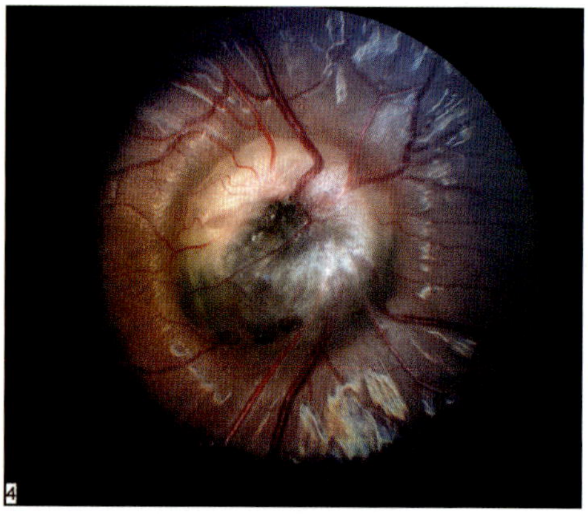

Figure 26-19 Melanocytoma of the optic disc and adjacent retina. *(Photograph courtesy of Scott Lambert, MD.)*

A retinoblastoma is a neuroblastic tumor, biologically similar to neuroblastoma and medulloblastoma. Diagnosis of retinoblastoma can usually be based on its ophthalmoscopic appearance. Intraocular retinoblastoma can exhibit a variety of growth patterns. With endophytic growth, it appears as a white to cream-colored mass that breaks through the internal limiting membrane (Fig 26-20B). Endophytic retinoblastoma is sometimes associated with vitreous seeding, in which individual cells or fragments of tumor tissue become separated from the main mass, as shown in Figure 26-21A. Vitreous seeds may be few and localized or so extensive that the clinical picture resembles endophthalmitis. Occasionally, malignant cells enter the anterior chamber and form a pseudohypopyon.

Exophytic tumors are usually yellow-white and occur in the subretinal space so that the overlying retinal vessels are commonly increased in caliber and tortuosity (Fig 26-21B). Exophytic retinoblastoma growth is often associated with subretinal fluid accumulation that can obscure the tumor and closely mimic the appearance of an exudative retinal detachment suggestive of advanced Coats disease. Retinoblastoma cells have the potential to implant on previously uninvolved retinal tissue and grow, thereby creating an impression of multicentricity in an eye with only a single primary tumor.

Large tumors often show signs of both endophytic and exophytic growth. Small retinoblastoma lesions appear as a grayish mass and are frequently confined between the internal and external limiting membranes. A third pattern, diffuse infiltrating growth retinoblastoma, is usually unilateral, nonhereditary, and found in children over 5 years old. The tumor presents with conjunctival injection, anterior chamber seeds, pseudohypopyon, large clumps of vitreous cells, and retinal infiltration of tumor. Because no distinct tumor mass is present, diagnostic confusion with inflammatory conditions is common.

Spontaneous regression of retinoblastoma is also possible and can be asymptomatic, resulting in the development of a benign retinocytoma, or it can be associated with inflammation and, ultimately, phthisis bulbi. In either case, the genetic implications are the same as for an individual with an active retinoblastoma.

Pretreatment evaluation of a patient with presumed retinoblastoma requires imaging of the head and orbits, which can confirm the diagnosis and can assist in evaluating possible extraocular extension and potential intracranial disease (Fig 26-22). MRI and

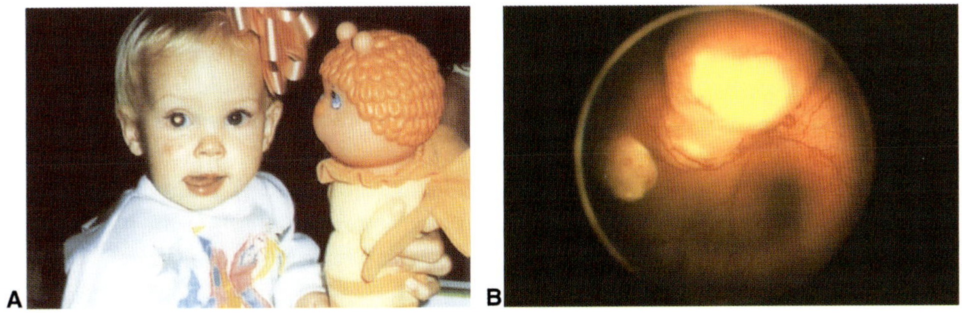

Figure 26-20 **A,** Leukocoria of the right eye shown in family photograph of a 1-year-old girl with retinoblastoma. **B,** Wide-angle fundus photograph showing multiple retinoblastoma lesions, left eye. *(Photograph courtesy of A. Linn Murphree, MD.)*

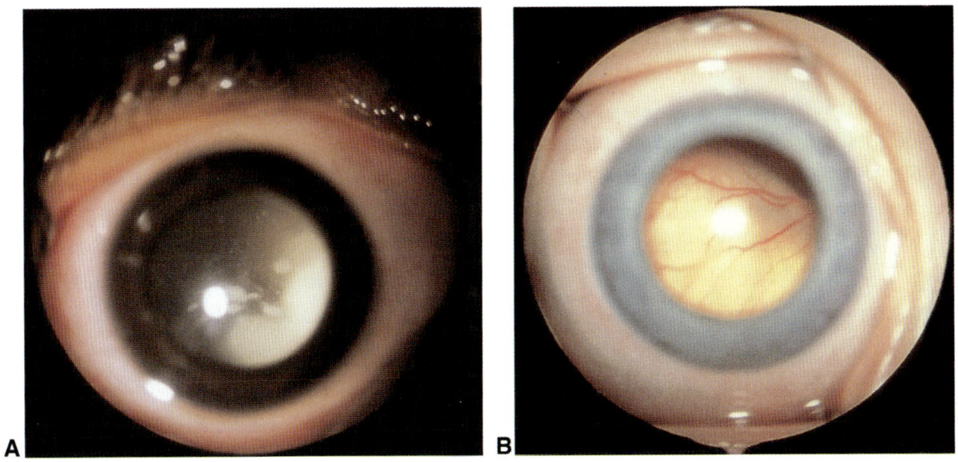

Figure 26-21 **A,** Endophytic retinoblastoma with vitreous seeding. **B,** Exophytic retinoblastoma with overlying detached retina.

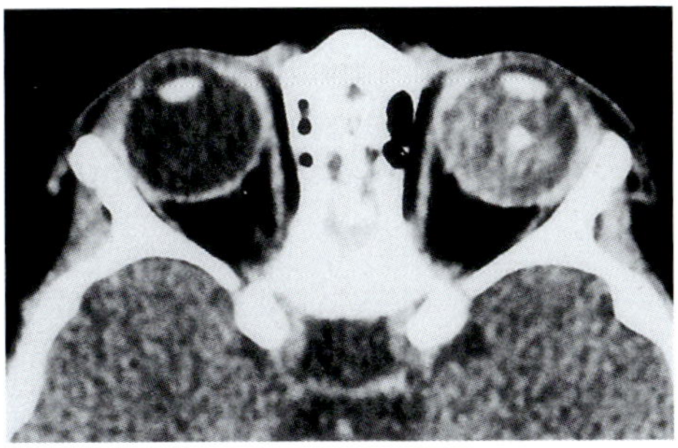

Figure 26-22 Axial CT image showing retinoblastoma filling most of the posterior segment of left eye, with localized calcification.

ultrasound, which avoid use of radiation, may be preferable to CT, because the risk of secondary tumors is high in many of these patients. Other, more invasive tests are reserved for atypical cases. Aspiration of ocular fluids for diagnostic testing should be performed only under the most unusual circumstances because such procedures can disseminate malignant cells.

The retinoblastoma gene *(RB1)* maps to a locus within the q14 band of chromosome 13 and codes for a protein, pRB, that functions as a suppressor of tumor formation. pRB is a nucleoprotein that binds to DNA and controls the cell cycle at the transition from the G1 to the S phase, thereby inhibiting cellular proliferation. Approximately 60% of retinoblastoma cases arise from somatic nonhereditary mutations of both alleles of *RB1* in a retinal cell. These mutations generally result in unifocal and unilateral tumors. In the other 40% of patients, a mutation in 1 of the 2 alleles of *RB1* either is inherited from an affected parent (10%) or occurs spontaneously in one of the gametes. A second somatic mutation occurs in one or more retinal cells, resulting in multicentric and usually bilateral tumor formation.

Genetic counseling for the families of retinoblastoma patients is complex and challenging (Table 26-2). Both of the patient's parents and all siblings should also be examined. In about 1% of cases, a parent may be found to have an unsuspected fundus lesion that represents a spontaneously regressed retinoblastoma or retinocytoma.

Genetic testing for retinoblastoma is available but has limitations. Karyotypic studies can identify only large deletions spanning 2 to 5 million base pairs, which account for only 3%–5% of retinoblastoma patients. Other direct and indirect methods can be used to detect smaller mutations; however, indirect methods require the presence of 2 or more affected family members, and the accuracy of these analyses greatly increases with examination of tumor-derived DNA, which is not available if the proband is being treated with methods other than enucleation. Direct methods are time consuming and costly and fail to find the mutation in up to 20% of cases. Preimplantation genetic testing can be performed, and in vitro fertilization techniques have been used to select embryos that are free from the germinal *RB1* mutation, successfully resulting in the birth of children unaffected by retinoblastoma.

The differential diagnosis of leukocoria is shown in Table 26-3. The most common retinal lesion simulating retinoblastoma is Coats disease. The presence of crystalline material, extensive subretinal fluid, and peripheral vascular abnormalities, combined with absence of calcium, suggests Coats disease. *Astrocytic hamartomas* and *hemangioblastomas* are benign retinal tumors that may simulate the appearance of small retinoblastomas. Both are usually associated with the neurocutaneous syndromes discussed in Chapter 27.

The characteristic histopathologic features of retinoblastoma include Flexner-Wintersteiner rosettes, which are usually present, and fleurettes, which are less common. Both represent limited degrees of retinal cellular differentiation. Homer-Wright rosettes are also frequently present but are less specific for retinoblastoma because they are common in other neuroblastic tumors. Calcification of varying extent is usually present.

Classification of retinoblastoma

The Reese-Ellsworth classification (Table 26-4) was originally developed to predict globe salvage after external beam radiotherapy. Although it is still useful for comparing

Table 26-2 Genetic Counseling for Retinoblastoma

If Parent:	Has Bilateral Retinoblastoma				Has Unilateral Retinoblastoma				Is Unaffected			
Chance of offspring having retinoblastoma	45% affected			55% unaffected	7%–15% affected			85%–93% unaffected	<1% affected			99% unaffected
Laterality	85% bilateral	15% unilateral		0%	85% bilateral	15% unilateral		0%	33% bilateral	67% unilateral		0%
Focality	100% multi-focal	96% multi-focal	4% uni-focal	0%	100% multi-focal	96% multi-focal	4% uni-focal	0%	100% multi-focal	15% multi-focal	85% uni-focal	0%
Chance of next sibling having retinoblastoma	45%	45%	45%	45%	45%	45%	45%	7%–15%	5%*	<1%*	<1%*	<1%

*If parent is a carrier, then 45%

Table created by David H. Abramson, MD.

Table 26-3 Differential Diagnosis of Leukocoria

Clinical Diagnosis in Suspected Retinoblastoma
Retinoblastoma
Persistent hyperplastic primary vitreous
Retinopathy of prematurity
Cataract
Coloboma of choroid or optic disc
Uveitis
Larval granulomatosis (toxocariasis)
Congenital retinal fold
Coats disease
Organizing vitreous hemorrhage
Retinal dysplasia
Corneal opacity
Familial exudative vitreoretinopathy (FEVR)
High myopia/anisometropia
Myelinated nerve fibers
Norrie disease
Retinal detachment

Table 26-4 Reese-Ellsworth Classification of Retinoblastoma

Group I
  a. Solitary tumor, less than 4 disc diameters in size, at or behind the equator
  b. Multiple tumors, none over 4 disc diameters in size, all at or behind the equator

Group II
  a. Solitary tumor, 4 to 10 disc diameters in size, at or behind the equator
  b. Multiple tumors, 4 to 10 disc diameters in size, behind the equator

Group III
  a. Any lesion anterior to the equator
  b. Solitary tumors larger than 10 disc diameters behind the equator

Group IV
  a. Multiple tumors, some larger than 10 disc diameters
  b. Any lesion extending anterior to the ora serrata

Group V
  a. Massive seeding involving over half the retina
  b. Vitreous seeding

contemporary treatment modalities to older ones, new classification schemes are emerging, such as the Philadelphia practical classification (Table 26-5), and the ABC classification (Table 26-6). No single new scheme has yet been widely accepted.

Management of retinoblastoma

The management of retinoblastoma has changed dramatically over the past decade and continues to evolve. External beam radiotherapy is seldom used as the primary treatment of intraocular retinoblastoma because of its high association with craniofacial deformity and secondary tumors in the field of radiation. Primary enucleation of eyes with advanced unilateral retinoblastoma is still recommended to avoid the side effects of systemic che-

Table 26-5 Philadelphia Practical Grouping System of Retinoblastoma Based on Clinical Features

Group	Abbreviation	Features	Success*
1	T	Tumor only†	100%
2	T + SRF	Tumor plus subretinal fluid	91%
3	T + FS	Tumor plus focal seeds a. SRS ≤ 3mm from tumor b. VS ≤ 3 mm from tumor	59%
4	T + DS	Tumor plus diffuse seeds a. SRS > 3 mm from tumor b. VS > 3 mm from tumor	12%
5	High risk	Tumor plus (any one) a. Neovascular glaucoma b. Opaque media from hemorrhage c. Invasion of post-laminar optic nerve, choroid (>2 mm) sclera, orbit or anterior chamber	NA

*Success after treatment with systemic chemotherapy with or without local consolidation is defined as avoidance of enucleation or need for external beam radiotherapy.
†Regardless of tumor number, size, or location.
DS = diffuse seeds, *FS* = focal seeds, *SRF* = subretinal fluid, *SRS* = subretinal seeds, *T* = tumor, *VS* = vitreous seeds, *NA* = not applicable because these patients had primarily enucleation.

Table 26-6 ABC Classification of Retinoblastoma

Group A	Small tumors (<3 mm—about 0.1 inch) confined to the retina
Group B	Larger tumors confined to the retina
Group C	Localized seeding of the vitreous or under the retina <6 mm (0.2 inch) from the original tumor
Group D	Widespread vitreous or subretinal seeding; may have total retinal detachment
Group E	No visual potential; eye cannot recover

motherapy when the likelihood of salvaging vision is low. Unnecessary manipulation of the globe should be avoided and a long segment of optic nerve obtained to avoid extraocular spread of the tumor.

Primary systemic chemotherapy (chemoreduction) followed by local therapy (consolidation) is now the most commonly used vision-sparing technique (Fig 26-23). Most studies of chemoreduction for retinoblastoma have employed vincristine, carboplatin, and an epipodophyllotoxin, either etoposide or teniposide. Others have added cyclosporine. The choice of agents as well as number and frequency of cycles varies from institution to institution. Chemotherapy is rarely successful when used alone, but in some cases, local therapy (cryotherapy, laser photocoagulation, thermotherapy, or plaque radiotherapy) can be used without chemotherapy. Side effects of chemoreduction treatment include low blood count, hair loss, hearing loss, renal toxicity, and neurologic and cardiac disturbances. Acute myelogenous leukemia has been reported after a chemoreduction regimen that included etoposide. Local administration of chemotherapy is being investigated, potentially minimizing systemic complications.

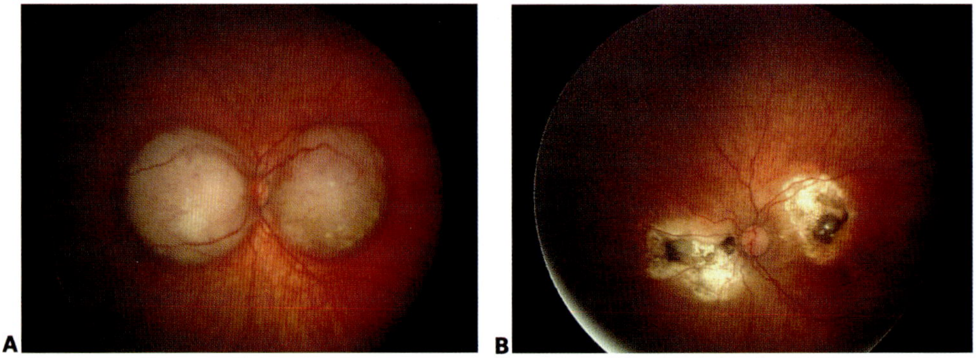

Figure 26-23 **A,** Left eye of infant with bilateral retinoblastoma. Two tumors straddle the optic nerve. Other small tumors are present in the periphery. **B,** After chemoreduction and careful laser consolidation, all tumors are nonviable. The child's vision was 20/25 at age 5 years.

Treated retinoblastoma sometimes disappears altogether, but more often it persists as a calcified mass (type 1, or cottage cheese, pattern) or a noncalcified, translucent grayish lesion (type 2, or fish flesh, pattern, which is difficult to distinguish from untreated tumor). Type 3 regression has elements of both types 1 and 2, and type 4 regression is a flat, atrophic scar. A child with treated retinoblastoma must be followed closely, with frequent examinations under anesthesia.

Extraocular retinoblastoma, although uncommon in the United States, is still problematic in developing countries, primarily due to delay in diagnosis. The 4 major types are optic nerve involvement, orbital invasion, CNS involvement, and distant metastasis. Treatment of extraocular retinoblastoma includes intensive multimodality chemotherapy, autologous hematopoietic stem cell rescue, and external beam radiation therapy. Exenteration is rarely necessary. Long-term, disease-free survival is possible if the CNS is not involved; otherwise, the prognosis is usually poor.

Patients with trilateral retinoblastoma have a primitive neuroectodermal tumor of the pineal gland or parasellar region, in addition to retinoblastoma. The risk of trilateral retinoblastoma is <0.5% and 5%–15% in patients with unilateral and bilateral retinoblastoma, respectively. Serial MRIs every 6 months are used to screen high-risk patients until age 5. Treatment includes systemic and intrathecal chemotherapy and external beam, stereotactic or gamma knife radiation therapy. Favorable responses have been obtained in some cases, but the prognosis is often poor.

Monitoring

Close monitoring of patients with retinoblastoma and their family members is crucial. Even patients with unilateral unifocal tumors have an almost 20% chance of developing retinoblastoma in their fellow eye. This risk is diminished with age and is low after age 24 months. If the retinoblastoma is the hereditary form, the patient and siblings should be examined every 4 months until age 3 or 4 years and then every 6 months until age 6 years. General anesthesia is indicated to obtain a thorough peripheral examination. Most children over age 8 years can be examined yearly in the office.

Nonocular tumors are common in patients with germinal mutations, estimated to occur with an incidence of 1% rate per year of life (eg, 10% prevalence by age 10, 30% by age 30). The incidence is higher for patients treated with external beam radiotherapy before age 1 year. The most common secondary tumors are osteogenic sarcoma of the skull and long bones, soft tissue sarcomas, cutaneous melanoma, breast cancer, lung cancer, brain tumors, and Hodgkin's lymphoma. Patients who develop second, nonocular tumors are at even greater risk for additional malignancies.

Abramson DH, Schefler AC. Update on Retinoblastoma. *Retina.* 2004:24(6):828–848

Gunduz K, Shields CL. Retinoblastoma update. *Focal Points: Clinical Modules for Ophthalmologists.* San Francisco: American Academy of Ophthalmology; 2005, module 7.

CHAPTER 27

Phakomatoses

The *phakomatoses*, or *neurocutaneous syndromes*, are a group of disorders featuring multiple discrete lesions of 1 or a few histologic types that are found in 2 or more organ systems, including the skin and central nervous system. The lesions are usually hamartomas (abnormal proliferations of tissues normally found in the involved organs). Each syndrome is defined not by the characteristics of the individual lesions but by their multiplicity or association with one another. Eye involvement is frequent and may constitute an important source of morbidity or provide information of critical importance to diagnosis. Four major disorders have traditionally been designated phakomatoses, and all have important eye manifestations:

- neurofibromatosis (von Recklinghausen disease)
- tuberous sclerosis (Bourneville disease)
- angiomatosis of the retina and cerebellum (von Hippel–Lindau disease)
- encephalofacial or encephalotrigeminal angiomatosis (Sturge-Weber syndrome)

Other conditions sometimes classified as phakomatoses include

- incontinentia pigmenti (Bloch-Sulzberger syndrome)
- ataxia-telangiectasia (Louis-Bar syndrome)
- racemose angioma (Wyburn-Mason syndrome)

Table 27-1 describes the features of the phakomatoses.

Korf BR: The phakomatoses. *Clin Dermatol.* 2005;23(1):78–84.

Neurofibromatosis

Persons with *neurofibromatosis (NF)*, or *von Recklinghausen disease*, manifest characteristic lesions composed of melanocytes or neuroglial cells, which are both primarily derivatives of neural crest mesenchyme. Although the melanocytic and glial lesions in NF are often called *hamartomas*, this designation is questionable in that most lesions do not become evident until years after birth and many are histologically indistinguishable from low-grade neoplasms originating in the same tissues.

NF has 2 distinct forms (NF1 and NF2) that are distinguished by differences in genetics, diagnostic criteria, morbidity, and treatment. Both are familial disorders that show autosomal dominant inheritance with very high penetrance (virtually 100% in NF1). However, a large percentage of cases (nearly half in NF1) are sporadic, presumably

Table 27-1 The Phakomatoses

Condition	Description	Associated Ocular Condition	Associated Conditions and Risks	Transmission
von Hippel–Lindau disease (retinal angiomatosis)	Retinal angioma supplied by dilated tortuous arteriole and venule; may be multiple	Retinal exudates, hemorrhages, retinal detachment, glaucoma	Cerebellar capillary hemangiomas, malformation of visceral organs	Autosomal dominant, chromosome 3p25
Sturge-Weber syndrome (encephalofacial angiomatosis)	Capillary hamartia (nevus flammeus) of skin, conjunctiva, episclera, and/or uveal tract, and of meninges	Glaucoma (especially with upper eyelid involvement by nevus flammeus)	Diffuse meningeal hemangioma with seizure disorder, hemiplegia or hemianopia, or mental retardation	Sporadic
Neurofibromatosis (von Recklinghausen disease)	Occasionally congenital, widespread hamartomas of peripheral nerves and tissue of neural crest derivation	Neurofibromas of eyelid and orbit, uveal melanocytic nevi, retinal glial hamartomas, congenital glaucoma, optic nerve glioma, absence of greater wing of sphenoid with pulsating exophthalmos	Similar hamartomas of central nervous system, peripheral and cranial nerves, gastrointestinal tract; malignant transformation possible	Autosomal dominant NF1: chromosome 17q11.2 NF2: chromosome 22q
Tuberous sclerosis (Bourneville disease)	Variable mental deficiency, seizures, and adenoma sebaceum	Angiofibromas of eyelid, skin; glial hamartomas of retina and optic disc	Adenoma sebaceum (angiofibromas), cerebral glial hamartomas	Autosomal dominant, chromosome 9q34
Ataxia-telangiectasia (Louis-Bar syndrome)	Progressive cerebellar ataxia, ocular and cutaneous telangiectasia, pulmonary infections	Conjunctival telangiectasia, anomalous ocular movements, and nystagmus	Dysarthria, coarse hair and skin, immunologic deficiency, and mental and growth retardation	Autosomal recessive, chromosome 11q22
Wyburn-Mason syndrome (racemose angioma)	Retinal and midbrain arteriovenous (A-V) communication (aneurysms and angiomas) and facial nevi	A-V communication (racemose angioma) of retina, with vision loss depending on location of A-V communication	A-V aneurysm at midbrain; intracranial calcification	Sporadic
Incontinentia pigmenti (Bloch-Sulzberger syndrome)	Cutaneous; dental, central nervous system, and ocular changes	ROP-like vasculopathy may progress to retinal detachment and retrolental membrane	"Splashed paint" hyperpigmented maculas, microcephaly, seizures, and mental deficiency	X-linked dominant

Modified from Isselbacher K, Braunwald E, Wilson JD, eds. *Harrison's Principles of Internal Medicine.* 13th ed. New York: McGraw-Hill; 1994:2207–2210.

reflecting the high rate of mutation known to be true for the responsible gene. The genetic locus of NF1 is on the long arm of chromosome 17, and that of NF2 is on the long arm of chromosome 22. The NF1 gene has been isolated and cloned. It appears to code for a protein involved in regulation of cellular proliferation.

Type 1 (NF1), sometimes called *peripheral neurofibromatosis*, is by far the more common, with a prevalence of 1 in 3000–5000. Details of NF1's clinical and pathologic manifestations follow.

Melanocytic Lesions

Almost all adults with NF1 have melanocytic lesions involving both the skin and the eye. The most common cutaneous expression, café-au-lait spots, appears clinically as flat, sharply demarcated, uniformly hyperpigmented macules of varying size and shape. At least a few are usually present at birth, but their number and size increase during the first decade of life. Clusters of small café-au-lait spots, or freckling, in the axillary or inguinal regions are particularly characteristic of NF1, occurring in a majority of patients over age 10 years.

Many unaffected people have 1 to 3 café-au-lait spots, but greater numbers are rare except in association with NF. In the past, NF was often diagnosed solely on the basis of multiple café-au-lait spots, but it is now recognized that a few persons with this finding never develop other stigmata of the disease and may have offspring with a similarly limited condition, suggesting the existence of a genetic disorder distinct from NF1. Currently, NF1 is diagnosed only when 2 or more criteria from the following group of 7 are met:

- 6 or more café-au-lait spots >5 mm in diameter in prepubescents or >15 mm in diameter in postpubescents
- 2 or more neurofibromas of any type or one plexiform neurofibroma
- freckling of axillary, inguinal, or other intertriginous areas
- optic nerve glioma
- 2 or more iris Lisch nodules
- a distinctive osseous lesion, such as sphenoid bone dysplasia or thinning of the long-bone cortex, with or without pseudarthrosis
- a first-degree relative with NF1, according to the above criteria

Neurofibromatosis. Conference Statement. National Institutes of Health Consensus Development Conference. *Arch Neurol.* 1988;45:575–578.

Occasionally, eyelid skin or conjunctiva is hyperpigmented in NF1, but melanocytic lesions of the uveal tract are far more common ocular manifestations. In the iris, these lesions take the form of small (usually ≤1 mm), sharply demarcated, dome-shaped excrescences known as *Lisch nodules* (Fig 27-1; see Fig 20-3). Clinically, Lisch nodules usually appear to have smooth surfaces and a translucent interior suggesting a gelatinous consistency, but in some people they look solid and wartlike. Color varies but can be described as tan in most cases. In heavily pigmented brown irides, the nodules tend to stand out as lighter nodules against the smooth, dark anterior surface and may be visible to the unaided eye. When overall iris stromal pigmentation is lighter, Lisch nodules are

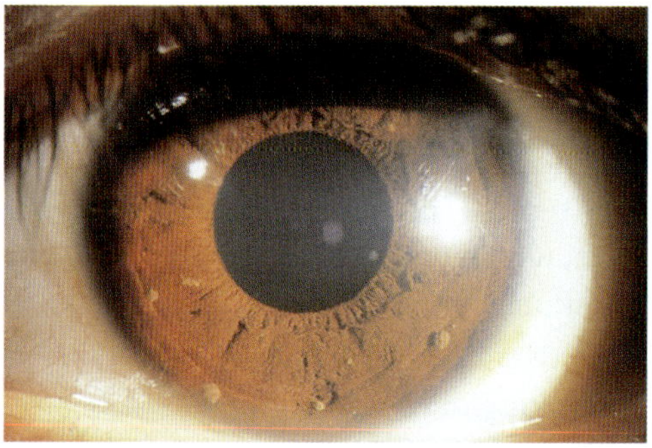

Figure 27-1 Lisch nodules of iris, left eye, in child with type 1 neurofibromatosis.

usually slightly darker than the rest of the iris but can be partly hidden within recesses in the stromal tissue and may be overlooked unless a slit lamp is used. They may be difficult to differentiate from small clumps of normal pigmented tissue, especially when they are few and the patient is less than fully cooperative. Histopathologically, the lesions consist primarily of uniform spindle-shaped, melanin-containing cells, indistinguishable from those found in iris nevi and low-grade spindle-cell melanomas.

Most Lisch nodules develop during childhood or adolescence. They are seen infrequently before age 3 years, appear in a majority of cases of NF1 between ages 5 and 10 years, and are present in nearly 100% of affected adults. The finding of 2 or more Lisch nodules is a diagnostic criterion for NF1, but an affected adult's eye typically has dozens and occasionally 100 or more (see also Chapter 20).

Choroidal lesions have been reported to occur in one third to one half of adults with NF1. These lesions are described as flat with indistinct borders and hyperpigmented in relation to the surrounding fundus but ranging from yellow-white to dark brown in color. Their number varies from 1 to 20 per eye, with each lesion typically 1 to 2 times the size of the optic disc. Direct histopathologic correlation for this clinical finding is lacking, but it is presumed to represent localized concentration of melanocytes similar to a choroidal nevus.

Neither the vision nor the health of the eye is affected by these lesions, regardless of their extent, except for the association with glaucoma in iris ectropion. People with NF1 are thought to be predisposed to uveal melanoma as well as a number of other malignant neoplasms. However, the incidence of iris, and especially choroidal, tumors is still quite low.

Glial Cell Lesions

Nodular neurofibromas

Among lesions of neuroglial origin in NF1, *nodular cutaneous* and *subcutaneous neurofibromas*, or *fibroma molluscum*, are by far the most common. These are soft papulonodules, often pedunculated, with color ranging from that of normal skin to violescent. They typically begin to appear in late childhood and increase in number throughout adolescence and adulthood; nearly all adults with NF1 have at least a few. In some cases, hundreds of these lesions are present, causing considerable disfigurement.

Plexiform neurofibromas

Of much greater clinical significance than nodular neurofibromas are the less common *plexiform neurofibromas*, which occur in approximately 30% of patients with NF1. These neurofibromas are very rarely seen in other contexts. The lesions appear clinically as extensive subcutaneous swellings with indistinct margins. Hyperpigmentation or hypertrichosis of the overlying skin is common, as is hypertrophy of underlying soft tissue and bone (regional gigantism). The consistency of plexiform neurofibromas is typically soft and not easily distinguished from that of normal tissue; the oft-repeated statement that they feel like a bag of worms applies in only a minority of cases.

Plexiform neurofibromas develop earlier than nodular lesions, frequently becoming evident in infancy or childhood. These neurofibromas often show considerable enlargement over time, resulting in severe disfigurement and functional impairment. Rarely, the lesions undergo malignant degeneration, producing a neurofibrosarcoma capable of widespread metastasis.

Approximately 10% of plexiform neurofibromas involve the face, commonly the upper eyelid and orbit. At onset, the involved upper eyelid is thicker than normal and usually appears mildly ptotic (Fig 27-2). Its inner surface may override the lower eyelid margin and lashes when the eye is closed. Characteristically, the greater involvement of its temporal portion gives the eyelid margin an S-shaped configuration and an overall appearance of an eyelid that is too big for the eye. The lesion undergoes considerable and sometimes massive growth during childhood and adolescence, although extension across the facial midline is rare. Complete ptosis may eventually result from the increasing bulk and weight of the upper eyelid. Irritation of the upper palpebral conjunctiva caused by rubbing against the lower lashes can create significant discomfort. Glaucoma in the ipsilateral eye is found in as many as half of cases.

Complete excision of a plexiform neurofibroma involving the eyelid is generally not possible. Treatment is directed toward the relief of specific symptoms and is likely to be partially successful at best. Distorted and chronically inflamed conjunctiva sometimes requires resection. Surgical debulking and frontalis suspension procedures can reduce ptosis sufficiently to permit binocular vision, but the condition is usually progressive.

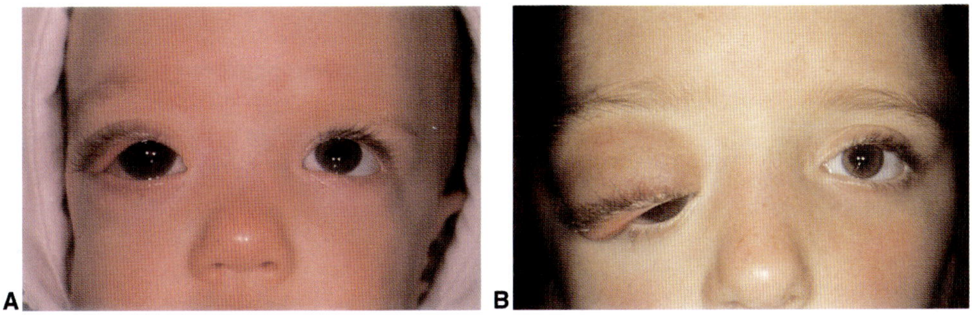

Figure 27-2 Plexiform neurofibroma involving the right upper eyelid, associated with ipsilateral buphthalmos, in girl with NF1. **A,** Age 8 months. **B,** Age 8 years.

Optic glioma

Low-grade pilocytic astrocytoma involving the optic nerve, chiasm, or both (optic glioma) is among the most characteristic and potentially serious complications of NF1. Symptomatic optic gliomas (ie, tumors producing significant visual loss, proptosis, or other complications) occur in 1%–5% of persons with NF1. When CT or MRI is performed prospectively on unselected NF1 patients, abnormalities of the optic nerve (often bilateral) or chiasm, indicating the presence of glioma, are found in approximately 15% of cases.

Typically, the entire orbital portion of an involved optic nerve shows cylindrical or fusiform enlargement (Fig 27-3). A relatively narrow central core usually differs from surrounding tissue because of the characteristic growth pattern of optic nerve glioma in NF1: most cellular proliferation occurs in the perineural intradural space (arachnoidal gliomatosis) associated with production of abundant mucinous material that gives this tissue the signal characteristics of water. This core shows higher density in CT; with MRI, the core shows higher density on T1-weighted images and lower density on T2-weighted images.

Exaggerated sinuousness or kinking of the optic nerve often occurs, creating an appearance of discontinuity or localized constriction on axial images. These appearances distinguish optic glioma from the principal differential diagnostic alternative, optic nerve sheath meningioma, which also occurs with increased frequency in NF. However, optic nerve sheath meningioma occurs much less commonly than optic glioma and rarely in childhood.

Gliomas involving the intracranial optic nerve or chiasm in NF1 produce enlargement of these structures on both CT and MRI and, frequently, abnormal signal intensity on MRI, which is now the preferred means of diagnosis. Associated contiguous involvement of the orbital portion of 1 or both optic nerves usually occurs, and extension into the optic tracts and posterior visual pathways is often evident, especially on MRI. Intraocular extension has also been reported.

Optic gliomas that become symptomatic in patients with NF1 nearly always do so before age 10 years, often apparently following a brief period of rapid enlargement. Even without treatment, some gliomas then appear to enter a phase of stability or much slower growth, and spontaneous improvement has been documented in a few cases.

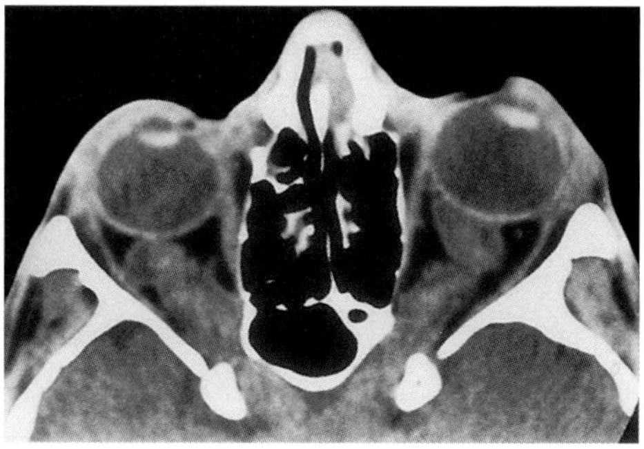

Figure 27-3 Axial CT image showing bilateral optic glioma with chiasmal involvement, associated with severe bilateral visual loss, in an adolescent boy with NF1. Note the relatively low density of tissue surrounding the central core of the enlarged optic nerve.

Tumors confined to the optic nerve at the time of clinical presentation infrequently extend into the chiasm subsequently and only rarely develop extradural extension or distant metastasis. Treatment remains controversial. Some authorities recommend complete excision through a transfrontal approach that preserves the globe but sacrifices any remaining vision on the involved side, but it has not been demonstrated that this approach improves the prognosis for sight in the other eye. Subtotal orbital excision for relief of proptosis can also be considered. New chemotherapy regimens are quite effective in halting growing masses, and radiation therapy can be useful, especially in cases of sudden vision loss or rapid growth.

In addition to bilateral visual loss, tumors primarily involving the chiasm may produce significant morbidity, including hydrocephalus and hypothalamic dysfunction leading to precocious puberty or hypopituitarism. Glioma of the chiasm carries a reported mortality rate of 50% or higher. In the past, most deaths occurred within months of diagnosis, but recent series show longer survival, reflecting earlier detection and improved management of complications, in addition to more effective treatment of the tumor itself with chemotherapy. Megavoltage radiation therapy appears to retard or reverse progression in many cases, but it is not firmly established that this therapy can substantially reduce the ultimate rate of tumor-related blindness and death, which may occur as late as 20 years after presentation.

Other neuroglial abnormalities

Abnormal proliferation of peripheral neuroglial or other neural crest–derived cells may occur in relation to deeper tissues and visceral organs as well as skin (spinal and gastrointestinal neurofibromas, pheochromocytoma). Prominence of corneal nerves, thought to represent glial hypertrophy, may be noted on slit-lamp examination in as many as 20% of cases. A frequent histopathologic finding in the choroid is the presence of so-called ovoid bodies, onionlike formations that appear to consist of hyperplastic Schwann cells surrounding peripheral nerve axons. Rarely, a localized neurofibroma develops within the orbit in association with NF. Retinal hamartomas indistinguishable from those seen in tuberous sclerosis have also been found in patients with NF1.

Other Manifestations

NF1 is associated with an increased, but still generally low, incidence of a number of conditions that cannot be explained by abnormal proliferation of neural crest–derived cells. These conditions include a variety of benign tumors that may involve skin or eye (juvenile xanthogranuloma, capillary hemangioma) and several forms of malignancy (leukemia, rhabdomyosarcoma, pheochromocytoma, Wilms tumor). Also relatively common are bony defects such as scoliosis, pseudarthrosis of the tibia, and hypoplasia of the sphenoid bone, which may result in ocular pulsation. Sphenoid dysplasia may be progressive and may be associated with neurofibromas in the ipsilateral superficial temporal fossa as well as in deep orbit. Neuroimaging should be obtained in any patient with ocular pulsations, neurofibromas in this area, or other reasons for clinical suspicion. A number of ill-defined abnormalities of the central nervous system (macrocephaly, aqueductal stenosis, seizures, and usually minor intellectual deficits) are also seen with increased frequency in patients with NF1.

The most significant ophthalmic disorder in this category is glaucoma, which is usually unilateral. In most cases, glaucoma is associated with ipsilateral plexiform neurofibroma of the upper eyelid or with the iris abnormality known as *congenital iris ectropion* (see Fig 20-9 and discussion in Chapter 20). Buphthalmos, or enlargement of the cornea and the globe as a whole, is seen if IOP is elevated during the first 2 years of life. In some cases, excessive growth of the eyeball may also be a manifestation of regional hypertrophy, at least in part. Corneal edema and high myopia can result from high pressure in early or later childhood.

The pathogenesis of glaucoma in NF1 is unknown. Abnormal trabecular meshwork development in some patients can lead to early-onset childhood or congenital glaucoma. In other patients, synechial closure of the angle may result from neurofibromatous tissue posterior to the iris or neurofibromatous infiltration of the angle directly. Medical management of the glaucoma can be attempted but frequently fails. A variety of surgical procedures have been employed with moderate success; achievement of adequate pressure control often requires several operations. Contributing to the poor prognosis are frequently associated, significant orbital and optic nerve abnormalities, as well as refractory amblyopia (anisometropic or deprivation).

A child or adult who appears to have any one of the abnormalities typically associated with NF1 should undergo an eye examination that includes the following:

- assessment of vision (acuity and color discrimination)
- pupillary light reaction, including careful scrutiny for relative afferent defect
- slit-lamp examination with particular attention to the iris
- ophthalmoscopy to identify disc pallor or edema and choroidal lesions
- measurement of IOP, when indicated by other findings

The discovery of Lisch nodules has been used to confirm the presence of NF1 in a patient with café-au-lait spots, and the absence of such nodules in an adult patient has been said to virtually rule out the diagnosis. However, the use of iris changes as a diagnostic marker for NF1 has been questioned. Iris changes in patients with known NF1 are more diverse than the classic descriptions of Lisch nodules, and interobserver reliability for the diagnosis of NF1 based on iris findings is often poor.

Although the role of routine screening with MRI remains controversial, abnormalities of vision, pupil function, or optic disc appearance indicate a need for neuroimaging studies to look for optic glioma. Preverbal children, in whom vision and visual fields cannot be accurately assessed, should have screening neuroimaging. An appropriate interval for periodic ophthalmic reassessment in childhood is 1–2 years unless a significant abnormality requires closer observation. New onset of significant eye involvement is less likely in adults, but blood pressure should be regularly monitored because of the risk of pheochromocytoma.

NF2 is less common than NF1 by a factor of at least 10. NF2 has been termed *central NF* and is diagnosed by the presence of bilateral acoustic neuromas (eighth nerve tumors) or by a first-degree relative with NF2 and presence of a unilateral acoustic neuroma, neurofibroma, meningioma, schwannoma, glioma, or early-onset cataract (posterior subcapsular cataract).

Patients with NF2 typically present in their teens to early adulthood with symptoms related to the eighth nerve tumor(s), including decreased hearing or tinnitus. Ocular findings may predate the onset of symptoms. Therefore, the alert ophthalmologist may be able to help diagnose the potential for central nervous system tumors before they become symptomatic. The most characteristic eye finding in NF2 is lens opacity, especially posterior subcapsular cataract or wedge cortical cataracts. Other, less common findings are retinal hamartoma and combined hamartomas of the retina and retinal pigment epithelium (RPE). Lisch nodules of the iris can occur in NF2 but are not expected.

Jacquemin C, Bosley TM, Liu D, et al. Reassessment of sphenoid dysplasia associated with neurofibromatosis type 1. *Am J Neuroradiol.* 2002;23:644–648.

Kaiser-Kupfer MI, Freidlin V, Datiles MB, et al. The association of posterior capsular lens opacities with bilateral acoustic neuromas in patients with neurofibromatosis type 2. *Arch Ophthalmol.* 1989;107:541–544.

Listernick R, Charrow J, Greenwald MJ, et al. Natural history of optic pathway tumors in children with neurofibromatosis type 1: a longitudinal study. *J Pediatr.* 1994;125:63–66.

Trovo-Marqui AB, Goloni-Bertollo EM, Teixeira MF, et al. Presence of the R1748X mutation in the NF1 gene in a Brazilian patient with ectropion uveae. *Ophthalmic Res.* 2004;36:349–352.

Tuberous Sclerosis

Tuberous sclerosis (TS), or *Bourneville disease,* is a familial disorder associated with a variety of abnormalities involving the skin, eye, central nervous system, and other organs. Estimates of the prevalence of TS range from as high as 1:6000 to 1:100,000 or lower. Two distinct genes giving rise to TS have been identified: *TSC1* at chromosome 9q34 and *TSC2* at chromosome 16p13.3. Transmission as an autosomal dominant trait has been documented in numerous pedigrees, but new mutations account for as many as 80% of cases.

The 3 classic findings, known as the Vogt triad, are mental retardation, seizures, and facial angiofibromas, although all 3 are present in only about 30% of patients with TS. The disease is characterized by benign tumor growth in multiple organs, predominantly the skin, brain, heart, kidney, and eye. Primary features of this disorder, any one of which is sufficient to diagnose TS, are

- facial angiofibroma
- ungual fibromas (multiple)
- cortical tuber
- subependymal nodule (giant cell astrocytoma)
- multiple subependymal nodules protruding into the ventricle
- multiple retinal astrocytomas

Several distinct skin lesions are characteristic of TS (Fig 27-4). The earliest cutaneous sign to appear is the white spot, or hypopigmented macule, which is present in almost all cases at birth or in infancy. These lesions are sharply demarcated, with a shape that

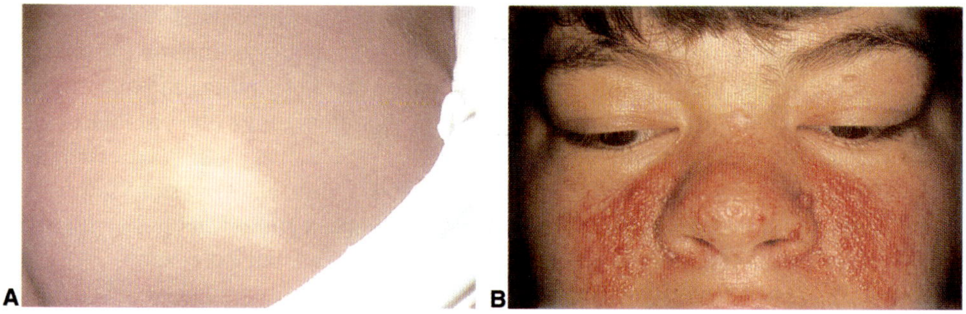

Figure 27-4 Cutaneous lesions of tuberous sclerosis. **A,** Hypopigmented macule. **B,** Adenoma sebaceum of the face.

often resembles an ash leaf. Ultraviolet light from a Wood's lamp increases the visibility of white spots in light-skinned people. Histopathologically, these spots have decreased melanin but normal numbers of melanocytes.

Facial angiofibromas often called *adenoma sebaceum* begin to appear in childhood and increase progressively in number; they are present in three quarters of adolescents and adults with TS. These lesions are often mistaken for common acne. Subungual and periungual fibromas are also common after puberty; gingival fibromas may occur as well. A thickened plaque of skin known as a shagreen patch, or collagenoma, occurs in approximately one quarter of cases, typically in the lumbosacral area. Plaques involving the forehead that sometimes extend into the eyelids may be present at birth.

Seizures occur in 80% of patients with TS, and they may be difficult to control. Severe mental retardation is present in 50% of patients, but intelligence is often normal. Characteristic findings in neuroimaging studies include nodular periventricular or basal ganglion calcifications (representing benign astrocytomas) and tuberous malformations of the cortex (Fig 27-5). Malignant astrocytomas occur infrequently. Obstruction of the foramen of Monro by tumor may produce hydrocephalus, and cardiac tumors (rhabdomyomas) can lead to early death or severe disability. Lesions of bone and kidney are common but usually produce no significant disturbance of function.

Hypopigmented lesions analogous to white spots of the skin are occasionally seen in the iris or choroid, but the most frequent and characteristic ocular manifestation of TS is the retinal phakoma (Fig 27-6). Pathologically, this growth arises from the innermost layer of the retina and is composed of nerve fibers and relatively undifferentiated cells that appear to be of glial origin; the growth is frequently called an *astrocytic hamartoma.* Phakomas can develop anywhere in the fundus but are usually found near the posterior pole, involving the retina, the optic disc, or both. They vary in size from about half to twice the diameter of the disc. Vision is rarely affected significantly.

Retinal phakomas usually have 1 of 2 distinct appearances, although intermediate forms can occur. The first type is typically found in very young children and is relatively flat with a smooth surface, indistinct margins, and gray-white color. These lesions are translucent to a degree that at times makes them difficult to detect ophthalmoscopically. The examiner can most easily locate them by tracing retinal vessels from the disc peripherally and scrutinizing points at which a vessel is partially obscured by overlying

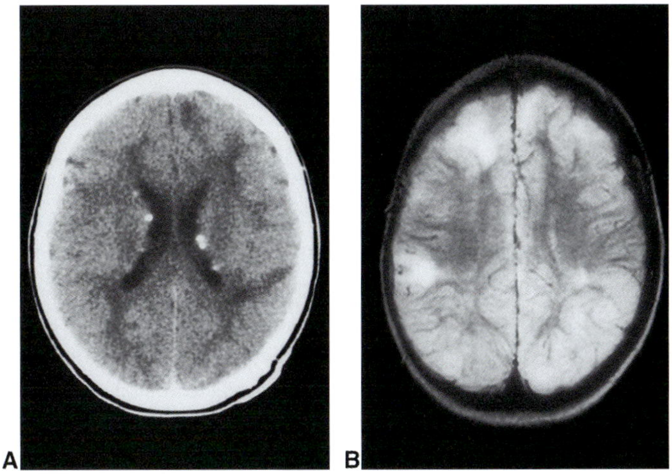

Figure 27-5 Brain lesions of tuberous sclerosis. **A,** Axial CT image showing small periventricular calcifications in the basal ganglia bilaterally. **B,** Axial T2-weighted MRI showing 2 tuberous malformations of the right hemisphere cortex.

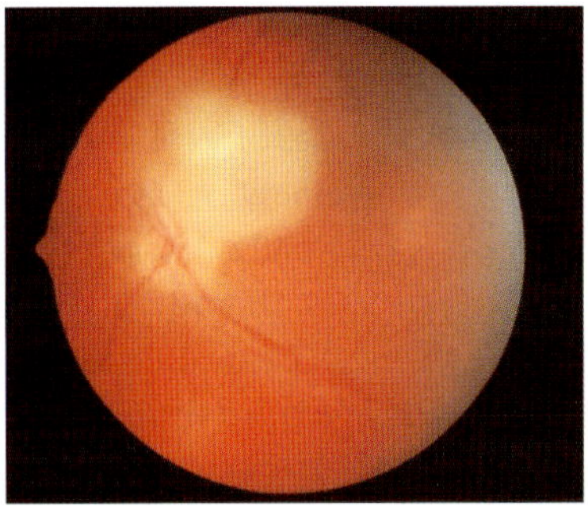

Figure 27-6 Fundus lesions of tuberous sclerosis, left eye. In addition to the large phakoma partially overlying the optic disc, a small hypopigmented lesion appears in the temporal macula, and a barely visible second phakoma partially obscures a retinal blood vessel near the edge of the photograph, directly below the disc.

tissue. The examiner can then perceive domelike elevations with the binocular indirect ophthalmoscope by carefully observing the surface light reflection while shifting viewing direction slightly. The second type of phakoma is sharply demarcated and more elevated than the first type, with an irregular surface that has been compared to a mulberry or a cluster of tapioca grains or fish eggs. These lesions are opaque, glistening, and yellow-white as a result of calcification. They are found relatively more often in older patients and on or adjacent to the optic disc. The term *giant drusen* has been applied to disc involvement by a mulberry phakoma because of its resemblance to the common but unrelated condition known as *drusen* (or *hyaline bodies*) of the optic nerve head.

The reported frequency of phakomas in persons with TS varies greatly, but data from recent series suggest that they are present in one third to more than one half of cases. One to several may be found in a single eye, and the rate of bilateral involvement is about 40%. There is no evidence that the number of lesions increases with age, although individual tumors have been documented to grow over time. Phakomas are not pathognomonic of TS; they occur occasionally in association with neurofibromatosis and in the eyes of unaffected persons.

Alcorn DM. Ocular oncology. *Ophthalmol Clin North Am.* 1999;12:2.

von Hippel–Lindau Disease

von Hippel–Lindau (VHL) disease, or *retinal angiomatosis,* is an autosomal dominantly inherited disorder manifesting both benign and malignant tumors of many organ systems. The most common abnormalities are vascular tumors *(hemangioblastomas)* of the retina and central nervous system, most often the cerebellum. These tumors have only limited proliferative capacity, but exudation across thin vessel walls in the lesions leads to the formation of fluid accumulations that may attain considerable size and compromise vital structures. Cysts and tumors occur frequently in numerous other organs, including the kidneys *(renal cell carcinoma)*, pancreas, liver, epididymis, and adrenal glands *(pheochromocytoma).* Despite its well-accepted classification as a neurocutaneous syndrome, VHL disease rarely has significant cutaneous manifestations, although café-au-lait spots and port-wine stains *(nevus flammeus)* are seen occasionally. Mental deficiency is not a feature of the disease. The *VHL* gene is a tumor suppressor found on chromosome 3. The prevalence of VHL is approximately 1 in 36,000 births. Associated malignant tumors make it a potentially fatal disease.

Pedigree studies suggest that ocular involvement occurs in most cases of VHL disease. (Identical eye disease without familial transmission or systemic involvement is 3 to 4 times more common than the complete syndrome.) The retinal lesions originally described by von Hippel usually become visible ophthalmoscopically between ages 10 and 35 years, with an average age of onset of 25 years, about a decade before the peak clinical incidence of cerebellar disease. Tumors are multiple in the same eye in about one third of cases and bilateral in as many as one half of cases. Tumors typically occur in the peripheral fundus, but lesions adjacent to the optic disc have also been described.

The incipient retinal lesion appears as a minor, nonspecific vascular anomaly or a small reddish dot in the fundus that gradually enlarges into a flat or slightly elevated grayish disc. The lesion ultimately acquires the fully developed appearance of a pink globular mass 1 to 3 or more disc diameters in size. The hallmark of the mature tumor is a pair of markedly dilated vessels (artery and vein) running between the lesion and the optic disc, indicating significant arteriovenous shunting (Fig 27-7). Recent observations suggest that characteristic paired or twin retinal vessels of normal caliber may be present before the tumor becomes visible.

Histopathologically, retinal angiomas consist of relatively well-formed capillaries; however, fluorescein angiography shows these vessels to be leaky. Transudation of fluid into the subretinal space causes lipid accumulation, retinal detachment, and consequent loss of vision in many involved eyes. Secondary degenerative changes, including cataract and glaucoma, often occur in blind eyes with long-standing retinal detachment; ultimately, enucleation may become necessary.

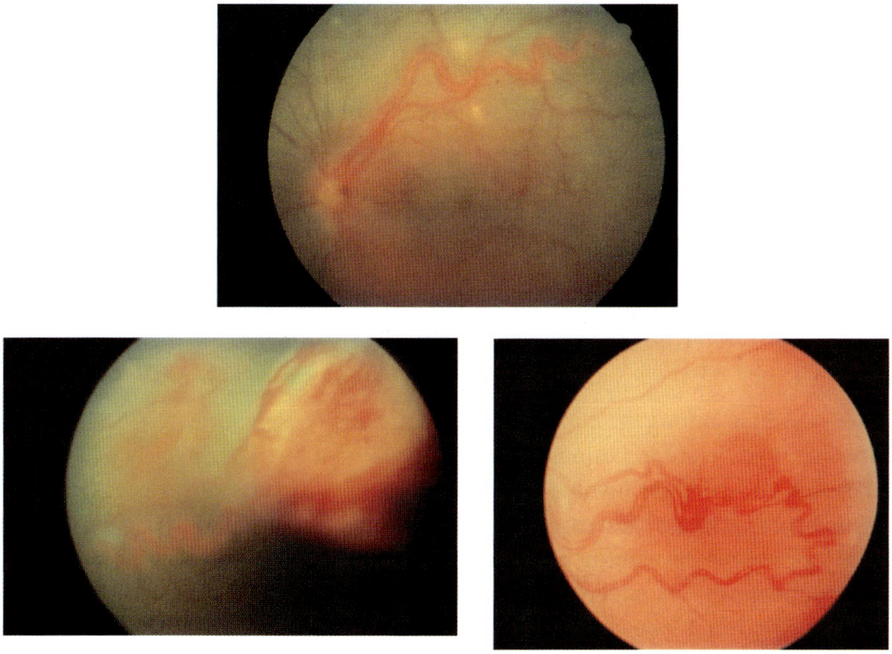

Figure 27-7 von Hippel–Lindau disease (retinal angiomatosis), left eye.

Retinal angiomas can be effectively treated with cryotherapy or laser photocoagulation in two thirds or more of cases, particularly when the lesions are still small. Multiple treatment sessions may be necessary to achieve complete success. Early diagnosis increases the likelihood of successful treatment, yet the ocular lesions of VHL are asymptomatic prior to retinal detachment. Therefore, children known to be at risk for the disease should undergo periodic ophthalmologic evaluation beginning at about age 5 years.

Systemically, early tumor diagnosis can significantly reduce morbidity and mortality. The Cambridge screening protocol recommends that patients with VHL undergo annual complete physical examination and dilated eye examinations, renal ultrasonography, and 24-hour urine collection for vanillylmandelic acids. These patients should undergo neuroimaging every 3 years to age 40 and every 5 years thereafter. At-risk relatives should also undergo thorough annual screening for the disorder. Molecular genetic testing has been suggested for patients with early-onset cerebellar hemangioblastoma (<30 years old), early-onset retinal angioma, or familial clear cell renal carcinoma.

Chang JH, Spraul CW, Lynn ML, et al. The two-stage mutation model in retinal hemangioblastoma. *Ophthalmic Genet.* 1998;19:123–130.

Sturge-Weber Syndrome

Sturge-Weber syndrome (SWS), or *encephalofacial angiomatosis*, consists of a facial cutaneous angioma (port-wine stain) with an ipsilateral leptomeningeal vascular malformation that typically results in the following:

- cerebral calcification
- seizures, which may show a jacksonian pattern, progressing from focal to grand mal
- focal neurologic deficits (hemianopia, hemiparesis)
- a highly variable degree of mental deficiency (with normal intelligence in many affected persons)

SWS is unique among the 4 major neurocutaneous syndromes in that it is not a genetically transmitted disorder. Lesions are always present at birth, however. The distribution of cutaneous and cerebral involvement suggests a disturbance very early in embryonic development (4–8 weeks' gestation), when primitive facial structures overlie the future occipital lobes of the developing brain. The prevalence of SWS is not reliably known.

Calcium deposits characteristic of SWS form after birth in brain parenchyma, usually involving the occipital lobe and varying portions of the parietal, temporal, and occasionally frontal lobes. Curvilinear densities, paralleling cerebral convolutions to produce the so-called railroad track sign, can be demonstrated by means of CT earlier and more consistently than by conventional radiographs, but these densities are often not detectable before age 2 years. MRI is less sensitive than CT for identifying calcification but may provide better delineation of other abnormalities associated with the angiomatous malformation that can confirm the diagnosis in very young children (Fig 27-8). These abnormalities include cerebral volume reduction, abnormal signal intensity in cortex and white matter, prominent deep venous system, and enlarged choroid plexus.

The Sturge-Weber skin lesion, which can be quite disfiguring, consists of dilated and excessively numerous but well-formed capillaries in the dermis. The lesion usually involves the forehead and upper eyelid on the same side as the cerebral vascular malformation, with varying extension to the ipsilateral lower eyelid and maxillary and mandib-

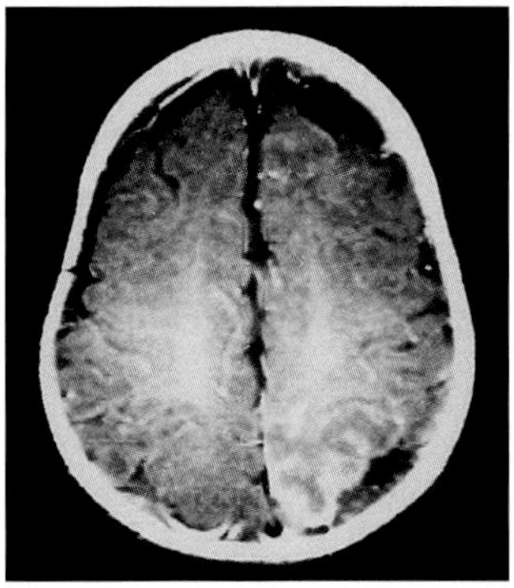

Figure 27-8 Axial gadolinium-enhanced T1-weighted MRI shows vascular malformation with underlying cortical atrophy in the left occipital lobe of a 4-month-old girl with Sturge-Weber syndrome.

ular regions (Fig 27-9). The sharply demarcated area of the port-wine nevus frequently does not conform to the distribution of the trigeminal divisions, and involvement of the contralateral face, the scalp, and the trunk and extremities is common. (The designation Klippel-Trénaunay-Weber syndrome is sometimes applied to cases with extensive lesions of the extremities, although this syndrome may not be a true phakomatosis.) Hypertrophy of soft tissue and bone underlying the angioma is common in childhood, and thickening of the involved skin (sometimes with a nodular pattern) may develop later in life. Treatment of affected skin with a pulsed dye laser has been shown to markedly reduce vascularity, considerably improving appearance without causing significant damage to dermal tissue.

Many children have a port-wine stain but do not have SWS.

Ocular Involvement

Any portion of the ocular circulation may be anomalous in SWS when the skin lesion involves the eyelids. Increased conjunctival vascularity commonly produces a pinkish discoloration. Frequently, an abnormal plexus of episcleral vessels appears, although it may be hidden by the overlying tissue of Tenon's layer. The retina sometimes shows tortuous vessels and arteriovenous communications.

The choroid is the site of the most significant, purely vascular anomaly of the eye associated with SWS. In a majority of cases of SWS with ocular involvement, increased numbers of well-formed choroidal vessels give the fundus a uniform bright red or red-orange color that has been compared to tomato catsup (Fig 27-10). Typically, the region of the posterior pole is involved; in some cases, there is gradual transition to a normal vascular pattern in the periphery, whereas in others the entire fundus seems to be affected.

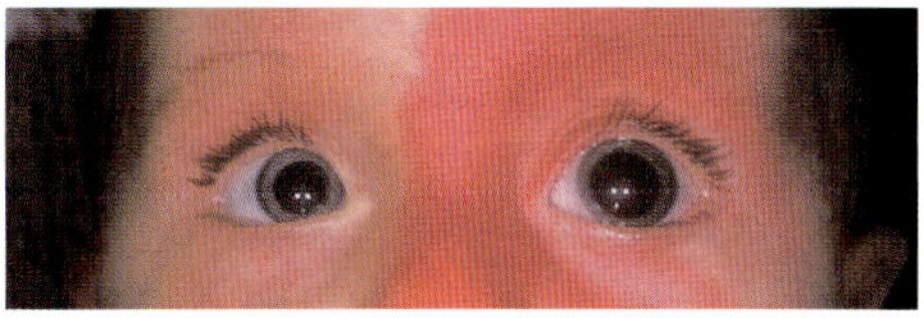

Figure 27-9 Facial port-wine nevus involving the left eyelids, associated with ipsilateral buphthalmos in an infant girl with Sturge-Weber syndrome.

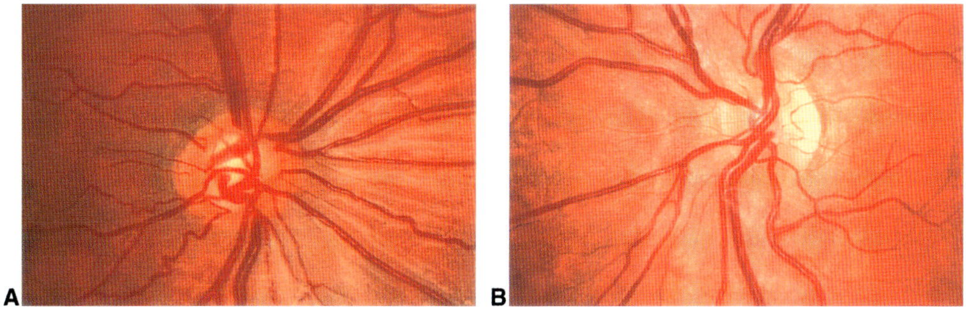

Figure 27-10 Fundus appearance in an adolescent boy with Sturge-Weber syndrome. **A,** Right eye. Note glaucomatous disc cupping and deeper red color of surrounding choroid, compared with normal fellow eye. **B,** Left eye.

Choroidal angiomatosis usually remains asymptomatic in childhood. During adolescence or adulthood, however, the choroid sometimes becomes markedly thickened. Degeneration or detachment of the overlying retina with severe visual loss may follow, but the frequency of this progression is not established. No treatment is known to effectively prevent or reverse such deterioration, although scattered application of laser photocoagulation, which has proven useful in the management of circumscribed choroidal angiomas not associated with SWS, may help.

Glaucoma is the most common and serious ocular complication, occurring in approximately half of cases. The cause of elevated IOP is uncertain but is likely secondary to elevated episcleral venous pressure, hyperemia of the ciliary body with hypersecretion of aqueous, or developmental anomaly of the anterior chamber angle. Involvement of the upper-lid skin seems to raise the likelihood of glaucoma. Onset of glaucoma can be at birth or later in childhood. If IOP is elevated during early infancy, enlargement of the cornea can occur.

Management

When SWS is first documented or suspected, a complete ophthalmic evaluation is essential, including measurement of IOP. Sedation or general anesthesia may be necessary for uncooperative children. Examination should be repeated periodically throughout childhood even if no ocular abnormality is initially detected. SWS glaucoma is difficult to treat, and there is no universally accepted treatment scheme. Initial therapy with topical drops can be effective, especially when onset occurs later. Surgery is indicated in early-onset cases and when medical treatment is inadequate. Adequate long-term pressure control can frequently be achieved, although multiple operations are typically necessary. Aqueous shunting devices, or setons, have shown promise in the management of otherwise intractable glaucoma in patients with SWS (see BCSC Section 10, *Glaucoma*). A particular hazard of glaucoma surgery in SWS is the risk of massive intraoperative or postoperative exudation or hemorrhage from anomalous choroidal vessels due to rapid ocular decompression. Special care must be taken with implanted drainage devices to prevent excessive early postoperative hypotony. Choroidal or subretinal fluid accumulation after surgery may be dramatic, but spontaneous resorption usually occurs within 1–2 weeks. Angle surgery in the form of goniotomy and trabeculotomy has been used successfully in some patients, presumably those whose glaucoma has some etiologic similarity to typical congenital glaucoma.

Eibschitz-Tsimhoni M, Lichter PR, Del Monte MA, et al. Assessing the need for posterior sclerotomy at the time of filtering surgery in patients with Sturge-Weber syndrome. *Ophthalmology.* 2003;110:1361–1363.

Thomas-Sohl KA, Vaslow DF, Maria BL. Sturge-Weber syndrome: a review. *Pediatr Neurol.* 2004;30:303–310.

Ataxia-Telangiectasia

Ataxia-telangiectasia (AT), or *Louis-Bar syndrome*, is an autosomal recessive disorder that primarily involves the central nervous system (particularly the cerebellum), the ocular surface, the skin, and the immune system. Although rare (prevalence is about 1:40,000), AT is thought to be the most common cause of progressive ataxia in early childhood. Truncal ataxia is usually noted during the second year of life, with subsequent development of dysarthria, dystonia, and choreoathetosis. Progressive deterioration of motor function leads to serious disability by age 10 years. Intellectual impairment, if present, is usually mild.

Recognition of ocular features is often the key to diagnosis of AT. Ocular motor abnormalities are found in many patients with AT and are frequently among the earliest manifestations. Characteristically, the ability to initiate saccades with preservation of vestibulo-ocular movements is poor, very similar to congenital ocular motor apraxia. Head thrusts are used to compensate for saccades. Strabismus and nystagmus may also be present.

Telangiectasia of the conjunctiva develops between the ages of 3 and 5 years. In one study, 91% of AT patients had conjunctival telangiectasia. Involvement is initially interpalpebral but away from the limbus, eventually becoming generalized (Fig 27-11). Similar, though less obvious, vessel changes can appear in the skin of the eyelids and other sun-exposed areas. A variety of skin changes that suggest accelerated aging are common in older children and adults with AT.

People with AT show greatly increased sensitivity to the tissue-damaging side effects of therapeutic radiation and many chemotherapeutic agents. Defective T-cell function in patients with AT is usually associated with hypoplasia of the thymus and decreased levels of circulating immunoglobulin. Recurrent respiratory tract infections are a serious problem, frequently causing death in adolescence or young adulthood even with optimal antimicrobial and supportive treatment. The increased susceptibility to various malignancies, particularly lymphomas and leukemias, contributes to early mortality in one third to one half of cases.

The causative gene in AT is called *ATM* and is found on chromosome 11. The gene product is required for cell survival after exposure to low labile iron concentrations and may have a role in treating Parkinson disease, as well as AT, in the future. The gene appears to play a role in some cancers as well. A new rapid test from peripheral blood can diagnose AT accurately. AT heterozygosity is present in an estimated 1%–3% of the population. Although gene carriers are generally healthy and cannot be identified except

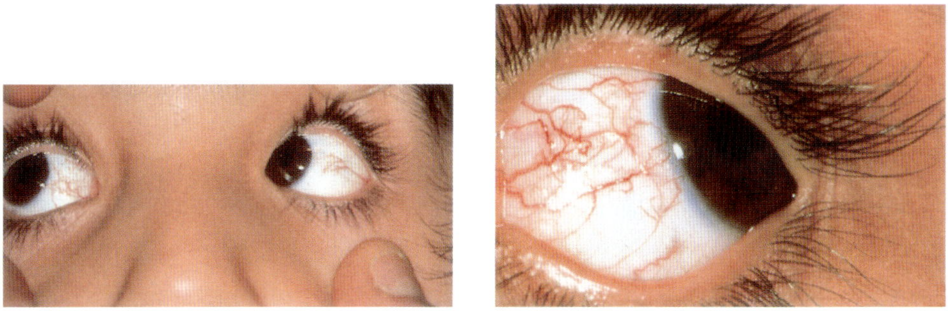

Figure 27-11 Abnormally dilated and tortuous conjunctival vessels in a child with ataxia-telangiectasia.

in the context of a known AT pedigree, they are at significantly increased risk for common forms of malignancy and show greater-than-normal sensitivity to radiation. In women heterozygous for the AT gene, breast cancer is about 7 times more frequent than in non-carriers and may account for nearly 10% of all cases in the United States.

Butch AW, Chun HH, Nahas SA, et al. Immunoassay to measure ataxia-telangiectasia mutated protein in cellular lysates. *Clin Chem.* 2004;50:2302–2308.

Farr AK, Shalev B, Crawford TO, et al. Ocular manifestations of ataxia-telangiectasia. *Am J Ophthalmol.* 2002;134:891–896.

Incontinentia Pigmenti

Incontinentia pigmenti (IP), or *Bloch-Sulzberger syndrome*, involves the skin, brain, and eyes and shows the unusual inheritance pattern of X-linked dominance with a presumed lethal effect on the hemizygous male fetus. Nearly all affected persons are female, with mother-to-daughter transmission in familial cases. BCSC Section 2, *Fundamentals and Principles of Ophthalmology*, details this inheritance pattern in the chapters on genetics.

The cutaneous manifestations of IP are distinctive. The skin usually appears normal at birth, but erythema and bullae develop during the first few days of life, usually on the extremities, and persist for weeks to months. A second distinct phase characterized by verrucous changes begins at about 2 months of age, subsiding after a few more months. Finally, clusters of small hyperpigmented macules in a characteristic splashed-paint distribution make their appearance, most prominently on the trunk (Fig 27-12).

Histopathologically, the early vesicular lesions show local accumulation of unusually large macrophages and eosinophils, accompanied by peripheral blood eosinophilia. In the lesions of the pigmentary stage, which persist for years before gradually fading, free melanin granules are found abnormally scattered in the dermis. Although present in all cases, skin involvement varies considerably in extent, occasionally being so limited that it is completely overlooked at one or more of its stages.

About one third of patients with IP have central nervous system problems that may include microcephaly, hydrocephalus, seizures, and varying degrees of mental deficiency. Dental abnormalities (missing and malformed teeth) are found in roughly two thirds of cases. Other, less common findings include scoliosis, skull deformities, cleft palate, and dwarfism.

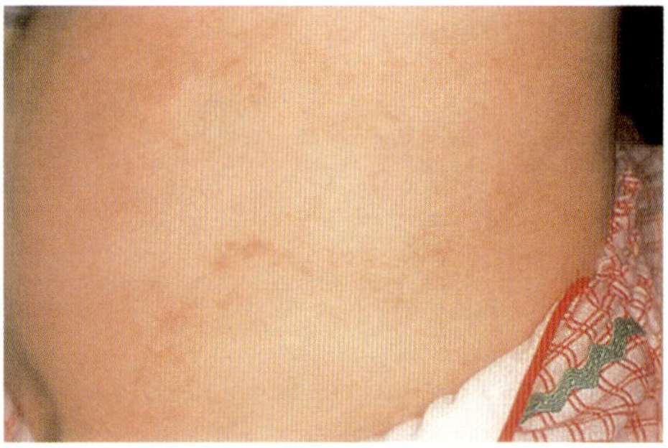

Figure 27-12 Pigmented skin lesions of incontinentia pigmenti.

Ocular involvement occurs in at least one quarter to one third of cases, typically in the form of a proliferative retinal vasculopathy that closely resembles retinopathy of prematurity. At birth, the only detectable abnormality may be incomplete peripheral retinal vascularization. Abnormal arteriovenous connections, microvascular abnormalities, and neovascular membranes develop at or near the junction of the vascular and avascular retina (Fig 27-13). Rapid progression sometimes leads to total retinal detachment and retrolental membrane formation (pseudoglioma) within the first few months of life. Other affected eyes show gradual deterioration over a period of several years; still others have proliferative lesions of limited extent that may persist for decades. Microphthalmos, cataract, glaucoma, optic atrophy, strabismus, and nystagmus occur occasionally, representing secondary consequences of end-stage retinopathy in most if not all cases.

The retinopathy of IP has been managed by photocoagulation or cryotherapy in a small number of cases, with varying degrees of reported success. Treatment is usually applied primarily to the avascular peripheral retina, as in the currently preferred approach to management of retinopathy of prematurity.

Catalano RA. Incontinentia pigmenti. *Am J Ophthalmol.* 1990;110:696–700.

Wyburn-Mason Syndrome

Wyburn-Mason syndrome, or *racemose angioma*, is a nonhereditary arteriovenous malformation of the eye and brain, typically involving the optic disc or retina and the midbrain. Skin lesions are present in a minority of cases. The complete syndrome is considerably less common than an isolated occurrence of similar ocular or intracranial disease.

Seizures, mental changes, hemiparesis, and papilledema may result from the central nervous system lesions, which are frequently a source of hemorrhage, unlike the hemangioma of SWS.

Ocular manifestations are unilateral and congenital but may progress somewhat during childhood. The typical lesion consists of markedly dilated and tortuous vessels that

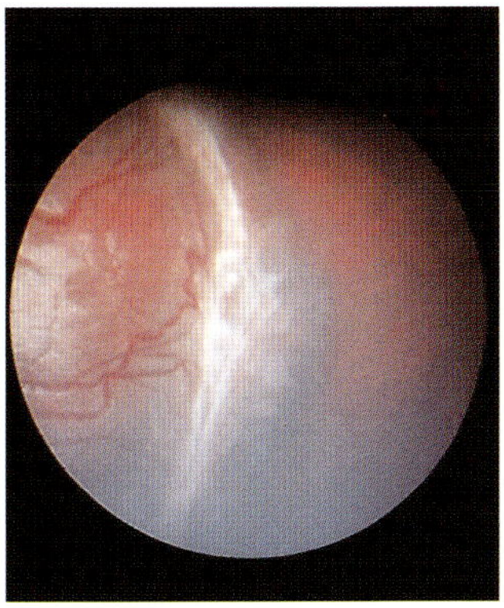

Figure 27-13 Vascular abnormalities of the temporal retina, right eye, in a 2-year-old child with incontinentia pigmenti. Note avascularity peripheral to the circumferential white vasoproliferative lesion, which showed profuse leakage on fluorescein angioscopy.

shunt blood flow directly from arteries to veins; these vessels do not leak fluid (Fig 27-14). Vision ranges from normal to markedly reduced in the involved eye, and intraocular hemorrhage and secondary neovascular glaucoma are possible complications. No treatment is indicated for primary lesions.

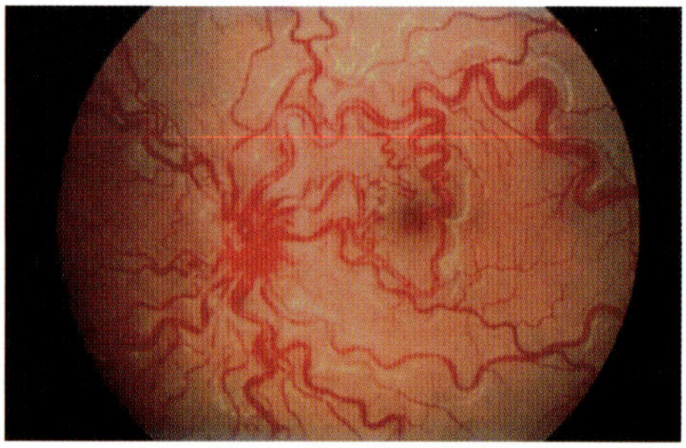

Figure 27-14 Racemose angioma of the retina, left eye.

CHAPTER 28

Craniofacial Malformations

Approach to the Child With Craniofacial Malformations

This chapter includes most of the common craniofacial conditions an ophthalmologist may encounter. A working knowledge of these conditions is important because these syndromes may primarily affect the eye or ocular adnexa and may induce secondary ocular complications. Some craniofacial malformations are the result of craniosynostosis; others are not.

Craniosynostosis

Craniosynostosis is the premature closure of 1 or more cranial sutures during the embryonic period or early childhood. Cranial sutures are present throughout the skull, which is divided into 2 parts, the *calvarium* and the *skull base*, via an imaginary line drawn from the supraorbital rims to the base of the occiput (Fig 28-1).

Bony growth of the skull occurs in osteoblastic centers located at the suture sites. Bone is laid down parallel and perpendicular to the direction of the suture. Premature suture closure prevents perpendicular growth but allows parallel growth. This pattern is termed *Virchow's law* and leads to clinically recognizable cranial bone deformations, all of which carry specific nomenclature (Fig 28-2). The following are important terms associated with craniosynostosis.

Plagiocephaly The term *plagiocephaly* literally means "oblique head." Most often it is the consequence of a unilateral coronal suture synostosis. On the synostotic, or fused suture, side, the forehead is retruded (depressed), the supraorbital rim is retruded, and the orbit is often higher than on the nonsynostotic side. Because of brain growth and necessary cranial vault expansion, the nonsynostotic side will, in contrast, display protrusion or bulging of the forehead, lower supraorbital rim, and often a lower orbit (Fig 28-3).

Oxy-, turri-, acrocephaly These terms all mean "tower head." The condition occurs most often with multiple suture closures, such as both coronals, the sagittal, and possibly the lambdoidals.

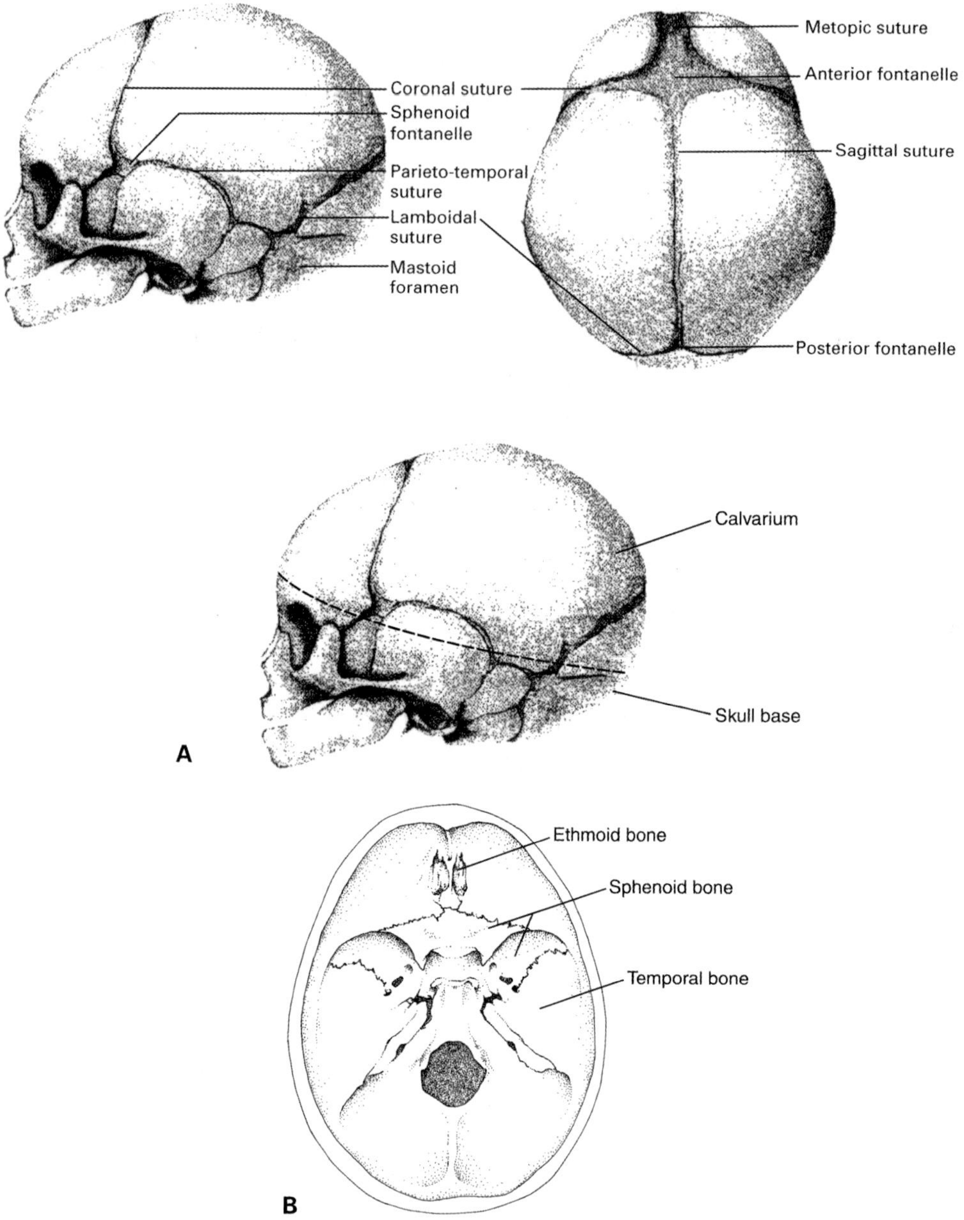

Figure 28-1 **A,** Normal sutures and fontanelles of the fetal skull. **B,** Adult cranial base, complete with sutures. *(Illustration by C. H. Wooley.)*

Brachycephaly "Short head"; specifically refers to growth in the anterior-posterior axis. Brachycephaly is often the result of bilateral closure of the coronal sutures. The forehead is most often wide and flat.

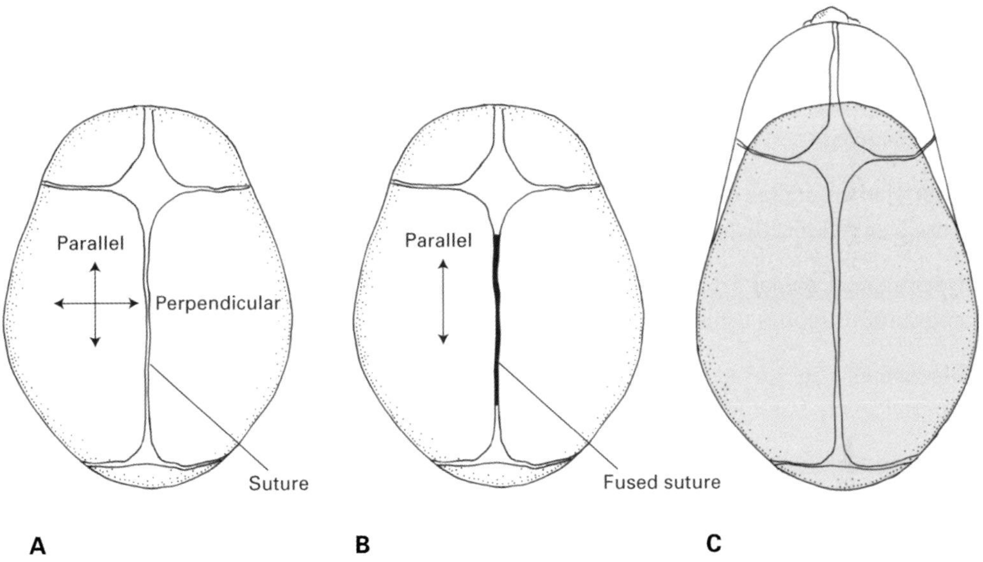

Figure 28-2 **A,** Normal sutures. Bone growth occurs at the suture, laid down parallel and perpendicular to the suture. **B,** Virchow's law. Prematurely fused sutures allow bone growth only in the parallel direction; perpendicular growth is inhibited. **C,** An example of Virchow's law. Closure of the sagittal suture produces scaphocephaly (boatlike skull) when compared to the normal skull (shaded area). *(Illustration by C. H. Wooley.)*

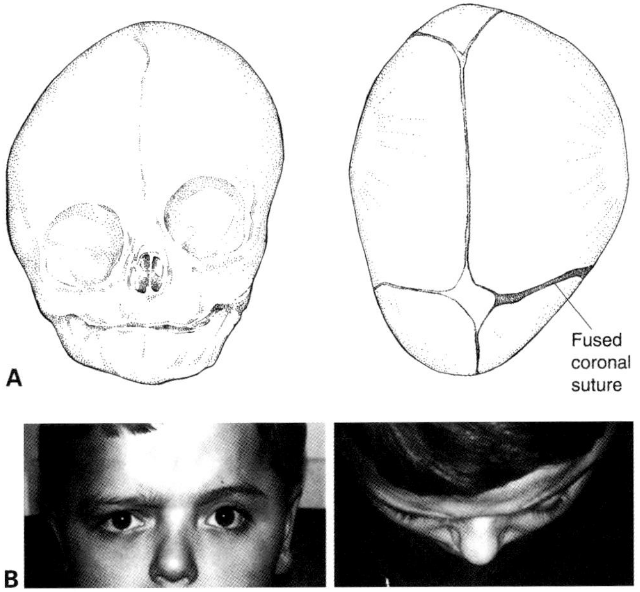

Figure 28-3 **A,** Fused coronal suture, with inhibition of perpendicular skull growth. **B,** Patient with left coronal synostosis. Note retruded left forehead, elevated brow, and wider interpalpebral fissure, with compensatory protrusion of the right forehead, with lower brow and narrowed interpalpebral fissure. *(Part A illustration by C. H. Wooley; part B courtesy of Jane Edmond, MD.)*

Scaphocephaly "Boat head." Scaphocephaly usually results from premature closure of the sagittal suture; the skull is thus long in the anterior-posterior axis and narrow bitemporally.

Dolichocephaly "Long head"; the skull shape is much like that in scaphocephaly.

Hypertelorism, orbital Excessive distance between the medial orbital walls. This diagnosis is made not clinically but rather radiographically.

Hypertelorism, ocular Excessive interpupillary distance when compared to standard nomograms; it implies orbital hypertelorism.

Telecanthus Increased distance between the medial canthi. This may be secondary to hypertelorism, but it can be a primary soft tissue abnormality.

Calvarial suture fusion impacts cranial shape and orbital development. Skull base suture fusion impacts facial and orbital development. In contrast to calvarial suture fusion, which causes different cranial deformations, skull base suture fusion causes just 1 constellation of abnormalities, midface hypoplasia, specifically consisting of the following:

- maxillary hypoplasia
- beak nose
- hypertelorism
- shallow orbits with proptosis and lagophthalmos
- high-arched palate with dental malocclusion
- relative mandibular prognathism (prominent-appearing jaw is due to retruded maxilla)

These abnormalities can range in severity from mild (eg, proptosis and mild, beak-shaped nose in families with undiagnosed Crouzon syndrome) to severe, in cases of skull base suture fusion (Fig 28-4).

Etiology of Craniosynostosis

Early suture fusion can occur sporadically as an isolated abnormality (eg, sagittal suture synostosis and most cases of unilateral coronal suture synostosis), or it can be associated with other abnormalities (eg, genetic syndromes, chromosomal anomalies, metabolic factors, in utero exposure to teratogens). The most frequently encountered group is the craniosynostosis syndromes, which are usually of autosomal dominant transmission (eg, Apert, Crouzon, Pfeiffer, Saethre-Chotzen syndromes). Common systemic features of the craniosynostosis syndromes include premature suture fusion of multiple calvarial sutures and skull base suture fusion, which results in midface hypoplasia. Syndactyly and brachydactyly, ranging in severity, are also hallmarks of these syndromes—with one notable exception: Crouzon syndrome.

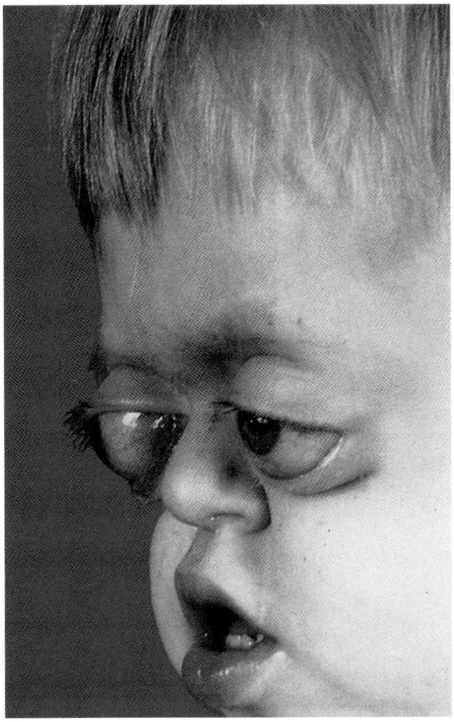

Figure 28-4 Note the manifestation of skull base suture fusion—namely, midface hypoplasia, in this child with Crouzon syndrome. *(Reproduced by permission from Miller MT. Ocular malformations in craniofacial malformations.* Int Ophthalmol Clin. *1984;24:148.)*

Craniosynostosis Syndromes

Crouzon Syndrome

Crouzon syndrome is the most common autosomal dominant craniosynostosis syndrome. Calvarial bone synostosis often includes both coronal sutures, resulting in a broad, retruded forehead; brachycephaly; and tower skull. The skull base sutures are also involved, which leads to varying degrees of midface retrusion. There is often marked variability of the skull and facial features, with milder cases escaping diagnosis through multiple generations. Hypertelorism and proptosis, with inferior scleral show (lower lid below limbus with scleral baring), are the most frequent features of Crouzon syndrome (Fig 28-5). Intelligence is usually normal. Findings are usually limited to the head. There are no obvious hand or foot abnormalities, such as those encountered in Apert and other craniosynostosis syndromes, which can greatly aid the clinician in diagnosing Crouzon. Elevated intracranial pressure is more common in Crouzon than in all other craniosynostosis syndromes. Over 30 mutations cause the Crouzon phenotype, all occurring on the fibroblast growth factor receptor-2 *(FGFR2)* gene on chromosome 10.

Apert Syndrome

Patients with Apert syndrome usually have both coronal sutures and the skull base suture fused, as well as others, and, because of marked skull and facial involvement, may look

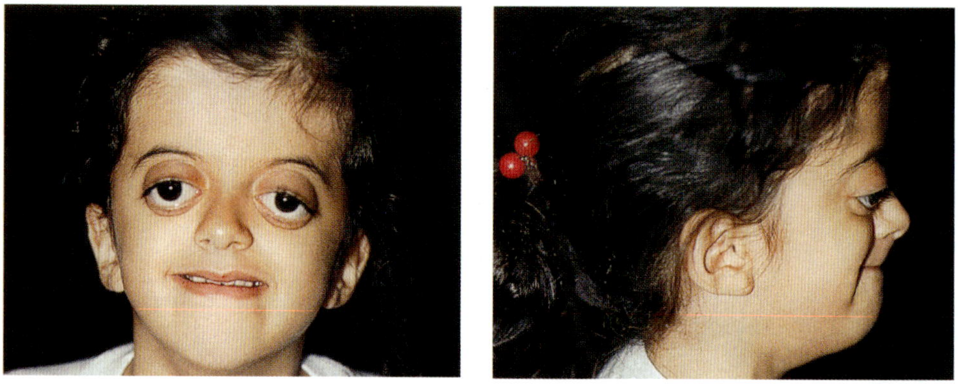

Figure 28-5 Crouzon disease. This patient evidences turribrachycephaly with forehead retrusion, proptosis, inferior scleral show, and a small, beak-like nose. Also visible is the emerging midface hypoplasia. *(Reproduced with permission from Katowitz J, ed.* Pediatric Oculoplastic Surgery. *New York: Springer; 2002:fig 31-23.)*

like Crouzon syndrome patients. However, a patient with the Apert syndrome displays an often extreme amount of syndactyly, causing all the digits (hands and feet) to be completely fused. Apert syndrome is likely to be associated with internal organ malformations (cardiovascular and genitourinary) and mental deficiency. The condition is autosomal dominant. Two mutations, both on the *FGFR2* gene on chromosome 10, account for most patients who carry this diagnosis (Fig 28-6).

Saethre-Chotzen Syndrome

In general, the features of Saethre-Chotzen syndrome are much milder than those of other craniosynostosis syndromes and therefore are often underdiagnosed. Early suture fusion is not a constant feature but, when present, typically involves 1 coronal suture (plagiocephaly), inducing an asymmetric face, a characteristic cited as a classic feature of Saethre-Chotzen syndrome. Other common features are ptosis, low hairline, and ear abnormalities. The hands and feet display slightly shortened digits (brachydactyly) and mild syndactyly. Intelligence is usually normal. The condition is autosomal dominant. Mutations in the *TWIST* gene on chromosome 7 cause the Saethre-Chotzen phenotype (Fig 28-7).

Ocular Complications

Proptosis

Proptosis (or exorbitism) in craniosynostosis results from the reduced volume of the bony orbital space that usually occurs in syndromes with coronal and/or skull base suture fusion. The severity of the proptosis in these patients is not uniform and frequently increases with age because of the impaired growth of the bony orbit.

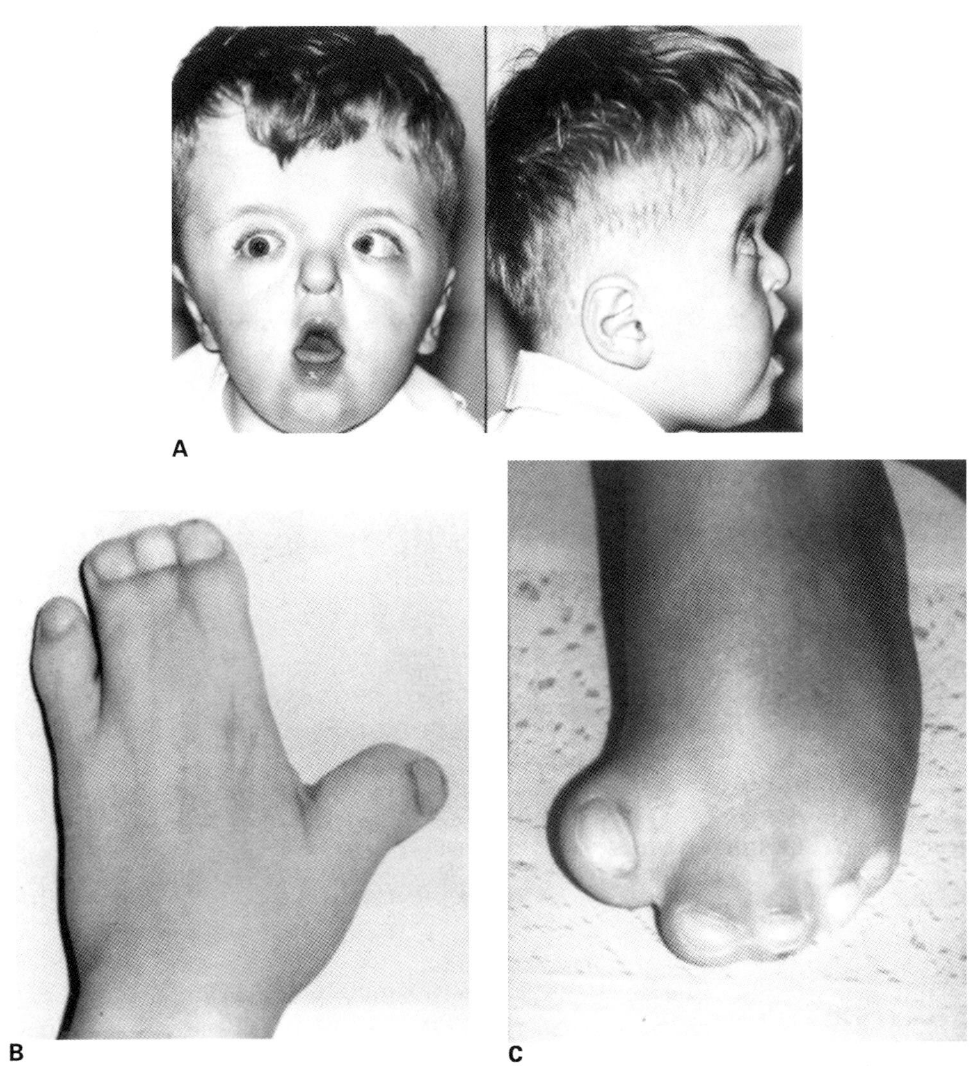

Figure 28-6 Patient with Apert syndrome. **A,** Note turribrachycephaly, forehead and superior orbital rim retrusion, maxillary hypoplasia, beak nose with depression of nasal bridge, and trapezoid-shaped mouth (common in infancy in Apert syndrome.) **B,** Extreme syndactyly of the digits; the thumb is spared but is broad and deviated. When all digits are fused, it is termed *mitten deformity.* **C,** Syndactyly of the toes analogous to that of the hands. *(Reproduced by permission from Cohen MM Jr, Maclean R.* Craniosynostosis: Diagnosis, Evaluation, and Management. *2nd ed. New York: Oxford University Press; 2000:figs 24-18, 24-46A, 24-51B.)*

Corneal Exposure

Because the eyelids may not close completely over the proptotic globes, corneal exposure may occur secondary to inadequate blink and/or nocturnal lagophthalmos, with possible development of exposure keratitis. Exposure keratitis, in the short term, can lead to punctate epithelial erosions, epithelial defects, and possible infectious keratitis. Scarring may result, which can cause vision loss. Aggressive lubrication is necessary to prevent

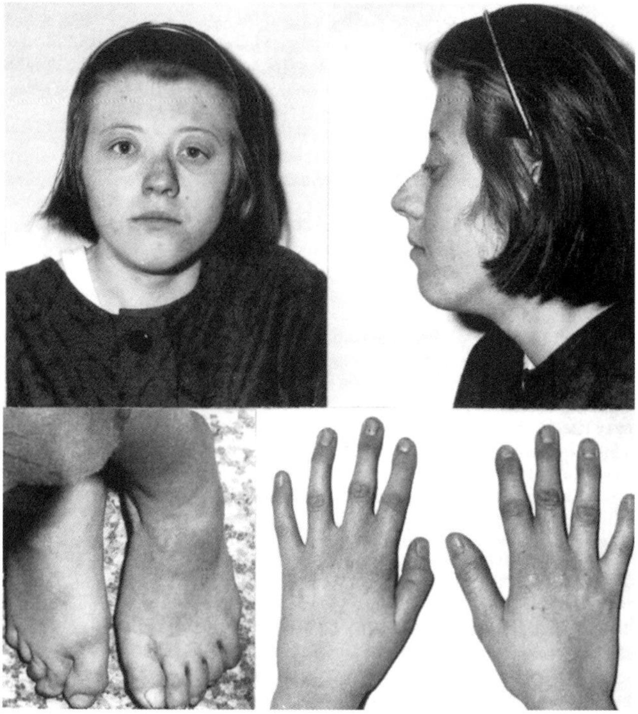

Figure 28-7 Patient with Saethre-Chotzen syndrome. Note the facial asymmetry, flat forehead, low-set hairline, mild left ptosis, classic lateral deviation in great toes, shortened toes, and partial syndactyly of fingers 2 and 3. *(Reproduced by permission from Cohen MM Jr, Maclean R.* Craniosynostosis: Diagnosis, Evaluation, and Management. *2nd ed. New York: Oxford University Press; 2000:fig 28-4.)*

corneal drying. Tarsorraphies can decrease the exposure. Surgically expanding the orbital volume, thereby eliminating the proptosis, is the treatment when the proptosis and exposure are severe and lubrication and tarsorraphies fail. These latter surgeries are performed by oculoplastic and plastic surgeons and neurosurgeons.

Globe Luxation

Patients with extremely shallow orbits may suffer globe luxation when their eyelids are manipulated or when there is increased pressure in the orbits, such as occurs with a Valsalva maneuver. The globe is luxated forward, with the eyelids falling behind the equator of the globe. The condition is very painful and can cause corneal exposure; it may also possibly compromise the blood supply to the globe, which is a medical emergency. Physicians and patients (or their caregivers) should quickly replace the globe behind the lids. The best technique for doing this is to place a finger and thumb over the conjunctiva within the interpalpebral fissure and exert gentle but firm pressure to reposition the globe; this technique does not damage the cornea. For recurrent luxation, the short-term solution is tarsorraphies; the long-term solution is orbit volume expansion by plastic surgeons.

Vision Loss

Patients with craniofacial syndromes commonly suffer vision loss due to a variety of causes: corneal scarring from exposure, uncorrected refractive errors, amblyopia, and optic nerve atrophy. Most cases of visual loss can be prevented.

Refractive errors

Patients with craniofacial syndromes are at higher risk for unusual refractive errors that can be amblyogenic if uncorrected.

Amblyopia

Amblyopia is common in patients with craniofacial syndromes and is secondary to high uncorrected refractive errors, anisometropia, and strabismus, all of which occur more frequently in these patients.

Strabismus

Patients with craniosynostosis show a variety of horizontal deviations in primary position; exotropia is the most frequent. The most consistent finding, however, is a marked V pattern, most commonly with a large exotropia on upgaze. This V pattern is often accompanied by a marked apparent overaction or pseudooveraction of the inferior oblique muscles, especially when 1 or both coronal sutures are synostosed, as occurs in plagiocephaly (unicoronal synostosis) and Apert and Crouzon syndromes (Fig 28-8). The apparent inferior oblique overaction on the side of the coronal suture fusion may be due to the following: orbital (and secondary globe) extortion, superior oblique trochlear retrusion (because of superior orbital rim retrusion), which induces superior oblique underaction and secondary inferior oblique overaction, and/or anomalous extraocular muscle insertions or agenesis, which occurs more frequently in craniofacial patients.

Optic Nerve Abnormalities

Papilledema can occur because of elevated intracranial pressure (ICP) secondary to the inability of the synostosed cranial vault to expand as the brain grows. That is, the intracranial contents are crowded and pressure elevates. Elevated ICP also can occur because of inherent brain abnormalities (eg, aqueductal stenosis) that give rise to hydrocephalus. Children with low-level chronic elevation of ICP may not complain of a headache but may still have papilledema. Chronic papilledema leads to optic atrophy and vision loss over time. Therefore, young patients with multiple sutures fused, such as Apert and Crouzon patients, should be examined yearly or biyearly. Optic nerve edema and/or atrophy can also occur secondary to optic nerve foramina synostosis, where the bony canal within the orbit stenoses. This is rare but has been described in patients with craniofacial syndromes.

Ocular Adnexa Abnormalities

Patients with craniosynostosis syndrome display more adnexal abnormalities than the isolated patient with suture fusion. Common abnormalities include orbital hypertelorism, telecanthus, abnormal slant of the palpebral fissures secondary to superior displacement

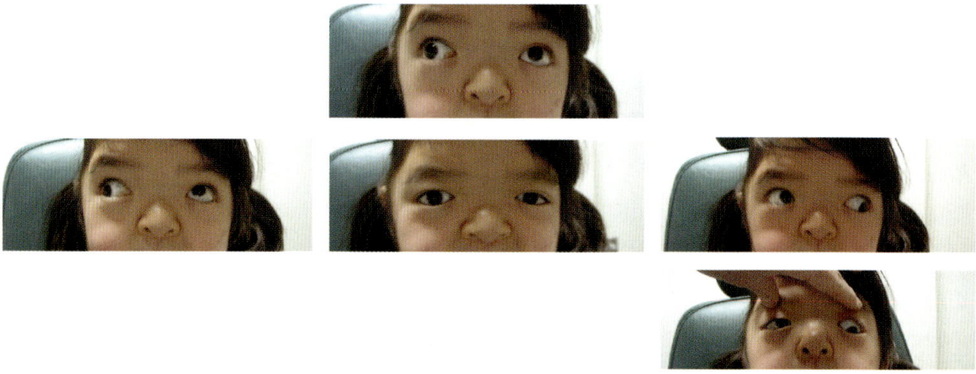

Figure 28-8 Patient with Apert syndrome. Note the good alignment in primary position with marked exotropia in upgaze (V pattern). Note marked elevation of adducted eyes (inferior oblique overaction) and lack of depression of adducted eye (superior oblique underaction). *(Photographs courtesy of John Simon, MD.)*

of the medial canthi, ptosis, and nasolacrimal apparatus abnormalities such as duct obstruction and punctal anomalies. Epiphora is a common finding in these patients and may be secondary to nasolacrimal apparatus abnormalities that produce obstruction, poor blink secondary to proptosis, obliquity of the palpebral fissures, or ocular irritation for corneal exposure.

Management

Reconstructive surgery for severe craniofacial malformation has undergone major advances in recent decades. This surgery is frequently extensive and involves en bloc movement of the facial structures. The status of the visual system should be documented preoperatively, with attention to vision, the lids and orbit, and the motility examination. Postoperatively, the function of the visual system should be reevaluated and appropriate treatment instituted.

In many centers, a specialized craniofacial team—comprising facial plastic surgeons, neurosurgeons, ophthalmologists, and oral surgeons—collaborates to determine the timing of the reconstructive surgery by prioritizing the child's multiple problems. Common surgical procedures include frontoorbital advancement; Le Fort II, or midface advancement; orbital hypertelorism repair; and a variety of jaw procedures. The first 2 procedures involve manipulation of the orbits and expansion of orbital volume.

In addition, reconstructive surgery that involves moving the orbits may significantly change the degree or type of strabismus, thereby modifying the indicated form of strabismus surgery. Another consideration is that improved binocular function may not be attainable in these patients because of their unusual and incomitant form of ocular muscle imbalance. Thus, early strabismus surgery may offer no particular advantage, and deferring treatment until craniofacial surgery is completed may be appropriate.

Cohen MM, MacLean RE. *Craniosynostosis: Diagnosis, Evaluation, and Management.* 2nd ed. New York: Oxford University Press; 2000.
Gorlin RJ, Cohen MM, Hennekam RCM. *Syndromes of the Head and Neck.* 4th ed. New York: Oxford University Press; 2001.
Katowitz J, ed. *Pediatric Oculoplastic Surgery.* New York: Springer-Verlag; 2002.
Rimoin DL, Connor JM, Pyeritz RE, et al. *Emery and Rimoin's Principles and Practice of Medical Genetics.* 4th ed. Vol 3. New York: Churchill Livingstone; 2001.

Nonsynostotic Craniofacial Conditions

Many craniofacial abnormalities do not involve synostosis. A few of particular importance to the ophthalmologist are discussed in the following sections.

Branchial Arch Syndromes

Branchial arch syndromes are caused by disruptions in the embryonic development of the first 2 branchial arches, which are responsible for the formation of the maxillary and mandibular bones, the ear, and facial musculature. The best known of these are *oculoauriculovertebral (OAV) spectrum*, which includes hemifacial microsomia and Goldenhar syndrome, and *Treacher Collins syndrome.*

Oculoauriculovertebral spectrum

There has been no firm agreement about the nomenclature involved with this condition, but most believe that hemifacial microsomia (HFM) is the forme fruste of the OAV spectrum. Hemifacial microsomia affects aural, oral, and mandibular growth. Patients with HFM may display, on the involved side, decreased jaw and cheek growth, ear abnormalities such as microtia or anotia (small or absent external ear), pretragal skin tags, deafness, and facial weakness (CN VII courses through the middle ear). Macrostomia can also occur. Hemifacial microsomia is usually unilateral but may be bilateral.

Patients with the OAV spectrum may have characteristic vertebral abnormalities such as hemivertebrae and vertebral hypoplasia. Patients may also have neurologic, cardiovascular, and genitourinary abnormalities.

Goldenhar syndrome Goldenhar syndrome is a more severe presentation of the OAV spectrum. Patients with Goldenhar syndrome have HFM (unilateral or bilateral) in addition to characteristic ophthalmic abnormalties. Most cases are sporadic.

Epibulbar and limbal dermoids are the ocular hallmarks of Goldenhar syndrome. Epibulbar dermoids (also termed *lipodermoids*) usually occur in the inferotemporal quadrant, covered by conjunctiva and often hidden by the lateral upper and lower lids. Limbal dermoids are reported more frequently than lipodermoids and can be bilateral (in approximately 25% of cases). They occasionally impinge on the visual axis but more commonly interfere with visual acuity by causing astigmatism; they can also cause anisometropic amblyopia. Upper eyelid coloboma may occur. Duane syndrome is more common in patients with Goldenhar syndrome than in the general population. Other abnormalities include microphthalmia, cataract, and iris abnormalities (Fig 28-9).

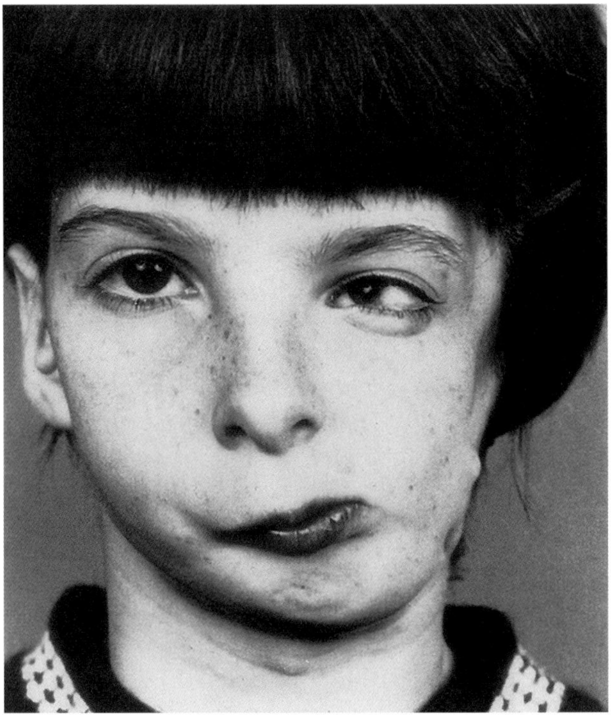

Figure 28-9 Hemifacial microsomia, Goldenhar variant. Patient has facial asymmetry, a hypoplastic left ear, an ear tag near the right ear, conjunctival lipodermoid in the left eye, and esotropia. Patient also has a left Duane syndrome.

Treacher Collins syndrome

Abnormal growth and development of the first and second branchial arch in Treacher Collins syndrome (mandibulofacial dysostosis) give rise to underdevelopment and even agenesis of the zygoma and malar eminences bilaterally. The cheeks and lateral orbital rims are depressed and the palpebral fissures slant downward because of lateral canthal dystopia. Pseudocolobomas (and, uncommonly, true colobomas) are found in the outer third of the lower lids. Meibomian glands may be absent. The cilia of the medial lower lid may be absent, medial to the pseudocoloboma. The ears are malformed and hearing loss is common. The mandible is typically hypoplastic, leading to micrognathia. Macrostomia is common. Intelligence is normal. The syndrome is autosomal dominant and displays variable expression (Fig 28-10).

Gorlin RJ, Cohen MM, Hennekam RCM. *Syndromes of the Head and Neck.* 4th ed. New York: Oxford University Press; 2001.

Rimoin DL, Connor JM, Pyeritz RE, et al. *Emery and Rimoin's Principles and Practice of Medical Genetics.* 4th ed. Vol 3. New York: Churchill Livingstone; 2001.

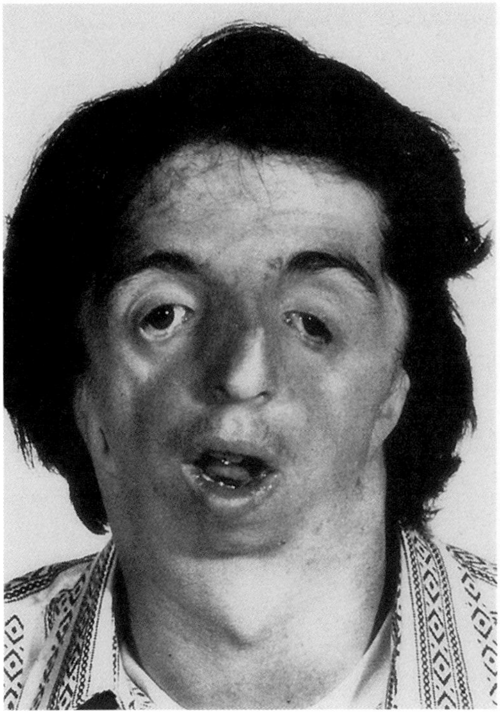

Figure 28-10 Mandibulofacial dysostosis (or Treacher Collins–Franceschetti syndrome). Note downward slant of palpebral fissure, low-set abnormal ears, notch or curving of the inferotemporal eyelid margin, and maxillary and mandibular hypoplasia. *(Reproduced by permission from Peyman GA, Sanders DR, Goldberg MF.* Principles and Practice of Ophthalmology. *Philadelphia: Saunders; 1980:2411.)*

Pierre Robin Sequence

The Pierre Robin sequence (also *anomaly, deformity*) is characterized by micrognathia, glossoptosis, and cleft palate. These abnormalities occur in a variety of syndromes, and associated ocular anomalies include retinal detachment, microphthalmos, congenital glaucoma, cataracts, and high myopia. The Pierre Robin sequence is a frequent finding in Stickler syndrome.

Fetal Alcohol Syndrome

Fetal alcohol syndrome is an example of a craniofacial condition caused by in utero exposure to a teratogen, in this case ethanol. A pattern of malformations has been observed in children born to women with a history of heavy alcohol use during pregnancy. Alcohol and other teratogens can produce a wide range of effects on the developing fetus, depending on consumption or dose, timing of intake, genetic background, and other factors. The presence of certain dysmorphic features, along with other symptoms and signs, has been designated *fetal alcohol syndrome* (Fig 28-11). The more consistent characteristics of fetal alcohol syndrome include facial abnormalities, with short palpebral fissures; a thin vermilion border of the upper lip; epicanthal folds; mental retardation (mild to severe); and small weight and height at birth that persist in the postnatal period.

Ocular involvement can include hypoplasia of the optic nerve head and increased tortuosity of retinal vasculature. Optic disc anomalies are the most common malformations of the fundus (up to 48%). Frequently, the disc is small, with sharp and often

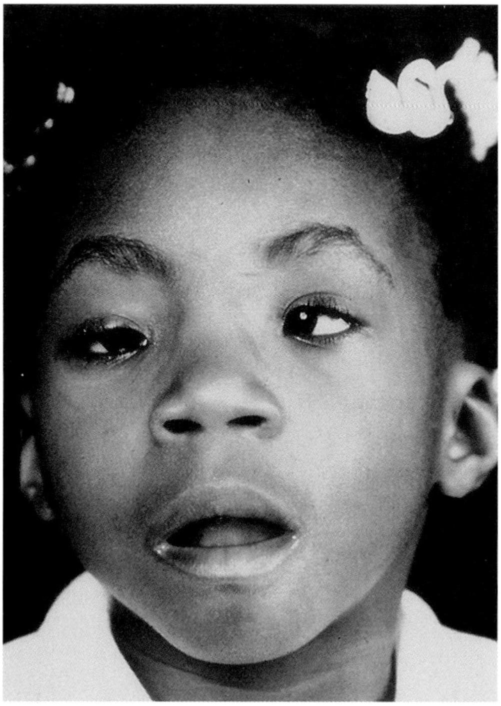

Figure 28-11 Fetal alcohol syndrome. Asymmetric ptosis; telecanthus; strabismus; long, flat philtrum; anteverted nostils. This child also had Peters anomaly of the left cornea and myopia of the right eye. *(Reproduced by permission from Miller MT. Fetal alcohol syndrome.* J Pediatr Ophthalmol Strabismus. *1981;18:6–15.)*

irregular margins; the condition may be unilateral or bilateral. A combination of anomalies of the optic disc and the retinal vessels is a typical finding in the fundus of a child with fetal alcohol syndrome.

Stromland K, Hellstrom A. Fetal alcohol syndrome—an ophthalmological and socioeducational prospective study. *Pediatrics.* 1996;97:845–850.

CHAPTER 29

Ocular Findings in Inborn Errors of Metabolism

With advances in ophthalmology and medicine over the past 50 years, and the elimination of infectious diseases and cataract as major causes of blindness in the United States and other industrialized countries, genetic and metabolic disorders affecting the eye have assumed a much larger role in visual impairment and blindness. Ophthalmologists must therefore learn more about the ophthalmic manifestations of genetic and metabolic disorders. Genetic disorders are also discussed in detail in BCSC Section 2, *Fundamentals and Principles of Ophthalmology.*

Inborn errors of metabolism are a group of disorders characterized by the genetic absence, either physical or functional, of 1 or more enzymes. This enzyme deficiency creates a block in one of the many metabolic or biochemical pathways critical to the normal growth, development, or functioning of the organism.

Inborn errors of metabolism are generally inherited as recessive disorders, either autosomal or X-linked. Germline mutations—that is, genetic errors of the gametes only—have been reported. The presence of half the normal quantity of an enzyme, as is expected in persons with 1 normal gene and 1 defective one, usually results in adequate metabolic function. Enzyme activity can be measured in suspected carriers: documentation of enzyme levels that are half normal is frequently diagnostic of the carrier state. Measurement of enzyme levels in fetal cells obtained through amniocentesis may allow prenatal detection of many of these metabolic conditions. The causative genes are known for many of these disorders, allowing preconception or prenatal testing in some cases.

Eye findings may be the earliest signs in a number of disorders, such as the neuronal ceroid lipofuscinoses, homocystinuria, and albinism. Early diagnosis of these conditions permits genetic counseling regarding the risk of recurrence in the family, as well as aiding in determining prognosis. Most important, many of these disorders now have treatments, which are more effective if instituted early. Consultation with a geneticist is warranted for any patient with ocular findings suggestive of an inborn error of metabolism.

Table 29-1 summarizes the common ophthalmic manifestations of the major inborn errors of metabolism that affect the eye. Evaluation of patients should include

- complete ocular and family history
- examination of other family members for additional evidence or findings that confirm the carrier state

Table 29-1 Ocular Findings in Mucopolysaccharidoses, Mucolipidoses, Lipidoses, Gangliosidoses, and Miscellaneous Disorders

Disease	Enzyme Deficiency	Corneal Clouding	Motility Disorders	Cherry-Red Spot	RPE Degeneration	Optic Atrophy	Other	Inheritance
Mucopolysaccharidoses								
MPH I H, I S Hurler (2528)* Scheie	α-iduronidase	+++	–	–	+++	+	glaucoma papilledema	AR
MPS II Hunter (30990)	iduronate sulfatase	–	–	–	++	+	–	XR
MPS III Sanfilippo (25290)	A: heparan *N*-sulfatase B: *N*-acetyl-α-D-glucosaminidase	+	–	–	++	rare	late blindness	AR
MPS IV Morquio (25300)	A: *N*-acetyl-galactosamine-6-sulfatase B: β-galactosidase	++	–	–	rare	rare	–	AR
MPS VI Maroteaux-Lamy (25320)	arylsulfatase B	++	–	–	–	+	papilledema glaucoma	AR
MPS VII Sly (25322)	β-glucuronidase	+	–	–	–	–	–	AR
Mucolipidoses								
Type I (25240) sialidosis (type 2) cherry-red-spot myoclonus syndrome	neuraminidase	–	+	+	+	–	hearing loss	AR
Type II I-cell disease (25250)	multiple lysosomal enzymes	++	–	–	–	–	Hurler-like	AR
Type III pseudo-Hurler polydystrophy (25260)	multiple lysosomal enzymes	+++	–	–	–	–	Hurler-like puffy eyelids (25260)	AR
Type IV (25265)	partial ganglioside sialidase	+++	–	–	++	+	photophobia	AR
Lipidoses								
Niemann-Pick disease (25720)	sphingomyelinase	+	nystagmus	+	–	+	eventual vision loss	AR
Fabry disease (30150)	α-galactosidase A	whorl-like	–	–	–	–	angiokeratoma, spokelike cataract, aneurysmal conjunctival vessels	XR
Gaucher disease (Type I 23080) (Type II 23090) (Type III 23100)	glucocerebrosidase	–	paralytic strabismus, looped saccades	–	+	–	pinguecula, conjunctival pigmentation	AR
Metachromatic leukodystrophy (25010)	arylsulfatase A	–	nystagmus	+	–	+	blindness, decreased pupil reaction	AR
Krabbe disease (24520)	galactocerebrosidase	–	nystagmus	rare	–	+	cortical blindness	AR
Fucosidosis (23000)	α-L-fucosidase	–	–	–	+	–	Hurler-like features, angiokeratoma tortuous conjunctival vessels	AR

Disease	Enzyme Deficiency	Conjunct. Tortuosity	Corneal Clouding	Motility Disorders	Cherry-Red Spot	RPE Degeneration	Optic Atrophy	High Myopia	Blindness	Inheritance
Gangliosidoses										
Generalized (GM_1) gangliosidosis										
(1) Type I (23050)	β-galactosidase A, B, and C	+	±	ET, nystagmus	50% of patients	–	+	+	+	AR
(2) Type II (23060) Derry disease juvenile GM_1	β-galactosidase B and C	–	–	ET, nystagmus	–	+	±	–	late	AR
(3) Type III (23065) adult GM_1	β-galactosidase (partial)	±	rare	–	–	–	–	–	–	AR
GM_2 gangliosidosis										
(1) Type I (27280) Tay-Sachs disease	hexosaminidase A	–	–	nystagmus, ophthalmoplegia	+	–	+	–	+	AR
(2) Type II (26880) Sandhoff disease	hexosaminidase A and B	–	rare	ET	+	–	±	–	+	AR
(3) Type III (23065) juvenile GM_2 Bernheimer-Seitelberger disease	hexosaminidase A (partial)	–	–	–	–	+	+	–	late	AR

Disease	Enzyme Deficiency	Corneal Clouding	Motility Disorders	Cherry-Red Spot	RPE Degeneration	Optic Atrophy	Other	Inheritance
Miscellaneous Disorders								
Galactosialidosis	β-galactosidase neuraminidase	+	–	+	–	+	dwarfism, seizures, coarse facies	AR
Ceroid lipofuscinosis (20420)								
Hagberg-Santavuori disease	PPT-1	–	+	Macular	+	+	blindness	AR
Jansky-Bielschowsky disease	PPT-1	–	+	bull's	+	+	blindness	AR
Spielmeyer-Vogt disease	unknown	–	+	eye	+	+	blindness	AR
Kufs disease	unknown	–	–	–	–	–		AR
Cystinosis (21980)	unknown	crystals	–	–	++	–	conjunctival crystals, renal problems	AR
Galactosemia (23040)	gal-1-PO_4 uridyl transferase	–	–	–	–	–	cataracts if not treated	AR
Mannosidosis (24850)	α-mannosidase	++	–	–	–	pallor, blurred margin	Hurler-like, spokelike cataract	AR
Homocystinuria (23620)	cystathionine β-synthase	–	–	–	+	–	dislocated lens, cataract	AR
Refsum disease (26650)	phytanic acid α-hydrolase	–	–	–	++	–	cataract, night blindness	AR

* These code numbers refer to the system developed by Victor McKusick (McKusick VA, Francomano CA, Antonarakis SE. *Mendelian Inheritance in Man: Catalogs of Autosomal Dominant, Autosomal Recessive, and X-Linked Phenotypes.* 10th ed. Baltimore: The Johns Hopkins University Press; 1992).

Plus (+) and minus (–) signs indicate the relative likelihood of occurrence of ocular findings in these systemic disorders.

- complete ocular examination focusing on the expected findings
- appropriate directed laboratory testing

Treatment

Many previously untreatable metabolic disorders now have treatment options, either through clinical trials or as standard of care. The earlier a patient is referred to a geneticist, the better the chance of a beneficial effect from such treatments. Treatments include, but are not limited to, enzyme replacement therapy [eg, mucopolysaccharidosis (MPS) I, Fabry], bone marrow or umbilical cord blood stem cell transplant (mucopolysaccharidoses and leukodystrophies), and dietary changes (eg, homocystinuria, Refsum disease). Gene therapy is on the horizon.

Some examples of treatable metabolic disorders with ocular findings follow. Classic homocystinuria is caused by cystathionine beta-synthase deficiency, which is usually detected shortly after birth. Milder forms may be diagnosed later in life. Dietary restriction of methionine and supplementation of folate, pyridoxine (vitamin B6), vitamin B12, and/or betaine (N,N,N-trimethylglycine) can markedly reduce plasma homocysteine levels and prevent progression of disease in homocystinuria. Most untreated patients with classic homocystinuria will develop mental retardation and ectopia lentis; thrombotic events will likely occur in 50% before age 30 years. The risk is greatly decreased by metabolic control; there is evidence that even increased axial eye length is affected favorably. In patients with cystinosis, systemic cysteamine can ameliorate renal disease and topical cysteamine eyedrops can prevent or reverse painful crystalline keratopathy.

Patients and families can also be reassured that much research is ongoing. In vitro studies of cells from albino mice have been successful in repairing the tyrosinase gene, allowing previously amelanotic cells to produce melanin, and early in vivo animal results look promising. Nonsteroidal anti-inflammatory agents have been shown to slow progression of disease in the Sandhoff disease mouse, whereas tamoxifen and vitamin E are beneficial in the mouse model of Niemann-Pick C. Gene therapy in Fabry mice using lentivirus vectors and in MPS I mice using adeno-associated virus vector has shown positive results. Transplantation of genetically modified bone marrow cells directly into the brains of MPS VII mice corrects the brain pathology, and using an adeno-associated virus vector, researchers have performed gene therapy intravitreally with improved retinal function. A clinical trial of gene therapy in the brains of children with late infantile neuronal ceroid lipofuscinosis is being planned. It is the responsibility of ophthalmologists to have a high suspicion for these devastating disorders in order to direct patients to the best treatment options as early as possible.

Alexeev V, Yoon K. Stable and inheritable changes in genotype and phenotype of albino melanocytes induced by an RNA-DNA oligonucleotide. *Nat Biotechnol.* 1998;16:1343–1346.

Hennig AK, Ogilvie JM, Ohlemiller KK, et al. AAV-mediated intravitreal gene therapy reduces lysosomal storage in the retinal pigment epithelium and improves retinal function in adult MPS VII mice. *Mol Ther.* 2004;10:106–116.

Khan AO, Latimer B. Successful use of topical cysteamine formulated from the oral preparation in a child with keratopathy secondary to cystinosis. *Am J Ophthalmol.* 2004;138:674–675.

Mulvihill A, O'Keeffe M, Yap S, et al. Ocular axial length in homocystinuria patients with and without ocular changes: effects of early treatment and biochemical control. *J AAPOS.* 2004;8:254–258.

OMIM (Online Mendelian Inheritance in Man). www.hgmp.mrc.ac.uk/omim/.

Vellodi A. Lysosomal storage disorders. *Br J Haematol.* 2005;128:413–431.

Yap S. Classical homocystinuria: vascular risk and its prevention. *J Inherit Metab Dis.* 2003; 26:259–265.

CHAPTER 30

Ocular Trauma in Childhood

Trauma is one of the most important causes of ocular morbidity in childhood. Only strabismus ranks higher in frequency among reasons for pediatric eye surgery, and only amblyopia is responsible for more early monocular vision loss. Children 11–15 years old have a particularly high incidence of severe eye injury compared with other age groups. Injured boys outnumber girls by a factor of 3 or 4 to 1.

Most ocular trauma in younger children occurs during casual play with other children. Older children and adolescents are most likely to be injured while participating in sports. A majority of serious childhood eye injuries could thus, in principle, be prevented by appropriate adult supervision and by regular use of protective eyewear for sports. Fireworks and BB guns are among the less frequent causes of pediatric ocular trauma, but they are likely to cause severe injuries.

American Academy of Pediatrics, Committee on Sports Medicine and Fitness; American Academy of Ophthalmology, Eye Health and Public Information Task Force. Protective eyewear for young athletes. *Ophthalmology.* 2004;111:60–63.

The management of eye trauma in very young patients requires several special considerations. First, the difficulty of evaluation and treatment is often considerably increased by inadequate cooperation. Even school-age children, stressed by the recent injury, may strenuously resist any approach to the eye. Overcoming the child's opposition by force risks exacerbating the damage caused by penetrating wounds or blunt impact. In a child older than 3 years, a forceful approach may make it exceedingly difficult to establish the rapport needed for subsequent treatment. Examination in cases likely to involve minor injury can be facilitated by instilling topical anesthetic and by giving the child a chance to calm down in quiet surroundings. When preliminary assessment indicates that prompt surgical treatment may be necessary, it is appropriate to defer detailed physical examination of the eye until the patient is in the operating room under general anesthesia.

A second issue in the care of children with eye trauma is the potential for the injury or its treatment to lead to visual loss from amblyopia. In children younger than 5 years, visual deprivation amblyopia associated with traumatic cataract or other media opacity may be more likely to cause severe long-term reduction of acuity than the original physical damage. Minimizing the interval between the injury and restoration of optimal media clarity and optics, including adequate aphakic refractive correction, must be a high priority. Monocular occlusion following injury should be kept to a minimum as well; the expected benefit from an occlusive dressing must be weighed against the risk of disturbing binocular function or inducing amblyopia.

Child Abuse

Although most eye injuries in childhood are accidental or innocently caused by other children, a significant portion results from physical abuse by adults. Child abuse is a pervasive problem in our society, with an estimated 2 million victims per year in the United States. Abusive behavior in a parent or other caregiver usually reflects temporary loss of control during a period of anger or stress rather than premeditated cruelty. Lack of knowledge of the proper way to care for or discipline a child is also a frequent contributing factor. In the relatively rare *Munchausen syndrome by proxy*, the child is physically harmed by a psychopathic parent to create signs of illness in an effort to manipulate medical care providers.

A reliable history is often difficult to obtain when child abuse has occurred. Suspicion should be aroused when repeated accounts of the circumstances of injury or histories obtained from different individuals are inconsistent or when the events described seem to conflict with the extent of injuries (eg, bruises on multiple aspects of the head after a fall) or with the child's developmental level (eg, a 2-month-old rolling off a bed or a 6-month-old climbing out of a high chair).

Any physician who suspects that child abuse might have occurred is required by law in every US state and Canadian province to report the incident to a designated governmental agency. Once this obligation has been discharged, the ophthalmologist is probably best advised to leave full investigation of the situation to appropriate specialists or authorities.

The presenting sign of child abuse involves the eye in approximately 5% of cases, and ocular manifestations are detected in the course of evaluating many others. Blunt trauma inflicted with fingers, fists, or implements such as belts or straps is the usual mechanism of nonaccidental injury to the ocular adnexa or anterior segment. Periorbital ecchymosis, subconjunctival hemorrhage, and hyphema should raise suspicion of recent abuse if the explanation provided is less than completely plausible. Cataract and lens dislocation may be signs of repeated injury or trauma inflicted more remotely in the past. A majority of rhegmatogenous retinal detachments that occur in childhood have a traumatic origin; abuse should be suspected when such a finding is encountered in a child without a history of injury or an apparent predisposing factor such as high myopia.

Shaking Injury

A unique complex of ocular, intracranial, and sometimes other injuries occurs in infants who have been abused by violent shaking. Because the essential features of what is now generally known as *shaken baby syndrome* were identified in the early 1970s, it has become widely recognized as one of the most important manifestations of child abuse.

Victims of shaking injury are always under 3 years old and usually under 12 months. When a reliable history is available, it typically involves a parent or other caregiver who shook an inconsolably crying baby in anger and frustration. Often, however, the only information provided is that the child's mental status deteriorated or that seizures or respiratory difficulty developed; or the involved caregiver may relate that an episode of relatively minor trauma occurred, such as a fall from a bed. Even without a supporting history, the diagnosis of shaken baby syndrome can still be made with confidence on the basis of characteristic clinical findings. It must be kept in mind, however, that answers to important questions concerning the timing and circumstances of injury and the identity of the perpetrator frequently cannot be inferred from medical evidence alone.

Intracranial injury in shaken infants almost always includes subdural hematoma, typically bilateral over the cerebral convexities or in the interhemispheric fissure. Evidence of subarachnoid bleeding is also often apparent. Although initial scans may be normal in many cases, cerebral parenchymal damage is manifest on neuroimaging, acutely as edema, ischemia, or contusion and in later stages as atrophy. These findings are thought to result from repetitive abrupt deceleration of the child's head as it whiplashes back and forth during the shaking episode. Some authorities, citing the frequency with which shaken baby syndrome victims also show evidence of having received blows to the head, think that impact is an essential component. Displacement of the brain in relation to the skull and dura mater ruptures bridging vessels, and compression against the cranial bones produces further damage. The infant's head is particularly vulnerable to such effects because of its relatively large mass in relation to the body and poor stabilization by neck muscles.

Ocular involvement

The most common ocular manifestation of shaking injury, present in a large majority of cases, is retinal hemorrhage. Preretinal, nerve fiber layer, deep retinal, or subretinal localization may be seen. Hemorrhages tend to be concentrated in or near the macular region but sometimes are so extensive that they occupy nearly the entire fundus (Fig 30-1). Vitreous hemorrhage may also develop, usually as a secondary phenomenon resulting from migration of blood that was initially intraretinal. Occasionally, the vitreous becomes almost completely opacified by dispersed hemorrhage within a few days of injury. Retinal hemorrhages in shaken infants resolve over a period ranging from 1 or 2 weeks to several months. Vitrectomy should be considered if amblyopia is likely.

Some eyes of shaken infants show evidence of retinal tissue disruption in addition to hemorrhage. Full-thickness perimacular folds in the neurosensory retina, typically with circumferential orientation around the macula that creates a craterlike appearance, are

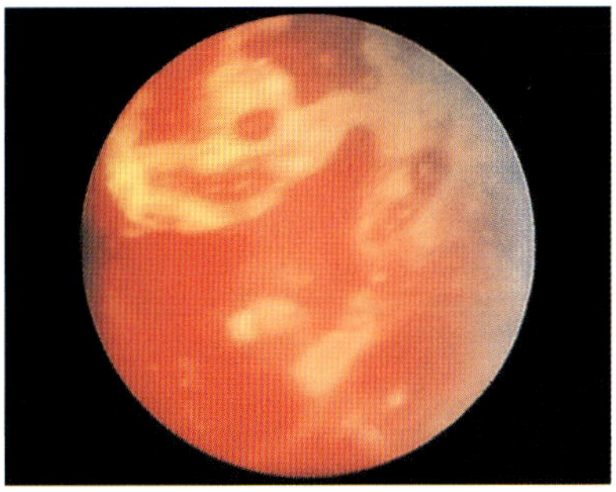

Figure 30-1 Extensive retinal hemorrhages, left eye, in a 2-month-old infant thought to have been violently shaken. Temporal portion of the disc is visible near the left edge of the photograph.

highly characteristic. Splitting of the retina (traumatic retinoschisis), either deep to the nerve fiber layer or superficial (involving only the internal limiting membrane), may create partially blood-filled cavities of considerable extent, also usually in the macular region (Fig 30-2). Full-thickness retinal breaks and detachment are rare. Retinal folds usually flatten out within a few weeks of injury, but schisis cavities can persist indefinitely.

A striking feature of shaken baby syndrome is the typical lack of external evidence of trauma. The ocular adnexa and anterior segments appear entirely normal. Occasionally, the trunk or extremities show bruises representing the imprint of the perpetrator's hands. In a minority of cases, broken ribs or characteristic metaphyseal fractures of the long bones result from forces generated during shaking. It must be kept in mind, however, that many shaken babies are also victims of other forms of abuse. In particular, signs of impact to the head must be carefully sought.

When extensive retinal hemorrhage accompanied by perimacular folds and schisis cavities is found in association with intracranial hemorrhage or other evidence of trauma to the brain in an infant, shaking injury can be diagnosed with confidence regardless of other circumstances. Extensive retinal hemorrhage without other ocular findings strongly suggests that intracranial injury has been caused by shaking, but alternative possibilities such as a coagulation disorder must be considered as well. Severe accidental head trauma (eg, sustained in a fall from a second-story level or a motor vehicle collision) is infrequently accompanied by retinal hemorrhage, which is virtually never extensive. Retinal hemorrhage is rare and has never been documented to be extensive following cardiopulmonary resuscitation by trained personnel. Spontaneous subarachnoid hemorrhage occurs rarely in young children and may be associated with some degree of intraocular bleeding. Retinal hemorrhages resulting from birth trauma are common in newborns but seldom persist beyond age 1 month.

Emerson MV, Pieramici DJ, Stoessel KM, et al. Incidence and rate of disappearance of retinal hemorrhage in newborns. *Ophthalmology*. 2001;108:36–39.

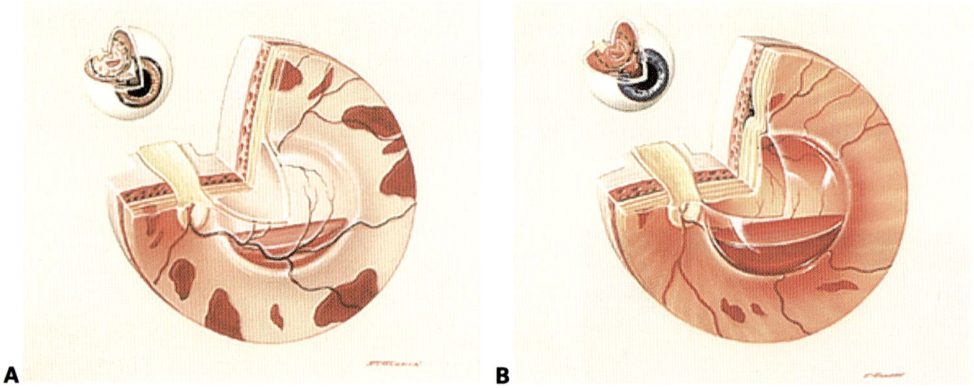

Figure 30-2 Traumatic retinoschisis. **A,** Deep splitting of the retina, typically associated with severe permanent visual impairment and loss of ERG b-wave. **B,** Superficial splitting, with separation of the internal limiting membrane and a full-thickness perimacular fold. Recovery of good vision is common. *(Reproduced by permission from Greenwald MJ. The shaken baby syndrome.* Semin Ophthalmol. *1990;5:202–213. Illustrations by S. Gordon.)*

Prognosis

In one large study, 29% of children with shaken baby syndrome died from their injuries. Poor visual and pupillary response were correlated with a higher risk of mortality. Survivors often suffered permanent impairment ranging from severe retardation and quadriparesis to mild learning disability and motor disturbances. Visual loss from traumatic retinoschisis, optic nerve damage, or cortical injury occurred in 20% of patients, but nearly complete recovery of vision was common. Dense vitreous hemorrhage, usually associated with deep traumatic retinoschisis, carried a poor prognosis for both vision and life. Vitrectomy should be deferred if bright-flash electroretinography shows loss of the b-wave.

McCabe CF, Donahue SP. Prognostic indicators for vision and mortality in shaken baby syndrome. *Arch Ophthalmol.* 2000;118:373–377.

Morad Y, Kim YM, Armstrong DC, et al. Correlation between retinal abnormalities and intracranial abnormalities in the shaken baby syndrome. *Am J Ophthalmol.* 2002;134:354–359.

Pierre-Kahn V, Roche O, Dureau P, et al. Ophthalmologic findings in suspected child abuse victims with subdural hematomas. *Ophthalmology.* 2003;110:1718–1723.

Superficial Injury

Corneal abrasion is one of the most common ocular injuries among children, as it is among older people. Use of a pressure patch to keep the eyelids closed so that an abrasion will heal faster is of questionable value for the preschool child. Obtaining and maintaining the desired effect is difficult in this age group, and if the patch loosens, contact between the cotton eye pad and the ocular surface may actually aggravate the problem. Even without patching, moderately large traumatic corneal epithelial defects usually heal within 1–2 days in young children. Use of topical cycloplegic drops and antibiotic ointment may help reduce discomfort and risk of infection.

Cigarette burns of the cornea are the most common thermal injuries to the ocular surface in childhood. Usually, these occur in the age range of 2–4 years and are accidental, not manifestations of abuse. These burns result from the toddler's running into a cigarette held at eye level by an adult. Despite the alarming initial white appearance of coagulated corneal epithelium, cigarette burns typically heal rapidly and without scarring. Treatment is the same as for mechanical abrasions.

Chemical burns in childhood are generally caused by organic solvents or soaps found in household cleaning agents. Even those involving almost total loss of corneal epithelium are likely to heal in a week or less with or without patching. Acid and alkali burns in children, as in adults, can be much more serious. The initial and most important step in management of all chemical injuries is copious irrigation and meticulous removal of any particulate matter from the conjunctival fornices. See also BCSC Section 8, *External Disease and Cornea.*

Corneal foreign bodies in children can sometimes be dislodged with a forceful stream of irrigating solution from a small bottle; sharp instruments can thus be avoided. When mechanical removal proves necessary, it is important that the patient not move during the procedure.

Penetrating Injury

Unless an adult has witnessed a traumatic incident, the history cannot be relied on to exclude the possibility of penetrating injury to the globe. The anterior segment and fundus must be thoroughly inspected in suspicious circumstances, using general anesthesia if necessary. An area of subconjunctival hemorrhage or chemosis or a small break in the skin of the eyelid may be the only surface manifestation of scleral perforation by a sharp-pointed object, such as a dart or scissors blade (Fig 30-3). Distortion of the pupil

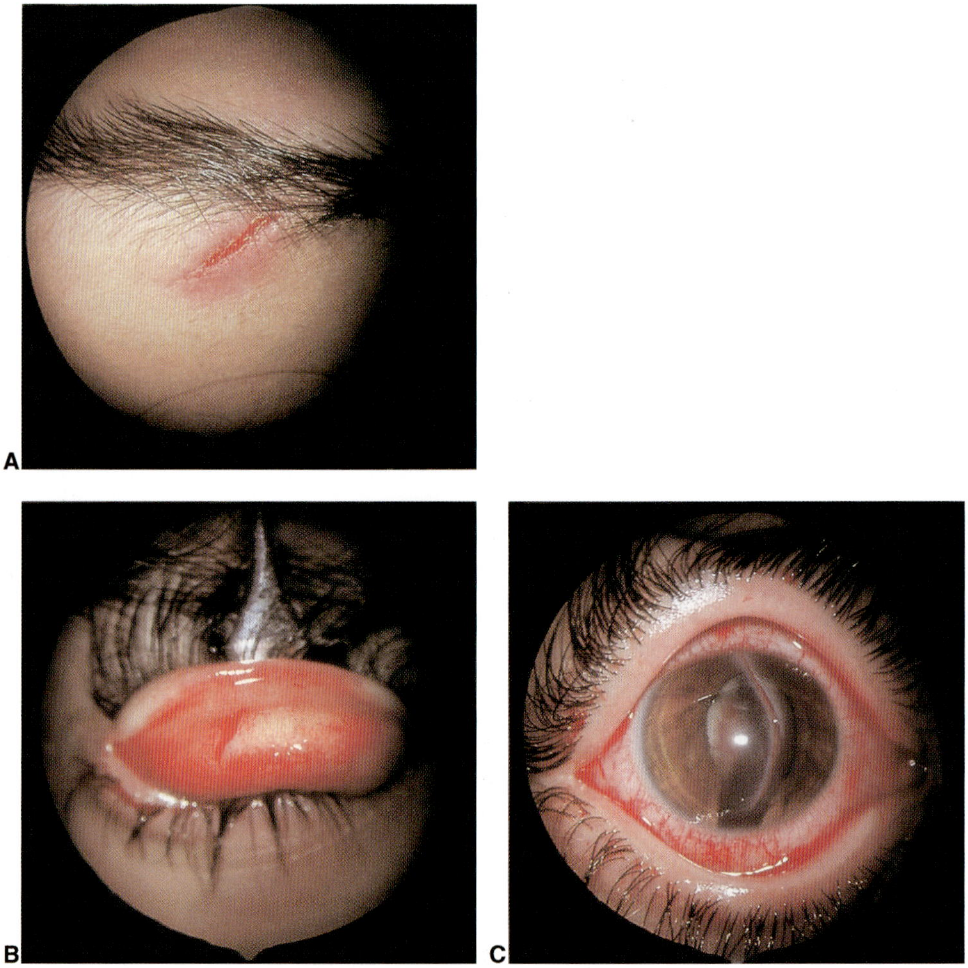

Figure 30-3 **A,** Small skin entry wound created by a thrown dart, right brow region, in a 7-year-old boy. **B,** Conjunctival exit wound indicates complete perforation of the eyelid. **C,** Extensive injury to the anterior segment of the same eye.

may be the most evident sign of a small corneal or limbal perforation. CT of the orbits should be considered if there is any reason to suspect an intraocular or deeply situated foreign body.

Corneoscleral lacerations in children are repaired according to the same principles as for adults. Corneal wounds heal relatively rapidly in very young patients, however, and sutures should be removed correspondingly early.

Fibrin clots often form quickly in the anterior chamber of a child's eye after a penetrating injury to the cornea, and these can simulate the appearance of fluffy cataractous lens cortex to a remarkable degree. To avoid unnecessarily rendering the eye aphakic (and thereby compromising visual rehabilitation), lens removal should not be performed in the course of primary wound repair unless the clinician is absolutely certain that the anterior capsule has been ruptured. Even if lens cortex is exposed, postponing cataract surgery for 1–2 weeks until severe posttraumatic inflammation has quieted down may result in a smoother recovery and reduced risk of complications, without significantly worsening the visual prognosis. See also BCSC Section 11, *Lens and Cataract.*

Small conjunctival lacerations are often self-sealing. Full-thickness eyelid lacerations should be repaired meticulously, and sedation or general anesthesia may be required, even in older children. Otherwise, working near the eyes with sharp instruments and draping the face to create a sterile field are likely to frighten the patient and add to the difficulty of the repair. Clearly superficial wounds can be repaired in the emergency room. Use of 6-0 plain gut or synthetic absorbable sutures is an acceptable alternative if the physician wishes to avoid the need for removal of nonabsorbable sutures.

Blunt Injury

Hyphema

The management of hyphema in infants and children requires special considerations. As with all forms of pediatric trauma, the precise occurrence that led to intraocular bleeding may be difficult to determine. The possibility of abuse must be considered, as must the possibility of nontraumatic etiology: retinoblastoma, juvenile xanthogranuloma of the iris, and bleeding diathesis resulting from leukemia or other blood dyscrasia are relatively rare but important causes of spontaneous hyphema during the early years of life. Ultrasonography or CT should be performed to rule out intraocular tumor in suspicious cases wherein the iris and fundus cannot be adequately seen, and a complete blood count should be performed routinely, with coagulation studies, if a bleeding disorder is suspected.

Intraocular pressure (IOP), an important parameter for therapeutic decision making with traumatic hyphema, is often difficult to monitor in the pediatric patient. The risks of inaccurate measurements and of further traumatizing the injured eye may outweigh the potential value of obtaining results in uncooperative children. With small amounts of blood pooling in the anterior chamber, concern about pressure tends to be greatest in patients with sickle cell trait or disease (Fig 30-4). Such patients may develop sickling in the anterior chamber, elevating IOP and retarding resorption of blood, or in the retinal circulation, causing vascular occlusion.

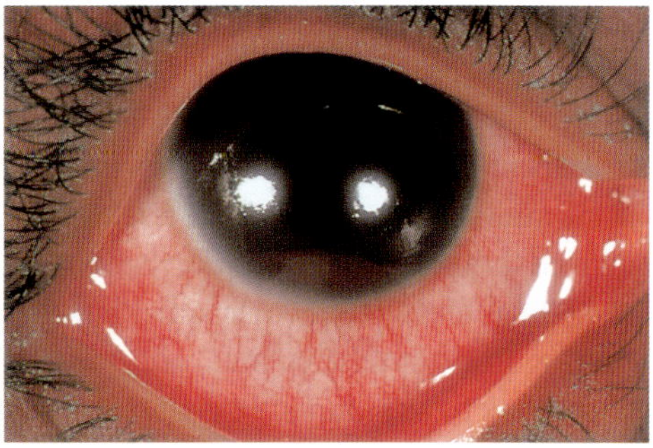

Figure 30-4 Small hyphema, right eye, in an adolescent girl with sickle trait. Note corneal edema resulting from high intraocular pressure.

It was once common practice to hospitalize all patients with hyphema and place them on bed rest with bilateral patching of the eyes. Such extreme restriction has never been shown to improve prognosis, however, and is likely to be unproductive in children. On the other hand, some decrease in normal childhood running, jumping, and rough play is both reasonable and appropriate. Hospitalization during the first 5 days after injury, when risk of rebleeding is greatest, remains justifiable and is one way to ensure the opportunity for daily follow-up evaluation. Outpatient management with daily, careful follow-up is an acceptable alternative.

Medical management of hyphema remains controversial in children as in adults. Many ophthalmologists routinely use cycloplegic and corticosteroid drops to facilitate fundus examination, improve comfort, and reduce the risk of inflammatory complications and possibly of rebleeding as well. The value of these topical agents is unproven, however, and some clinicians prefer to use them selectively for control of pain or obvious inflammation or avoid them altogether to minimize manipulation of the eye. Pressure-lowering medication is appropriate for eyes known or strongly suspected to be hypertensive. Aspirin-containing compounds should be scrupulously avoided because of their antiplatelet action.

Oral administration of an antifibrinolytic agent (ε-aminocaproic acid, 50 mg/kg every 4 hours to a maximum of 30 g daily; or tranexamic acid, 25 mg/kg every 8 hours to a maximum of 4.5 g daily, for 5 days) has been shown to reduce the incidence of rebleeding in traumatic hyphema. However, 1 study found an insignificant decrease in the incidence of rebleeding among patients treated with tranexamic acid; gastric upset and hypotension may be significant side effects of oral ε-aminocaproic acid. Recently, topical aminocaproic acid has been demonstrated to be an effective alternative. Oral prednisolone has also been advocated in a dosage of 0.75 mg/kg/day in 2 divided doses (to a maximum of 40 mg/day in children).

Surgical evacuation of hyphema is usually performed in adults when early corneal blood staining is detected or when significant IOP elevation has persisted for 5–7 days. The difficulty of detecting early blood staining in a child and the risk that corneal staining may cause severe deprivation amblyopia, coupled with the problems of accurately measuring IOP, justify earlier surgical intervention whenever a total hyphema persists for 4–5 days. Various operative techniques have been employed; none has been shown to offer particular advantages in childhood.

Late glaucoma is a potential complication of traumatic hyphema in children, as in adults, and may present no symptoms. Gonioscopy can be performed after the eye has healed and the child can cooperate. Routine annual follow-up should be continued in children who are found to have an angle recession. It is important to remember that children with hyphemas may also have other significant injuries, including damage to the retina and optic nerve.

Pieramici DJ, Goldberg MF, Melia M, et al. A phase III, multicenter, randomized, placebo-controlled clinical trial of topical aminocaproic acid (Caprogel) in the management of traumatic hyphema. *Ophthalmology.* 2003;110:2106–2112.

Walton W, Von Hagen S, Grigorian R, et al. Management of traumatic hyphema. *Surv Ophthalmol.* 2002;47:297–334.

Orbital Fractures

Children, like adults, may sustain isolated fractures of orbital bone after blunt impact in the region of the eye. Careful examination of the eye is important to rule out associated ocular damage. CT should be performed to evaluate the fracture and possible associated injuries. The involvement of other specialties, including otolaryngology and neurosurgery, may be helpful in some cases. If there is severe enophthalmos or if the eye movements are extremely compromised, consideration should be given to primary repair of orbital fractures during the first 2 weeks following injury. In many cases, however, the motility will recover or strabismus surgery can be considered after several months if it proves necessary.

The most common orbital fracture in early childhood involves the orbital roof, which is rarely fractured in older patients. Isolated roof fractures typically result from impact to the brow region in a fall, often from a height of only a few feet. The principal external manifestation is hematoma in the upper eyelid (Fig 30-5). For further discussion of diagnosis and management of orbital trauma, see Chapter 10 of this book and BCSC Section 7, *Orbit, Eyelids, and Lacrimal System.*

A

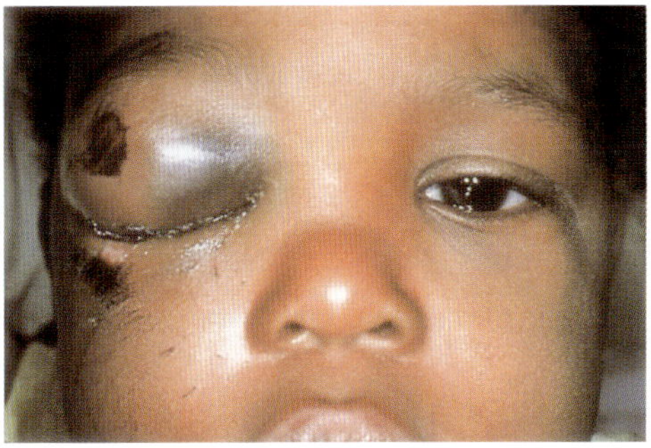

B

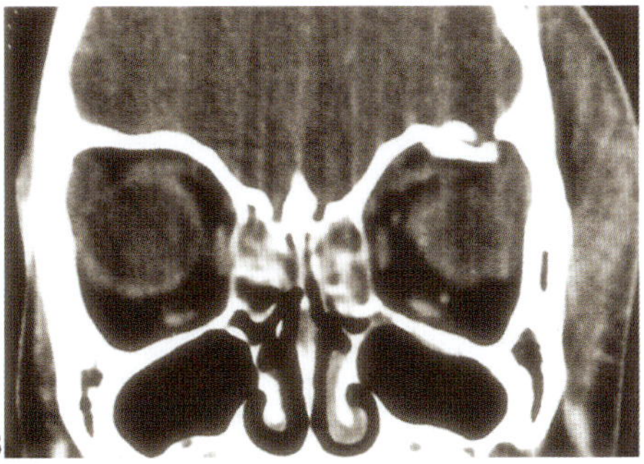

Figure 30-5 Orbital roof fracture in infants who fell with frontal impact. **A,** Marked right upper eyelid swelling from hematoma originating in the superior orbit adjacent to a linear fracture. **B,** Coronal CT image of a different patient, showing a bone fragment displaced into the left orbit.

Bansagi ZC, Meyer DR. Internal orbital fractures in the pediatric age group: characterization and management. *Ophthalmology.* 2000;107:829–836.

Burnstine MA. Clinical recommendations for repair of isolated orbital floor fractures: an evidence-based analysis. *Ophthalmology.* 2002;109:1207–1210.

Jordan DR, Allen LH, White J, et al. Intervention within days for some orbital floor fractures: the white-eyed blowout. *Ophthal Plast Reconstr Surg.* 1998;14:379–390.

CHAPTER 31

Decreased Vision in Infants and Children

When an infant has not developed good visual attention or ability to fixate and follow objects by age 3–4 months, several causes must be considered. Many of these causes are covered elsewhere in this volume, in the chapters on cataracts, glaucoma, retinal disorders, and malformations. Some ocular abnormalities are relatively easily diagnosed by standard ophthalmic examinations. Others, however, are subtle and difficult to detect.

Normal Visual Development

Visual development is a highly complex maturation process. Structural changes occur in both the eye and the central nervous system. Laboratory and clinical research has shown that normal vision develops as a result of both genetic coding and experience in a normal visual environment.

Vision in the infant usually is assessed qualitatively by clinical appraisal as well as by psychophysical tests such as *optokinetic nystagmus (OKN)* responses, or *visually evoked cortical potentials* (*VEP;* also known as *visual evoked responses, VER*), and preferential looking techniques. A blink reflex to bright light should be present several days after birth. The pupillary light reflex is usually present after 31 weeks' gestation, but it can be difficult to evaluate because of miosis in the newborn.

At about 6 weeks of age, the normal baby should be able to make and maintain eye contact with other humans and react with facial expressions. Infants 2–3 months old should be interested in bright objects. Premature infants can be expected to reach these landmarks later, depending on their degree of prematurity.

Disconjugate eye movements may be noted initially, but these should not persist after age 4 months. Skew deviation and *sunsetting* (tonic downward deviation of both eyes) have been observed as transient deviations in the newborn period. Signs of actual poor visual development include wandering eye movements, lack of response to familiar faces and objects, and nystagmus. Staring at bright lights and forceful rubbing of the eyes in an otherwise visually disinterested infant *(oculodigital reflex)* are other signs of poor visual development and suggest an ocular cause for the deficiency.

Weinacht S, Kind C, Monting JS, et al. Visual development in preterm and full-term infants: a prospective masked study. *Invest Ophthalmol Vis Sci.* 1999;40:346–353.

Approach to the Infant With Decreased Vision

A careful history, beginning with a review of vision problems in the family, is essential. If the patient is male, the possibility of an X-linked disorder should be explored. If a sibling has a similar condition not present in previous generations, an autosomal recessive disease is suggested.

Details of the pregnancy should be reviewed: important factors include maternal infection, radiation, drugs, or trauma. Perinatal problems including prematurity, intrauterine growth retardation, fetal distress, bradycardia, meconium staining, and oxygen deprivation are important. The clinician also should inquire about the presence of systemic abnormalities or delayed developmental milestones.

Examination of the infant must include special attention to visual fixation, crispness and equality of pupillary light responses, ocular alignment and motility, and the presence of nystagmus or roving eye movements. A detailed fundus examination also is necessary.

An infant with a normal but immature visual system may be unresponsive to even a very bright light, a state indistinguishable from blindness. By moving a red light horizontally or vertically in front of the infant, the clinician can sometimes elicit a fixation-and-following response in an otherwise unresponsive baby.

Pupillary responses are sluggish with anterior visual pathway disease such as optic nerve hypoplasia or atrophy, optic nerve coloboma, and morning glory disc anomaly. Paradoxical pupillary phenomenon (constriction to darkness) implies diffuse retinal disease such as cone dystrophy or optic nerve hypoplasia. Pupillary responses are normal in infants with cortical visual impairment.

Nystagmus (a rhythmic pendular or jerk movement pattern) as an indicator of decreased vision usually begins at age 2–3 months, not at birth. Nystagmus implies the presence of at least some visual function (nystagmus does not occur in total blindness). In contrast, roving eye movements suggest total or near-total blindness. Both of these conditions are different from congenital motor nystagmus (no organic eye abnormality), which is associated with only a mild to moderate reduction in visual acuity. Chapter 12 discusses nystagmus in detail.

Visual deficits in 1 or both eyes can cause abnormal binocular alignment. In an infant younger than 1 year, the most common misalignment is exotropia. Beyond the age of 1 year, esotropia is more common.

When an infant presents with poor vision and ocular structures that appear normal, a number of retinal disorders should be considered, including Leber congenital amaurosis, achromatopsia, blue-cone monochromatism, and X-linked or autosomal recessive congenital stationary night blindness. Electroretinography (ERG) can aid in the diagnosis of these disorders, and some investigators advocate ERG testing for all infants with visual inattentiveness and normal eye structures. Other researchers think that, in infancy, ERGs should be reserved only for patients thought to have Leber congenital amaurosis. Obtaining quality ERGs in infants is difficult, and the examiner must be aware of the normal developmental variations that show up in these electrophysiologic tests in the first year of life. Serial testing may be important before definitive diagnostic and prognostic information is provided.

For infants with low vision, additional testing might include VEP, ultrasonography, CT, or MRI. In some cases, specialized laboratory studies are indicated; these should be obtained in consultation with a pediatric neurologist, an endocrinologist, a neurosurgeon, and a geneticist.

The most common causes of reduced vision in infants are listed here, and most are discussed individually in the following sections:

- anterior segment anomalies
- glaucoma
- cataract
- optic nerve hypoplasia
- optic atrophy
- Leber congenital amaurosis
- achromatopsia (rod monochromatism)
- congenital infection syndrome/TORCH syndrome
- cortical visual impairment
- delay in visual maturation
- retinopathy of prematurity (see Chapter 24)
- X-linked retinoschisis (see Chapter 24)
- congenital motor nystagmus (see Chapter 12)
- albinism (see Chapter 24)
- coloboma (see Chapters 20 and 25)

Anterior Segment Anomalies, Glaucoma, Cataract

The common feature of childhood anterior segment anomalies, glaucoma, and cataract is stimulus deprivation severe enough to result in permanently reduced vision. Complete ptosis and lens or corneal opacification (eg, Peters anomaly, sclerocornea, glaucoma) are prominent among the causes. Even with only partial loss of clarity, image degradation can be significant and result in amblyopia.

If the condition is unilateral or not of comparable severity in both eyes, an additional component of inhibition of the more disadvantaged eye is present. Although some of these abnormalities often are beyond correction, prompt attention to the remediable ones is required during the critical window (within several weeks of birth). See also Chapters 6, 19, 21, and 22.

Optic Nerve Hypoplasia

Disturbed optic nerve development can range from a minimal decrease in size to complete absence of the nerve (aplasia), causing varying degrees of reduced visual function in infants. In hypoplasia, the optic disc appears somewhat pale and small and may be circumscribed by a yellow-white ring, surrounded by pigmentation. This encircling ring has been described clinically as the *double ring sign*. It is not apparent in every case.

The condition can be unilateral or bilateral, and there is no sex predilection. When hypoplasia is unilateral, strabismus is often present, and one element of partial loss may be secondary to a superimposed amblyopia. Nystagmus frequently accompanies severe bilateral involvement.

A relative afferent pupillary defect usually is present with asymmetrical involvement, and the ERG usually appears normal. The VEP is subnormal, reflecting the disturbed conduction of visual impulses via the optic nerve. Imaging studies may demonstrate a small optic foramen or optic nerve.

Optic nerve hypoplasia is associated with other developmental abnormalities, including hydrocephalus, hydranencephaly, anencephaly, and congenital tumors of the anterior visual pathways. The brain may be affected by midline defects, including agenesis of the septum pellucidum, malformations of the corpus callosum, and enlargement of the chiasmal cistern.

The *de Morsier syndrome (septo-optic dysplasia)* includes optic nerve hypoplasia, absence of the septum pellucidum, agenesis of the corpus callosum, and pituitary dwarfism. Endocrine abnormalities may occur when the midline defect extends into the hypothalamus, with resulting panhypopituitarism, growth hormone deficiency, diabetes insipidus, and hypoglycemia. Recent studies have identified ectopia or absence of the posterior pituitary gland, revealed on MRI, as a predictor of endocrine abnormalities in patients with optic nerve hypoplasia.

Neuroimaging is recommended for children with bilateral optic nerve hypoplasia. When the condition is unilateral, the incidence of midline brain abnormalities is much smaller, but many neurologists would obtain such studies in this instance also.

The cause of optic nerve hypoplasia remains unknown. Maternal ingestion of phenytoin, quinine, and LSD has been implicated. Optic nerve hypoplasia is common in infants with fetal alcohol syndrome and has been reported in the offspring of mothers with diabetes. Another postulated cause of optic nerve hypoplasia is degeneration of ganglion cell axons due to an insult occurring prior to the 13th week of gestation. See also Chapter 25.

Hellstrom A, Wiklund LM, Svensson E. The clinical and morphologic spectrum of optic nerve hypoplasia. *J AAPOS.* 1999;3:212–220.

Weiss AH, Kelly JP. Acuity, ophthalmoscopy, and visually evoked potentials in the prediction of visual outcome in infants with bilateral optic nerve hypoplasia. *J AAPOS.* 2003;7:108–115.

Optic Atrophy

Various inherited and noninherited conditions can cause *optic atrophy.* Congenital and acquired forms occur and can be an isolated defect or a facet of systemic disease.

Secondary optic atrophy has been attributed to hydrocephalus, brain tumors, perinatal hypoxia, central nervous system malformations such as porencephaly, and toxins (eg, lead, quinine, and methyl alcohol) and has been associated with metabolic storage diseases and with trauma, including child abuse. See Chapter 25.

Leber Congenital Amaurosis

Leber congenital amaurosis is responsible for an estimated 10% of cases of congenital blindness. Infants with this condition may have severe visual impairment at birth, although the visual deficit is noted more typically at age 2–3 months with the onset of a coarse, searching sensory nystagmus. The pupillary reactions to direct light are poor, and the pupils may paradoxically constrict in the dark. The oculodigital habit is common, with gouging of the eyes by a finger or fist in an effort to induce entoptic stimulation of the retina. The inheritance pattern is autosomal recessive.

Initially, the fundus can appear completely normal, although a diffuse pigmentary change, optic nerve pallor, or both may be noted. A blond fundus and an atrophic appearance of the macula are additional characteristics. With time, optic atrophy, narrowing of the retinal vessels, and diffuse retinal pigmentary changes indistinguishable from retinitis pigmentosa develop. Other findings include cataracts, hyperopia, and glaucoma.

The ERG appears abnormal, showing either completely flat or low voltage, and the base value of the electro-oculogram is low, with no rise after light adaptation. Such a result may not be clearly distinguishable from normal in an infant younger than 12–15 months. Histologic examination reveals severe disorganization or absence of the rods and cones.

Associated neurologic conditions include abnormal electroencephalogram results, microcephaly, hydrocephaly, seizures, and other cerebral abnormalities. Possible associated skeletal changes are acrocephaly, hemifacial hypoplasia, polydactyly, kyphoscoliosis, arachnodactyly, and osteoporosis. Muscular hypotony and kidney abnormalities with oligophrenia also may occur. See also Chapter 24.

Dharmaraj S, Leroy BP, Sohocki MM, et al. The phenotype of Leber congenital amaurosis in patients with AIPL1 mutations. *Arch Ophthalmol.* 2004;122:1029–1037.

Hanein S, Perrault I, Gerber S, et al. Leber congenital amaurosis: comprehensive survey of the genetic heterogeneity, refinement of the clinical definition, and genotype-phenotype correlations as a strategy for molecular diagnosis. *Hum Mutat.* 2004;23:306–317.

Achromatopsia

Achromatopsia (rod monochromatism) is a retinal disorder characterized by total color blindness, with all colors perceived as varying brightnesses of gray. The condition is inherited as an autosomal recessive trait. Photophobia of varying degree, nystagmus, and visual acuity in the 20/200 range are common. The degree of nystagmus may decrease at near fixation, giving better visual acuity than at distance.

Fundus examination usually is normal when the child is young, although an abnormal foveal reflex may develop later. A central scotoma can be demonstrated. The ERG usually shows a normal scotopic recording and an abnormal photopic response. The electro-oculogram typically appears normal.

Histopathologic examination reveals a markedly reduced population of cones. Those that are present are often abnormally structured. The rods are normal. The condition is nonprogressive and has no associated neurologic abnormalities. See also Chapter 24.

Congenital Infection Syndrome/TORCH Syndrome

Congenital infection syndrome/TORCH syndrome is characterized by a marked reduction in visual acuity that is often associated with congenital infections (primarily toxoplasmosis, rubella, cytomegalovirus, herpes simplex, and syphilis) and with severe disruption of the visual pathways from encephalitis, meningitis, arachnoiditis, optic neuritis, and sometimes chorioretinitis. Chapter 17 discusses these conditions in detail.

Cortical Visual Impairment

Infants with *cortical visual impairment* demonstrate varying degrees of visual attentiveness. Both the family and the ophthalmologist may be uncertain as to whether the baby can see. Examination reveals normal ocular structures, normal pupillary responses, and searching eye movements.

The ERG appears normal; the VEP may be normal or subnormal. Neuroimaging may reveal changes such as atrophy and porencephaly in the occipital (striate or parastriate) cortex, damage to the optic radiations, or periventricular leukomalacia. This last condition is a prominent cause of visual impairment in children born prematurely. In some cases, no such findings are present and the prognosis may be more favorable.

Cortical visual impairment may be congenital or acquired. Prenatal and perinatal causes include intrauterine infection (see Chapter 17), cerebral dysgenesis, asphyxia, intracranial hemorrhage, hydrocephalus, and infection. Acquired causes include trauma and child abuse (see Chapter 30), shunt malfunction, meningitis, and encephalitis.

Cortical visual impairment may be transient or permanent and can be an isolated finding or associated with multiple neurologic handicaps. Descending optic atrophy (transsynaptic degeneration) may coexist.

Brodsky MC, Fray KJ, Glasier CM. Perinatal cortical and subcortical visual loss: mechanisms of injury and associated ophthalmologic signs. *Ophthalmology.* 2002;109:85–94.

Good WV. Development of a quantitative method to measure vision in children with chronic cortical visual impairment. *Trans Am Ophthalmol Soc.* 2001;99:253–269.

Delay in Visual Maturation

Sometimes, when eye examination results are totally normal but fixation is poor, the problem is merely delayed maturation of the visual system. In such children, neurologic examination results may be normal except for poor visual attention. Some patients, however, have evidence of other neurologic impairment. The problem is especially common in children with other developmental disabilities.

If the infant's visual behavior does not begin to progress toward normal within a few months, further investigation is warranted. Visually evoked cortical potentials recorded very early in life may initially be abnormal; this determination is more valid as the child approaches 12 months of age. Such testing can be omitted when the infant's visual behavior is clearly progressing toward normal.

Acquired Vision Loss Later in Childhood

When a child with normal visual development in infancy subsequently loses vision, the search for a treatable disorder is of paramount concern. Table 31-1 lists many of the conditions that can lead to acquired amaurosis. Amblyopia, the most prevalent cause of treatable vision loss in children, is discussed in Chapter 5 and elsewhere in this volume.

Table 31-1 Acquired Childhood Amaurosis

Congenital Malformations
- Congenital hydrocephalus
- Encephalocele, particularly occipital type

Tumors
- Retinoblastoma
- Optic glioma
- Perioptic meningioma
- Craniopharyngioma
- Chiasmal glioma
- Posterior and intraventricular tumors when complicated by hydrocephalus

Neurodegenerative Diseases: Abiotrophies
- Cerebral storage disease
- Gangliosidoses, particularly Tay-Sachs disease (infantile amaurotic familial idiocy), Sandhoff disease, generalized gangliosidosis
- Other lipidoses and ceroid lipofuscinoses, particularly the late-onset amaurotic familial idiocies such as those of Jansky-Bielschowsky and of Spielmeyer-Vogt
- Mucopolysaccharidoses, particularly Hurler syndrome and Hunter syndrome
- Leukodystrophies (dysmyelination disorders), particularly metachromatic leukodystrophy and Canavan disease
- Demyelinating scleroses (myelinoclastic diseases), especially Schilder disease and Devic neuromyelitis optica
- Special types: Dawson disease, Leigh disease, Bassen-Kornzweig syndrome, Refsum disease
- Retinal degenerations of obscure pathogenesis: retinitis pigmentosa and its variants, and Leber congenital type
- Optic atrophies of obscure pathogenesis: congenital autosomal recessive type, infantile and congenital autosomal dominant types, Leber disease, and atrophies associated with hereditary ataxias—the types of Behr, of Marie, and of Sager-Brown

Infectious or Inflammatory Processes
- Encephalitis, especially in the prenatal infection syndromes due to *Toxoplasma gondii,* cytomegalovirus, rubella virus, *Treponema pallidum*
- Meningitis; arachnoiditis
- Optic neuritis
- Chorioretinitis

Hematologic Disorders
- Leukemia with CNS involvement

Vascular and Circulatory Disorders
- Collagen vascular diseases
- Arteriovenous malformations: intracerebral hemorrhage, subarachnoid hemorrhage

Trauma
- Contusion or avulsion of optic nerves or chiasm
- Cerebral contusion or laceration
- Intracerebral, subarachnoid, or subdural hemorrhage

Drugs and Toxins
- Lead
- Quinine
- Methyl alcohol

Adapted from Nelson LB, Calhoun JH, Harley RD, eds. *Pediatric Ophthalmology.* 3rd ed. Philadelphia: Saunders; 1991.

Table 31-2 Sources of Information on Low Vision

American Foundation for the Blind, 11 Penn Plaza, Ste 300, New York, NY 10001; (212) 502-7600 or (800) 232-5463; www.afb.org. For the publication *Reach Out and Teach: Meeting the Training Needs of Parents of Visually and Multiply Handicapped Young Children* by KA Ferrell, PhD (AFB, 1985), call (800) 232-3044.

American Printing House for the Blind (APH), 1839 Frankfort Avenue, PO Box 6085, Louisville, KY 40206-0085; (502) 895-2405 or (800) 223-1839; www.aph.org. Large-print and braille books, tapes, and talking computer software, and low vision aids.

Family Support America, 205 W. Randolph St, Ste 2222, Chicago, IL 60606; (312) 338-0900; www.familysupportamerica.org. Identifies parent support groups all over the country.

Lighthouse for the Blind, Lighthouse Center for Education, Information, and Resource Service: (800) 829-0500. Independent organizations in every state; check local directories for listings.

National Association of Parents of Children With Visual Impairments (NAPVI), PO Box 317, Watertown, MA 02471; (800) 562-6265; www.spedex.com/napvi. Some areas have a state organization as well; NAPVI can direct the parent.

National Association for the Visually Handicapped (NAVH). West Coast office: 3201 Balboa St, San Francisco, CA 94121, (415) 221-3201; East Coast office: 22 West 21st St, 6th floor, New York, NY 10010, (212) 889-3141; www.navh.org. Large-print textbooks, library material on request. Sources of information and guidance on resources for the visually handicapped.

National Information Center for Children and Youth With Handicaps (NICCYH), PO Box 1492, Washington, DC 20013; (800) 695-0285.

National Library Service for the Blind and Physically Handicapped (NLS), Library of Congress, 1291 Taylor St NW, Washington, DC 20011; (202) 707-5100 or (800) 424-8567. Books and magazines in braille and audio.

National Organization for Albinism and Hypopigmentation (NOAH), PO Box 959, East Hampstead, NH 03826-0959; (800) 473-2310; www.albinism.org.

Prevent Blindness America, 211 West Wacker Drive, Ste 1700, Chicago, IL 60606; (800) 331-2020; www.preventblindness.com.

Recording for the Blind & Dyslexic, 20 Roszel Road, Princeton, NJ 08540; (866) RFBD-585 [(866) 732-3585]; www.rfbd.org.

Retinoblastoma Support News (newsletter for families of children with retinoblastoma) and *Parent to Parent* (newsletter for families of blind or visually impaired or multihandicapped children). Published by Institute for Families, PO Box 54700, mail stop 111, Los Angeles, CA 90054-0700; (323) 669-4649; www.instituteforfamilies.org.

National Toll-Free Numbers

- **American Council of the Blind** (800) 424-8666
- **Better Hearing Institute** (800) 327-9355 (800-EAR-WELL)
- **Epilepsy Information Line** (800) 332-1000 [(800) EFA-1000]
- **Cystic Fibrosis Foundation** (800) 344-4823
- **National Down Syndrome Society** (800) 221-4602
- **Down Syndrome Information Center** (888) 999-3759
- **National Easter Seal Society** (800) 221-6827
- **National Health Information Center** (800) 336-4797
- **Spina Bifida** (800) 621-3141
- **United Cerebral Palsy Association** (800) 872-5827
- **National Fragile X Foundation** (800) 688-8765
- **American Kidney Fund** (800) 638-8299
- **The Arc of the United States** (formerly Association for Retarded Citizens) (800) 433-5255
- **Sickle Cell Association** (800) 421-8453
- **Retina International** (formerly International Retinitis Pigmentosa Association) (800) 344-4877

Sources of Large-Print Books

- **New York Times Large Print Weekly**, 229 West 43rd Street, New York, NY 10036; (800) 631-2580
- **Library for the Blind and Physically Handicapped**, Free Library of Philadelphia, 919 Walnut St, Philadelphia, PA 19107-5289; (800) 222-1754
- **Reader's Digest Large Print**, PO Box 8177, Red Oak, IA 51591-1177; (800) 807-2780

Childhood cataract acquired as a developmental, familial, traumatic, or metabolic disorder is discussed in Chapter 22.

Vision screening programs in schools, primary care medical offices, and community outreach programs should be supported and monitored. Visual recovery often is directly related to early, accurate detection of the visual loss. For patients whose visual function could be helped or enhanced by visual rehabilitation, the Academy provides the SmartSight website: http://one.aao.org/SmartSight. Table 31-2 also lists resources for further information.

Hutcheson KA, Drack AV. Diagnosis and management of the infant who does not see. *Focal Points: Clinical Modules for Ophthalmologists.* San Francisco: American Academy of Ophthalmology; 1998, module 12.

Basic Texts

Pediatric Ophthalmology and Strabismus

Brodsky MC, Baker RS, Hamed LM. *Pediatric Neuro-Ophthalmology.* New York: Springer-Verlag; 1996.

Buckley EG, Freedman S, Shields MB. *Atlas of Ophthalmic Surgery.* Vol III: *Strabismus and Glaucoma.* St Louis: Mosby; 1995.

Calhoun JH, Nelson LB, Harley RD. *Atlas of Pediatric Ophthalmic Surgery.* Philadelphia: Saunders; 1987.

Cibis GW, Tongue AC, Stass-Isern ML. *Decision Making in Pediatric Ophthalmology.* St Louis: Decker; 1993.

Del Monte MA, Archer SM. *Atlas of Pediatric Ophthalmology and Strabismus Surgery.* New York: Churchill Livingstone; 1993.

Helveston EM. *Surgical Management of Strabismus: An Atlas of Strabismus Surgery.* 4th ed. St Louis: Mosby; 1993.

Helveston EM, Ellis FD. *Pediatric Ophthalmology Practice.* 2nd ed. St Louis: Mosby; 1984.

Isenberg SJ, ed. *The Eye in Infancy.* 2nd ed. St Louis: Mosby-Year Book; 1994.

Jones KL. *Smith's Recognizable Patterns of Human Malformation.* 5th ed. Philadelphia: Saunders; 1997.

Leigh RJ, Zee DS. *The Neurology of Eye Movements.* 3rd ed. New York: Oxford; 1999.

Miller NR, Newman NJ. *Walsh and Hoyt's Clinical Neuro-Ophthalmology.* 5th ed. Baltimore: Williams & Wilkins; 1999.

Nelson LB, Olitsky SE, Harley RD, eds. *Harley's Pediatric Ophthalmology.* 5th ed. Philadelphia: Lippincott Williams & Wilkins; 2005.

Pratt-Johnson JA, Tillson G. *Management of Strabismus and Amblyopia: A Practical Guide.* 2nd ed. New York: Thieme; 2001.

Renie WA, ed. *Goldberg's Genetic and Metabolic Eye Disease.* 2nd ed. Boston: Little, Brown & Co; 1986.

Spencer WH, ed. *Ophthalmic Pathology: An Atlas and Textbook.* 4th ed. Philadelphia: Saunders; 1996.

Tasman W, Jaeger EA, eds. *Duane's Clinical Ophthalmology* [CD-ROM set]. Lippincott Williams & Wilkins; 2002.

Taylor D. *Pediatric Ophthalmology.* 2nd ed. Cambridge, MA: Blackwell Science; 1997.

von Haam E, Helveston EM. *Strabismus: A Decision Making Approach.* St Louis: Mosby; 1994.

von Noorden GK. *Binocular Vision and Ocular Motility: Theory and Management of Strabismus.* 6th ed. St Louis: Mosby; 2002.

von Noorden GK. *von Noorden–Maumenee's Atlas of Strabismus.* 4th ed. St Louis: Mosby; 1983.

Wright KW, ed. *Color Atlas of Stabismus Surgery: Strategies and Techniques.* 2nd ed. *Strabismus.* Torrance, CA: Wright; 2000.

Wright KW, Spiegel PH, eds. *Pediatric Ophthalmology and Strabismus.* 2nd ed. New York: Springer; 2002.

Related Academy Materials

Focal Points: Clinical Modules for Ophthalmologists

Beck AD, Lynch MG. Pediatric glaucoma (Module 5, 1997).
Curnyn KM, Longest C. Why do kids do that? (Module 6, 2006).
Dunn JP. Uveitis in children (Module 4, 1995).
Haldi BA, Mets MB. Nonsurgical treatments of strabismus (Module 4, 1997).
Hertle RW, Kowal LM, Yeates KO. The ophthalmologist and learning disabilities (Module 2, 2005).
Hutcheson KA, Drack AV. Diagnosis and management of the infant who does not see (Module 12, 1998).
Keech RV. Practical management of amblyopia (Module 2, 2000).
Levin AV. The ocular findings in child abuse (Module 7, 1998).
Mets MB, Noffke AS. Ocular infections of the external eye and cornea in children (Module 2, 2002).
Meyer DR. Congenital ptosis (Module 2, 2001).
Quinn GE, Young TL. Retinopathy of prematurity (Module 11, 2001).
Robb RM. Nasolacrimal duct obstruction in children (Module 8, 2004).
Ruttum MS. Childhood cataracts (Module 1, 1996).
Silkiss RZ. Craniofacial anomalies (Module 11, 1992).
Suh DW. Acquired esotropia in children and adults (excluding pediatric accommodative esotropia) (Module 10, 2003).
Wilson ME. Exotropia (Module 11, 1995).
Wilson ME. Management of aphakia in childhood (Module 1, 1999).
Wygnanski-Jaffe T, Levin AV. Introductory genetics for the ophthalmologist (Module 5, 2005).

Publications

Lane SS, Skuta GL, eds. *ProVision: Preferred Responses in Ophthalmology*, Series 3 (Self-Assessment Program, 1999; reviewed for currency 2001).
Plager DA, ed. *Strabismus Surgery: Basic and Advanced Strategies.* Written by Buckley EG, Plager DA, Repka MX, Wilson ME, with contributions by Parks MM, von Noorden GK. American Academy of Ophthalmology Monograph Series No. 17. New York: Oxford University Press; 2004.
Skuta GL, ed. *ProVision: Preferred Responses in Ophthalmology*, Series 2 (Self-Assessment Program, 1996; reviewed for currency 2001).
Wilson FM II, ed. *Practical Ophthalmology: A Manual for Beginning Residents.* 5th ed. (2005).

Preferred Practice Patterns/Ophthalmic Technology Assessments

PPP Committee, Pediatric Ophthalmology Panel. *Amblyopia* (2002).
PPP Committee, Pediatric Ophthalmology Panel. *Esotropia and Exotropia* (2002).
PPP Committee, Pediatric Ophthalmology Panel. *Pediatric Eye Evalutions* (2002).
Ophthalmic Technology Assessment Committee. *Strabismus Surgery for Adults* (2003).

Policy Statement

Learning Disabilities, Dyslexia, and Vision. A Joint Statement of the American Academy of Pediatrics, American Association for Pediatric Ophthalmology and Strabismus, and American Academy of Ophthalmology, 1998. Available at www.aao.org.

Academy MOC Essentials

MOC Exam Study Guide: Comprehensive Ophthalmology and Practice Emphasis Areas (2005).
MOC Exam Self-Assessment: Core Ophthalmic Knowledge and Practice Emphasis Areas (2005).

Specialty Clinical Updates Online

Lambert SC, Tychsen L. *Advances in Surgical Management, Part I* (Module 1, 2002).
Parsa CF. *Papillorenal Syndrome and Associated PAX2 Mutations* (Module 6, 2003).
Repka MX, Alcorn DM, West CE. *Advances in Medical Management* (Module 2, 2003).
Repka MX, Tychsen L, West CE. *Advances in Diagnosis* (Module 3, 2003).
West CE. *Advances in Basic Science, Disease Etiology, and Risk Factors* (Module 5, 2003).
West CE, Repka MX, Brandt JD. *Advances in Surgical Management, 2* (Module 4, 2003).

Multimedia

Demer JL, Lambert SR, Tychsen L. *LEO Clinical Update Course on Pediatric Ophthalmology and Strabismus* (CD-ROM, 2003).
Johns KL, ed. *Eye Care Skills: Presentations for Physicians and Other Health Care Professionals* (CD-ROM, 2005).

Continuing Ophthalmic Video Education

Price RL, Beauchamp GR. *Strabismus Surgery: Oblique Procedures* (1989; reviewed for currency 2004).
Price RL, Beauchamp GR. *Strabismus Surgery: Rectus Recession and Resection* (1989; reviewed for currency 2004).
Reinecke RD. *Nystagmus: Fundamentals of Clinical Evaluation* (2000; reviewed for currency 2004).
Wilson ME. *Ocular Motility Evaluation of Strabismus and Myasthenia Gravis* (1993; reviewed for currency 2004).

To order any of these materials, please call the Academy's Customer Service number at (415) 561-8540, or order online at www.aao.org.

Credit Reporting Form

Basic and Clinical Science Course, 2008–2009
Section 6

The American Academy of Ophthalmology is accredited by the Accreditation Council for Continuing Medical Education to provide continuing medical education for physicians.

The American Academy of Ophthalmology designates this educational activity for a maximum of 40 *AMA PRA Category 1 Credits*™. Physicians should only claim credit commensurate with the extent of their participation in the activity.

If you wish to claim continuing medical education credit for your study of this Section, you may claim your credit online or fill in the required forms and mail or fax them to the Academy.

To use the forms:

1. Complete the study questions and mark your answers on the Section Completion Form.
2. Complete the Section Evaluation.
3. Fill in and sign the statement below.
4. Return this page and the required forms by mail or fax to the CME Registrar (see below).

To claim credit online:

1. Log on to the Academy website (www.aao.org/cme).
2. Select Review/Claim CME.
3. Follow the instructions.

Important: These completed forms or the online claim must be received at the Academy by June 2011.

I hereby certify that I have spent _____ (up to 40) hours of study on the curriculum of this Section and that I have completed the study questions.

Signature: ____
Date

Name: ____

Address: ____

City and State: ______________________ Zip: ______________________

Telephone: (_______) ______________________ Academy Member ID# ______________
area code

Please return completed forms to:
American Academy of Ophthalmology
P.O. Box 7424
San Francisco, CA 94120-7424
Attn: CME Registrar, Customer Service

Or you may fax them to: 415-561-8575

2008–2009
Section Completion Form

Basic and Clinical Science Course

Answer Sheet for Section 6

Question	Answer	Question	Answer	Question	Answer
1	a b c d	18	a b c d	35	a b c d
2	a b c d	19	a b c d	36	a b c d
3	a b c d	20	a b c d	37	a b c d
4	a b c d	21	a b c d	38	a b c d e
5	a b c d e	22	a b c d	39	a b c d
6	a b c d e	23	a b c d	40	a b c d
7	a b c d	24	a b c d	41	a b c d
8	a b c d e	25	a b c d	42	a b c d
9	a b c d	26	a b c d	43	a b c d
10	a b c d	27	a b c d	44	a b c d
11	a b c d	28	a b c d	45	a b c d
12	a b c d	29	a b c d e	46	a b c d
13	a b c d e	30	a b c d	47	a b c d
14	a b c d	31	a b c d	48	a b c d
15	a b c d	32	a b c d	49	a b c d
16	a b c d	33	a b c d e	50	a b c d
17	a b c d	34	a b c d e		

Section Evaluation

Please complete this CME questionnaire.

1. To what degree will you use knowledge from BCSC Section 6 in your practice?

   ☐ Regularly

   ☐ Sometimes

   ☐ Rarely

2. Please review the stated objectives for BCSC Section 6. How effective was the material at meeting those objectives?

   ☐ All objectives were met.

   ☐ Most objectives were met.

   ☐ Some objectives were met.

   ☐ Few or no objectives were met.

3. To what degree is BCSC Section 6 likely to have a positive impact on health outcomes of your patients?

   ☐ Extremely likely

   ☐ Highly likely

   ☐ Somewhat likely

   ☐ Not at all likely

4. After you review the stated objectives for BCSC Section 6, please let us know of any additional knowledge, skills, or information useful to your practice that were acquired but were not included in the objectives. [Optional]

5. Was BCSC Section 6 free of commercial bias?

   ☐ Yes

   ☐ No

6. If you selected "No" in the previous question, please comment. [Optional]

7. Please tell us what might improve the applicability of BCSC to your practice. [Optional]

Study Questions

Although a concerted effort has been made to avoid ambiguity and redundancy in these questions, the authors recognize that differences of opinion may occur regarding the "best" answer. The discussions are provided to demonstrate the rationale used to derive the answer. They may also be helpful in confirming that your approach to the problem was correct or, if necessary, in fixing the principle in your memory.

1. A 6-month-old full-term healthy infant is brought in by his parents for an evaluation of esotropia. The parents state that the crossing started at approximately 6 weeks of life and has become constant over the past few months. On examination, fixation is central, steady, and maintained in each eye. The deviation measures 50 prism diopters by alternate cover testing. The child does not voluntarily abduct either eye. The anterior segment and fundus examination is normal. The cycloplegic refraction is +1.50 sphere OU. The next appropriate step would be
   a. to prescribe glasses containing +1.50 sphere OU
   b. surgery for the full measured deviation
   c. neuroimaging
   d. observation

2. A 9-month-old girl has been observed to have abnormal movement of her right eye. It started shortly after birth and has been stable over time. On examination, the child displays good vision in each eye. She has a small, 10° left face turn. With this face turn, her eyes are straight. The right eye moves normally. However, the left eye demonstrates a complete inability to abduct past the midline. In forced primary position, there is an esotropia of 20 prism diopters in magnitude. The remainder of her examination is normal. Her cycloplegic refraction is +1.00 sphere OU. The next step in the treatment and evaluation should be
   a. neurologic evaluation with neuroimaging
   b. prescription of the full cycloplegic refraction
   c. observation only
   d. strabismus surgery for the deviation in primary position

3. A 3-year-old boy initially presented with an esotropia of approximately 6 weeks' duration. He was placed into his full cycloplegic refraction of +3.00 sphere OU. He returns for a repeat evaluation. At that time, his vision is equal in each eye. With his glasses in place, his distance deviation measures 20 prism diopters and his near deviation measures 45 prism diopters. Which of the following is not likely to be beneficial in the management of this child?
   a. a repeat cycloplegic refraction
   b. strabismus surgery
   c. addition of a bifocal lens with a +3.00 OU
   d. prism adaptation

4. All of the following are true of strengthening procedures *except*
   a. They include advancing the insertion, especially if the muscle has been previously recessed.
   b. They include tucking, especially on the superior oblique muscle.
   c. They are especially useful for the inferior oblique muscle.
   d. They may produce an iatrogenic Brown syndrome.

5. Changes in eyelid position after strabismus surgery
   a. are especially common after inferior rectus recession
   b. rarely occur after inferior oblique recession
   c. can be addressed by release of the lower lid retractors
   d. include advancement of the lower lid after inferior rectus resection
   e. All of the above are true.

6. Which statement about the inferior rectus muscle is *not* true?
   a. It is rarely involved in thyroid myopathy.
   b. It is connected to the lower lid by Lockwood's ligament.
   c. Its actions are depression, extorsion, and adduction.
   d. It runs between the globe and the inferior oblique muscle.
   e. Its yoke muscle is the superior oblique.

7. Brown syndrome is usually distinguishable from monocular elevation deficiency by
   a. exotropia in upgaze in Brown syndrome
   b. exotropia in downgaze in Brown syndrome
   c. hypotropia of the affected eye in primary position in monocular elevation deficiency
   d. a negative forced duction test for elevation in monocular elevation deficiency

8. All of the following are possible causes of papilledema and a sixth nerve palsy *except*
   a. diabetes
   b. dural AVM
   c. cranial venous thrombosis
   d. pseudotumor
   e. sleep apnea

9. Which of the following statements is *true*?
   a. The superior oblique muscle affects horizontal rotation of the eye.
   b. The Harada-Ito procedure is useful in the treatment of Brown syndrome.
   c. Limited motility from orbital floor fractures is always due to restriction.
   d. Dissociated vertical deviation (DVD) follows Hering's law.

10. The normal growth and development of the human eye includes all of the following *except*
    a. a 4-mm increase in axial length of the eye during the first 6 months of life
    b. a corneal diameter of 10.5 mm at birth, increasing to 12 mm by age 2
    c. an increase in corneal power during the first 6 months of life
    d. a dramatic decrease in lens power over the first year of life

11. In Duane syndrome,
    a. type 3 is associated with the largest face turns
    b. exotropia in gaze away from the affected eye of a unilateral case can sometimes be seen
    c. lateral rectus resection should be included in the treatment of Duane syndrome with esotropia
    d. upshoots and downshoots are manifestations of severe oblique muscle dysfunction

12. Which of the following statements about congenital motor nystagmus is *not* true?
    a. There can be a sensory component.
    b. The purpose of surgery is to move the null zone closer to the primary position.
    c. This type of nystagmus is compatible with good vision.
    d. For surgery to be effective, the preferred eye should not be included in the operation.

13. Tucking the superior oblique tendon
    a. is appropriate to correct superior oblique muscle palsy
    b. can result in Brown syndrome
    c. is the procedure of choice when the symptoms and measurements indicate principally a torsional misalignment
    d. (a) and (b)
    e. (b) and (c)

14. Which of the following procedures is not typically employed as the initial surgery for congenital lacrimal system obstruction?
    a. simple probing
    b. balloon catheter dilation
    c. fracture of the inferior turbinate
    d. dacryocystorhinostomy

15. In the treatment of toxoplasmic retinitis, it is reasonable to use steroids as part of the regimen under which of the following conditions?
    a. Central vision is not threatened; that is, the lesion is small and peripheral.
    b. Concomitant antimicrobial coverage is used.
    c. The steroids are given as a depot injection.
    d. Steroids are contraindicated for this organism.

16. A 5-year-old child presents with a dense unilateral cataract noted by the parents 1 week previously. There has been no trauma to the eye. The child is orthophoric, B-scan shows no posterior segment pathology, and corneal diameters are noted to be 12 mm in each eye. The most likely etiology for this cataract is
    a. posterior lenticonus
    b. persistent fetal vasculature (PFV) (formerly *persistent hyperplastic primary vitreous, PHPV*)
    c. congenital nuclear cataract
    d. lamellar cataract (zonular)

17. For the child in question 16, what is the most appropriate advice to give the parents regarding surgery and prognosis?
    a. No educated prediction of vision potential can or should be given.
    b. Surgery is not indicated because visual potential is so poor for a dense congenital cataract in a 5-year-old.
    c. Although visual potential is undoubtedly poor, surgery should be attempted because there is little to lose.
    d. Surgery should be performed because the visual potential is often good.

18. A 2-year-old child with a history of prematurity and cerebral palsy is brought in for evaluation of possible ocular torticollis. The child maintains a frequent head posture of tilting to the left. He can sit unaided but is not crawling or walking. On examination, his vision is central, steady, maintained OD and central, steady, not maintained OS. There is a constant 45 left esotropia, and bilateral inferior oblique muscle overaction is greater OS than OD. Which of the following best explains the torticollis?
    a. It is nonocular.
    b. It is due to congenital bilateral superior oblique palsies.
    c. It is an effort to avoid the left inferior oblique overaction.
    d. It is due to a V pattern.

19. All of the following are true of complications following strabismus surgery *except*
    a. The most common complication is unsatisfactory alignment.
    b. Diplopia after surgery is especially common if there is undercorrection.
    c. Perforation of the sclera is rarely followed by serious complications.
    d. Anterior segment ischemia can occur after surgery on 2 rectus muscles.

20. Which of the following types of juvenile idiopathic arthritis is least likely to have associated uveitis?
    a. oligoarthritis
    b. RF-negative polyarthritis
    c. enthesis-related arthritis
    d. systemic arthritis

21. Commonly accepted treatment regimens in children with juvenile idiopathic arthritis (JIA) include all of the following *except*
    a. treatment of uveitis with topical or periocular steroids and cycloplegic agents
    b. treatment of glaucoma with aqueous shunting procedures
    c. treatment of cataract with lensectomy and intraocular lens implantation
    d. treatment of band keratopathy with a chelation procedure

22. Which of the following statements about the genetics of retinoblastoma is *false*?
    a. The retinoblastoma gene codes for a tumor suppressor protein.
    b. Genetic testing for retinoblastoma has eliminated the need for serial examinations of the siblings of affected children.
    c. Approximately 60% of retinoblastoma cases arise from somatic nonhereditary mutations.
    d. In vitro fertilization techniques have been used to select embryos that are free from the germinal retinoblastoma mutation, successfully resulting in the birth of children unaffected by retinoblastoma.

23. Regarding the treatment of retinoblastoma, which of the following is *true*?
    a. The preferred pretreatment imaging modality is MRI or ultrasound of the head and orbits.
    b. The primary treatment of intraocular retinoblastoma is external beam irradiation.
    c. Enucleation is no longer an appropriate treatment for retinoblastoma.
    d. Systemic chemotherapy is used only for patients with extraocular extension of retinoblastoma.

24. All of the following are characteristic of hyphema in childhood *except*
    a. It is more commonly seen in patients with sickle cell trait.
    b. It occurs spontaneously in juvenile xanthogranuloma.
    c. Management should include gonioscopy.
    d. It should be evacuated if total and lasting more than 5 days.

25. A 3-year-old boy initially presented with a new-onset esotropia and was given his full cycloplegic refraction. On a return evaluation 2 months later, he is found to have 20/20 vision in his right eye and 20/60 vision in his left eye. In his glasses, he continues to have a left esotropia of 30 prism diopters. The next step in treatment could likely include any of the following *except*
    a. part-time patching of the right eye for 2 hours a day
    b. full-time occlusion of the right eye
    c. atropine drops instilled into the right eye twice each day
    d. strabismus surgery of the left eye

26. Trabeculotomy or goniotomy is the procedure of choice for which of the following mechanisms of childhood glaucoma?
    a. Axenfeld-Rieger syndrome
    b. primary congenital glaucoma
    c. Lowe syndrome
    d. aphakic glaucoma

27. In planning surgery for strabismus,
    a. visual acuity of the deviating eye is not an important consideration
    b. the surgeon should weaken the superior obliques if they overact and there is an associated A pattern
    c. the procedure should include asymmetric weakening of the lateral recti if there is an exotropia worse to 1 side
    d. the procedure should always include weakening restricted muscles

28. A 2-month-old boy presents with epiphora, photophobia, and a band of cloudiness of the right cornea that does not obscure the pupil. Appropriate evaluation should include
    a. corneal biopsy with oil red O stain
    b. examination under anesthesia, with IOP measurement at the end of the case
    c. refraction
    d. conjunctival scraping for chlamydia

29. Which of the following statements regarding the pathophysiology of amblyopia is true?
    a. Changes in the nerve fiber layer of the retina are characteristic of strabismic amblyopia.
    b. The cells in the medial geniculate body corresponding to the amblyopic eye may be smaller and less intensely staining than those corresponding to the sound eye.
    c. The visual acuity of an amblyopic eye may be better when measured in the presence of contour interaction than if measured with isolated optotypes.
    d. The most significant change in the visual cortex of an amblyopic patient is loss of binocular cells, cells that are responsive to stimulation from either eye.
    e. The sensitive period for the development of deprivation amblyopia begins earlier and lasts longer than that for strabismic or anisometropic amblyopia.

30. A 1-year-old child has a 3-month history of intermittent, rapid, asymmetrical, fine nystagmus. Ophthalmic and neurologic examination results are otherwise normal. Further evaluation should include MRI of the
    a. cerebellum
    b. chiasmal area
    c. brain stem
    d. foramen magnum

31. Which of the following is *not* a major criterion for the diagnosis of neurofibromatosis type 1?
    a. sphenoid wing dysplasia
    b. posterior subcapsular cataract
    c. single plexiform neurofibroma
    d. optic nerve glioma

32. Which of the following is true concerning retinal angiomas associated with von Hippel–Lindau disease?
    a. Their peak clinical incidence coincides with the peak incidence of cerebellar hemangioblastomas.
    b. The tumors are rarely bilateral.
    c. Vision loss is usually secondary to lipid accumulation and serous retinal detachment.
    d. Cryotherapy, laser photocoagulation, or both are ineffective in the treatment of these lesions.

33. An obese 30-year-old female complains of transient visual obscurations, headaches, and diplopia, which is worse at distance viewing. All of the following are consistent findings in the patient *except*
    a. papilledema
    b. increased intracranial pressure
    c. partial third nerve palsy
    d. visual field defects
    e. cranial venous thrombosis

34. A 15-year-old obese female presents with a long-standing history of exotropia and wants to have the condition surgically corrected. Her examination is remarkable only for 30 D exotropia at distance and 25 D exotropia at near, as well as marked optic nerve head elevation. The first thing you would do is
    a. schedule a lateral rectus recession
    b. schedule a lumbar puncture and make sure to check the opening pressure
    c. schedule an ophthalmic ultrasound
    d. schedule an MR angiography and MR venography
    e. schedule a sleep study

35. The most characteristic motility abnormality associated with craniosynostosis syndromes is
    a. esotropia
    b. exotropia
    c. V pattern
    d. A pattern

36. Crouzon syndrome is *not* associated with
    a. autosomal dominant inheritance
    b. syndactyly
    c. midface retrusion
    d. premature suture fusion

37. Goldenhar syndrome includes all of the following findings *except*
    a. cleft palate
    b. epibulbar dermoids
    c. Duane syndrome
    d. lid notching

38. Which antibiotic should be given for suspected neonatal *Neisseria* conjunctivitis?
    a. intravenous ceftriaxone
    b. intravenous penicillin
    c. oral amoxicillin
    d. topical gentamicin
    e. topical ciprofloxacin

39. Which is a feature of orbital, not preseptal, cellulitis?
    a. eyelid edema
    b. tenderness to palpation
    c. proptosis
    d. conjunctivitis

40. A 2-year-old girl is brought in for examination because her mother and brother have neurofibromatosis type 1 and the family wishes to determine whether this child is also affected. Her ocular examination results are normal. Which of the following statements is *true*?
    a. The absence of Brushfield spots means that the child is unaffected.
    b. Optic nerve gliomas in neurofibromatosis usually develop in infancy, so this child is unlikely to be affected by this complication.
    c. The absence of Lisch nodules does not mean that the child is unaffected.
    d. The child should undergo examination under sedation to check intraocular pressure.

41. Which of the following topical glaucoma preparations is contraindicated for infants?
    a. timolol (Timoptic)
    b. betaxolol (Betoptic)
    c. dorzolamide (Trusopt)
    d. brimonidine (Alphagan)

42. Overcorrections following strabismus surgery
    a. can be avoided with adjustable sutures
    b. can occur when the resected muscle slips or is lost after surgery
    c. are less common than undercorrections
    d. frequently cause diplopia in young children

43. Scleral perforations during strabismus surgery in children
    a. are frequently followed by retinal detachment
    b. are frequently treated with laser therapy or cryopexy
    c. occur in about 10% of strabismus surgeries
    d. frequently cause postoperative endophthalmitis

44. Localized conjunctival injection and chemosis noted several days postoperatively at the site of eye muscle surgery may be caused by
    a. suture allergy
    b. poor closure of the conjunctival wound
    c. conjunctival inclusion cyst
    d. all of the above

45. Anterior segment ischemia following eye muscle surgery
    a. is especially common following muscle transposition procedures
    b. can occur following surgery on 2 rectus muscles
    c. typically presents with iritis and an irregular pupil
    d. all of the above

46. Botulinum toxin is particularly useful for
    a. large-angle exotropia
    b. mechanical restrictions
    c. small residual angles following strabismus surgery
    d. dissociated vertical deviations

47. A 3-year-old boy was brought to the emergency room following an injury to the right eye. The history states that he wandered too close when his father was practicing his golf swing. The lids are ecchymotic and cannot be opened. The child is inconsolably terrified. You should
    a. call Child Protective Service
    b. get a papoose board to restrain the child and open the lids with a speculum to investigate for ocular injury
    c. prepare the child for an examination under anesthesia
    d. send the child home for reexamination in several days, when the swelling has subsided

48. All of the following are characteristic of the shaken baby syndrome *except*
    a. the child is younger than 12 months
    b. parenchymal brain damage and intracranial hemorrhage are common
    c. ocular adnexae and anterior segments are typically involved
    d. retinal hemorrhage is typical, especially in the posterior pole

49. All of the following suggest an occult perforating injury *except*
    a. an eyelid laceration with intact conjunctiva
    b. an irregular pupil
    c. loss of ocular rotations
    d. All of the above suggest perforation.

50. Hyphema following blunt trauma in a child
    a. should be treated on an inpatient basis, with bilateral patching and bed rest
    b. should be treated with long-acting cycloplegics and topical steroids on an outpatient basis
    c. is more common in children with sickle cell hemoglobin
    d. should be evacuated if a total hyphema in a young child persists more than 4 or 5 days

Answers

1. **b.** The time of onset, the age at evaluation, and the large-angle deviation are all consistent with a diagnosis of infantile, or congenital, esotropia. The onset shortly after birth, the magnitude of the deviation, and the small refractive error are not consistent with a diagnosis of accommodative esotropia. Therefore, glasses would be unlikely to have any significant effect on the crossing. Although the child appears to be unable to abduct either eye, the apparent abduction deficit is secondary to cross-fixation in a child with a large esotropia and good vision in each eye. Given the diagnosis and the age of the child, spontaneous resolution of the deviation is unlikely, and therefore observation is no longer warranted.
2. **c.** The child demonstrates the typical findings of Duane syndrome. Duane syndrome occurs more commonly in girls and affects the left eye more frequently than the right. Parents often state that the normal eye moves too much compared to the affected side. The large abduction deficit may raise the suspicion of a unilateral sixth nerve palsy. However, if this were a sixth nerve palsy, the expected deviation in primary position would be much larger, given the extent of the abduction deficit. The child is able to align her eyes with a small face turn. Therefore, strabismus surgery is not indicated and the child can simply be observed.
3. **c.** A repeat cycloplegic refraction may find additional hyperopia, which, when corrected, may further improve his alignment. Because the deviation is too large to allow for the development of fusion, strabismus surgery is indicated. Prism adaptation may be helpful in determining the amount of surgery to perform. A bifocal add may improve the near deviation but would not decrease either the distance or near deviation enough to allow the patient to develop fusion and therefore is not indicated.
4. **c.** Inferior oblique strengthening is rarely performed. All other choices are true of strengthening procedures.
5. **e.** All are correct.
6. **a.** It is commonly involved in thyroid myopathy.
7. **a.** Exotropia in upgaze was described by Brown as an essential feature of this syndrome, although it is not prominent in every case. A horizontal deviation in other gazes, unless coexisting as a separate entity, is not a feature of either disorder. Hypotropia in primary position is present in monocular elevation deficiency, but the most severe cases of Brown syndrome show this as well. Because "monocular elevation deficiency" includes both pareses and restrictive conditions, the forced duction test can be positive and therefore not always a distinction.
8. **a.** Although a sixth nerve palsy is common in diabetes, papilledema is not common. Diabetic papillitis is an entity, but it should not be confused with true papilledema.
9. **a.** The superior and inferior oblique muscles contribute to abduction of the eye, although their vertical and torsional effects are antagonistic. The Harada-Ito procedure is employed in cases of bilateral superior oblique muscle paralysis with a prominent torsional imbalance. Its use in Brown syndrome would probably worsen the condition. The findings in DVD are opposite to those expected from Hering's law.
10. **c.** The cornea flattens during the first year of life, resulting in a decrease in corneal power.

11. **b.** This finding is a feature differentiating type 1 Duane syndrome from sixth cranial nerve paralysis. Despite the often profound rotation defects in type 3 Duane syndrome, compensatory head positions tend to be modest. Tightening the lateral rectus muscle would, in most cases, tend to exaggerate the effects of co-contraction. Upshoots and downshoots are generally considered to be effects of co-contraction, despite some limited electromyographic evidence of oblique muscle dysfunction.

12. **d.** The null zone is determined by the preferred eye. Moving the null zone closer to the primary position reduces the need for a compensatory head position and is a principal goal of the surgery. Many cases of congenital motor nystagmus have a sensory visual defect.

13. **d.** Tucking is a tightening procedure intended to improve superior oblique muscle action. Because all of the tendon fibers are included in the procedure, tucking cannot be employed selectively only for the torsional component of the deviation. Tucking too much or too close to the trochlea can hinder the movement of the tendon through that structure; hence, tucking generally is performed in the portion of the tendon adjacent to the nasal border of the superior rectus muscle or more distally.

14. **d.** Dacryocystorhinostomy usually is reserved for cases that do not respond to other surgical procedures. Although simple probing, repeated if necessary, is the most common first surgical approach, many surgeons combine this with balloon catheter dilation and/or inferior turbinate initially in all cases or in cases presenting for treatment late.

15. **b.** Steroids can be used to combat the intraocular inflammation caused by *Toxoplasmosis.* The steroids should be given only if appropriate concomitant antimicrobial coverage of the offending organism is used. The steroids should never be given as a depot injection. Small peripheral non–sight-threatening lesions usually do not require treatment of any kind.

16. **a.** Acquired unilateral cataracts in full-size eyes are due almost exclusively to posterior lenticonus or trauma. Both PFV and congenital nuclear cataracts are associated with microcornea. Lamellar cataracts are always bilateral.

17. **d.** In general, posterior lenticonus behaves as an acquired cataract, and therefore the visual potential is often good. The additional fact that the child has not developed strabismus is a point in favor of this not being a long-standing, visually significant cataract with dense amblyopia.

18. **a.** This child has esotropia associated with significant cerebral palsy and motor delays. Although it is often not possible to perform cover testing in various positions of gaze, simple observation ususally establishes that there is no fusional position (no head posture where the eyes are sufficiently aligned to allow for a degree of binocular function). Primary inferior oblique overaction is common in childhood esotropia and is not due to superior oblique palsies. Because the child is right eye dominant and nonfusing, he suppresses the left eye and has no reason to try to avoid the left inferior oblique overaction. Children with V-pattern esotropia who have binocular function use a chin-down posture, not a head tilt. In this case, the torticollis is nonocular and is likely another muscular manifestation of the cerebral palsy.

19. **b.** Diplopia is more common with overcorrections. Perforation of the sclera usually causes a chorioretinal scar with no visual sequela.

20. **d.** Uveitis is most common in children with RF-negative oligoarthritis, but it is also seen in children with RF-negative polyarthritis and enthesis-related arthritis. It is rare in children with systemic arthritis.

21. **c.** Although lensectomy is an accepted procedure for treating visually significant cataracts in children with JIA, intraocular lens implantation in children with JIA remains controversial.

22. **b.** Genetic testing for retinoblastoma is available but limited.

23. **a.** MRI and ultrasound are preferred over CT for imaging because they avoid the use of radiation. Primary systemic chemotherapy (chemoreduction) followed by local therapy (consolidation) is now the most commonly used vision-sparing technique for treating retinoblastoma. External beam irradiation is avoided because it is associated with an increased risk of second tumors. Enucleation is still commonly used to treat eyes with poor visual potential.

24. **a.** Hyphema is more dangerous with sickle cell trait, or disease, because of sickling in the anterior chamber or in the retinal circulation, but it is not more common in such patients.

25. **d.** Given the moderate level of amblyopia that is present, full-time occlusion, part-time occlusion, and atropine penalization are all likely to be effective. Strabismus surgery should be deferred until the vision is improved in the left eye.

26. **b.** Angle surgery, either trabeculotomy or goniotomy, is the procedure of choice for primary congenital glaucoma.

27. **d.** Restriction should always be considered at surgery because there is no other way to address the diminished rotation in the opposite field. Visual acuity is important in that surgery should be preferentially performed on the poorer seeing eye if the vision is very poor. Superior oblique weakening is a very potent and somewhat unpredictable procedure that can cause torsional diplopia in older patients. Asymmetric weakening may be indicated in incomitant strabismus, but only if there is no restriction.

28. **c.** The classic presentation for congenital glaucoma is epiphora, light sensitivity, and hazy cornea. Chlamydial infections are normally transmitted from the mother and are present soon after birth. IOP should be measured at the beginning of the examination under anesthesia because anesthesia has a rapid lowering effect on IOP. Refraction might show a myopic anisometropia, which helps confirm the diagnosis and which may require treatment to prevent amblyopia.

29. **e.** The critical period for the development of deprivation begins earlier and lasts longer than that for strabismic or anisometropic amblyopia. Furthermore, a shorter period of time is necessary for visual deprivation to cause amblyopia than is the case for strabismic or anisometropic amblyopia. Evidence that the retina is involved in amblyopia is inconclusive. The lateral geniculate body, not the medial geniculate body, is involved in amblyopia. The visual acuity of an amblyopic patient worsens with contour interaction (crowding). The most significant cortical change in amblyopia is loss of cells responsive to stimulation from the amblyopic eye.

30. **b.** Spasmus nutans is a bilateral, often very asymmetrical, fine horizontal nystagmus. The nystagmus can be intermittent and difficult to see. It normally is idiopathic starting at about age 3–4 months and resolves by age 3–4 years. The nystagmus can be seen in patients who have gliomas of the chiasm. These cases are always associated with decreased vision and optic atrophy. However, because these findings can be subtle in a very young baby, neuroimaging is often recommended when the diagnosis is uncertain.

31. **b.** Posterior subcapsular or wedge cortical lens opacities are associated with neurofibromatosis type 2 and are not a feature of type 1. Other major criteria for neurofibromatosis type 1 include the presence of 2 or more Lisch nodules, 6 or more café-au-lait spots, axillary or inguinal freckling, and a family history of a first-degree relative with neurofibromatosis type 1.

32. **c.** Retinal angiomas are often located in the peripheral fundus and may be asymptomatic when small. As the lesion grows, its capillaries may become more incompetent and allow for transudation of fluid. If the retinal edema and exudates are extensive enough to involve the macula, vision becomes compromised. The peak incidence of retinal angioma occurs a decade before its cerebellar counterpart. The tumors are bilateral in up to 50% of cases. Treatment with cryotherapy or laser photocoagulation may be especially efficacious with smaller lesions.
33. **c.** A third nerve palsy would not cause double vision that would be worse at distance. That type of diplopia would be due to a sixth nerve palsy, which would be consistent with papilledema, increased intracranial pressure, and visual field defects due to either pseudotumor or mass lesion in the brain. A cranial venous thrombosis can mimic an orbital pseudotumor.
34. **c.** Schedule an ophthalmic ultrasound. The physician is obligated to find an etiology for the marked optic nerve head elevation in both eyes. Papilledema due to increased intracranial pressure from a number of lesions would most likely cause a sixth nerve palsy, which would not result in exotropia. The most likely etiology for the asymptomatic finding of optic nerve head elevation would be optic nerve head drusen. These can be readily discovered on an ophthalmic ultrasound or also on a CT scan, with particular attention to axial sections through the optic nerve globe junction.
35. **c.** Stated in the chapter is the occurrence of orbital extorsion and secondary apparent inferior oblique overaction (IOOA).
36. **b.** The main difference between the phenotype of Crouzon vs other craniofacial syndromes (especially Apert) is that Crouzon patients do not have hand or foot deformities.
37. **a.** Cleft palate was *not* discussed among the findings for Goldenhar syndrome; all the others were.
38. **a.** If untreated, children affected with *Neisseria gonorrhoeae* conjunctivitis can develop life-threatening complications, such as sepsis and meningitis. Antibiotic therapy should therefore be systemic. Topical medications may be used as an adjunct but should certainly not be considered primary therapy. Although intravenous penicillin was once considered the treatment of choice of *Neisseria* infections, resistant strains have made ceftriaxone a better choice. Fluoroquinolones should be avoided in this age group because of potential bone toxicity.
39. **c.** Preseptal cellulitis is an inflammatory process of the tissues anterior to the orbital septum that can occur secondary to trauma, severe conjunctivitis, or upper-respiratory or sinus infection. Orbital cellulitis is an infection of the orbit involving the tissues posterior to the orbital septum. Both may present with eyelid edema and tenderness to palpation, but proptosis is not a feature of preseptal cellulitis. Full ocular motility and absence of pain on eye movement help distinguish preseptal from orbital cellulitis.
40. **c.** Brushfield spots are seen in Down syndrome, not neurofibromatosis. Optic nerve gliomas associated with neurofibromatosis generally develop in the first 1–2 decades of life, rarely in toddlerhood. Glaucoma with neurofibromatosis is seen in association with plexiform neurofibromas of the eyelids (a secondary form of glaucoma); in the absence of a lid lesion, there is no reason to suspect that this child has elevated IOP and no reason to sedate her to measure IOP. Lisch nodules eventually develop in over 90% of patients with neurofibromatosis type 1, but they are rarely present in early childhood. Lisch nodules are, therefore, a sensitive, but not a specific, finding for neurofibromatosis at this age.
41. **d.** Brimonidine (Alphagan) has been associated with CNS depression that can be marked in children under 3 years of age, and therefore it should not be used in this age group.

42. **c.** Undercorrections are much more common than overcorrections. Overcorrections can occur after suture adjustment. Slippage of a resected muscle causes an undercorrection. Although definitely an issue in adults, diplopia is not a problem in young children.

43. **b.** Retinal detachments (especially in children) and endophthalmitis are rare even in cases with known scleral perforation. Although the incidence was as high as 10% in the 1970s, spatulated needles have made the complication much less common recently. Most surgeons recommend cryopexy or laser therapy, although some do not.

44. **d.** They all can present in this fashion.

45. **d.** Transposition procedures and other surgeries involving 3 or more rectus muscles pose a special risk of anterior segment ischemia. Such ischemia can occur even following 2-muscle surgery, although typically in elderly patients with poor circulation or blood dyscrasias. Iritis and sector iris atrophy are characteristic of anterior segment ischemia.

46. **c.** Botulinum has been shown to be relatively ineffective in the other conditions listed but can often resolve a small residual angle strabismus in the first few months following surgery.

47. **c.** The presentation does not suggest child abuse. Forcing an examination in a terrified child with a possibly ruptured globe risks further injury. Sending the child home is inappropriate because he may have suffered serious ocular damage.

48. **c.** Adnexae and anterior segments are typically uninvolved. The other choices are characteristic of the syndrome.

49. **d.** A sharp object can perforate the sclera posterior to the conjunctival cul-de-sac through a lid laceration. Other choices are typical of perforating injuries.

50. **d.** Hospitalization, patching, bed rest, cycloplegia, and steroids are all controversial in the treatment of hyphemas, which should be individualized according to the risk of complications. Hyphemas are not more common in sickle cell disease or trait, but they are more dangerous because of impeded resorption and risk of retinal vascular occlusion. Because of the risk of corneal blood staining and the difficulty obtaining accurate pressure measurements, total hyphemas in young children should be evacuated in this time frame.

Index

(*i* = image; *t* = table)